MASTERCASES
Spine Surgery

MasterCases
Spine Surgery

Alexander R. Vaccaro, M.D.
Professor
Co-Director, Delaware Valley Regional Spinal Cord Injury Center
Co-Chief, Spinal Surgery
Thomas Jefferson University and the Rothman Institute
Philadelphia, Pennsylvannia

Todd J. Albert, M.D
Associate Professor and Vice Chairman, Department of Orthopaedics
Co-Chief, Spinal Surgery
Thomas Jefferson University and the Rothman Institute
Philadelphia, Pennsylvannia

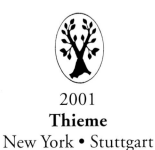

2001
Thieme
New York • Stuttgart

Thieme New York
333 Seventh Avenue
New York, NY 10001

Consulting Medical Editor: Esther Gumpert
Editor: Kathleen P. Lyons
Assistant Editor: Todd Warnock
Production Editor: David Stewart
Director, Production and Manufacturing: Anne Vinnicombe
Marketing Director: Phyllis D. Gold
Sales Manager: Ross Lumpkin
Chief Financial Officer: Peter van Woerden
President: Brian D. Scanlan
Compositor: Compset, Inc.
Printer: Grafiche Fover

MasterCases: Spine Surgery
Alexander R. Vaccaro, M.D.
Todd J. Albert, M.D.

Library of Congress Cataloging-in-Publication Data

MasterCases: spine surgery / [edited by] Alexander R. Vaccaro, Todd J. Albert.
    p. ; cm.
    Includes bibliographical references and index.
    ISBN 0-86577-924-4 (TNY)—ISBN 3131259914 (GTV)
    1. Spine—Surgery—Case studies. 2. Spine—Wounds and injuries—Case studies. I. Title: Spine surgery. II. Vaccaro, Alexander R. III. Albert, Todd J.
    [DNLM: 1. Spinal Diseases—therapy—Case Report. 2. Spinal Injuries—therapy—Case Report. 3. Spine—surgery—Case Report. WE 725 M423 2001]
    RD768 .M386 2001
    617.5'6059—dc21
                                                                            00-059941

Important note: Medical knowledge is ever-changing. As new research and clinical experience broaden our knowledge, changes in treatment and drug therapy may be required. The authors and the editors of the material herein have consulted sources believed to be reliable in their efforts to provide information that is complete and in accord with the standards accepted at the time of publication. However, in view of the possibility of human error by the authors, editors, or publisher of the work herein, or changes in medical knowledge, neither the authors, editors, publisher, nor any other party who has been involved in the preparation of this work, warrants that the information contained herein is in every respect accurate or complete, and they are not responsible for any errors or omissions or for the results obtained from use of such information. Readers are encouraged to confirm the information contained herein with other sources. For example, readers are advised to check the product information sheet included in the package of each drug they plan to administer to be certain that the information contained in this publication is accurate and that changes have not been made in the recommended dose or in the contraindications for administration. This recommendation is of particular importance in connection with new or infrequently used drugs.

Some of the product names, patents, and registered designs referred to in this book are in fact registered trademarks or proprietary names even though specific reference to this fact is not always made in the text. Therefore, the appearance of a name without designation as proprietary is not to be construed as a representation by the publisher that it is in the public domain.

Printed in Italy

5 4 3 2 1

TNY ISBN 0-86577-924-4
GTV ISBN 3-13-125991-4

CONTENTS

Foreword by Steven R. Garfin . . . . **ix**

Preface . . . . **xi**

Contributors . . . . **xii**

SECTION I: DEGENERATIVE CONDITIONS

CASE 1. Axial Neck Pain: Nonoperative Approach,
Terrence P. Sheehan **3**

CASE 2. Whiplash Injuries: Nonoperative Approach,
Kanwaldeep S. Sidhu and Jeffrey S. Fischgrund **10**

CASE 3. Cervical Spondylosis—Soft Disc Herniation: Anterior
Approach, *Joseph M. Kowalski, Steven C. Ludwig, and
Scott D. Boden* **18**

CASE 4. Cervical Spondylosis—Soft Disc Herniation: Posterior
Approach, *Steven C. Ludwig, Joseph M. Kowalski, and
Scott D. Boden* **27**

CASE 5. Cervical Spondylosis—Myelopathy: Anterior Approach,
Bradford L. Currier and Michael J. Yaszemski **35**

CASE 6. Cervical Spondylosis—Myelopathy: Posterior Approach,
Bradford L. Currier and Michael J. Yaszemski **45**

CASE 7. Thoracic Disc Herniation: Anterior Approach,
Douglas M. Ehrler and Alexander R. Vaccaro **52**

CASE 8. Thoracic Disc Herniation: Posterior Approach,
Douglas M. Ehrler and Alexander R. Vaccaro **61**

CASE 9. Thoracic Disc Herniations: Minimally Invasive Approach,
Srdjan Mirkovic **68**

CASE 10. Axial Low Back Pain: Nonoperative Approach,
Mitchell K. Freedman **78**

CASE 11. Lumbar Degenerative Disc Disease—Axial Back Pain:
Anterior Approach, *Stephen D. Kuslich* **84**

CASE 12. Lumbar Degenerative Disc Disease—Axial Back Pain:
Posterior Approach, *Stephen D. Kuslich* **93**

CASE 13. Lumbar Spinal Stenosis without Instability, *John A.
McCulloch* **100**

CASE 14. Lumbar Degenerative Spondylolisthesis, *Eeric Truumees
and Harry N. Herkowitz* **109**

CASE 15. Lumbar Degenerative Scoliosis with Spinal Stenosis,
Eeric Truumees and Harry N. Herkowitz **119**

CASE 16. Microdiscectomy, Arthroscopic Discectomy, Chymopapain
Injection, *John A. McCulloch* **129**

CASE 17. Lumbar Degenerative Disc Disease—Axial Low Back Pain:
Minimally Invasive Laparoscopic Approach, *John D. Tydings,
Alexander R. Vaccaro, and Philip Minotti* **136**

CASE 18. Recurrent Lumbar Disc Herniation, *R. Scott Meyer and Steven R. Garfin* **143**

CASE 19. Intradural Disc Herniation—Lumbar Spine, *Kush Singh and Alexander R. Vaccaro* **150**

CASE 20. Spinal Meningeal or Perineural Cysts, *Alexander R. Vaccaro, Kern Singh, and Janet C. Donohue* **157**

CASE 21. Iatrogenic Lumbar Instability, *Robert J. Benz and Steven R. Garfin* **163**

CASE 22. Management of Failed Back Surgery Syndrome, *Christopher C. Annunziata, William C. Lauerman, and Samuel W. Wiesel* **172**

CASE 23. Sacroiliac Joint Dysfunction, *Jeffrey B. Kleiner and Michael R. Moore* **179**

SECTION II: INFLAMMATORY DISORDERS

CASE 24. Rheumatoid Arthritis Cranial–C1/C2 Disease, *Seth M. Zeidman and Thomas B. Ducker* **189**

CASE 25. Osteomyelitis—Cervical Spine, Thoracic Spine, Lumbar Spine, *M. Darryl Antonacci and Frank J. Eismont* **199**

CASE 26. Postoperative Lumbar Discitis, *Alan S. Hilibrand* **208**

CASE 27. Ankylosing Spondylitis—Cervical Osteotomy, *Alok D. Sharan, Alexander R. Vaccaro, and Todd J. Albert* **215**

CASE 28. Postoperative Spinal Wound Infections, *Steven C. Ludwig, Joseph M. Kowalski, and John G. Heller* **220**

SECTION III: METABOLIC DISEASE

CASE 29. Pagetoid Disease of the Spine, *Jeffrey S. Fischgrund* **231**

CASE 30. Circumferential Surgery for Ossification of the Posterior Longitudinal Ligament in the Cervical Spine, *Nancy E. Epstein* **239**

CASE 31. Transthoracic and Transabdominal Approach to T9 to T12 Ossification of the Posterior Longitudinal Ligament with Herniated Disc/Stenosis, *Nancy E. Epstein* **247**

CASE 32. Diffuse Idiopathic Skeletal Hyperostosis, *Donal B. Rose and Jeffrey D. Klein* **255**

CASE 33. Osteoporotic Fractures of the Spine, *Amir Matityahu, Jeffrey D. Klein, and Frank J. Schwab* **262**

CASE 34. Spinal Deformity in the Presence of Osteogenesis Imperfecta, *Fabien D. Bitan, Georges Finidori, Marianne Pouliquen, and Gilda Forseter* **269**

SECTION IV: TRAUMA

CASE 35. Spinal Cord Injury: Pharmacologic and Nonoperative
Management, *Terrence P. Sheehan* **281**

CASE 36. Traumatic Injuries of the Occipitocervical Junction,
*David L. Kramer, Suken A. Shah, Gregg R. Klein,
Alexander R. Vaccaro, and Jerome M. Cotler* **288**

CASE 37. Bilateral Cervical Facet Joint Dislocation without
Neurologic Deficit, *Gregg R. Klein, Suken A. Shah, and
Alexander R. Vaccaro* **297**

CASE 38. Fixed Traumatic Atlantoaxial Rotatory Deformity,
Suken A. Shah, Alexander R. Vaccaro, and Carl E. Becker II . **305**

CASE 39. Thoracolumbar Trauma with or without Neurologic Deficit,
Glenn R. Rechtine II and Michael J. Bolesta **313**

CASE 40. Low Lumbar Fracture with or without Neurologic
Deficit, *Thomas D. Kramer and Alan M. Levine* **320**

CASE 41. Sacral Fractures, *Kirkham B. Wood and Francis Denis* **329**

CASE 42. Gunshot Wounds—Cervical Spine, Thoracic Spine,
Lumbar Spine, *Robert F. Heary and Christopher M. Bono* . . **336**

SECTION V: SPINAL NEOPLASMS

CASE 43. Primary Tumor—Cervical Spine, Thoracic Spine, Lumbar
Spine, *Takuya Fujita, Norio Kawahara, and Katsuro Tomita* **345**

CASE 44. Primary Tumor of the Cervical Spine, *Jed S. Vanichkachorn
and Alexander R. Vaccaro* **354**

CASE 45. Spinal Cord Herniation, *Erol Veznedaroglu and Gregory J.
Przybylski* **360**

CASE 46. Metastatic Disease—Cervical Spine, Thoracic Spine,
Lumbar Spine, *Joseph M. Kowalski, Steven C. Ludwig, and
John G. Heller* **366**

CASE 47. Spinal Intradural Intramedullary and Extramedullary
Tumors, *Michael K. Rosner, James M. Ecklund, and Seth M.
Zeidman* **378**

SECTION VI: ADULT AND PEDIATRIC DEFORMITY

CASE 48. Congenital Scoliosis, *Paul E. Savas, Peter G. Gabos, and
Alexander R. Vaccaro* **391**

CASE 49. Adolescent Idiopathic Scoliosis, *Peter G. Gabos* **401**

CASE 50. Kyphosis—Round-Back Deformity, Scheuermann's Kyphosis,
Gregory V. Hahn, Peter O. Newton, and Dennis R. Wenger . . **411**

CASE 51. Postlaminectomy Kyphosis, *Todd J. Albert and Alexander R.
Vaccaro* **420**

CASE 52. Fixed Pelvic Obliquity, *Jean-Pierre C. Farcy, Brian D. Hoffman, and Frank J. Schwab* **426**

CASE 53. Klippel-Feil Syndrome, *Peter O. Newton* **435**

CASE 54. Chiari Malformations, *William Mitchell and Gregory J. Przybylski* **443**

CASE 55. Diastematomyelia, *James S. Harrop, Leslie N. Sutton, and Gregory J. Przybylski* **450**

CASE 56. Spinal Deformity in Myelodysplasia—Lumbar Kyphectomy, *Mohammad E. Majd, Richard T. Holt, and Joseph L. Richey* . **455**

CASE 57. Adult Scoliosis, *David B. Cohen and John P. Kostuik* **464**

CASE 58. Adult Isthmic Spondylolisthesis, *Geoffrey J. Coldham and Edward N. Hanley, Jr.* **471**

CASE 59. Achondroplasia—Cervical Postlaminectomy Kyphosis, *Jeffrey L. Bush, David Horn, and Alexander R. Vaccaro* **479**

CASE 60. Postradiation Spinal Deformity, *Alan S. Hilibrand* **484**

SECTION VII: MISCELLANEOUS

CASE 61. Persistent Spinal Fluid Leakage Following Spinal Surgery, *Jeffrey D. Coe* **495**

CASE 62. Syringomyelia and Scoliosis, *Kirkham B. Wood and Francis Denis* **502**

CASE 63. Vascular Malformations of the Spinal Cord, *James S. Harrop and Gregory J. Przybylski* **509**

INDEX **517**

FOREWORD

Master has multiple possible definitions. As a noun it can be used to describe "a person whose teaching one accepts or follows," "a workman qualified to teach apprentices and carry on his trade independently," or "a man eminently skilled in something, as in occupation, art, or science." It can also function as an adjective as "being master, or exercising mastery," "being a master of some occupation, art," "eminently skilled," or to "become adept in."

A dictionary definition of *teaching* is "imparting knowledge of, or skill in" an area. In the usual higher education system, as well as most texts, this is done in a didactic, relatively structured fashion, beginning with historical information. In medicine texts in particular, this often begins with the anatomy of, and pathophysiology, diagnosis, and treatment options for, specific disorders. However, medical education, and particularly surgical training, do not follow that classic route. As Oliver William Holmes stated in *Scholastic and Bedside Teaching*, "the bedside is always the true center of medical teaching. . . . The most essential part of a student's instruction is obtained, as I believe, not in the lecture room, but at the bedside." Medical clerkships, residencies, and grand rounds are organized in this manner. Patients are the nidus for understanding a medical problem. Additionally, in medical school, teaching is passed down the line, as the ability to explain and teach improves our ability to understand. Joubert stated in 1842, "to teach is to learn twice."

In *MASTERCASES: Spine Surgery*, Drs. Vaccaro and Albert and the authors have incorporated all of the above. Using methods we as physicians are familiar with in education, each of these concisely written, well-focused chapters starts with a patient— a typical patient with a history and physical. Each chapter introduces us to the problem in the normal medical fashion, presenting a patient and the work-up. This is followed by a short description of the diagnosis and treatment and well written discussion sections. Highlights of the diagnosis (pearls) and potential difficulties (pitfalls) in making the diagnosis and providing treatment are called out by the authors and listed in the margins to emphasize critical points. This is the manner in which we are accustomed to learning. These well-written chapters, in all areas of spine, draw the reader in through a patient (reminding us of one of our own) and then proceeding in a logical, thoughtful, manner as we do in the outpatient and inpatient settings. As Thomas Mann wrote, in *Magic Mountain*, "order and simplification are the first steps towards the mastery of a subject."

The authors are a mix of older "masters" and their students or younger colleagues who impart knowledge in a distilled fashion. This also is a manner we are used to from grand and ward rounds, where junior faculty or residents present a case and discuss the problem, before it is culled down further by the appropriate senior faculty. The chapter presentations are uniform, easy to follow, appropriately illustrated, and provide useful references. For a text that has been in the process for a period of time, it is up to date, in both wording and illustrations—like a recent grand rounds presentation.

I commend Drs. Vaccaro and Albert for organizing the text, soliciting top rate authors and co-authors, and developing a structure that is different than most texts. It is easy to read and follow, is up to date, yet will be useful for many years. It is written in a fashion that does not target any particular audience, but encompasses information that should be of interest to the spine specialist, general orthopaedists, neurosurgeons, and other physicians and health care providers that treat spinal disorders, as well as residents and students. *As usual, great job Alex and Todd.*

Steven R. Garfin, M.D.
Professor and Chair, Department of Orthopaedics
University of California San Diego Medical Center
San Diego, California

PREFACE

Over the last decade, a plethora of reference textbooks concerning the management of spinal disorders have inundated the medical marketplace. These issues have been presented in single- or multivolume textbooks, written by surgeons prominent in their respective fields, concerning the global treatment of a particular spinal disorder. As our clinical and academic responsibilities grow, surgeons have been afforded less and less time to wade through the voluminous resources available to them, especially when specific detailed information is needed in the care of particular patient disorders. The *MasterCases* series is an innovative approach to medical education in which the treating physician presents useful, practical information packaged in a case history format for quick reference and ease of digestion and application. The variety of pathologies discussed and the book's organization allows the spinal physician to compare the issues encountered in daily patient management with specific patient case histories, and to explore the common and not so common differential diagnoses and treatment alternatives for managing a particular spinal disorder effectively. Easy-to-read tables are provided to serve as a quick reference for review of different treatment alternatives and their advantages and disadvantages. Experts in the field of spinal science illustrate the highlights of particular spinal disorders that they manage on a frequent basis. The diverse topic range includes degenerative disorders of the cervical and thoracolumbar spine, sacral iliac joint dysfunction. inflammation spinal disease, metabolic disorders, contemporary trauma management, spinal neoplasms, and adult and pediatric deformities.

The book is intended to be a useful tool for an active practicing spinal clinician who wants to maintain a general level of proficiency in the standard nonoperative and operative treatment of a diverse group of spinal conditions. It is also a valuable teaching aid, through its structural and comprehensive organization, for the resident or fellow interested in spinal care.

Alexander R. Vaccaro, M.D.
Todd J. Albert, M.D.

CONTRIBUTORS

Todd J. Albert, M.D.
Associate Professor and Vice
　Chairman
Department of Orthopaedics;
Co-Chief, Spinal Surgery
Thomas Jefferson University and the
　Rothman Institute
Philadelphia, Pennsylvania

Christopher C. Annunziata, M.D.
Instructor
Department of Orthopaedic Surgery
Georgetown University Hospital
Washington, District of Columbia

M. Darryl Antonacci, M.D.
Director, Spine Diagnostic and
　Treatment Center
Assistant Professor of Orthopaedic
　Surgery
Department of Orthopaedic Surgery
Graduate Hospital
Philadelphia, Pennsylvania

Carl E. Becker II, M.D.
Clinical Instructor
Department of Orthopaedic Surgery
Jefferson Medical College
Thomas Jefferson University
Philadelphia, Pennsylvania

Robert J. Benz, M.D.
Spine Fellow
Department of Orthopaedic Surgery
Institute of Spine Care
Syracuse, New York

Fabien D. Bitan, M.D.
Department of Orthopaedic Surgery
Spine Institute
Beth Israel Medical Center
New York, New York

Scott D. Boden, M.D.
Associate Professor
Department of Orthopaedic Surgery
Emory University School of Medicine
Decatur, Georgia

Michael J. Bolesta, M.D.
Assistant Professor
Department of Orthopaedic Surgery
University of Texas Southwestern
　Medical Center
Dallas, Texas

Christopher M. Bono, M.D.
Resident
Department of Orthopaedic Surgery
UMDNJ-New Jersey Medical School
Newark, New Jersey

Jeffrey L. Bush, B.S.
Medical Student
Jefferson Medical College
Philadelphia, Pennsylvania

Jeffrey D. Coe, M.D.
Medical Director
Center for Spine Deformity and
　Injury
Los Gatos, California

David B. Cohen, M.D.
Assistant Professor
Department of Orthopaedic Surgery
Johns Hopkins University
Baltimore, Maryland

Geoffrey J. Coldham, M.B.C.H.B.
Department of Orthopaedic Surgery
Middlemore Hospital
South Auckland, New Zealand

Jerome M. Cotler, M.D.
Professor
Department of Orthopaedic Surgery
Jefferson Medical College
Thomas Jefferson University
Philadelphia, Pennsylvania

Bradford L. Currier, M.D.
Associate Professor
Department of Orthopaedic Surgery
Mayo Clinic
Rochester, Minnesota

Francis Denis, M.D.
Clinical Professor, Spine Surgeon
Department of Orthopaedic Surgery
University of Minnesota
Minneapolis, Minnesota

Janet C. Donohue, M.D.
Trauma Fellow, Orthopaedic Surgery
Cooper Medical Center
Camden, New Jersey

Thomas B. Ducker, M.D.
Professor
Department of Neurosurgery
Johns Hopkins Hospital
Baltimore, Maryland

James M. Ecklund, M.D.
Assistant Professor
Department of Neurosurgery
Walter Reed Army Medical Center
Washington, District of Columbia

Douglas M. Ehrler, M.D.
Assistant Clinical Professor
Northeastern Ohio University
　College of Medicine
Rootstown, Ohio;
Department of Orthopaedic Surgery
Orthopaedic Multispeciality
　Network, Inc.
Canton, Ohio

Frank J. Eismont, M.D.
Professor and Vice Chairman
Department of Orthopaedic Surgery
and Rehabilitation
University of Miami School of
Medicine
Miami, Florida

Nancy E. Epstein, M.D.
Clinical Associate Professor of
Surgery (Neurosurgery)
Department of Neurosurgery
Cornell University Medical College
New York, New York

Jean-Pierre C. Farcy, M.D.
Director, Brooklyn Spine Center;
Department of Orthopaedic Surgery
Maimonides Medical Center
Brooklyn, New York

Georges Finidori, M.D.
Department of Pediatric
Orthopaedic Surgery
Hospital des Enfants Malades
Paris, France

Jeffrey S. Fischgrund, M.D.
Orthopaedic Surgeon
Department of Orthopaedic Surgery
William Beaumont Hospital
Southfield, Michigan

Gilda Forseter, F.N.P.
Department of Orthopaedic Surgery
Spine Institute
Beth Israel Medical Center
New York, New York

Mitchell K. Freedman, D.O.
Physiatrist
Rothman Institute at Jefferson
Philadelphia, Pennsylvania

Takuya Fujita, M.D.
Assistant Professor
Department of Orthopaedic Surgery
Kanazawa University School of
Medicine
Ishikawa, Japan

Peter G. Gabos, M.D.
Assistant Clinical Professor of
Orthopaedic Surgery
Jefferson Medical College;
Attending Pediatric Orthopaedic
Surgeon
Thomas Jefferson University Hospital
Philadelphia, Pennsylvania

Steven R. Garfin, M.D.
Professor and Chair
Department of Orthopaedic Surgery
University of California San Diego
San Diego, California

Gregory V. Hahn, M.D.
Department of Orthopaedic Surgery
Children's Hospital of San Diego
San Diego, California

Edward N. Hanley, Jr., M.D.
Department of Orthopaedic Surgery
Carolinas Medical Center
Charlotte, North Carolina

James S. Harrop, M.D.
Resident
Department of Neurosurgery
Jefferson Medical College
Philadelphia, Pennsylvania

Robert F. Heary, M.D.
Assistant Professor
Department of Neurosurgery
UMDNJ-New Jersey Medical
School
Newark, New Jersey

John G. Heller, M.D.
Associate Professor
Director, Orthopaedic Surgery
The Emory Spine Center
Decatur, Georgia

Harry N. Herkowitz, M.D.
Section of Spinal Surgery
Department of Orthopaedic Surgery
William Beaumont Hospital
Royal Oak, Michigan

Alan S. Hilibrand, M.D.
Assistant Professor
Department of Orthopaedic Surgery
Jefferson Medical College
Thomas Jefferson University
Philadelphia, Pennsylvania

Brian D. Hoffman, M.D.
Resident
Department of Orthopaedic Surgery
Maimonides Medical Center
Brooklyn, New York

Richard T. Holt, M.D.
Assistant Professor
Division of Orthopaedic Surgery
University of Kentucky
Lexington, Kentucky

David Horn, M.D.
Department of Orthopaedic Surgery
Children's Hospital of Pennsylvania
Philadelphia, Pennsylvania

Norio Kawahara, M.D.
Associate Professor
Department of Orthopaedic Surgery
Kanazawa University School of
Medicine
Ishikawa, Japan

Gregg R. Klein, M.D.
Resident
Department of Orthopaedic Surgery
Jefferson Medical College
Thomas Jefferson University
Philadelphia, Pennsylvania

Jeffrey D. Klein, M.D.
Instructor
Department of Orthopaedic Surgery
NYU School of Medicine, Hospital
for Joint Diseases
Maimonides Medical Center
Brooklyn, New York

Jeffrey B. Kleiner, M.D.
Orthopaedic Spine Surgeon
Spine Consultants
Aurora, Colorado

John P. Kostuik, M.D.
Professor
Department of Orthopaedic Surgery
Johns Hopkins University
Baltimore, Maryland

Joseph M. Kowalski, M.D.
Clinical Instructor
Department of Orthopaedic Surgery
Emory University School of
  Medicine
Decatur, Georgia

David L. Kramer, M.D.
Orthopaedic Spinal Surgeon
Danbury Orthopaedics
Danbury, Connecticut

Thomas D. Kramer, M.D.
Clinical Instructor
Department of Orthopaedic Surgery
University of Pittsburgh School of
  Medicine;
Staff Orthopaedic Surgeon
St. Francis Medical Center
Pittsburgh, Pennsylvania

Stephen D. Kuslich, M.D.
St. Croix Orthopaedics
Stillwater, Minnesota

William C. Lauerman, M.D.
Associate Professor
Chief, Division of Spinal Surgery
Department of Orthopaedic Surgery
Georgetown University Hospital
Washington, District of Columbia

Alan M. Levine, M.D.
Director, The Cancer Institute
Sinai Hospital of Baltimore;
Professor of Orthopaedic Surgery
University of Maryland
Baltimore, Maryland

Steven C. Ludwig, M.D.
Assistant Professor, Spine
Department of Orthopaedics and
  Rehabilitation
Penn State Hershey Medical Center
Hershey, Pennsylvania

Mohammad E. Majd, M.D.
Spine Surgery, PSC
Louisville, Kentucky

Amir Matityahu, M.D.
Resident
Department of Orthopaedic Surgery
Maimonides Medical Center
Brooklyn, New York

John A. McCulloch, M.D.
Professor
Department of Orthopaedic Surgery
Northeastern Ohio Universities,
  College of Medicine
Akron, Ohio

R. Scott Meyer, M.D.
Assistant Professor
Department of Orthopaedic Surgery
University of California San Diego
San Diego, California

Philip Minotti, M.D.
Orthopaedic Resident
Thomas Jefferson University
Philadelphia, Pennsylvania

Srdjan Mirkovic, M.D.
Assistant Clinical Professor
Department of Orthopaedic Surgery
Northwestern Memorial Hospital
Chicago, Illinois

William Mitchell, M.D.
Resident
Department of Neurosurgery
Jefferson Medical College
Philadelphia, Pennsylvania

Michael R. Moore, M.D.
Assistant Clinical Instructor
Department of Orthopaedic Surgery
University of Colorado Health
  Sciences Center
Boulder, Colorado

Peter O. Newton, M.D.
Assistant Clinical Professor
Department of Orthopaedic Surgery
University of California San Diego
San Diego, California

Marianne Pouliquen, M.D.
Department of Pediatric
  Orthopaedic Surgery
Hospital des Enfants Malades
Paris, France

Gregory J. Przybylski, M.D.
Assistant Professor
Department of Neurosurgery
Jefferson Medical College
Philadelphia, Pennsylvania

Joseph L. Richey, M.D.
Director of Spine Care
Redding Orthopaedic Center
Redding, California

Glenn R. Rechtine II, M.D.
Professor
Chief of Spinal Surgery
Department of Orthopaedics and
  Rehabilitation
University of Florida College of
  Medicine
Gainesville, Florida

Donal B. Rose, M.D.
Resident
Department of Orthopaedic Surgery
Maimonides Medical Center
Brooklyn, New York

Michael K. Rosner, M.D.
Chief Resident
Department of Neurosurgery
Walter Reed Army Medical Center
Washington, District of Columbia

Paul E. Savas, M.D.
Spine Fellow
The Rothman Institute
Thomas Jefferson University
    Hospital
Philadelphia, Pennsylvania

Frank J. Schwab, M.D.
Attending Orthopaedic Surgeon
Department of Orthopaedic Surgery
Maimonides Medical Center
Brooklyn, New York

Suken A. Shah, M.D.
Attending Pediatric Orthopaedic
    Surgeon
Alfred I. DuPont Hospital for
    Children
Wilmington, Delaware;
Clinical Instructor of Orthopaedic
    Surgery
Jefferson Medical College
Philadelphia, Pennsylvania

Alok D. Sharan, M.D.
Orthopaedic Resident
Albany Medical Center
Albany, New York

Terrence P. Sheehan, M.D.
Assistant Professor
Department of Physical Medicine
    and Rehabilitation
Kessler Institute for Rehabilitation
West Orange, New Jersey

Kanwaldeep S. Sidhu, M.D.
Orthopaedic Surgeon
Department of Orthopaedic Surgery
St. John Hospital and Medical
    Center
Detroit, Michigan

Kern Singh, M.D.
Orthopaedic Resident
Rush Presbyterian Medical Center
Chicago, Illinois

Kush Singh, B.S.
Medical Student
Jefferson Medical College
Philadelphia, Pennsylvania

Leslie N. Sutton, M.D.
Professor
Department of Neurosurgery
Children's Hospital of Pennsylvania
Philadelphia, Pennsylvania

Katsuro Tomita, M.D.
Professor and Chairman
Department of Orthopaedic Surgery
Kanazawa University School of
    Medicine
Ishikawa, Japan

Eeric Truumees, M.D.
Attending Spine Surgeon
Department of Orthopaedic Surgery
William Beaumont Hospital
Royal Oak, Michigan

John D. Tydings, M.D.
Spinal Surgeon
Lawrenceville, New Jersey

Alexander R. Vaccaro, M.D.
Professor
Co-Director, Delaware Valley
    Regional Spinal Cord Injury
    Center;
Co-Chief, Spinal Surgery
Thomas Jefferson University and the
    Rothman Institute
Philadelphia, Pennsylvania

Jed S. Vanichkachorn, M.D.
Clinical Instructor
Department of Orthopaedic Surgery
Jefferson Medical College
Thomas Jefferson University
Philadelphia, Pennsylvania

Erol Veznedaroglu, M.D.
Resident
Department of Neurosurgery
Jefferson Medical College
Philadelphia, Pennsylvania

Dennis R. Wenger, M.D.
Director, Pediatric Orthopaedics
Children's Hospital of San Diego;
Clinical Professor of Orthopaedic
    Surgery
University of California San Diego
San Diego, California

Samuel W. Wiesel, M.D.
Professor and Chairman
Department of Orthopaedic Surgery
Georgetown University Hospital
Washington, District of Columbia

Kirkham B. Wood, M.D.
Associate Professor
Department of Orthopaedic Surgery
University of Minnesota, Twin
    Cities Spine Center
Minneapolis, Minnesota

Michael J. Yaszemski, M.D.
Associate Professor
Department of Orthopaedic Surgery
Mayo Clinic
Rochester, Minnesota

Seth M. Zeidman, M.D.
Chief, Division of Complex Spinal
    Neurosurgery
Department of Neurosurgery
Strong Memorial Hospital
Rochester, New York

To my wife and children, Max, Alex, and Juliana, who without their loving support and devotion, a project of this magnitude could not have been possible.

Alexander Vaccaro

To the memory of my wife Lauren. Her support and love sustain me still.

Todd Albert

Section I

Degenerative Conditions

Case 1

Axial Neck Pain: Nonoperative Approach

Terrence P. Sheehan

History and Physical Examination

A 38-year-old man without a significant past medical history presented to the out-patient injured workers clinic for evaluation of neck and shoulder pain. The patient reported the onset of left posterior neck pain 1 week prior to his visit, after lifting office furniture as part of his usual work routine. He was unsure of specific weakness because he was favoring the arm, but he did feel that power and endurance were reduced when using the affected arm. A cervical spine film taken at that time revealed degenerative changes but no fracture. The patient noted no numbness or tingling in the right upper extremity or bilateral lower extremities, no bowel or bladder dys-

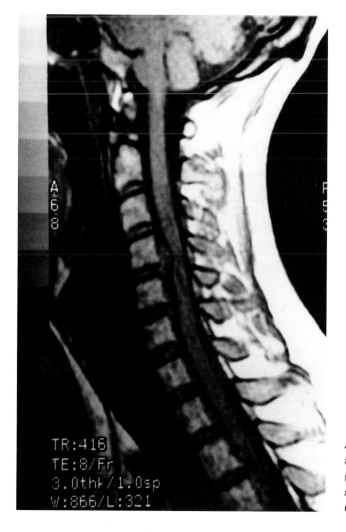

Figure 1–1. A sagittal magnetic resonance imaging (MRI) of the cervical spine reveals a moderate-sized C4/C5 disc herniation.

function, and no balance or gait disturbance. He had no prior history of neck pain symptoms, trauma, or history of work-related injuries. He did report tobacco use.

On directed physical examination, he appeared to hold his neck stiffly, with his head to the right. He had reduced range of motion in all planes of flexion, extension, lateral bending, and rotation, with increased pain with any motion to the left and with rotation to the right. There was palpable spasm in bilateral cervical paraspinals and the left middle trapezius. There were multiple tender points but no specific trigger points in these muscles. Spurling's maneuver was positive on the left with radiation of pain into the left proximal upper extremity, and Lhermitte's sign was negative. Examination of the shoulders revealed no joint laxity or rotator cuff impingement. Provocative testing for impingement of the neurovascular structures in the thoracic outlet was negative. On manual muscle testing of the upper extremities and lower extremities, the strength was graded as 5/5 except for 4+/5 for left elbow flexion. The sensory examination revealed no abnormalities in all four extremities. On reflex testing, the left biceps reflex was depressed and asymmetric when compared to the right. There was no Hoffmann sign and the plantar reflexes were down-going (negative Babinski).

Radiologic Findings

Plain X-ray

Degenerative disc disease with decreased height at the C4/C5 level and mild foraminal stenosis at this level were found on plain X-ray. A sagittal magnetic resonance imaging (MRI) of the cervical spine revealed a moderate-sized disc herniation at the C4/C5 level (Fig. 1–1).

Diagnosis

Cervical sprain and strain. Myofacial pain. Left C5 radiculopathy.

Nonoperative Management

Initial management entails both diagnostic workup and symptom relief. Electrodiagnostic studies were ordered at 21 days postinjury to evaluate for left cervical radiculopathy. The patient was prescribed nonsteroidal antiinflammatory drugs (NSAIDs) and a muscle relaxant. The narcotics were discontinued. The side effects and precautions were reviewed. A course of physical therapy was initiated 2 to 3 times per week. The therapy prescription included initial trials of modalities such as moist heat and cold, and a trial of gentle manual traction. The therapy prescription also detailed a progression to myofacial release of the cervical paraspinals and bilateral upper extremities with focus on the left middle trapezeii and left rhomboids as tolerated. Development of a home self-administered flexibility program 1 to 2 times per day was also requested. The goals of therapy were to restore full range of motion (ROM) and flexibility to the neck and shoulders. The patient and therapist were instructed to discontinue the program and have the patient reevaluated if the pain increased or further neurologic symptoms developed. A cervical pillow was prescribed for use during sleep. The patient was kept off work, with instructions to inquire

- In the evaluation of neck pain, the examiner needs to thoroughly test the upper and lower extremity reflexes and include the Hoffmann and plantar reflexes. Diffuse hyperreflexia (especially in the lower extremities), positive Hoffmann, and the presence of an abnormal gait indicate the presence of a cervical myelopathy.
- Diagnostic studies are complementary to the information gathered from the history and physical examination. Studies have demonstrated significant abnormalities (i.e., diffuse degenerative changes, disc herniation, foraminal stenosis) in asymptomatic populations; thus, clinical correlation and interpretation are the mainstay in formulating a diagnosis and treatment plan.
- Cervical manipulation should not be used in the spondolytic cervical spine with or without associated radiculopathy. This activity is usually performed with high- and/or low-velocity thrusting and thus raises the risk of potentially serious neurologic complications.

about sedentary light duty positions available from the employer as a possible transition for return to full work duty.

Discussion

Clinical Assessment of Axial Neck Pain

Initial assessment of the patient with neck pain begins with a detailed history. An account of the onset and progression of symptoms should first be obtained. The predominant symptom (e.g., pain, spasm, numbness, tingling) should be identified and the relevant history should include quality, timing, frequency, and duration. This history helps form the differential diagnosis and plan the management course. Previsit diagrams are useful for revealing patient symptom locations and patterns. To formulate a treatment plan, it is helpful to know which medications (e.g., narcotics, muscle relaxants) were used and which treatments (e.g., heat, cold, therapies) provided relief.

A review of systems needs to be made. This can be done efficiently with previsit checklists. In axial neck pain, a history of myelopathic symptoms such as bowel and bladder dysfunction, gait dysfunction, lower extremity stiffness, spasms, and weakness needs to be obtained. The symptoms of other systemic processes including other neurologic diseases, infection, malignancy, and inflammatory processes should also be reviewed prior to initiating a treatment plan.

The physical examination begins with observation of the position of the head, neck, shoulders, and upper extremities. With the neck and shoulders exposed, bony and muscular asymmetries are noted. Asymmetries in shoulder height and scapular position are a sign of restricted muscle lengthening and limited movement. Inspection for muscular atrophy helps to date the injury. From history and observation, the suspected pain originators are noted and should be examined last as the exam can exacerbate the irritated structures. Thus, the noninvolved extremities, spine, and portions of the trunk are examined first. The examination of the neck begins with palpation of the base of the skull and then proceeds to the bony cervical spine segments. The cervical paraspinals, anterior neck, and posterior shoulder muscles are palpated for tender points and trigger points. Tender points are areas in the muscle that are localized with deep digital palpation. Trigger points are similar, except that both local and referred symptoms are elicited. Cervical and axillary lymph node examination is done at this point. Range of motion of the cervical spine is first done passively by the examiner then actively assisted by the patient to determine current functional motion. An understanding of the prime movers for each active motion of the cervical spine localizes the elicited pain complaints to specific muscle groups and the possible involved root level. The examiner should use a standard convenient scale for cervical spine motion analysis so that initial exams and response to treatment can be correlated on follow-up.

Important provocative maneuvers for the neck are Lhermitte's sign, Spurling's sign, and cervical distraction. Lhermitte's sign is obtained when flexing the neck causes electric-like sensations down the spine. A positive test may indicate spinal cord compression and/or tethering. Spurling's maneuver is performed by combining lateral flexion, posterior rotation, and axial compression through the head. This test reduces the diameter of the neural foramen and a positive test produces radiation of symptoms into the ipsilateral shoulder and often down the arm. It is often present in severe cervical spondylosis and is a test that is specific for acute radiculopathy. Lastly, in the cervical distraction test, the patient is examined in the supine position. The examiner applies gentle manual traction to the cervical spine through the craniocervical junction. The reduction of symptoms occurs in a positive test. A positive sign is often associated with acute disc involvement.

The manual muscle test (MMT) is the most valuable tool for determining root-level involvement and thus radiculopathy. This scale was originally adopted and standardized by the British Medical Research Council in 1943 and is the international standard for motor strength testing used by clinicians. However, it does have certain flaws. It should be understood that the 0 to 5 intervals are an ordinal scale (e.g., the interval 2 to 3 does not numerically equal the interval 3 to 4) and thus lacks precision as a scientific measure. The MMT is also unable to discriminate the range of strengths described as normal; thus, it is a rather subjective measure. Despite these shortcomings it works well in the clinical setting. It is important that the clinician have appropriate training to perform the testing properly. For example, when testing the extensor carpi radialis (C6), the antigravity position (0–2) is tested first with the elbow extended and the forearm in midpronation (neutral); for gravity testing (3) the forearm is in full pronation; and for resistance testing (4–5) the forearm is in full pronation on a table, the proximal joint (elbow) is fixed, and the force is applied to the fifth metacarpal and is directed toward the radial side. When properly performed, the MMT is more specific for detecting the root-level injury than the sensory testing. The muscles need to be tested in more than one peripheral nerve distribution to identify a root-level injury as opposed to a mononeuropathy [e.g., for the C7 root level, elbow extension (radial n.) and forearm pronation (median n.) strengths are tested].

The sensory examination is essential but involves subjective processing by the patient and thus has limited reliability and reproducibility. A dermatomal pattern of decreased/lost sensation or hyperpathia to light touch and/or sharp touch is tested and indicates specific root injury. The examiners should know the dermatomal patterns and recommended points for testing. Deep tendon reflexes (DTRs) are another important part of the examination of the patient with axial neck pain. Any grade of reflex can be normal if symmetric bilaterally; thus, it is the evaluation for asymmetry that is important in identifying radiculopathy. Reflex testing is more sensitive in the lower extremities than in the upper extremities for exposing root-level injury.

Diagnostic Tests in Axial Neck Pain

Diagnostic tests must be correlated with the history and physical examination. Imaging studies are used to define the anatomy, and electrodiagnostic studies are used to define peripheral nerve physiology. They both complement the information gathered from the history and physical examination. Plain X-rays are helpful as an initial test in patients presenting with neck pain, especially if trauma is involved. In trauma cases and when instability is suspected, flexion-extension and atlantoaxial views are needed in addition to the routine anteriorposterior, oblique, and lateral views. Degenerative changes commonly occur after the age of 40 in both symptomatic and asymptomatic populations, which limits the usefulness of X-rays. The entire spinal cord, nerve roots, ligaments, and soft tissues can be visualized by MRI. It is the imaging method of choice for patients with possible neurologic compromise and for those unresponsive to initial conservative measures. Studies have demonstrated significant abnormalities (e.g., disc herniation, foraminal stenosis) in asymptomatic populations, and thus clinical correlation and interpretation are challenging. Electrodiagnostic studies have two components: the nerve conduction portion used to identify slowing or loss of impulse conduction of the limb sensory and motor nerves, and the electromyogram (EMG) used to identify disruption of the nerve-muscle interface of the specific limb muscles. Injuries to sensory or motor fibers can be diagnosed. These studies give information on the pathophysiology from the nerve root to the nerve-muscle interface. They do not give the cause of the nerve-root/nerve injury. Studies are done at least 18 to 21 days after the onset of symptoms, as this is the time when denervation (fibrillation potentials and positive sharp waves) is detected in the root-level specific muscle. When done by the seasoned electromyographer, these studies are also useful in detecting the chronicity of the injury. The abnormalities that are found can persist after clinical symptoms have resolved, and thus they are not helpful in defining recovery.

Treatment in Axial Neck Pain

Few controlled trials of neck pain have been performed investigating the treatment of neck pain, including that associated with cervical radiculopathy. The "pain originator" is thought to be the compression of the nerve root initiating an inflammatory process. It is in this inflammatory milieu that the chemical mediators of pain ignite the cascade of muscle spasm, cervical immobilization, and local and referred dysesthesias. These symptoms then cause more pain and dysfunction until the chain is broken. Treatment can begin with local icing and NSAIDs. NSAIDs are often beneficial for some pain relief, but are unlikely to affect nerve root inflammation because of poor penetration. Oral steroids have been reported to be effective in acute (e.g., the first 7 to 10 days) radiculopathy at doses of 60 mg/day of prednisone for 1 week followed by a brief methylprednisolone taper. There are no controlled trials to confirm the efficacy of oral steroids in the treatment of radiculopathy. Other classes of medications for symptom relief include muscle relaxants and low-dose tricyclic antidepressants. These have common sedative side effects and they are best taken at bedtime to enhance rest and provide relief of pain and spasm. Narcotics have a finite role at the onset of pain and should be used sparingly and for a limited course, usually until physical measures are implemented. If pain control is inadequate to permit remobilization after 10 days to 2 weeks, the option of more invasive cervical injection techniques such as epidural steroids, intraarticular corticosteroid injections to the cervical zygapophyseal joint, and selective nerve blocks can be considered. These techniques have been inadequately studied and they pose increased risks to the patient. These treatment options, like the others, should not be used in isolation but as one step in the program of symptom relief and functional remobilization.

Physical Measures

In axial neck pain associated with acute radiculopathy, the principal goal during the acute phase of rehabilitation is to reduce pain and inflammation. During the initial painful inflammatory phase, modalities such as heat, cold, and electrical stimulation are effective. The use of moist heat for muscle relaxation can alleviate cervical tension and facilitate effective focal passive muscle stretch. The muscle stretch can be soothing, and it is the initial step in restoring proper movement patterns in the cervical segments. The use of cold to dull the pain, particularly during the initial inflammatory phase and after therapeutic stretch activity, is also effective. Cold results in vasoconstriction and decreases the release of chemical pain mediators such as prostaglandins. It reduces conduction along pain fibers. Both heat and cold modalities are easily transferred to the home self-administered program for symptomatic relief. Electrical stimulation of the muscle in spasm can also provide relaxation and relief, but its mechanism is poorly understood. Ultrasound, because of its deep heating properties, can be irritating to the inflamed tissue and should be avoided. Massage is effective in restoring mobility and improving circulation. Once the patient is past the acute phase, the use of modalities should be limited, and progression to restoring motion and strength should be the focus.

As inflammation and pain diminishes, there is a progression to remobilization and strengthening of the cervical structures. This restorative phase emphasizes restoring functional range of motion through soft tissue release and resetting the head-neck-shoulder biomechanics through a balanced strengthening program of the cervicothoracic musculature. This mobilization is done through therapist-administered passive mobilization techniques (e.g., Maitland technique) and therapist-directed active mobilization techniques performed by the patient (e.g., McKenzie method). It should be understood that the passive techniques produce short-lived results and that it is the progression to the active independent program that produces the long-term benefits. The therapy is a training course; the patient becomes competent with the learned techniques so that at its conclusion the patient is independent with the maintenance program. Spinal stabilization through strengthening of the cervicothoracic musculature should occur after pain-free flexibility of the soft tissues has been restored. No resistive strengthening exercises are done during acute radiculopathy. The therapist and patient progress initially to single plane (e.g., lateral flexion) isometric contractions as tolerated without pain. They move to isotonic contractions in multiple planes. Strengthening of the scapula stabilizers and the bilateral upper extremities is a significant part of this program.

The patient is subsequently transitioned to a home maintenance program for retaining the flexibility, postural controls, and strength achieved during the treatment. It is during this transition that environmental and behavioral issues are addressed and modifications to prevent recurrence and exacerbations are implemented.

Alternative Methods of Management

Type of Management	Advantages	Disadvantages	Comments
Medications			
Narcotics	Acute phase pain relief	Addictive, ineffective for neuropathic pain	Avoid, brief course if needed
Nonsteroidal antiinflammatory drugs (NSAIDs)	Pain and spasm relief	GI side effects, poor penetration of nerve root	Usually helpful throughout course
Oral steroids	Dampens inflammation	Systemic side effects, efficacy unproven	Avoid, may be helpful with acute radiculopathy

Continued on next page

Continued

Type of Management	Advantages	Disadvantages	Comments
Muscle relaxants	Spasm relief, rest enhancement	Sedative	Helpful with initial rest and sleep
Tricyclic low-dose antidepressant	Rest/sleep enhancement	Sedative	Helpful with initial rest and sleep
Physical Measures			
Cervical collar	Reminder to limit motion in acute phase	Awkward, slows functional progression	Avoid
Manual traction	Diagnostic, brief relief	Therapist dependent	Helpful
Mechanical traction	Nerve root decompression	Cumbersome	Avoid
Cervical manipulation	Soft tissue release, pain relief	Neurologic risks	Caution
Massage		Therapist dependent	Helpful
Modalities			
Heat	Pain and spasm relief, enhances flexibility	Irritating to inflamed tissues	Effective
Cold	Inflammation reduction, pain relief	Stiffens soft tissues, nerve irritation	Effective
Electrical stimulation	Spasm reduction, soothing	Therapist dependent	Effective
Ultrasound	None	Enhances inflammation	Do not use with acute inflammation
Physical Therapy			
Passive	Early tissue mobilization, spasm and pain reduction	Short-lived response, therapist dependent	Standard
Active assisted	Tissue mobilization	Initially uncomfortable	Standard
Strengthening	Maintains the resetting of cervical biomechanics	Patient dependent, behavior modification	Not during acute radiculopathy

Suggested Readings

Braddom RL. Management of common cervical pain syndromes. In: De Lisa JA, ed. Rehabilitation Medicine: Principles and Practice, 2nd ed., p. 1038. Philadelphia: JB Lippincott, 1993.

Cailliet R. Neck and upper arm pain. In: Soft Tissue Pain and Disability, 2nd ed., pp. 123–167. Philadelphia: FA Davis, 1991.

Ellenberg M, Honet JC. Clinical pearls in cervical radiculopathy. Phys Med Rehab Clin North Am 1996; 7:487–505.

Malanga GA. The diagnosis and treatment of cervical radiculopathy. Med Sci Sports Exerc 1997; 29(suppl 7):S236–S245.

Case 2

Whiplash Injuries: Nonoperative Approach

Kanwaldeep S. Sidhu and Jeffrey S. Fischgrund

History and Physical Examination

A 29-year-old woman presented with complaints of neck pain 2 months after a motor vehicle accident. She reported being a restrained driver who was rear-ended at a stoplight by a second vehicle traveling at approximately 35 mph. She was initially seen in the emergency room, where radiographs were negative, and she was diagnosed as having a cervical strain. Her symptoms now include pain in the cervical area with radiation to the posterior occiput and trapezius and distally to the upper thoracic spine. She also complains of headaches and limited range of motion of the neck. She denies any weakness or paresthesias in the upper extremities. Physical

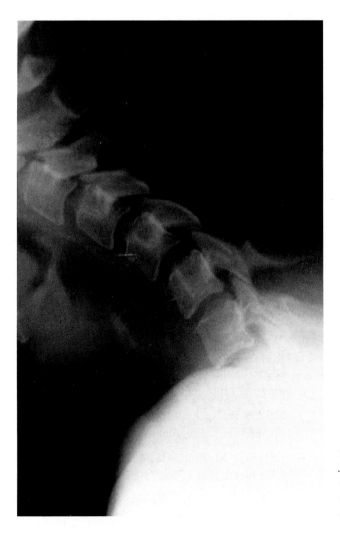

Figure 2–1. A lateral plain flexion radiograph of the cervical spine revealing no evidence of pathologic cervical subluxation.

examination revealed limited range of motion of the cervical spine upon flexion, and rotation. She was neurologically intact in both upper and lower extremities without any myelopathic signs.

Radiologic Findings

Radiographs of the cervical spine revealed flattening of cervical lordosis. There was no evidence of any fractures. The soft tissue shadow measurements were within normal limits. A flexion lateral plain radiograph revealed no significant subluxation (Fig. 2–1).

Discussion

Soft tissue injuries to the cervical spine are a common source of disability after motor vehicle accidents. Rear-ending automobile accidents are typically associated with whiplash. The term "whiplash" was first described by Crowe in 1928. It lacks precise definition, and has typically been used to define the initial injury and subsequent sequelae associated with the acceleration-extension of the head and neck during a rear-impact collision. Simply stated, it is a musculoligamentous sprain of the cervical region.

It is estimated that over 250,000 cervical whiplash injuries occur every year in the United States. Although symptoms associated with most of these injuries will be self-limiting over 4 to 6 weeks, a significant percentage may go on to chronic pain syndromes and litigation. These injuries can account for up to 85% of compensated claims from litigation associated with motor vehicle accidents. Up to 25% of patients may have chronic neck pain after a whiplash injury, and 10 to 15% may have severe disabling symptoms.

History and Physical Examination

The typical history involves a front-seat driver/passenger involved in a rear-impact collision. Symptoms such as neck pain may not be severe initially at the time of impact. Within 48 to 72 hours, most patients complain of neck pain and stiffness. Other associated symptoms include headaches, visual and memory disturbances, weakness, paresthesias, and dysesthesias of the upper extremities (Table 2–1).

Historical data that may be useful for diagnosis and treatment include speed of impact, presence or absence of headrests, and whether the patient was wearing a seat belt. Seat belts have saved countless lives by preventing life-threatening injuries; however, the incidence of cervical strain such as that associated with whiplash, has increased since their use. A 3-year study in Scotland found that the number of cervical strains associated with automobile accidents doubled since the introduction of mandatory seat belt laws. The U.S. National Highway Transportation Safety Administration found that the rate of whiplash injuries in drivers of vehicles with headrests was 10% lower than in drivers of vehicles without head restraints. In addition, fixed headrests worked better than adjustable head restraints in minimizing injury.

Identification of risk factors for poor prognosis after whiplash injury is important. Preexisting degenerative changes in the cervical spine and/or prior neck

Table 2–1
Whiplash Injury Symptoms and Frequency of Occurrence

Symptom	Frequency (%)
Neck pain	88–100
Headache	54–66
Shoulder pain	40–42
Dizziness	17–25
Paresthesias	13–62
Visual disturbance	8–21
Auditory disturbances	4–18

surgery may be important in the appropriate diagnosis and treatment of symptoms associated with whiplash that may be refractory to standard treatment protocols.

The Quebec Task Force on Whiplash-Associated Disorders recommended a classification for whiplash injuries based on clinical presentation (Table 2–2).

According to the above classification, Norris and Watt (1983) concluded that 43% of the whiplash patients in their study corresponded to Quebec grade I, 29% to grade II, 12% to grade III, and 6% to grade IV. Burke and colleagues (1992), in their series, concluded that 41% of the patients were in grade I, 56% in grade II, and only 3% in grade IV.

Radiologic Findings

Most patients presenting with whiplash symptoms either have normal cervical spine radiographs or show degenerative changes physiologic for age. Widening of the prevertebral soft tissue shadow may indicate underlying hematoma. Laceration of the anterior longitudinal ligament secondary to hyperextension may result in hematoma formation. If ligamentous injury is suspected, then flexion-extension radiographs or magnetic resonance imaging (MRI) may be the study of choice.

Magnetic resonance imaging is an ideal tool to assess the degree of soft tissue damage associated with cervical trauma. In the absence of neurologic deficit, the role of computed tomography (CT) or MRI in an acute injury setting is minimal.

Table 2–2
Proposed Clinical Classification of Whiplash-Associated Disorders

Grade	Clinical Presentation[a]
0	No complaint about the neck/no physical sign(s)
I	Neck complaint of pain, stiffness, tenderness only No physical sign(s)
II	Neck complaint AND musculoskeletal sign(s)[b]
III	Neck complaint AND neurologic sign(s)[c]
IV	Neck complaint AND fracture/dislocation

[a]Symptoms and disorders that can be manifest in all grades including deafness, dizziness, tinnitus, headache, memory loss, dysphagia, and temporomandibular joint pain.
[b]Musculoskeletal signs include decreased range of motion and point tenderness.
[c]Neurologic signs include decreased or absent deep tendon reflexes, weakness, and sensory deficits.

Bone scans typically do not have a role in acute diagnosis or treatment of whiplash disorders. They may be useful to look for occult cervical fractures. Such fractures, however, may be better evaluated by CT scans.

Other diagnostic studies, such as discography and facet blocks, may be useful in pinpointing the source of chronic neck pain after whiplash injuries. However, they have no role in acute treatment.

Nonoperative Management

Most patients with whiplash injuries do well with nonoperative management. The natural history of whiplash is that 75% of the patients will improve spontaneously. However, more than 25% of the patients may suffer from persistent pain at 1 year after injury. Surgical intervention is reserved for patients with fractures, disc herniations, or instability that is not amenable to nonoperative measures.

Treatment for whiplash injuries must be tailored to the severity of injury and the individual symptoms. Initial management is the same as that for any other musculoligamentous sprain, and depending on severity, may include rest, immobilization, and medications. Rigid cervical collars are uncomfortable and are rarely indicated. The use of a soft collar may reduce pain, provide support, and minimize motion associated with activities of daily living. Immobilization should be limited to 2 to 3 weeks so as to avoid dependence and muscle atrophy. The use of a cold pack for the first 48 to 72 hours may decrease swelling and inflammation. After that, moist heat may provide symptomatic relief.

Pharmacologic intervention may include antiinflammatories, analgesics, and muscle relaxers. The use of long-term narcotics should be minimized.

After the initial pain and spasms has subsided, patients should be weaned off medications, and started into a mobilization and exercise program. An initial program of isometric exercises may be better tolerated than aggressive physical therapy and traction. Patients should be instructed to go through a regimen of flexion, extension, and rotation exercises within their limits of pain tolerance several times a day. Formal physical therapy, for 8 to 12 sessions, may be beneficial for select patients who need a structured treatment protocol for compliance. This should preferably be done within 2 weeks of injury. Mealy and colleagues compared two treatment modalities in 61 patients with whiplash: collar immobilization and active exercises. They reported a superior outcome at 8 weeks in the active exercise group. McKinney (1989) reported on 126 patients with whiplash treated one of three ways: mobilization, physiotherapy, and no treatment. He concluded that a mobilization regimen was superior to physiotherapy or no treatment. Pennie and Agambar (1990) compared rest in a soft collar/unsupervised mobilization to early traction/physiotherapy in 135 whiplash patients. They reported no difference in outcome between the two groups at 5 months after injury. Borchgrevink and colleagues (1998) conducted a single-blind randomized trial for treatment of acute whiplash. Two different treatment regimens were used within the first 14 days after injury. Group I patients were encouraged to resume normal daily life activities, whereas group II patients were given time off from work and were immobilized in a soft collar. At 6-month follow-up, the outcome was better for patients in group I than in group II.

Injection therapy with either saline, lidocaine, or corticosteroids has no role in acute treatment. Select studies have postulated that in patients with chronic pain after whiplash injuries, the cervical zygapophyseal joints may be responsible. Lord and colleagues (1996) conducted a double-blind study on 68 patients with chronic whiplash symptoms using placebo-controlled local anesthetic blocks. Patients underwent injections of two different local anesthetics and placebo (saline) in random order and under double-blind conditions. The authors concluded that the overall prevalence of cervical facet joint pain was 60% in patients with chronic neck pain after whiplash. The authors suggested that most headaches in whiplash patients are associated with C2/C3 zygapophyseal joint dysfunction. Such injections should be used sparingly in clinical practice because of the discomfort associated with the procedure itself and lack of proven efficacy over the natural history of the disease.

The role of methylprednisolone in treatment of spinal cord injury is well established. However, its role in the treatment of musculoligamentous sprains is more controversial. Pettersson and Toolanen (1998) reported a prospective, randomized, double-blind study comparing high-dose methylprednisolone with placebo. The steroids were administered within 8 hours of whiplash injury. At 6-month follow-up, there was a statistically significant difference in outcome between the two groups regarding number of sick days and sick leave profile. The authors concluded that high-dose methylprednisolone may be beneficial for acute treatment of whiplash. However, because the patient sample size in this study was small, we do not recommend high-dose intravenous steroids for treatment of acute whiplash at this time. Intraarticular facet injections of steroids have not been shown to be helpful for patients with chronic whiplash syndrome.

Pulsed electromagnetic therapy has been shown to have antiinflammatory effects and promote healing. Foley-Nolan and colleagues (1992) reported a double-blind randomized study on the effect of pulsed electromagnetic therapy (PEMT) on 40 patients with whiplash. Half the patients were treated with PEMT, and the remaining with placebo. At 2- and 4-week follow-up, the PEMT group had statistically significant improvement in pain compared to the placebo group. The improved outcomes continued at 12-week follow-up. The authors concluded that pulsed electromagnetic therapy has a beneficial effect in the treatment of acute whiplash.

Prognosis

The prognosis for most patients with whiplash injuries is good. The symptoms are often self-limiting and resolve spontaneously within 4 to 6 weeks. Up to 25% of the patients have persistent symptoms lasting for more than a year. Norris and Watt (1983) analyzed 61 patients with whiplash injuries to develop indicators of prognosis. They concluded that factors that indicate a poor prognosis include presence of objective neurologic signs, stiffness of the neck, muscle spasm, and preexisting degenerative spondylosis. A 10-year follow-up was reported by Gargan and Bannister (1990) on 43 patients with whiplash injuries. Older patients had a worse prognosis, and symptom recovery plateaued at 2 years. At 10.8-year follow-up, 12% had continued severe symptoms. Hohl (1974) reported retrospectively on 146 patients with whiplash injuries. Poor prognosis in this series was associated with numbness and/or pain in an upper extremity, sharp reversal of the cervical lordosis on radiographs, restricted motion on flexion extension views, need for cervical collar for more than 12 weeks, need for home traction, and repeat course of physical therapy because of symptom recurrence. Degenerative changes developed in 39% of patients who prior to injury had no cervical degeneration.

Alternative Methods of Management

Alternative methods of treatment may include manipulative therapy and acupuncture. Due to lack of data from prospective randomized trials involving the use of such treatments, nontraditional therapies are not discussed here.

Type of Management	Advantages	Disadvantages
Nonsteroidal antiinflammatory drugs (NSAIDs) and home exercise regimen	Efficacious for most patients with self-limiting symptoms; low cost; available to all patients	Side effects of medications; compliance with medication regimen and participation with home exercises
Physical therapy	Structured regimen of exercises over a 3- to 4-week period; includes local modalities and instructions regarding home exercises	High cost; needs time commitment for participation; transportation to the physical therapy facility may be an issue with some patients
Immobilization	May provide symptomatic short-term relief	Deconditioning of muscles with prolonged use and dependency
Narcotics and muscle relaxers	Efficacious for severe pain and muscle spasms	Potential for addiction; side effects of medication
Injections	May provide relief of symptoms in small percentage of chronic whiplash patients	Invasive procedure; no long-term prospective randomized trials supporting efficacy
Pulsed electromagnetic fields (PEMF)	May have some benefit in reducing inflammation and promoting soft tissue healing	Lacks proven efficacy over natural history of the disease; no large prospective randomized trials

Suggested Readings

Barancik JL, Kramer CF, Thode HC. Epidemiology of Motor Vehicle Injuries in Suffolk County, New York Before Enactment of the New York Senate Seatbelt Use Law. DOT HS 807 638. Washington, DC: US Department of Transportation, National Highway Safety Administration, 1989.

Barnsley L, Lord S, Bogduk N. Whiplash injury—a clinical review. Pain 1994; 58:283–307.

Barnsley L, Lord SM, Wallis BJ, et al. Lack of effect of intraarticular corticosteroids for chronic pain in the cervical zygapophyseal joints. N Engl J Med 1994; 330:1047–1050.

Barnsley L, Lord SM, Wallis B, et al. The prevalence of chronic cervical zygapophyseal joint pain after whiplash. Spine 1995; 20(1):20–26.

Barton D, Allen M, Finlay D, et al. Evaluation of whiplash injuries by technetium 99m isotope scanning. Arch Emerg Med 1992; 10:197–202.

Boden SD, McCowin PR, Davis DO, et al. Abnormal magnetic-resonance scans of the cervical spine in asymptomatic subjects. J Bone Joint Surg 1990; 72A:1178–1184.

Borchgrevink GE, Kaasa A, McDonagh D, et al. Acute treatment of whiplash neck sprain injuries. A randomized trial of treatment during the first 14 days after a car accident. Spine 1998; 23:25–31.

Borchgrevink GE, Smevik O, Nordby A, et al. MR imaging and radiography of patients with cervical hyperextension-flexion injuries after car accidents. Acta Radiol 1995; 36:425–428.

Bracken MD, Shepard MJ, Collins WF, et al. A randomized controlled trial of methylprednisolone or naloxone in the treatment of acute spinal cord injury. N Engl J Med 1990; 332:1405–1411.

Burke JP, Orton HP, West J, et al. Whiplash and its effect on the visual system. Graefes Arch Clin Exp Ophthalmol 1992; 230:335–339.

Byrn C, Olsson I, Falkheden L, et al. Subcutaneous sterile water injections for chronic neck and shoulder pain following whiplash injuries. Lancet 1993; 341(8843):449–452.

Crowe H. Injuries to the cervical spine. Presentation to the annual meeting of the Western Orthopaedic Association, San Francisco, 1928.

Daffner RH. Evaluation of cervical cerebral injuries. Semin Roentgenol 1992; 27:239–253.

Deans GT, Magalliard JN, Kerr M, et al. Neck sprain—a major cause of disability following car accidents. Injury 1987; 18:10–12.

Foley-Nolan D, Moore K, Codd M, et al. Low energy high frequency pulsed electromagnetic therapy for acute whiplash injuries. A double blind randomized controlled study. Scand J Rehabil Med 1992; 24(1):51–59.

Gargan MF, Bannister GC. Long term prognosis of soft tissue injuries of the neck. J Bone Joint Surg 1990; 72B:901–903.

Gunzburg R, Szpalski M. Whiplash Injuries: Current Concepts in Prevention, Diagnosis and Treatment of the Cervical Whiplash Syndrome. Philadelphia: Lippincott-Raven, 1998.

Hildingsson C, Toolanen G. Outcome after soft tissue injury of the cervical spine. A prospective study of 93 car accident victims. Acta Orthop Scand 1990; 61:357–359.

Hirsch S, Hirsch P, Hiramoto H, et al. Whiplash syndrome: fact or fiction. Orthop Clin North Am 1988; 19(4):791–795.

Hohl M. Soft tissue injuries of the neck in automobile accidents. J Bone Joint Surg 1974; 56A(8):1675–1682.

Jolliffe VM. Soft tissue injury of the cervical spine: consider the nature of the accident. BMJ 1993; 307:439–440.

LaRocca HL. Cervical spine syndrome: diagnosis, treatment, and long term outcome. In: Frymoyer JW, Ducker TB, Hadler NM, et al. The Adult Spine, pp. 1051–1062. New York: Raven Press, 1991.

Liebermann JS. Cervical soft tissue injuries and cervical disc disease. In: Liebermann JS, ed. Principles of Physical Medicine and Rehabilitation in the Musculoskeletal Disease, pp. 263–286. New York: Grune and Stratton, 1981.

Lord SM, Barnsley L, Wallis BJ, et al. Chronic cervical azygapophyseal joint pain after whiplash. A placebo controlled prevalence study. Spine 1996; 21(15):1737–1745.

Martin DH. The acute traumatic central cord syndrome. In: Gunzburg R, Szpalski M, eds. Whiplash Injuries: Current Concepts in Prevention, Diagnosis and Treatment of the Cervical Whiplash Syndrome, pp. 129–134. Philadelphia: Lippincott-Raven, 1998.

McKinney LA. Early mobilization and outcome in acute sprains of the neck. BMJ 1989; 299:106–108.

Mealy K, Brennan H, Fenelon GC. Early mobilization of acute whiplash injuries. BMJ 1986; 292:656–657.

Nagele M, Koch W, Kaden B. Rofo Fortschr Geb Rontgenstr neuen bildgeb Verfahr. ROFO 1992; 157:222–228.

Norris SH, Watt I. The prognosis of neck injuries resulting from rear end vehicle collisions. J Bone Joint Surg 1983; 605B:608–611.

Pennie BH, Agambar LJ. Whiplash injuries: a trial of early management. J Bone Joint Surg 1990; 72B:277–279.

Pennie L. Prevertebral hematoma in cervical spine injuries. AJR 1981; 136:553–561.

Pettersson K, Hildingsson C, Toolanen G, et al. Disc pathology after whiplash injury: a prospective magnetic resonance imaging and clinical investigation. Spine 1997; 22(3):283–288.

Pettersson K, Toolanen G. High dose methylprednisolone prevents excessive sick leave after whiplash injury. A prospective, randomized, double blind study. Spine 1998; 23(9):984–989.

Provinciali L, Baroni L, Wallis BJ, et al. Multimodal treatment to prevent late whiplash syndrome. Scand J Rehabil Med 1996; 28(2):105–111.

Schneider RC, Sherry G, Pantek H. The syndrome acute central cervical spine cord injury. J Neurosurg 1954; 11:546–577.

Spitzer WO, Skovron ML, Salmi LR, et al. Scientific monolograph of the Quebec Task Force on whiplash-associated disorders: redefining "whiplash" and its management. Spine 1995; 20:1S–73S.

Stewart JR. Statistical Evaluation of the Effectiveness of FMVSS 202: Head Restraints. Task 3 report 2:1-1-A-10, DOT HS 8 02014. Chapel Hill, NC: Highway Research Center, University of North Carolina, 1980.

Szpalski M, Gunzburg R, Soeur M, et al. Pharmacologic interventions in whiplash associated disorders. In: Gunsburg R, Szpalski M, eds. Whiplash Injuries: Current Concepts in Prevention, Diagnosis and Treatment of the Cervical Whiplash Syndrome, pp. 175–182. Philadelphia: Lippincott-Raven, 1998.

Taylor JR, Finch PM. Neck sprain. Aust Fam Physician 1993; 22:1623–1625.

Turbridge RJ. The Long Term Effect of Seat Belt Legislation on Road User Injury Patterns. Research report 239. Crowthorne, UK: Transport and Road Research Laboratory, 1989.

Case 3
Cervical Spondylosis—Soft Disc Herniation: Anterior Approach

Joseph M. Kowalski, Steven C. Ludwig, and Scott D. Boden

History and Physical Examination

A 42-year-old woman presented with a 10-week history of suboccipital headaches, bilateral shoulder pain, and paresthesias. She had no antecedent trauma or previous neck symptoms. She received short-lived relief with the use of antiinflammatory medications and physical therapy to stretch and strengthen her shoulder and neck muscles. Her ability to work as an clerical administrator was significantly impaired,

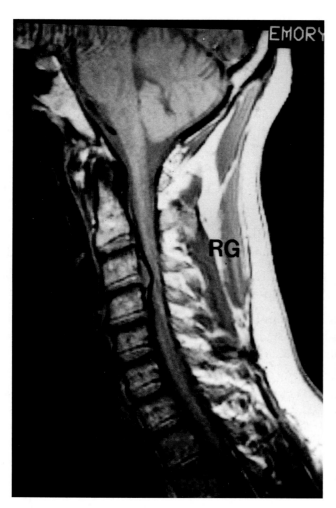

Figure 3–1. Sagittal magnetic resonance imaging (MRI) demonstrating large posterior disc herniation at C3/C4 with elevation of posterior longitudinal ligament (PLL) and compression of dural sac and spinal cord.

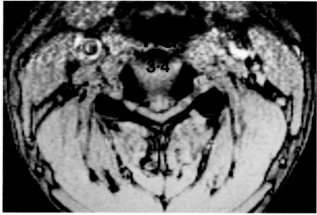

Figure 3–2. Axial MRI demonstrating larger central posterior disc herniation at C3/C4 with compression of dural sac and cord.

and wearing a cervical collar at night no longer provided adequate rest. She had no gait or dexterity disturbances and denied bowel or bladder dysfunction. There was mild limitation of cervical spine range of motion due to neck pain. Pinprick sensation was present but decreased over her posterior neck area bilaterally. Deep tendon reflexes in the upper and lower extremity were graded as 3+ and brisk and motor strength was graded as 5/5 in both upper and lower extremities. She had a reproduction of symptoms with Spurling's maneuver on the left side and did not have a Babinski sign, clonus, or Hoffmann sign. Axial distraction improved her symptoms.

Radiologic Findings

Plain roentgenograms of the cervical spine were unremarkable. Magnetic resonance imaging (MRI) revealed a large central disc herniation at C3/C4 with compression of the dural sac and spinal cord (Figs. 3–1 and 3–2).

Diagnosis

Myeloradiculopathy involving the fourth cervical nerve root from herniation of the C3/C4 nucleus pulposus.

Surgical Management

The patient was positioned supine on a standard operating table and her head placed on a horseshoe-shaped headrest. General anesthesia and endotracheal intubation was performed and a folded sheet was placed between the shoulder blades allowing the neck to be slightly extended. Evidence of spinal instability, spinal cord compromise, or exacerbation of symptoms with neck extension requires fiberoptic nasotracheal intubation with the patient awake and with the neck in a neutral position. Another folded sheet was placed under the patient's right iliac crest, elevating the bone graft harvest site. Her upper extremities were tucked at her sides and her shoulders were pulled distally and taped to the table. This maneuver allowed for better visualization of the lower cervical spine on lateral intraoperative radiographs. Leads to monitor evoked potentials were applied by the monitoring technician, and the head of the table was slightly elevated 15 degrees to reduce venous engorgement. One gram of cefazolin was administered intravenously, and the skin of the neck and right anterior iliac crest was prepared with a betadine solution and draped with an iodinated adhesive skin barrier and multiple layers of sheets.

A slightly curved transverse incision was made in a skin crease on the left side of the neck starting from the midline at the upper end of the thyroid cartilage. Sharp dissection was used to continue the dissection to the level of the platysma muscle. Meticulous hemostasis was maintained throughout the dissection with electrocautery. A self-retaining retractor was placed, and the platysma muscle was identified and divided transversely with a scalpel blade. The plane beneath the platysma was bluntly developed to further mobilize it and enhance exposure. Superficial veins were cauterized through a combination of monopolar and bipolar techniques and larger tributaries ligated with 2-0 absorbable suture. The medial border of the sternocleidomastoid muscle was identified and the pulse of the carotid artery defined the location of the sheath. We used the interval between the carotid sheath laterally and the strap muscles with cervical viscera medially. The superficial layer of the deep

PEARL

- The clinician must correlate symptoms, objective findings, and imaging findings to confirm the diagnosis. The spinal cord and nerve roots may be compressed by a variety of tissues from any direction and one must identify the precise cause of nerve root or spinal cord impingement. These include soft disc herniations, osteophytes ("hard discs"), the ligamentum flavum, ossified posterior longitudinal ligament, tumors, and tumor-like processes to list a few. Myelography and postmyelography computed tomography (CT) may be used in place of or in addition to MRI to better evaluate the osseous anatomy, the course of the nerve root, and the status of the spinal canal. Each nerve root must be traced from the cord out through the foramen. The space available for the cord and the presence of congenital and acquired stenosis need to be appreciated, as does effacement or compression of the dural sac and spinal cord.

PITFALL

- Cervical spondylosis is a ubiquitous process and is apparent on imaging studies in approximately 15 to 20% of asymptomatic patients under 40 years of age and in 95% of men over 60 to 65 years of age. Patients may be treated for shoulder disease or carpal tunnel syndrome without an accurate diagnosis or appropriate workup. The patient may undergo extensive physical therapy, injections, and even surgery for shoulder, hand, or arm pain when the underlying culprit is cervical spine pathology. The converse may also be true.

cervical fascia was incised longitudinally along the sternocleidomastoid muscle. Two hand-held retractors were placed medially and laterally to maintain the plane of dissection. Gentle spreading of tissues with Metzenbaum scissors and bipolar cautery allowed passage through this plane to the pretracheal fascia with minimal bleeding.

The prominences of the intervertebral discs were palpated with the fingertip and the carotid tubercle of the C6 transverse process was gently palpated laterally. The prevertebral fascia was split in the midline with electrocautery and the longus colli muscle gently stripped laterally 2 to 3 mm to expose the anterior longitudinal ligament and intervertebral disc area. A 22-gauge spinal needle was bent in bayonet fashion and placed in the C3/C4 disc space anteriorly and the hand-held retractors were removed. A lateral roentgenogram was obtained to confirm the level. The spinal needle was removed and the anterior aspect of the disc was stripped of the longus colli with a neuro-Frazier suction tip and electrocautery around the anterolateral corners of the vertebral bodies of C3 and C4. Dissection too far laterally could cause injury to the vertebral artery or vein and potentially cause injury to the sympathetic chain, leading to Horner's syndrome. Transverse self-retaining retractors were placed to maintain the exposure. The smooth tips of the transverse blades were well seated beneath the longus colli muscles to minimize trauma to the trachea and esophagus medially and carotid sheath laterally.

A narrow Leksell rongeur was used to remove the anterior lip of the inferior edge of C3. Bone wax was used to stop any excessive osseous bleeding points. A no. 15 scalpel blade was used to incise the intervertebral disc at the attachment to the endplates. The scalpel blade was inserted laterally at the edge of the vertebrae with the cutting edge directed toward the midline. It was then passed parallel to the disc space and withdrawn prior to reaching the opposite side. Another pass was made starting on the opposite side with the cutting edge directed toward the midline. A pituitary rongeur was used to extract loose disc material and a straight 0 curette was further used to clean the anterior disc space, taking care not to violate the vertebral endplates or posterior annulus. The uncinate processes were identified at the posterolateral aspect of the disc space and used to define the lateral limits of the exposure. A medium Cobb elevator was then placed in the disc space and rotated slightly to allow distraction and loosen a stiff interspace. Unicortical threaded distraction screws (14 mm) were placed in the midline at the upper end of the C3 body and midpoint of the C4 vertebral body to allow for placement of the distraction device. Care was taken to place the pins far enough away from the C3/C4 disc space to allow for endplate decortication. The disc space was gently distracted 2 to 4 mm, allowing for better visualization of the posterior annulus and uncovertebral joints.

The remaining disc material and posterior annulus was gently resected using straight and curved 0 and 00 curettes, taking care to preserve the posterior longitudinal ligament. The large nuclear herniation was visualized and removed with a pituitary rongeur. The posterior longitudinal ligament (PLL) was probed with a nerve hook, and no defects were found. The PLL was flush with the back of the vertebral bodies and a small nerve hook was used to probe beyond the posterior margins of the vertebral bodies to ensure that no residual fragments remained. Sometimes it is necessary to release the PLL to make certain that the offending disc fragment is removed.

A 4-mm high-speed burr was used to remove the superior and inferior cartilaginous endplates to punctate bleeding bone. Structural integrity of the subchondral bone was maintained whenever possible to reduce risk of disc space collapse after graft placement. A small ridge of posterior cortex was left to prevent posterior graft migration. The height of the space created measured 7 mm.

The right iliac crest bone graft site was previously exposed while awaiting the localizing radiograph. The skin was injected with 0.25% Marcaine and a dilute epinephrine solution (1:500,000) to provide additional hemostasis and a degree of immediate postoperative analgesia. The white line of the external abdominal fascia was identified. Care was taken to stay two fingerbreadths (5 cm) posterior to the anterior superior iliac spine to minimize risk to the lateral femoral cutaneous nerve. The fascia was divided with electrocautery and subperiosteal dissection of both the inner and outer tables of ilium was performed. Malleable retractors were placed to protect the soft tissues. An oscillating saw with parallel dual blades 7 mm apart was used to cut the graft. A curved $\frac{1}{4}$-inch osteotome was used to remove the tricortical graft and thrombin-soaked Gelfoam was packed into the graft site.

The depth required to allow 2 mm of countersink of the graft site was calculated, and the oscillating saw was used to trim the graft to the appropriate depth. The wound was irrigated copiously with bacteriostatic saline. The graft was placed into the prepared interspace with the cortical surface facing anteriorly and recessed 2 mm with a bone tamp. The distraction was removed and a small Kocher clamp was used to test graft stability. Additional autologous bone was packed around the sides and anterior to the tricortical graft. Care was taken not to introduce anything into the intervertebral space that could potentially impinge the spinal canal posteriorly. The remainder of the distraction apparatus was removed, bone wax placed into the two pin holes, and the self-retaining retractors removed. Radiographs were obtained prior to wound closure to confirm accurate graft placement. The wounds were then closed in layers. A cervical drain was placed beneath the platysma. A cervical collar was applied, and the patient was awakened, extubated, and a brief neurologic examination of the upper and lower extremities was performed.

Postoperative Management

A liquid diet is started on the day following surgery and advanced as tolerated by the patient. A soft cervical collar is worn for 6 to 12 weeks, and radiographs are repeated at 6 weeks to evaluate graft position and flexion/extension views at 12 weeks to look for evidence of nonunion. Nonsteroidal antiinflammatory drugs (NSAIDs) are discontinued 2 weeks prior to surgery and not used in the postoperative period due to the potential effects on bone healing and increased risk of nonunion.

Discussion

Cervical spondylosis is a ubiquitous process and is apparent on imaging studies in approximately 15 to 20% of asymptomatic patients under 40 years of age and in 95% of men over 60 to 65 years of age. Degenerative changes occur most frequently at the C5/C6, C6/C7, and C4/C5 levels and correspond to the most common levels of cervical disc herniation. The mechanical and chemical responses to a herniated disc incite a predominantly local inflammatory response, leading to the syndrome of radiculopathy. Gradual resorption of the disc material and mediators breaks the cycle and can lead to resolution of the radiculopathy syndrome. Gore and colleagues (1987) reported that 50% of 205 patients with unilateral arm pain had persistent radicular pain at 15-year follow-up after receiving nonsurgical care. Lees and Turner (1963) followed 51 patients with cervical spondylosis for 2 to 19 years and found that 45% had a single episode of pain, 30% had intermittent episodes, and 25% had persistent pain.

Upper cervical disc herniations typically produce axial neck pain and headaches. Mixed or vague complaints related to the upper extremities may be present. Herniations at lower levels usually follow a dermatomal pattern. The C4/C5 disc encroaches the C5 nerve root, producing shoulder pain. Weakness of the biceps brachii may be evident with a diminished biceps reflex. Sensory testing may not reveal a significant deficit due to the overlapping and variable C5 dermatome on the neck, shoulder, and arm. Shoulder pathology and C5 radiculopathy may both have shoulder pain and weak shoulder abductors and external rotators. Physical examination should readily differentiate the two. The C5/C6 disc typically involves the C6 nerve root, causing pain, paresthesias, and decreased sensation in the shoulder, arm, and radial forearm toward the thumb and index finger. Weakness of the radial wrist extensors and biceps muscles with diminution of the brachioradialis reflex may be present. The C6/C7 disc involves the C7 nerve root, causing pain in the posterior arm, forearm, and middle and ring fingers with decreased sensation on physical examination. Weakness of the wrist flexors, long finger extensors, and triceps muscle with decreased deep tendon reflex may be elicited. The C7/T1 disc compromises the C8 nerve root, causing pain and paresthesias in the posterior shoulder, arm, and ulnar forearm to small and ring fingers. Associated sensory deficits and weakness of long finger flexors may be evident. This level is less commonly involved in cervical disc disease and lesions affecting the brachial plexus, for example, Pancoast tumor and peripheral nerve entrapment, should be investigated. There exists sufficient variability of innervation in some patients that the above patterns may not hold true.

Initial treatment of radiculopathy includes a combination of activity modification, rest, and collar immobilization. Medications including analgesics, NSAIDs, and muscle relaxants may be helpful in the acute setting. Patient active physical therapy modalities with or without traction are useful adjuncts, but there are no data to suggest that any of these conservative methods influence the natural history of cervical disc degeneration other than alleviating the acute symptoms.

Surgical treatment is indicated in those patients with the correct clinical diagnosis with symptoms refractory to nonsurgical care. Confirmatory evidence of disc herniation at the corresponding level on myelogram, CT scan, CT myelogram, or MRI is essential.

Soft disc herniations occur most commonly at the posterolateral edge of the annulus fibrosis adjacent to the posterior longitudinal ligament. Herniations may also occur laterally into the foramen or centrally (straight posterior), and may even herniate through the PLL. It is sometimes necessary to incise the PLL, perform a foraminotomy, or remove a portion of the vertebral body to access a portion of disc that has migrated out of view.

An anterior cervical discectomy and fusion (ACDF) with autogenous tricortical iliac crest bone graft is currently the most commonly used surgical technique for one-level cervical disc disease. Most ACDF techniques are variations of those described by Smith and Robinson (1955), Bailey and Badgley (1960), or Cloward (1958). The anterior approach provides access to the offending disc fragment, and the placement of a structural graft allows for restoration of disc space height and alignment and increases foraminal and spinal canal dimensions. Other surgical options for soft cervical disc herniations are a posterior laminoforaminotomy or anterior cervical discectomy without fusion. Although both techniques may gain access to the offending disc herniation, neither allows for restoration of disc space and neuroforaminal height or stabilization of the motion segment.

Grafting

The osteoinductive, osteoconductive, and structural properties of autogenous tricortical iliac crest bone graft currently makes this the best option for graft material. The reported fusion rate is 89 to 97% for one-level arthrodesis with no internal fixation. The rate of pseudarthrosis ranges from 17 to 27% with two- or three-level arthrodesis, and even higher with four levels.

A variety of graft configurations have been described as well, each having advocates and opponents (Fig. 3–3). There is general agreement that autogenous structural grafts should be at least 5 mm thick and allow 2- to 4-mm distraction of preoperative disc space height to reduce risk of graft resorption.

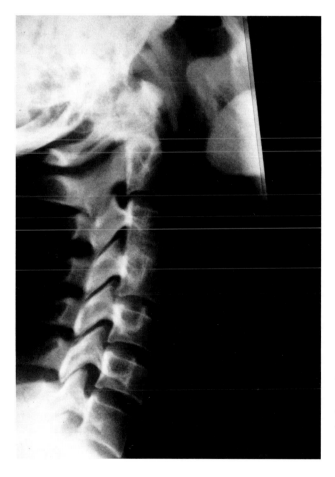

Figure 3–3. Lateral cervical radiograph 13 months after surgery showing graft position and incorporation with trabeculation across the graft-vertebra interface.

Alternative Methods of Management

Type of Management	Advantages	Disadvantages	Comments
Anterior cervical discectomy with fusion	Directly addresses pathology of disc herniation or osteophytes Indirectly decompresses foramen and spinal canal by distraction of disc space Stabilizes motion segment may alleviate axial neck pain Minimizes manipulation of spinal cord and nerve roots	Morbidity associated with anterior neck approach, e.g., dysphagia Risk to cervical viscera, recurrent laryngeal nerve, thoracic duct Morbidity of bone graft site Risk of nonunion, especially with multiple levels and smokers Postoperative immobilization Slower return to activities	Allograft may be acceptable substitute to minimize bone graft harvest-site morbidity Internal fixation may be necessary for multilevel and smokers
Anterior cervical discectomy without fusion	Directly addresses pathology of disc herniation or osteophytes No bone graft harvest-site morbidity	Does not restore neuroforaminal height Does not predictably stabilize the motion segment, despite significant rates of autofusion Poorer results in patients with spondylosis Risk of developing disc space collapse and kyphosis May develop significant neck pain	Seldom performed Assumes successful results occur with pseudarthroses Not recommended until better long-term studies are performed
Posterior laminotomy and foraminotomy	May directly address disc herniation Minimal posterior neck dissection and no need for postoperative orthosis Avoids morbidities associated with anterior neck approach, e.g., dysphagia, and risks of injury to anterior neck structures	Potential for nerve root injury with overzealous retraction and mobilization Does not stabilize motion segment Potential for iatrogenic instability	Limited indications; optimal candidate is young patient with soft unilateral posterolateral disc herniation with minimal spondylosis

Complications

Complications related to the exposure can involve any of the pertinent anatomy. Thorough knowledge of the anatomy and meticulous surgical technique with careful placement of retractors is required to minimize injury. Fortunately, transient sore throat and hoarseness remain the most common complications related to the exposure and typically resolve within 1 to 2 weeks. Neurologic injury remains a devastating but fortunately rare occurrence. The incidence of spinal cord injury is less than 0.1%. Nerve root injury from overzealous manipulation during decompression may manifest itself as persistent radiculopathy, and the true incidence is unknown. Dural tears are rarely encountered in soft disc disease but are more common in hard disc disease and ossification of the PLL. They need to be repaired or covered with fibrin glue, a muscle, or fascial graft with cerebrospinal fluid (CSF) diversion.

Bone graft intrusion or extrusion may occur as well as graft collapse or nonunion. Bone graft harvest site morbidity is commonly cited in the literature. Hematoma, infection, persistent pain, and cosmetic deformity are common to both iliac crest and fibular graft harvesting. These can be reduced with careful surgical technique and should not be relegated to the most inexperienced person on the surgical team.

Herniations or symptoms at other levels may reflect clinical judgment and not true complications. These events play a definite role in patient outcome and reoperation rate.

In summary, disc herniations causing myelopathy or radiculopathy can be safely addressed from the anterior approach. Predictable results with regard to pain relief and stabilization of the motion segment can be expected in the majority of patients.

Suggested Readings

An HS, Evanich CJ, Nowick BH, et al. Ideal thickness of Smith-Robinson graft for anterior cervical fusion: a cadaveric study with computed tomography correlation. Spine 1993; 18:2043–2047.

Bailey RW, Badgley CE. Stabilization of the cervical spine by anterior fusion. J Bone Joint Surg 1960; 42:565–594.

Boden SD, McCowin PR, Davis DO, Dina TS, Mark AS, Wiesel SW. Abnormal magnetic resonance scans of the cervical spine in asymptomatic subjects: a prospective investigation. J Bone Joint Surg 1990; 72A:1178–1184.

Bohlman HH, Emery SE, Goodfellow DB, Jones PK. Robinson anterior cervical discectomy and arthrodesis of cervical radiculopathy. J Bone Joint Surg 1993; 75A:1298–1307.

Cloward RB. The anterior approach for removal of ruptured cervical disc. J Neurosurg 1958; 15:602–614.

Fellrath RF, Hanley EN. Anterior cervical discectomy and arthrodesis for radiculopathy. In: The Cervical Spine Research Society Editorial Committee, eds. The Cervical Spine, pp. 785–798. Philadelphia: Lippincott-Raven, 1998.

Gore DR, Sepic SB. Anterior cervical fusion for degenerated or protruded discs. A review of one hundred forty-six patients. Spine 1984; 9:667–671.

Gore DR, Sepic SB, Gardner GM. Roentgenographic findings of the cervical spine in asymptomatic people. Spine 1986; 11:521.

Gore DR, Sepic SB, Garner G, Murray M. Neck pain. A long-term follow-up of 205 patients. Spine 1987; 12:1–5.

Gore DR, Sepic SB. Anterior discectomy and fusion for painful cervical disc disease. A report of 50 patients with an average follow-up of 21 years. Spine 1998; 23:2047–2051.

Lees F, Turner JW. Natural history and progression of cervical spondylosis. BMJ 1963; 5:1607.

Martin GJ, Boden SD, Titus L. BMP-2 reverses the inhibitory effect of ketorolac on posterolateral lumbar intertransverse process spine fusion. Spine 1999; 24:2188–2194.

Simmons EH, Bhalla SK, Butt WP. Anterior cervical discectomy and fusion. A clinical and biomechanical study with eight-year follow-up. With a note on discography: technique and interpretation of results. J Bone Joint Surg 1969; 51B(2): 225–237.

Smith GW, Robinson RA. Anterolateral disc removal and interbody fusion for cervical disc syndrome. Bull. Johns Hopkins Hosp. 1955; 96:223–224.

Whitecloud TS. Complications of anterior cervical fusion. Instr Course Lect 1978; 27:223–227.

Zdeblick TA, Ducker TB. The use of freeze-dried allograft for anterior cervical fusions. Spine 1991; 16:726–729.

Case 4

Cervical Spondylosis—Soft Disc Herniation: Posterior Approach

Steven C. Ludwig, Joseph M. Kowalski, and Scott D. Boden

History and Physical Examination

A 38-year-old, right-hand-dominant man presented with an 8-week history of left arm pain that radiated along the top of the shoulder to the midportion of the lateral aspect of the upper arm. The patient admitted to a minimal amount of neck pain along with numbness and paresthesias in the same distribution as his arm pain. He denied any history of trauma, upper or lower extremity weakness, gait imbalance, or bowel or bladder changes. On physical examination the patient had a slightly limited cervical range of motion secondary to pain. Motor strength was 5/5, except for 4+/5 testing of the left deltoid muscle. Sensation to pinprick was diminished along the C5 dermatome. The left biceps reflex was diminished compared to the contralateral side. All other upper and lower extremity reflexes were normal. The

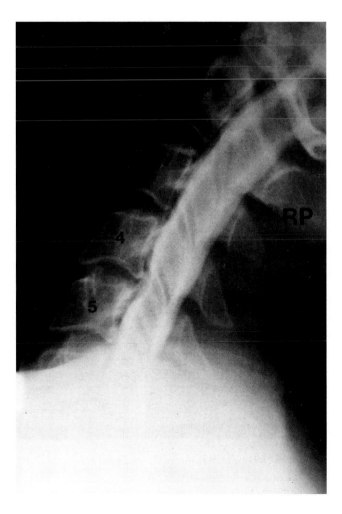

Figure 4–1. Lateral cervical myelogram revealing narrowing of the dye column at the C4/C5 level.

PEARLS

- To ensure a good surgical result and the relief of radicular arm pain, the patient's clinical history and physical examination should correlate with the advanced radiographic imaging studies (CT myelogram or MRI).
- Careful examination of intraoperative radiographs should be performed to confirm the appropriate surgical level.
- Following the laminoforaminotomy, the nerve root should demonstrate marked "looseness" in mobility when palpated in all directions.

patient exhibited a positive Spurling's sign, but failed to reveal a Hoffmann's sign, clonus, or Babinski's sign. Nonoperative treatment, including soft collar immobilization, nonsteroidal antiinflammatory drugs (NSAIDs), and physical therapy, failed to alleviate the patient's symptoms. A selective left-sided C5 nerve root injection initially ameliorated the patient's radicular arm pain for several days; however, it gradually returned to baseline soon thereafter.

Radiologic Findings

Radiographic analysis of the cervical spine included anteroposterior, lateral, oblique, and lateral flexion/extension views. The lateral cervical myelogram revealed narrowing of the dye column at the C4/C5 interspace (Fig. 4–1). Figure 4–2 demonstrates a postmyelogram computed tomograpy (CT) through the C4/C5 level. Transaxial magnetic resonance imaging (MRI) views at the C4/C5 level revealed a left-sided fragment of herniated nucleus pulposus posterolaterally within the spinal canal and neuroforamen (Fig. 4–3). Figure 4–4 demonstrates two large fragments that were removed following a C4/C5 laminoforaminotomy.

Diagnosis

Cervical radiculopathy secondary to posterolateral soft disc herniation. Since there was minimal evidence of osteophyte formation, the radiculopathy was considered to be solely due to the herniated nucleus pulposus on the left side at the C4/C5 level.

Surgical Management

The indication for operative intervention was the persistence of left-sided C5 radicular arm pain despite nonoperative treatment. A left-sided C4/C5 laminoforaminotomy was performed. The goal of the operation was to alleviate the right-sided radicular arm pain.

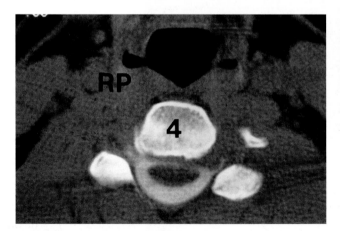

Figure 4–2. Postmyelogram computed tomography at the C4/C5 level demonstrating a significant left-sided posterolateral soft disc herniation.

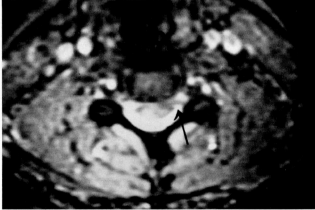

Figure 4–3. A T2-weighted transaxial magnetic resonance imaging (MRI) view of the C4/C5 level revealing herniated nucleus pulposus posterolaterally (arrow).

PITFALLS

• Avoid performing a posterior laminoforaminotomy in a patient with a central disc herniation, which would require retraction of the dura and spinal cord with the potential for catastrophic neurologic complications.

• To prevent iatrogenic instability, resection of the facet joint and capsular stripping should be limited to less than 50% of the facet.

• When removing the herniated disc through the foraminotomy, beware that the nerve root has both dorsal and ventral segments. Do not mistake the ventral segment for the herniated disc.

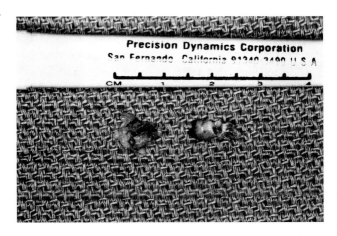

Figure 4–4. Two large disc fragments removed following the left-sided C4/C5 laminoforaminotomy.

The patient was taken to the operating room and general endotracheal anesthesia was administered. General anesthesia is preferred to local with sedation because it allows for better airway control and hemodynamic monitoring. The patient was then placed in the prone position with the head stabilized in Mayfield tongs. The patient's neck was then slightly flexed and the table placed in 20 degrees of reverse Trendelenburg. These maneuvers position the cervical spine parallel to the floor, which minimizes epidural venous congestion as well as the risk of venous air embolism. The shoulders were taped back to improve radiographic visualization of the lower cervical spine to ascertain the correct operative level. Fiberoptic headlight intensification and loupe magnification were worn to improve visualization.

The next step was identification of the posterior surface anatomy. The C2 and C7 spinous processes are the most prominent landmarks in the posterior cervical spine. The skin was first injected with a combination of a local anesthetic and hemostatic agent (e.g., epinephrine) to obtain postoperative analgesia and to decrease intraoperative blood loss. A midline approach to the posterior cervical spine was performed from just above the C4 spinous process to just below the C5 spinous process. The incision was carried down to the level of the fascia. A unilateral subperiosteal dissection was performed, and care was taken not to disturb the interspinous ligaments. A Kocher clamp was then placed on the spinous process, and a lateral cervical radiograph was obtained to verify the correct C4/C5 surgical level. The paraspinal muscles were held back with a self-retaining retractor and care was taken during the exposure to keep the C4/C5 facet capsules intact.

The ligamentum flavum at the primary interspace was gently dissected with a 3-0 curette off of the inferior aspect of the C5 superior laminar arch and from the superior aspect of the inferior C4 laminar arch. A 1-mm Kerrison punch was then used to create a circular laminotomy of approximately 8 mm in diameter. Half of this laminotomy was made on the superior lamina of C5 and the other half was made on the inferior lamina of C4, forming the circular portion of a keyhole. To determine the pathway required for the decompression of the C5 nerve root, a fine dental probe was placed through the laminotomy and into the C4/C5 foramen. Because the nerve root exits between the two laminae, partial excision of the medial aspect of the facet joint was performed. A 3-mm diamond tip burr was used to thin the outer cortical table of the medial aspect of the facet over the C5 nerve root. Once the cortical rim was thinned, a 2-mm Kerrison rongeur was used to remove the bone overlying the C5 nerve root. Adequate lateral decompression of the nerve root required approximately 5 mm of nerve root exposure. Cranial to caudal exposure was extended from the C4 to the C5 pedicle. Care was taken not to excise greater than 50% of the C4/C5 facet joint, to prevent iatrogenic instability. Based on gentle probing around the shoulder, axilla, and foramen of the nerve root, it was apparent that the C5 nerve root was not adequately decompressed.

As apparent on the patient's preoperative MRI scan, a large posterolateral disc fragment was impinging of the C5 nerve root. For many soft disc herniations, bony decompression thorough laminotomy and foraminotomy is adequate. However, due to the diminished mobility of the nerve root, it was thought that the C5 nerve root was not adequately decompressed. The vascular cuff enveloping the nerve root was then removed with bipolar electrocautery to explore both the root and soft disc. The anterior and posterior C5 roots were visualized and mobilized superiorly with a microhook. The C4/C5 disc herniation was seen in the axilla of the root under the C5 ventral branch still contained by the posterior annulus. With the root carefully protected, a no. 11 scalpel blade was used to incise the annulus over the apex of the disc protrusion. This then allowed a substantial portion of the C4/C5 disc to extrude. A small pituitary rongeur was used to remove the disc fragment. Following disc removal, the C5 nerve root was found to have increased mobility when palpated in all directions. Hemostasis was achieved via bipolar electrocautery and Gelfoam. The wound was copiously irrigated with bacteriostatic saline. There was no need for a postoperative drain. The fascia of the paraspinal muscles was approximated with interrupted no. 1 resorbable suture. The subcutaneous tissue was closed with 2-0 resorbable suture, and the skin was closed with 3-0 suture in a running subcuticular fashion. Because stability had not been compromised, a rigid orthosis was not necessary; however, the patient was placed in a soft collar postoperatively to provide initial comfort.

Postoperative Management

The patient was encouraged to ambulate the day of surgery. Routine perioperative antibiotics were administered for 24 hours. If a drain is used, it can be removed 24 hours following surgery. The patient was discharged from the hospital on postoperative day 1. The patient was told to take the soft collar off within the first 3 to 5 days following surgery.

Strenuous activities and heavy labor were restricted for a minimum of 6 to 8 weeks to allow for soft tissue healing. Isometric neck exercises were initiated at 4 weeks following surgery and progressed as tolerated. The patient was able to return to light office duties 2 weeks postoperatively.

Immediately following surgery the patient had diminution of his radicular arm pain. At 8 weeks, the patient returned to his laboring position with dramatic improvement of his radicular pain and neck discomfort. At 6-month and 2-year follow-up, the patient had complete relief of his right-sided radicular arm pain.

Discussion

The symptoms of cervical disc disease with radiculopathy may develop insidiously or acutely. Patients may complain of neck, interscapular, suboccipital, and, most importantly, upper extremity pain radiating in a specific nerve root distribution. Of paramount importance is the need to rule out cervical myelopathy, which can coexist with radiculopathy.

Indications for the elective surgical treatment of cervical radiculopathy include pain that is persistent in a radicular distribution and is unresponsive to conservative treatment for a minimum of 6 weeks. Indications for considering urgent surgical intervention include major debilitating neurologic deficits (C5-deltoid or C8-hand intrinsic) nerve root involvement, progressive neurologic deficit, or presence of concomitant myelopathy. Regardless of the indication, it is essential to correlate the patient's pain and objective findings with the specific radiographic abnormality. Following the decision to proceed with surgery, the appropriate operative approach needs to be selected.

In this case the patient had unremitting right-sided radiculopathy associated with reflex, motor, and sensory deficits in a well-defined C5 nerve root distribution. Moreover, advanced radiographic imaging studies including an MRI and CT myelogram correlated with the patient's clinical examination. The patient had a "soft" posterolateral herniated nucleus pulposus with minimal spondylitic changes. Because the patient had minimal neck symptoms and desired to return to work as soon as possible without the restriction of prolonged orthosis wear, a posterior C4/C5 laminoforaminotomy was the procedure chosen.

The posterior laminoforaminotomy as described by Spurling and Scoville (1944) is a less versatile procedure as compared to the anterior cervical discectomy and fusion. It is useful only in very specific clinical scenarios, which include a unilateral, posterolateral herniated disc with limited foraminal stenosis at one or more levels; patients who had previous anterior neck surgery; salvage for failed anterior cervical procedures; and patients with technical limitations of the anterior approach (e.g., C2/C3 and C7/T1 discectomies, and patients with short, thick necks).

The advantage of this procedure over the anterior approach is that it avoids potential injury to the trachea, esophagus, recurrent laryngeal nerve, and pseudarthrosis. The posterior approach also eliminates the morbidity associated with harvesting an iliac crest bone graft. It is an excellent choice in patients who have limited neck pain and in those with multilevel involvement. Because no arthrodesis is involved, there is no requirement for a postoperative orthosis, and patients may be able to return to their activities of daily living faster. The disadvantages of performing a posterior laminoforaminotomy are that it lacks neuroforaminal distraction as well as segmental stabilization. Moreover, since the nerve root must be routinely checked for mobility once decompressed, the potential of nerve root injury must be kept in mind.

In the patient described earlier, the nerve root was not felt to be adequately decompressed after the laminoforaminotomy was performed. Because the surgical probe could not comfortably slip between the tissues around the nerve root and bony foramen, the nerve root needed to be directly inspected. At this point in the operation if the nerve root was loose superiorly, laterally, and medially, and fine instruments were passed easily around the shoulder and axilla of the nerve root as well as out laterally, the foraminotomy would have been complete. However, when adequate decompression is not apparent, further exploration for the nerve root is indicated. When inspecting the nerve root, it is important to realize that the nerve root's dural sheath is divided into ventral and dorsal sections. Therefore, care should be taken when lifting up the dorsal section of the nerve root not to mistake the ventral section of the nerve root for the herniated disc. In this case an annular incision was made with a no. 11 scalpel blade, with care taken not to involve the dura of the nerve root sheath. The incision of the annulus was associated with a significant extrusion of disc material. Following removal of the disc material, the mobility of the nerve root was rechecked and demonstrated increased mobility of the root when palpated in all directions.

Typically, patients will experience relief of their radicular arm pain following surgery and are discharged from the hospital in 1 to 2 days. Most patients are discharged without any form of immobilization; however, some prefer to wear a soft collar for a few days or weeks. The relief of arm pain, lack of complications, and rapid return to normal activity compare favorably to anterior surgery.

Alternative Methods of Management

When reviewing the results of surgical treatment for cervical radiculopathy, it becomes apparent that many investigators do not distinguish among surgical treatments for radiculopathy, myelopathy, soft/hard disc herniation, single/multilevel disease, or central/posterolateral herniations. In addition, a standardized outcomes measurement has not been employed. In light of these limitations, it is extremely difficult to determine the best surgical approach for a specific cervical problem.

Currently, controversy exists about the surgical management of a soft posterolateral cervical disc herniation. Because decompression of the cervical spinal cord and nerve roots can be accomplished through either an anterior or posterior approach, alternatives to a posterior laminoforaminotomy include anterior cervical decompression with or without a fusion.

Anterior cervical discectomy and fusion as first described by Robinson and Smith (1958) is an extremely versatile surgical procedure for the treatment of a herniated cervical disc. There are numerous reports of excellent clinical results for the surgical management of cervical radiculopathy secondary to spondylosis (hard disc herniation) and central as well as posterolateral herniated discs. The primary goal is to reestablish the disc space height, thus indirectly distracting the neuroforamen and relieving nerve root compression. The surgical fusion allows for nerve root compression secondary to osteophytes reabsorbing, thus relieving nerve root compression. Although less reliable, an anterior cervical decompression and fusion may be the procedure of choice for palliating axial neck pain associated with primary radicular symptoms.

Another surgical option for the treatment of a posterolateral soft disc herniation is an anterior cervical decompression without fusion. This procedure eliminates the morbidity associated with harvesting an iliac crest bone graft. There are few reports in patients who lack spondylosis of good to excellent results with high rates of autofusion.

Both anterior and posterior surgical approaches play a role in the management of cervical radiculopathy. Thus, it is imperative to determine which patients are most likely to benefit from either an anterior or posterior approach. Location (central versus posterolateral disc herniation) and type of pathology (soft versus hard disc), spinal morphometry, body habitus, the presence of significant axial neck pain, and surgeon preference all play a pivotal role in a surgeon's decision-making algorithm. Making the appropriate surgical management decision will optimize the patient's outcome and minimize the rate of complications.

Type of Management	Advantages	Disadvantages	Comments
Posterior laminoforaminotomy	Overall fewer complications Avoids injuries to anterior soft tissue structures: carotid artery, jugular vein, trachea, esophagus, sympathetic chain, dysphonia, dysphagia, hematoma, pseudarthrosis Avoids morbidity of bone graft harvesting No postoperative orthosis Potential for faster return to activities	Limited indications Potential for the creation of iatrogenic instability Potential for nerve root injury with overzealous retraction and mobilization Inability to stabilize a spinal segment	Optimal candidate: young patient with soft unilateral posterolateral herniated nucleus pulposus (HNP), at one or more levels with minimal spondylosis and axial neck pain May also be a reasonable approach in patients with posterolateral HNP at C2/C3, C7/T1, and in those with short, thick necks
Anterior cervical discectomy without fusion	Eliminates the morbidity associated with iliac crest bone graft harvesting Significant rates of autofusion reported	Does not allow for neuroforaminal distraction or segmental stabilization Poor results seen in patients with spondylosis Risk of developing kyphotic deformity Development of significant neck pain reported	Seldom performed, assumes successful results occur with pseudarthroses Should not be recommended until better long-term studies are available
Anterior cervical discectomy and fusion	Most versatile procedure, considered to be the "gold standard" by most orthopaedic spine surgeons Avoids manipulation of the spinal cord and nerve roots Allows for neuroforaminal distraction, segmental stabilization May alleviate axial neck pain	Morbidity associated with an anterior approach, iliac crest bone graft harvest, pseudarthrosis Development of junctional accelerated degenerative disc disease Multilevel fusions have been shown to have a lower fusion rate when compared to single-level fusions Requirse postoperative immobilization Slower return to activities	Excellent alternative method of management

Complications

The complication rate in performing a posterior laminoforaminotomy for a soft posterolateral cervical disc herniation is low. Complications include failure to operate at the correct level, dural tear, nerve root injury, inadequate foraminotomy, and the creation of iatrogenic instability. As the surgeon improves and develops the skill of performing a laminoforaminotomy, these complications should diminish.

Overzealous nerve root retraction for removal of disc material should be avoided to prevent neurologic injuries. Typically, nerve root injury results from direct mechanical injury; thus, forcing instruments into the foraminal zone should be avoided. To ensure neurologic decompression, gentle palpation of the nerve root for "looseness" is necessary.

Dural tears, which are uncommon, should be repaired using 4-0 suture. If closure is not possible, the use of blood-soaked Gelfoam may allow for self-healing and prevent leakage of cerebrospinal fluid. Fibrin glue may be used as a supplement, and tight closure of the fascia without drains is required.

If decompression of the nerve root requires an extensive facetectomy (>50%), the surgeon must be aware of the potential for causing iatrogenic instability. Thus, a concomitant arthrodesis should be considered when this situation arises.

Suggested Readings

Henderson CM, Hennessy RG, Shuey HM, Shackelford EG. Posterior-lateral foraminotomy as an exclusive operative technique for cervical radiculopathy: a review of 846 consecutively operated cases. Neurosurgery 1983; 13:504.

Herkowitz HN, Kurz LT, Overholt DP. Surgical management of cervical soft disc herniation: a comparison between the anterior and posterior approach. Spine 1990; 15(10):1026.

Robinson RA, Smith GW. The treatment of certain cervical spine disorders by anterior removal of the intervertebral disc and Interbody fusion. J Bone Joint Surg 1958; 40:607–624.

Rothman RH, Simeone FA. The Spine, 3d ed., p. 608. Philadelphia: WB Saunders, 1992.

Spurling RG, Scoville WB. Lateral rupture of the cervical intervertebral disc. Surg Gynecol Obstet 1944; 78:350–358.

Zdeblick TA, Zou D, Warden KE, et al. Cervical stability after foraminotomy. J Bone Joint Surg 1992; 74A:22.

Zeidman SM, Ducker TB. Posterior cervical laminoforaminotomy for radiculopathy: review of 172 cases. Neurosurgery 1993; 33:356.

Case 5

Cervical Spondylosis—Myelopathy: Anterior Approach

Bradford L. Currier and Michael J. Yaszemski

History and Physical Examination

A 36-year-old man who works as a machinist presented with complaints of progressive gait unsteadiness, bilateral lower extremity weakness, sensory loss, and bowel and bladder dysfunction. His symptoms began 4 months before presentation when he fell off the back of a three-wheel all-terrain vehicle. He complained of three to four episodes of urinary incontinence and one episode of fecal incontinence. He denied upper extremity pain or numbness. He had long-standing moderate mechanical neck pain.

On examination, he walked with a markedly spastic, wide-based gait, and his station was grossly unsteady. It was not possible for him to walk on his toes or heels or tandem walk because of his unsteadiness. He had severe spasticity in his lower extremities and mild spasticity in his upper extremities. He had mild to moderate loss of pinprick sensation distal to the C7 dermatome. His strength was normal in all

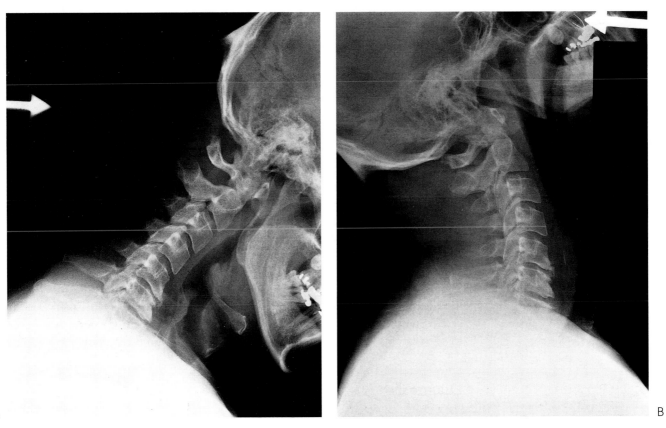

A   B

Figure 5–1. Flexion (A) and extension (B) preoperative lateral radiographs of the cervical spine show spondylosis primarily at the C5/C6 and C6/C7 interspaces with narrowing of the anteroposterior (AP) diameter of the spinal canal at these levels. The spine is stable.

muscle groups of the upper extremities except for his finger flexors and interossei, which had 4/5 strength. All lower extremity muscle groups had 4/5 strength. His biceps reflex was normal, the brachioradialis and triceps reflexes were decreased bilaterally, and he had moderate hyperreflexia of his knee jerk and ankle jerk. He had an inverted radial reflex (spastic contraction of the finger flexors and paradoxically diminished brachioradialis reflex elicited by tapping on the distal brachioradialis tendon, indicative of spinal cord compression at the C6 level). Hoffmann's sign (flexion of the thumb and index fingers elicited by flicking the long finger distal interphalangeal joint into extension, indicative of an upper motor neuron lesion) was present bilaterally and his toes had an extensor response on testing Babinski's reflex. He had sustained clonus at the ankles bilaterally. The scapulohumeral reflex (brisk scapular elevation with abduction of the humerus elicited by tapping the acromion, indicative of high cervical spinal cord compression) was not present. The jaw jerk reflex was normal (closure of the mouth caused by contraction of the masseter and temporalis muscles elicited by tapping a finger placed on the chin of a subject whose mouth is resting slightly open). A hyperactive jaw jerk reflex suggests an upper motor neuron lesion above the foramen magnum or systemic disease; a hypoactive reflex suggests pathology of the trigeminal nerve. Cervical range of motion (ROM) was mildly restricted in flexion and extension and the latter caused significant neck pain. Spurling's maneuver was negative. Waddell's score was 0/5.

Radiologic Findings

Cervical radiographs including flexion and extension films (Fig. 5–1) demonstrated spondylosis primarily at the C5/C6 and C6/C7 interspaces with narrowing of the anteroposterior (AP) diameter of the spinal canal at these levels. The spine was stable, and the alignment was normal with preserved cervical lordosis. The two radiographic measurements that are of importance are the developmental anteroposterior diameter (DAD) and the spondylotic anteroposterior diameter (SAD). The DAD is the distance from the posterior vertebral body margin at its cephalocaudal midpoint to the spinolaminar line of the same vertebra. The SAD is the narrowest distance from the posterior extent of an osteophyte to the spinolaminar line, measured on a plain radiograph. The SAD, when measured on a magnetic resonance imaging (MRI), has the most anterior extent of the ligamentum flavum as its posterior measurement point. The SAD provides a more realistic assessment of the actual space available for the cord at the spinal level of interest.

An MRI (Fig. 5–2) demonstrated spinal stenosis from the C5/C6 to C6/C7 disc spaces. The remainder of the spinal canal was congenitally narrow but not significantly stenotic. There was a high signal within the substance of the cord at the C6/C7 level secondary to myelomalacia from the stenosis. A preoperative computed tomography (CT) myelogram (Fig. 5–3) confirmed that the C5/C6 level was severely stenotic from spondylosis and showed that the C6/C7 level was severely stenotic from a large central disc herniation as well as an osteophyte.

Diagnosis

Cervical spondylosis and stenosis C5/C6 and C6/C7 with moderately severe cervical myelopathy.

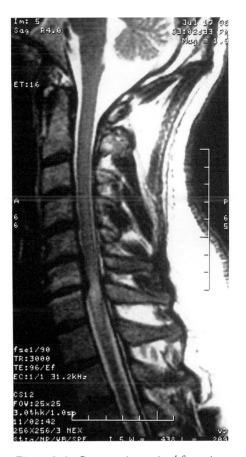

Figure 5–2. Preoperative sagittal fast spin echo T2-weighted magnetic resonance imaging (MRI) demonstrates spinal stenosis from the C5/C6 to C6/C7 disc spaces. The remainder of the spinal canal is congenitally narrow but not stenotic. There is a high signal within the substance of the cord at the C6/C7 level secondary to myelomalacia from the stenosis.

Surgical Management

The patient was positioned supine on the operating table and intubated with minimal neck extension; general anesthesia was induced. Through a left-sided transverse skin incision, the anterior cervical spine was exposed. The platysma was incised in line with its fibers and the deep cervical and pretracheal fascia were incised medial to the sternomastoid and carotid sheath, respectively. The prevertebral fascia was incised bluntly with a Kitner sponge and the midline was identified between the two longus coli muscles. A radiograph confirmed the location. The longus coli muscles were elevated off the spine using an insulated monopolar cautery (with the tip bent 90 degrees) and a Cobb elevator. Caspar self-retaining toothed retractors were placed beneath the longus coli muscles. Caspar distraction screws were placed into the C5 and C7 vertebral bodies in the midline, and the distraction apparatus was placed over

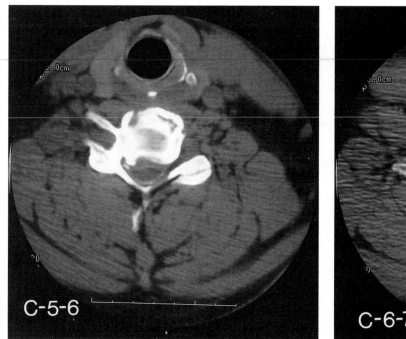
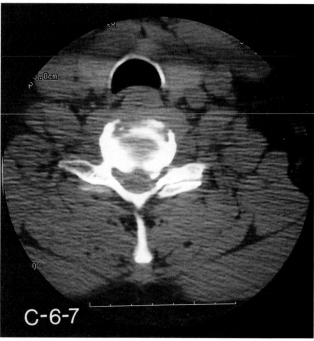

Figure 5–3. Preoperative computed tomography (CT) myelogram. The C5/C6 level (A) is severely stenotic from spondylosis. The C6/C7 level (B) is severely stenotic from a large central disc herniation as well as an osteophyte.

the screws. Smooth Caspar retractor blades were placed on a self-retaining retractor and held in place above and below the distraction screws for cephalocaudad exposure. The distance between the screws was measured to monitor and minimize the amount of distraction applied between C5 and C7. Mild distraction was applied and discectomies were performed at C5/C6 and C6/C7. Somatosensory evoked potential (SSEP) monitoring was performed throughout the case and it showed no changes. The discs were completely excised out to the uncinate processes bilaterally and the posterior longitudinal ligament was exposed at both levels. A large Leksell rongeur was placed in the discectomy sites at both levels and used to remove a trough in the midline of the C6 vertebral body, 16 to 18 mm wide. A high-speed drill excised the posterior portion of the body of C6 back to a thin eggshell of cortex. A small curette gently elevated the thinned posterior cortex of C6 away from the posterior longitudinal ligament. The high-speed drill burred the C5 and C7 endplates back to bleeding parallel surfaces, leaving small, thin lips of bone posteriorly.

Tiny curettes and a thin footplate 2-mm Kerrison were used to carefully remove osteophytes from the posterior-inferior aspect of the C5 and the posterior-superior aspect of the C7 vertebral bodies by elevating the thin lip of bone anteriorly. These instruments were also used to open the foramina of the C6 and C7 nerve roots bilaterally. A portion of the posterior longitudinal ligament was excised to confirm that disc material had not extruded posterior to the ligament. The anterior osteophytes on C5 and C7 were excised with a rongeur, creating a smooth, level surface for the instrumentation. A fresh frozen tricortical iliac crest graft was cut to fit the slightly distracted space and it was impacted into position, flush with the anterior aspects of C5 and C7. The size of the corpectomy defect was used to determine the appropriate-size Ventral Cervical Stabilization System (DePuy Acromed, Cleveland,

OH), which was fixed to the anterior aspects of C5 and C7 with 14-mm self-tapping bone screws. The C5 and C7 platforms were positioned on the respective vertebral bodies by placing the small posterior fins of the platforms adjacent to the endplates. The transverse connector was secured to the rods in a location that would allow 3 mm of implant settling. The locking screws were placed within the bone screws to lock the screws to the plate and expand the tips of the bone screws. The wound was copiously irrigated and then closed over a drain.

Postoperative Management

The patient was mobilized in a hard collar for 2 months and gradually weaned from the collar during the third postoperative month. During the weaning period he was instructed to perform isometric neck exercises three times per day. Radiographs were taken during his hospitalization (Fig. 5–4) and 3 months postoperatively (Fig. 5–5). The latter films demonstrated that the implant had

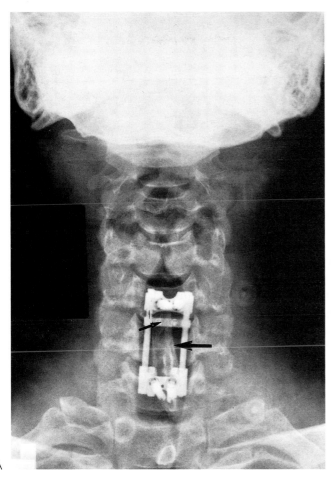
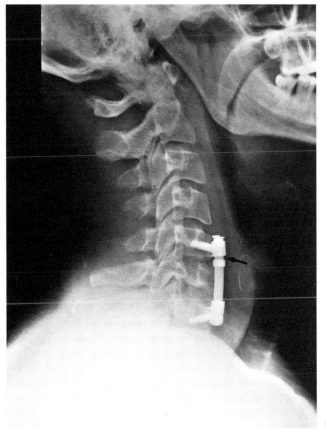

A

B

Figure 5–4. Plain cervical radiographs taken shortly after surgery. AP (A) shows the tricortical iliac crest graft in place (large arrow). The platforms of the dynamic implant are secured to the C5 and C7 vertebral bodies with screws. The two rods are joined by the platforms and a connector (small arrow). The lower platform is fixed to the rods but the upper platform is free to slide down the rods to the level of the connector as the fusion construct settles. The lateral radiograph (B) demonstrates the gap (arrow) between the upper platform and the connector, which represents the distance that the implant can collapse. The rods are contoured into lordosis so that the alignment of the spine will theoretically be maintained as it settles.

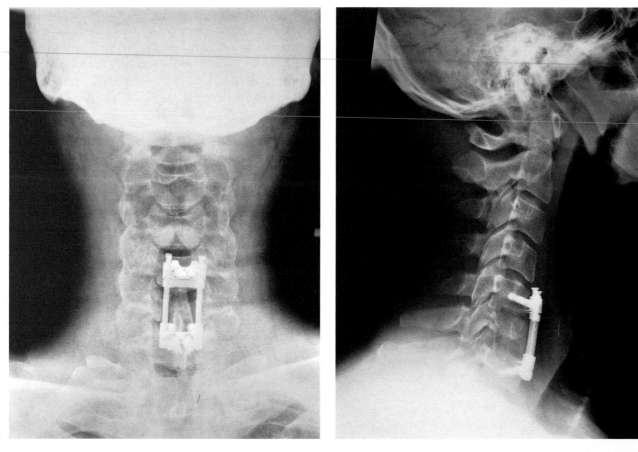

Figure 5–5. Plain cervical radiographs taken 3 months after surgery. AP (A) and lateral (B) views demonstrate that the implant has settled as planned and the graft has healed in good position.

allowed the spine to settle 3 mm as planned and the graft had healed. Graft healing was confirmed with tomograms and flexion/extension films. An MRI (Fig. 5–6) performed 5 months following surgery due to a continued sense of lower extremity weakness showed that the cord was adequately decompressed but there was still an area of increased T2 signal within the cord. The new symptoms resolved and the patient was able to return to work. He managed the residual spasticity with baclofen and Valium.

Discussion

Overall, about 70 to 85% of patients undergoing surgery for myelopathy can expect to improve, whereas less than 50% of patients treated nonoperatively will improve. The MRI findings of severe stenosis with cord deformity and high T2 signal within the cord are not good prognostic signs and can portend a poor result. It is best to counsel such patients that the surgery is being undertaken to prevent further deterioration and that any improvement in neurologic function is a bonus.

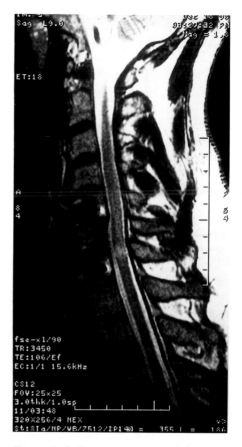

Figure 5–6. Postoperative sagittal fast spin echo T2-weighed MRI demonstrates that decompression is adequate. We could have removed a bit more of the inferior aspect of the C5 body but the cord is no longer deformed and it is surrounded by cerebrospinal fluid (CSF). The high signal within the cord at C6/C7 is still present.

Alternative Methods of Management

Nonoperative care is a reasonable option for patients who are poor surgical candidates because of medical comorbidities, severe and fixed neurologic compromise, or rapidly progressive neurologic deficits. Nonoperative treatment consists of a soft collar, nonsteroidal antiinflammatory drugs, and physical therapy.

We chose to decompress and fuse our patient's spine anteriorly because the pathology was located anteriorly, the stenosis was isolated to two levels, and he had severe spondylosis associated with neck pain. There are advantages and disadvantages associated with approaching the spine anteriorly or posteriorly. Laminectomy or laminoplasty would avoid all of the problems associated with a fusion including pseudarthrosis, graft migration or collapse, hardware complications, donor site problems, and bracing. Laminoplasty and laminectomy both work by indirectly decompressing the cord and therefore require a lordotic spine to allow the cord to drift away

PEARLS

- A transverse skin incision is markedly more cosmetically appealing. A three- and even four-level anterior cervical body decompression can be accomplished through a transverse incision if adequate care is taken to develop the tissue planes during the exposure.
- Releasing retractors from time to time is helpful in preventing tissue necrosis.
- To position the vertical cervical retractors over the desired levels, a sponge placed above or below the smooth retractor block can move the retractors over the levels of interest.
- Identification of the midline can be accomplished by marking the midline point between the longus colli muscles or removing the entire disc out to the uncinate processes bilaterally to establish the lateral borders of the decompression.

PITFALL

- Educate the patient thoroughly on the expectations of surgery. Certain subgroups of patients are at risk for a poor neurologic outcome. Patients with marked cord flattening and those with high signal within the cord on T2-weighted images are less likely to have a good outcome.

from the anterior osteophytes and disc. The difference in success rate between a laminoplasty and a laminectomy is presumably due to the higher risk of postoperative instability associated with a laminectomy. The main disadvantage of a posterior decompression in this case is that it cannot be expected to improve neck pain; in fact, it could even aggravate the symptom. A laminoplasty would have led to postoperative stiffness much like the two-level anterior fusion that we performed. Although a laminectomy does not lead to loss of motion, it has the potential to cause late instability. A laminectomy could be combined with a posterior instrumented fusion to avoid the problem of instability and to address the neck pain, but that procedure would require fusing more levels than a two-level anterior procedure.

A posterior decompression and fusion would have been the best option if the patient's congenital stenosis had caused significant cord deformity over at least three segments. Most surgeons prefer the anterior approach with stenosis over two segments and the posterior approach with stenosis over four or more segments. A laminoplasty would have been the best option if there was stenosis over at least three levels and the patient had no significant neck pain or instability. A laminectomy would have been the best option if there was multilevel stenosis, no neck pain or instability, or if the patient was elderly, with comorbidities necessitating the simplest, quickest procedure.

There are several anterior decompression options to consider. An anterior discectomy and fusion of the C5/C6 and C6/C7 disc spaces could have been performed, if a bony ridge was not present behind the vertebral body, using Smith-Robinson, Cloward, or keystone grafts instead of a strut graft. The two procedures are quite comparable. Theoretically the fusion rate is higher with a strut graft because only two sites need to fuse rather than four interfaces, but that point has never been proven conclusively.

The graft options include tricortical iliac crest or fibula and can be either autologous or cadaver bone. A single-level anterior cervical discectomy and fusion (ACDF) will eventually heal with the same pseudarthrosis rate regardless of whether the bone is autograft or allograft, although the former will heal more rapidly. A two-level ACDF will heal more predictably if the graft is autologous. It remains to be seen whether a dynamic implant changes the healing rate of bone graft.

The role of instrumentation is evolving. It is technically easier and faster to perform a decompression and fusion without instrumentation, and hardware problems will be obviated. When instrumentation is used, however, the fusion rate is higher, graft dislodgment and collapse are less likely, and rehabilitation is faster.

There are several options for instrumenting the cervical spine anteriorly. Doh and Heller (1998) recently reported a series comparing the fusion rates in multilevel corpectomies involving three levels. The fusion rate after a noninstrumented strut graft fusion immobilized with a halo was 85%, the rate for a long bridging plate was only 62%, all 11 patients treated with an anterior and posterior fusion healed, and 91% of the cases treated with a short anterior buttress plate fused. Vaccaro and colleagues (1998) recently reported a high rate of graft dislodgment with long anterior bridging plates. Dynamic anterior plates have just recently been introduced, and long-term clinical results are not known. These devices have the theoretical advantages of controlling graft settling while maintaining lordosis.

Type of Management	Advantages	Disadvantages
Anterior	Direct removal of structures causing compression Elimination of dynamic compression and instability Deformity correction Effective with kyphotic deformity Better neck pain relief	Technically demanding Pseudarthrosis Graft migration Hardware complications Graft donor-site problems Postoperative bracing required More complications with longer fusions
Posterior	Indicated for multilevel stenosis Loss of motion: laminectomy < laminoplasty < fusion Technical difficulty: laminectomy < laminoplasty < fusion Bracing requirements: laminectomy < laminoplasty < fusion Lower complication rate than multilevel anterior cervical discectomy and fusion (ACDF)	Indirect decompression Not effective with kyphotic alignment (unless lordosis restored and instrumented fusion done) Poor results with limited decompression Does not help neck pain unless combined with a fusion Potential for postoperative instability: laminectomy > laminoplasty > fusion Posterior fusion: donor-site problems, pseudarthrosis, hardware complications
Anterior discectomy without fusion	No graft/hardware problems Shorter operative time Less immediate postoperative pain	May lead to kyphosis May cause neck pain Will not relieve neck pain May narrow neural foramina Not appropriate for multilevel stenosis Fusion rate lower than ACDF (70%) Appropriate only when compression located at disc space
Anterior discectomy and fusion with or without instrumentation	Maintains lordosis May improve neck pain Maintains height of foramen Higher fusion rate than ACD	Technically more demanding Graft may dislodge Graft donor-site problems Accelerated adjacent segment degeneration Pseudarthrosis rate increases with number of levels Appropriate only when compression located at disc space Potential hardware problems
Anterior corpectomy and fusion with or without instrumentation	Same as ACDF Allows decompression behind vertebral body Graft must heal at only two sites	Same as ACDF except allows decompression behind vertebral body
No instrumentation	Technically easier No hardware problems Shorter operative time Lower hospital costs	Lower fusion rate than instrumented construct More rigid bracing required (halo may be needed) Slower rehabilitation May be slower return to work (higher overall cost) Higher rate of graft dislodgment
Posterior fusion and instrumentation	High fusion rate Lower hardware failure for long fusions	Not Food and Drug Administration (FDA) approved Technically more demanding than anterior instrumentation
Long anterior bridging plate	Easy to apply	High rate of hardware failure (long fusions) Prevents graft settling High pseudarthrosis rate High rate of graft dislodgment

Continued on next page

43

Continued

Type of Management	Advantages	Disadvantages
Short anterior buttress plate	Technically easiest to apply Higher fusion rate than bridging plate Allows graft settling Low rate of hardware failure	Lower fusion rate than anterior/posterior fusion Theoretically higher risk of graft dislodgment than dynamic plate or anterior/posterior May allow spine to settle into kyphosis
Long anterior dynamic plate	Theoretically allows controlled settling of graft Theoretically maintains lordosis Theoretically higher fusion rate Theoretically lower rate of hardware failure	Technically more demanding Higher initial cost than other implants Benefits not yet proven

Suggested Readings

Bertalanffy H, Eggert HR. Clinical long-term results of anterior discectomy without fusion for treatment of cervical radiculopathy and myelopathy. A follow-up of 164 cases. Acta Neurochir 1988; 90:127–135.

Crandall PH, Gregorius FK. Long-term follow-up of surgical treatment of cervical spondylotic myelopathy. Spine 1977; 2:139–146.

Doh E-S, Heller JG. Multi-level anterior cervical reconstruction: comparison of surgical techniques and results. Presented at the Cervical Spine Research Society, 26th annual meeting, Atlanta, December 3–5, 1998.

Emery SE, Bohlman HH, Bolesta MJ, et al. Anterior cervical decompression and arthrodesis for the treatment of cervical spondylotic myelopathy. J Bone Joint Surg 1998; 80A:941–951.

Fessler RG, Steck JC, Giovanini MA. Anterior cervical corpectomy for cervical spondylotic myelopathy. Neurosurgery 1998; 43:257–265.

Herkowitz HN. A comparison of anterior cervical fusion, cervical laminectomy and cervical laminoplasty for the surgical management of multiple level spondylotic myelopathy. Spine 1988; 13:774–780.

Kawakami M, Tamaki T, Yoshida M, et al. Axial symptoms and cervical alignment after cervical anterior spinal fusion for patients with cervical myelopathy. J Spinal Disord 1999; 12:50–56.

Naderi S, Ozgen S, Pamir MN, et al. Cervical spondylotic myelopathy: surgical results and factors affecting prognosis. Neurosurgery 1998; 43:43–49.

Vaccaro A, Balderston RA. Anterior plate instrumentation for disorders of the sub-axial cervical spine. Clin Orthop 1997; 335:112–121.

Vaccaro A, Falatyn SP, Scuderi GJ, et al. Early failure of long segment anterior cervical plate fixation. J Spinal Disord 1998; 11:410–415.

Vanichkachorn JS, Vaccaro AR, Silveri CP, Albert TA. Anterior junctional plate in the cervical spine. Spine 1998; 23:2462–2467.

Case 6

Cervical Spondylosis—Myelopathy: Posterior Approach

Bradford L. Currier and Michael J. Yaszemski

History and Physical Examination

A 65-year-old man presented with complaints of bilateral hand numbness, hand weakness, and incoordination of his gait. His hand symptoms were constant, progressive, and worse on the right side. He denied bowel and bladder dysfunction, upper extremity pain, or lower extremity symptoms except for the gait disturbance. He complained of a generalized electric shock sensation in his trunk and extremities occasionally when he flexed his neck (Lhermitte's sign). He had long-standing moderate mechanical neck pain.

On examination, he walked with a broad-based gait and had mild spasticity of his lower extremities. He had no motor weakness, and sensation was normal except for global diminution of light touch sensation in his hands. He had moderate hyperreflexia of all deep tendon reflexes except for the brachioradialis reflexes, which were decreased bilaterally. He had an inverted radial reflex (spastic contraction of the finger flexors and paradoxically diminished brachioradialis reflex elicited by tapping on the distal brachioradialis tendon, indicative of spinal cord compression at the C6 level). Hoffmann's sign (flexion of the thumb and index fingers elicited by flicking the long finger distal interphalangeal joint into extension, indicative of an upper motor neuron

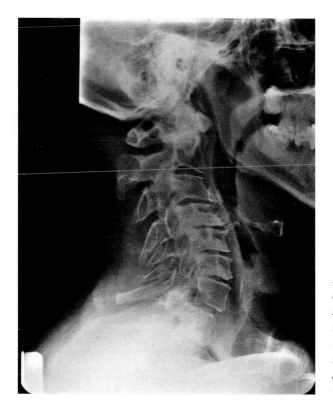

Figure 6–1. Lateral radiograph of the cervical spine showing a swan-neck deformity with C2/C4 kyphosis and C4/T1 lordosis. There is also 2 mm of subluxation at C2/C3 and 3 mm of subluxation at C7/T1.

lesion) was present bilaterally and his toes had an extensor response on testing Babinski's reflex. The scapulohumeral reflex (brisk scapular elevation with abduction of the humerus elicited by tapping the acromion, indicative of high cervical spinal cord compression) was not present. The jaw jerk reflex (closure of the mouth caused by contraction of the masseter and temporalis muscles elicited by tapping a finger placed on the chin of a subject whose mouth is resting slightly open, a hyperactive reflex suggests an upper motor neuron lesion above the foramen magnum or systemic disease; a hypoactive reflex suggests pathology of the trigeminal nerve) was normal.

Radiologic Findings

A lateral radiograph of the cervical spine (Fig. 6–1) demonstrated widespread spondylosis and a mild swan-neck deformity (upper cervical kyphosis and middle and lower cervical lordosis, usually seen as a complication of a destabilizing posterior decompression but occurring spontaneously in this case). The patient had 2 mm of subluxation of C2/C3 and 3 mm of subluxation of C7/T1.

Magnetic resonance imaging (MRI) of the cervical spine (Fig. 6–2) demonstrated severe spondylosis with spinal stenosis including the C4/C6 levels. The subarachnoid space was completely obliterated with flattening of the spinal cord throughout the area of stenosis. There were areas of increased T2 signal within the cord indicative of myelomalacia.

Diagnosis

Cervical myelopathy secondary to cervical spondylosis and spinal stenosis with spontaneous swan neck deformity and mild subluxation C2/C3 and C7/T1.

Surgical Management

Under general anesthesia, a Mayfield pinion head holder was applied and the patient was gently transferred to the prone position on the operating table. The position of

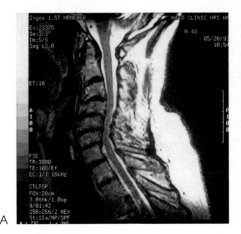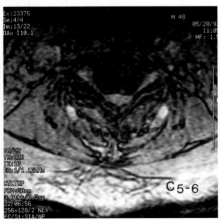

Figure 6–2. Magnetic resonance imaging (MRI) of cervical spine before decompression. Sagittal fast spin echo T2-weighted image (A) shows C4 to C7 cord compromise and high signal changes within the cord primarily at the C4/C5 level. Axial fast spin echo T2-weighted image (B) demonstrates the severe stenosis at the C5/C6 level.

the spine was verified with a cross-table radiograph using the image intensifier. Somatosensory evoked potential (SSEP) monitoring was used throughout the case for monitoring the function of the spinal cord. The cervical spine was approached through a posterior midline incision. The ligamentum nuchae was incised and the posterior elements of C2/T1 were exposed subperiosteally out to the lateral aspect of the facet joints bilaterally. A laminectomy was performed from C3 to C7 by using a large Leksell rongeur, with care taken to avoid placing any aspect of the instrument under the lamina during bone removal. The ligamentum flavum was easily peeled off the dura after bone removal. A thin footplate Kerrison rongeur was used to widen the laminectomy to the lateral border of the thecal sac (at the medial margin of the facet joints). Bleeding was controlled with bipolar coagulation and Gelfoam. Foraminotomies were not performed because the patient had no evidence of radiculopathy. Corticocancellous bone graft was harvested from the posterior ilium. The medial aspect of the pars interarticularis of C2 was identified with a nerve hook and a burr was used to create an entrance point in the C2 lamina for insertion of a screw. The trajectory of each C2 pars interarticularis screw was planned using a preoperative computed tomography (CT) scan, a lateral radiograph taken with an image intensifier, and the landmarks identified intraoperatively.

A 2-mm drill bit was attached to a T-handle chuck and it was slowly advanced into the pars interarticularis of C2 using an oscillating hand motion under image intensifier control with the medial wall of the pars under direct vision. The trajectory of the drill bit was medial and cephalad. The drill was advanced 20 mm into C2 and a 3.5-mm tap was used to create threads for a screw. The hole was gently palpated with a fine ball-tipped probe to confirm that the walls of the hole had not been breached. A small laminotomy was performed at C7/T1 to allow us to identify the medial and cephalad borders of the T1 pedicle. The trajectory and dimensions of the T1 pedicle screw were planned using the preoperative CT and the intraoperative landmarks. The patient's shoulders prevented a useful lateral radiograph at this location. A burr was used to create an entrance hole for the screw, and the hole was prepared using the same technique used for C2 except that the cephalad-caudad angle of the drill bit was determined by choosing a direction perpendicular to the C7/T2 laminae. The mobility of the spine was increased by removing cartilage from the facet joints of C2/T1 with a curette to reduce the swan neck deformity.

The ideal entrance point for each lateral mass screw was marked on the spine from C3 to C7. The points chosen were 1 mm medial to the center of each lateral mass. A plate template was chosen based on the location of the C2 and T1 screw holes and the intervening lateral mass screw entrance points. The template was contoured to fit the spine anatomy while attempting to reduce the deformity and place the spine in physiologic alignment. A plate of the same size was contoured to match the template and then twisted to accommodate the medial direction of the C2 pars and T1 pedicle screws and the lateral direction of the intervening lateral mass screws. Cancellous bone graft was placed in the facet joints, and the plate was secured to C2 and T1 with cortical screws. The drill guide was placed in the hole of the plate closest to the ideal entrance point of the C3 lateral mass screw, and the hole was drilled using the image intensifier to check the trajectory and length of the screw in the sagittal plane. The trajectory of the drill bit was approximately 30 degrees lateral and 15 to 30 degrees cephalad (An technique), to avoid the vertebral artery, nerve root, spinal cord, and facet joints. Bicortical holes were drilled using a power instrument to a depth of approximately 16 mm as determined by the preoperative CT scan, the lateral image, and the intraoperative findings when the ball-tipped probe was placed within each hole. The holes were tapped and lateral mass screws were placed at each level from C3 to C7. A similar procedure was carried out on the opposite side of the spine. Additional bone graft was placed lateral to the plates, and the wound was closed in layers over a drain. A hard collar was applied, the Mayfield pinion was removed, and the patient was transferred to the postanesthesia recovery room.

Postoperative Management

The drains were removed on the day after surgery. A postoperative CT scan (Fig. 6–3) was taken and it confirmed that the hardware was in a good position. The patient was mobilized in the collar and he was discharged from the hospital 5 days after surgery. He noted that his hands felt more normal immediately after surgery and his neurologic status continued to gradually improve over the next year. Radiographs (Fig. 6–4) were taken 3 months after surgery and demonstrated that the fusion was healing well and the construct was stable.

Discussion

Nonoperative care is a reasonable option for patients with cervical myelopathy who are poor surgical candidates because of medical comorbidities; severe, fixed neurologic compromise, or rapidly progressive neurologic deficits. The majority of patients with cervical spondylotic myelopathy will have a gradual deterioration in

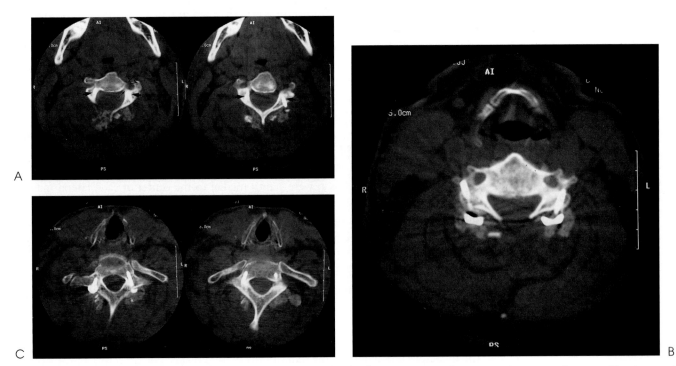

Figure 6–3. Postoperative computed tomography (CT) scan taken shortly after surgery to confirm appropriate screw placement. Two images of C2 (A) demonstrate the screws properly placed within the pars interarticularis bilaterally (large solid arrows). The vertebral arteries are in close proximity to the screw tips (open arrow). The pedicles of C2 (small arrow) are more medially directed than the pars interarticularis and screws placed within the pedicles would have a more lateral starting point and more medial trajectory. Bicortical lateral mass screws in C5 (B) exit anteriorly at the level of the posterior tubercle and course lateral to the vertebral arteries. Two images of T1 (C) demonstrate the medial trajectory of the screws within the pedicles.

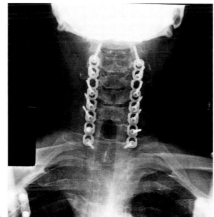

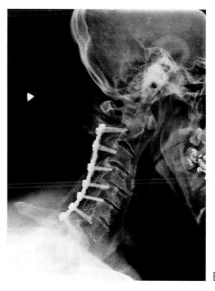

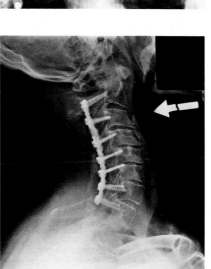

A

B

C

Figure 6–4. Plain films of the cervical spine taken 3 months after surgery. Anteroposterior (AP) radiograph (A) shows that the screw trajectory is medial at C2 and T1 and lateral in the intervening C3 to C7 lateral masses. The C7 lateral mass is frequently too small for lateral mass screws, and pedicle screws are usually more appropriate at that level. Flexion (B) and extension (C) lateral radiographs show that the fusion has healed in acceptable alignment. It was not possible to completely reduce the upper cervical kyphosis without an anterior approach but the spine is lordotic through the area that was decompressed and the alignment should remain stable.

their function without surgical decompression. Nonoperative treatment consists of a soft collar, nonsteroidal antiinflammatory drugs, and physical therapy.

We chose to decompress and fuse our patient's spine posteriorly because he had multilevel stenosis and required a long fusion due to the swan-neck deformity and the preexisting subluxation at C2/C3 and C7/T1. An anterior decompression and fusion could have been performed as a stand-alone procedure or combined with a posterior instrumented fusion. An anterior decompression and fusion would directly remove the cord compression and would eliminate any dynamic compression caused by instability. It would allow the deformity to be corrected and would have a reasonable chance of improving neck pain. An anterior procedure is technically demanding, however, and has a higher complication rate than a posterior decompression with or without a fusion.

The posterior decompression options include laminectomy with or without fusion and laminoplasty. A laminectomy in this case, however, almost certainly would have led to progressive swan-neck deformity and cervical instability because of the preexisting spinal alignment. A laminectomy is contraindicated in cases with kyphosis of the cervical spine because the procedure is an indirect means of decompressing the cord when the pathology is located anteriorly. The cord is draped over the anterior osteophytes when the spine is kyphotic and it cannot drift back away from the osteophytes unless lordosis can be achieved and maintained.

PEARLS

- The sagittal alignment of the cervical spine is the most critical piece of information used to decide whether to decompress the spine anteriorly or posteriorly. If the cord is compressed anteriorly and the spine alignment is neutral or kyphotic, a posterior approach will not decompress the cord unless it is combined with an instrumented fusion that restores and maintains lordosis.
- Flexion and extension films are important to obtain in that they may identify potentially unstable areas and mandate a fusion.
- If foraminotomies are necessary, excising less than 30 to 50% of the facet joint will minimize the risk of postoperative instability if a fusion is not performed.
- With long posterior cervical instrumented fusions, prepare the screw holes that are least forgiving first and then build the construct around them. One of the limitations of our current generation of implants is that the screw holes in the plates constrain the location of the bone screws and may force the surgeon to place a screw in a suboptimal position.

PITFALLS

- Regardless of the posterior surgical technique chosen, the surgeon must be meticulous and avoid any retraction or compression of the spinal cord.
- The lower aspect of any posterior internal fixation device is under high stress at the cervicothoracic junction and it may prove to be desirable to carry the fusion down into the upper thoracic spine to avoid implant failure and pseudarthrosis.

A laminoplasty is a good option for decompression in the setting of multilevel stenosis when the spine is stable and the alignment is lordotic. There are many variations of this procedure, but all of the techniques share the concept of enlarging the spinal canal dimensions while leaving the posterior elements of the spine partially intact as protection for the cord and structural support to prevent instability. A common form of the procedure is performed by creating longitudinal troughs with a high-speed drill on both sides of the spine from C3 to C7 at the junction of the lamina and facet joints. One of the troughs is cut completely down to the dura and the opposite side is drilled down to the anterior cortex of the lamina. The ligamentum flavum is sectioned at C2/C3 and C7/T1 and the lamina is opened like a book by creating a greenstick fracture on one side of the lamina. The "door" is held open by small strut grafts, sutures, or plates, and the wound is closed over the open door. Laminoplasty is not as technically demanding as an instrumented fusion but it is more difficult than a laminectomy. The results of laminoplasty are somewhat better than laminectomy in most series, whereas the long-term results of laminectomy with instrumented fusion are unknown.

The posterior fusion used in this patient relieved his axial pain and fortunately he did not sustain any of the potential complications of the procedure. The procedure was technically demanding, the patient required a brace postoperatively, and he lost a moderate amount of cervical motion. We believe that the long-term results of the procedure will offset the disadvantages and justify the additional risks of the operation, but long-term data are lacking to statistically validate this.

Alternative Methods of Management

Type of Management	Advantages	Disadvantages
Anterior	Direct removal of structures causing compression Elimination of dynamic compression and instability Deformity correction Effective with kyphotic deformity Better neck pain relief	Technically demanding Pseudarthrosis Graft migration Hardware complications Graft donor-site problems Postoperative bracing required More complications with longer fusions
Posterior	Indicated for multilevel stenosis Loss of motion: laminectomy < laminoplasty < fusion Technical difficulty: laminectomy < laminoplasty < fusion Bracing requirements: laminectomy < laminoplasty < fusion Lower complication rate than multilevel anterior cervical discectomy and fusion (ACDF)	Indirect decompression Not effective with kyphotic alignment (unless lordosis restored and instrumented fusion done) Poor results with limited decompression Does not help neck pain unless combined with a fusion Potential for postoperative instability: laminectomy > laminoplasty > fusion Posterior fusion: donor-site problems, pseudarthrosis, hardware complications

Continued on next page

Continued

Type of Management	Advantages	Disadvantages
Laminectomy	Technically easiest No brace No fusion/bone graft/hardware problems No bracing No loss of motion	Greater potential for postoperative instability and recurrent neurologic deterioration Does not help neck pain Not indicated with kyphotic alignment
Laminectomy with fusion	Prevents postoperative instability Maintenance of lordosis and stability may lead to better long-term neurologic results than laminectomy alone May help neck pain Can be used with kyphotic alignment if lordosis can be restored and maintained	Bone graft/fusion/hardware complications Bracing required Technically demanding Results unproven Loss of motion
Laminoplasty	Not as technically demanding as instrumented fusion Less risk of postoperative instability and swan-neck deformity Better long-term results than laminectomy	More technically demanding than laminectomy Not helpful for neck pain Not indicated with kyphotic alignment Door of laminoplasty may close or fracture and cause recurrent neurologic loss More loss of motion than laminectomy

Suggested Readings

Abumi K, Kaneda K, Shono Y, et al. One-stage posterior decompression and reconstruction of the cervical spine by using pedicle screw fixation systems. J Neurosurg 1999; 90:19–26.

Albert TJ, Klein GR, Joffe D, Vaccaro AR. Use of cervicothoracic junction pedicle screws for reconstruction of complex cervical spine pathology. Spine 1998; 23:1596–1599.

Albert TJ, Vaccaro AR. Post laminectomy kyphosis. Spine 1998; 23:2738–2745.

Epstein JA. The surgical management of cervical spinal stenosis, spondylosis, and myeloradiculopathy by means of the posterior approach. Spine 1988; 13:864–869.

Herkowitz HN. A comparison of anterior cervical fusion, cervical laminectomy and cervical laminoplasty for the surgical management of multiple level spondylotic myelopathy. Spine 1988; 13:774–780.

Yonenobu K, Yamamoto T, Ono K. Laminoplasty for myelopathy: indications, results, outcome, and complications. In: Clark CE, ed. The Cervical Spine, pp. 849–864. New York: Lippincott-Raven, 1997.

Case 7
Thoracic Disc Herniation: Anterior Approach

Douglas M. Ehrler and Alexander R. Vaccaro

History and Physical Examination

A 52-year-old woman presented with a chief complaint of midback pain for the previous 4 weeks. The pain started insidiously with no history of trauma. It now radiates down to her low back, and in a band-like fashion across into her chest wall. The pain is constantly present, including at rest and at night, and increases in intensity with coughing or sneezing. She has also noticed weakness in her legs, which has increased over the past 2 weeks. She denies fever or chills, weight loss, leg pain, numbness, or bowel or bladder changes. She has received no treatment and has only seen her primary care physician, who referred her. Past medical history is significant for controlled hypertension.

Physical examination reveals a well-nourished, well-developed female, 5'7" tall, weighing 145 lbs. She walks slightly dragging her right leg. She has normal balance. She lacks 20 inches with attempted toe touching and has 20 degrees of lateral bending limited by midthoracic pain. Motor testing reveals right L3 = 5/5, L4 = 4/5, L5 = 4/5, and S1 = 3/5. Left leg is L3 = 5/5, L4 = 5/5, L5 = 4/5, and S1 = 4/5. Deep tendon reflexes (DTRs) are bilateral patella 4/4 and Achilles 3/4. Babinski's signs

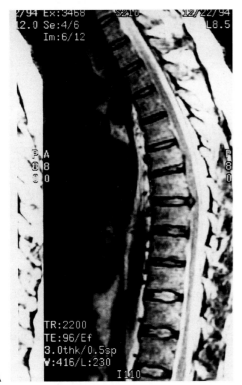

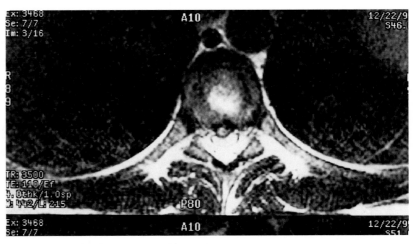

Figure 7–1. Sagittal magnetic resonance imaging (MRI) (A) demonstrating a thoracic disc herniation (TDH) at T7/T8 with ventral spinal cord compression. Axial MRI image (B) of the same TDH.

are up-going bilaterally, and there is sustained clonus on the right and 3 to 4 beats on the left. Straight leg raise (SLR) is negative. Sensory, vascular, rectal, and upper extremity exam is within normal limits.

Radiologic Findings

Plain radiographs of the entire spine demonstrate no abnormalities. Magnetic resonance imaging (MRI) demonstrates a central thoracic disc herniation (TDH) at T7/T8 (Fig. 7–1). A myelogram of the same area has a filling defect posterior to the T7/T8 disc space (Fig. 7–2). A postmyelogram computed tomography (CT) scan demonstrates the disc herniation with compression of the subarachnoid space (Fig. 7–3).

Diagnosis

The patient was diagnosed with a soft central disc herniation at T7/T8 with resultant myelopathy. The disc herniation was suggested by her history of atraumatic

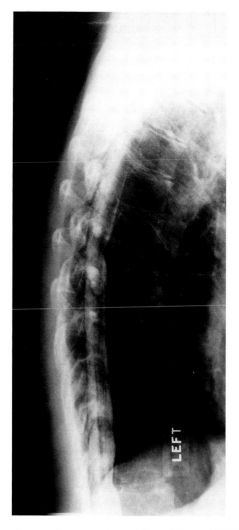

Figure 7–2. Thoracic myelogram demonstrating a filling defect at T7/T8.

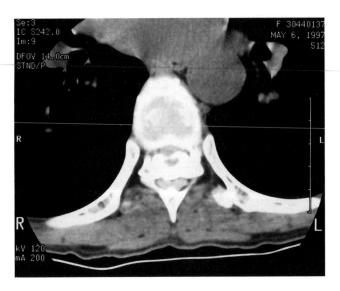

Figure 7–3. Postmyelogram computed tomography (CT) of a T7/T8 thoracic disc herniation with resultant ventral compression.

midback pain radiating to her low back and anterior chest wall, and by her subjective leg weakness. Leg weakness, hyperreflexia, and upper motor neuron (UMN) findings on physical exam supported this. The TDH was confirmed by the MRI images, the filling defect on the myelogram, and the subarachnoid compression on the postmyelogram CT scan. It was designated soft due to a lack of extravertebral calcification.

Surgical Management

After the diagnosis, prognosis, and treatment plans were explained to the patient, she decided to proceed with surgical management. The patient was taken to the operating room and induction of anesthesia with a double-lumen endotracheal tube was performed. Spinal cord monitoring leads were attached to the patient. Pneumatic compression boots were applied to her calves. She was placed in a right lateral decubitus position (left side up). This position was held with the use of a beanbag. The approximate level of herniation was placed over the break in the table. All pressure points were padded, including an axillary roll. A pillow was placed between the arms and legs and both were further padded with blankets. A safety belt was put on and a warming blanket applied to the lower half of the body. The table was flexed and then leveled to orient the patient's thorax parallel to the floor. The lateral chest, back, and iliac crest were prepared and draped. One gram of cefazolin was given intravenously.

At this time under loupe magnification an incision on top of the eighth rib was made from the lateral edge of the paraspinal muscles to the tip of the costal cartilage. Electrocautery was used to divide the subcutaneous tissue and the underlying muscle down to the rib. The periosteum of the rib was incised along the length of the incision. A periosteal elevator was used to strip the outer surface and a Doyen rib dissector was used to strip the undersurface of the rib, separating it from the underlying endothoracic fascia and pleura. The rib was resected with a rib shear and the cut edges were smoothed with a rongeur. The parietal pleura was lifted up and incised. The pleural incision was extended the length of the wound with scissors. A rib retractor was inserted. The lung was deflated and retracted medially and superiorly. A malleable C-shaped retractor, wrapped in a moist sponge, was placed in the chest and used as a self-retainer for the lung. A spinal needle was inserted in the T7/T8 disc and confirmed with a radiograph. The parietal pleura was incised longitudinally over the seventh and eighth vertebral bodies. The segmental vessels over each body were identified, dissected with a right-angled hemostat, and preserved. A Cobb elevator was used to retract the parietal pleura posteriorly, and electrocautery used to subperiosteally strip it off each vertebral body. Care was taken not to damage the sympathetic chain.

Once exposure and hemostasis were achieved, the eighth rib head over the T7/T8 interspace was identified. A 3-mm high-speed burr was used to remove the rib head. The exiting nerve root was then identified and traced back to the neuroforamen. Using both the burr and Kerrison rongeurs, the T8 transverse process and pedicle were removed. This step allowed visualization of the dural sac. The burr was then used to remove the inferior quarter of the T7 body and the superior quarter of the T8 body, maintaining the posterior wall of each. This created a box anterior to the spinal canal with only a thin rim of bone and annulus anterior to the cord. Forward- and reverse-angle curettes were used to manipulate the vertebral endplates and annulus into the formed cavity. Any disc material around the spinal cord was then gently teased away from it in an anterior direction. These maneuvers were done across the entire disc space until the contralateral pedicle was reached. Epidural bleeding was controlled with a bipolar. Great care was taken not to retract or manipulate the cord in any manner. Once a thorough decompression was achieved, the box was measured with a caliper and a piece of the harvested rib was cut to match this defect. The rib was gently impacted lengthwise into the cancellous bone of T7 and T8.

The chest cavity was then copiously irrigated. The parietal pleura was closed over the vertebral bodies and the lung expanded. A chest tube was placed superior to the incision in the midaxillary line. Five heavy absorbable sutures were placed around the seventh and ninth ribs. A rib approximator assisted in closing the space, and the sutures were tied. The periosteum of the rib bed, muscle fascia, and subcutaneous layer were closed with absorbable suture. The skin was closed with staples. A postoperative lateral X-ray (Fig. 7–4), CT scan (Fig. 7–5), and CT reconstruction (Fig. 7–6) are shown.

Postoperative Management

The patient was admitted to the intensive care unit (ICU) overnight. Morphine, administered by patient-controlled anesthesia (PCA), was used for pain. On postoperative day 1, the patient was transferred to a room and began ambulating in the hall. On postop day 2 the chest tube was removed and prophylactic antibiotics discontinued. Ambulation and incentive spirometry were encouraged. Pneumatic compression stockings were used while the patient was in bed. The patient was discharged on postop day 4.

The wound healed uneventfully. Skin staples were removed 15 days after surgery. The patient's midthoracic back pain had resolved by 3 weeks postop. Lower extremity strength returned to 5/5 for all roots by 8 weeks. The patient complained of some mild pain along the incision but had no pain with deep breathing or coughing.

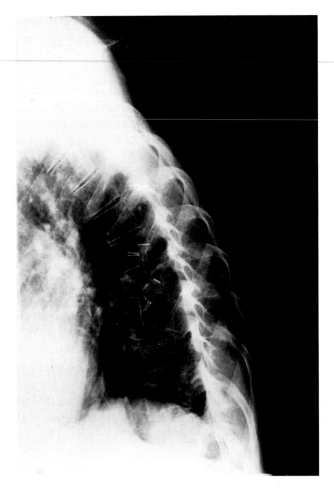

Figure 7–4. Postoperative lateral radiograph of a transthoracic discectomy.

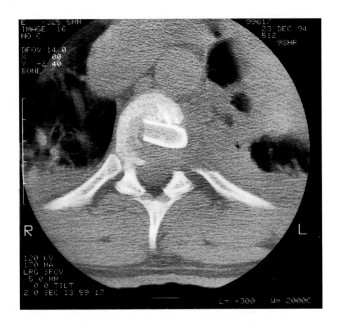

Figure 7–5. Computed tomography (CT) image demonstrating thoracic decompression and rib graft placement.

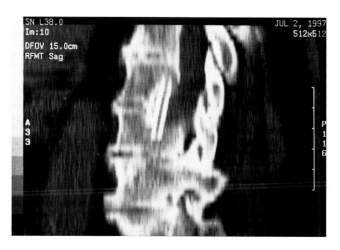

Figure 7–6. Computed tomography (CT) reconstruction of rib graft after transthoracic discectomy.

Discussion

Thoracic disc herniations (TDHs) are rare abnormalities in the spine. The incidence of clinically significant herniations is approximately 1/1,000,000 per year. They account for 0.25 to 0.75% of all spinal disc herniations. Eighty percent of patients present between their third and fifth decade of life. Male to female ratio is 1.5 : 1. Sixty-six percent occur between T8 and T11, with a peak at T9/T10 (26%). A history of torsional or twisting trauma is associated in 25% of cases. The low incidence is due to the limited mobility of the thoracic spine, small intervertebral discs, rib and sternal stability, and facet orientation. Thirty-seven percent of asymptomatic patients have a TDH on MRI. TDHs are classified by level, consistency (hard or soft), and location (central, centrolateral, lateral, or intradural). Seventy to ninety percent are central or centrolateral.

There are no characteristic signs or symptoms of a TDH. The most common presenting symptom is pain (49–70%). The pain can be localized as thoracic, axial, or radicular. Sensory impairment occurs in 24 to 61% of patients and ranges from dysesthesias/paresthesias to complete loss in the chest, groin, or legs. Motor impairment ranges from 17 to 61%. Any one or a combination of these symptoms can be present. Physical exam may reveal few signs of profound neurologic compromise involving sensory and or motor function. UMN signs such as weakness, hyperreflexia, spasticity, clonus, or Babinski sign may be present. A TDH at C7/T1 or T1/T2 may produce a Horner's syndrome (miosis, ptosis, anhidrosis) from preganglionic sympathetic fiber injury. A herniation at these levels may also mimic cervical degenerative disc disease. Midthoracic disc herniation may present as a Brown-Séquard syndrome, whereas low TDHs can present as conus medullaris syndrome.

Any radiographic evaluation of the spine should begin with plain X-rays, which can detect bone destruction as well as indirect evidence of TDH. The signs of disc degeneration include loss of disc space height, osteophyte formation, kyphosis, and calcification in the disc or spinal canal. Disc space calcification can occur in up to 70% of TDHs and signifies that the disc may be adherent to the cord. Intraspinal calcification is strongly suspicious for intrathecal extension of a TDH. MRI is now the diagnostic study of choice for TDHs. Its advantages are that of multiplanar imaging, identification of disc dehydration, lack of ionizing radiation, demonstration of marrow changes, and soft tissue definition, and it is noninvasive. It does have difficulty distinguishing between hard and soft disc herniations and detecting asymptomatic lesions and it overestimates cord compression.

A TDH can produce signs and symptoms by vascular occlusion or mechanical compression. The midthoracic region from T4 to T9 is termed the watershed zone due to its poor vascular supply. Any compression in that area can diminish an already tenuous blood supply. Further, despite the relative small size of the thoracic cord, its cord to canal area ratio is the largest of the entire spine.

The most agreed upon absolute indication for surgical intervention is severe static or progressive myelopathy. The presence of either indicates a poor prognosis. Mild static or improving myelopathy may be treated conservatively. However, some feel that this is an indication for surgical intervention. Radicular pain is initially treated conservatively, with surgical intervention only if medical means fail. Mild and moderate motor dysfunction can be treated conservatively, but severe static or progressive deficits should be treated surgically. Conservative treatment consists of steroidal and nonsteroidal inflammatory drugs, steroid injections, and controlled physical therapy concentrating on stretching, strengthening, controlled hyperextension exercises, and education. The judicious use of narcotics is also acceptable.

The transthoracic approach is the most versatile and can be used from T4 to the thoracolumbar junction. It allows excellent visualization for central and centrolateral hard and soft disc herniations. It is the preferred approach for multilevel disease, kyphosis (Scheuermann's), and TDHs that have migrated behind the vertebral body. The advantages are excellent visualization of the anterior and anterior lateral cord, direct exposure, access across the midline, ability to perform a fusion, and lack of cord manipulation. Disadvantages include limited intradural access, diaphragmatic takedown to expose the thoracolumbar junction, and the possible need of a thoracic surgeon to assist.

An incision is made directly over the rib to be resected. This rib corresponds to the caudad vertebral body adjacent to the disc to be removed. For T2 to T10, the rib articulates with the superior aspect and transverse process of the similarly numbered vertebra and the inferior aspect of the cephalad vertebra. Thus, for a T7/T8 TDH, the eighth rib is resected. After subperiosteal dissection of the rib, it is resected, taking care not to tear the underlying pleura. If this occurs, it is repaired or incorporated into the pleural incision. A finger inserted under the pleura can protect the lung during this step.

After placement of a rib retractor, the left lung is selectively deflated. A wide, malleable, C-shaped retractor that is covered with a moist sponge is a convenient self-retainer for the lung. Care must be taken not to exert excessive pressure on the mediastinum that would affect cardiac output. After incising the parietal pleura over the vertebral bodies, the segmental vessels must be identified. They are located in the midportion of the body. Ligation of these vessels is usually well tolerated if necessary. Sacrificed vessels should be kept to a minimum. They should be ligated anterior (proximal) to the foramen to allow retrograde flow through the intercostal artery. Also, by ligating them in the midportion, they are easily controlled if a clip or suture becomes loose. If a coronal plane abnormality is present, the arteries should be ligated on the convexity.

A burr is used to remove the rib head, transverse process, and caudal pedicle. A drill is less traumatic to the cord by avoiding the mechanical trauma that is associated with the repetitive insertion, removal, and recoil when using a Kerrison rongeur. A small burr is preferred to decrease the moment arm from the center of rotation to the cutting surface as well as the mass of the burr bit, thus minimize jumping. The cavity created in the two adjacent vertebrae allows the disc and bony endplates to be removed from around the cord without manipulation. Curettes are used for this step. A Kerrison should only be used if it can be safely inserted without displacing the cord. It is essential that the decompression be complete across the entire disc space. During the entire decompression absolute diligence must be maintained not to manipulate or stimulate the cord in any manner.

After decompression, the spine is usually stable because two-thirds of the body, both facets, and the posterior structures are still intact. Nonetheless, the resected rib is often fashioned as a graft to be inserted in the area of the partial corpectomy. The wound is copiously irrigated and closed as previously described.

The results for a transthoracic removal of TDHs are consistently good.

There is no single approach that is universally accepted for the removal of a TDH. In choosing an approach, one must consider the disc level, consistency, relation to the spinal cord, dural attachment, patient's medical condition, and surgeon's experience. Surgical principles common to any approach are (1) minimal spinal cord manipulation, (2) preservation of bony architecture, and (3) thorough decompression. Alternative approaches include costotransversectomy, and lateral extracavitary, transpedicular, and thoracoscopic techniques.

The costotransversectomy approach begins by placing the patient in a prone position. A curvilinear incision is made longitudinally with its apex centered 6 to 8 cm lateral to the desired level. This may be centered closer to the midline depending on the level and the surgeon's preference. Depending on the level, the trapezius, latissimus dorsi, or rhomboids are divided. Erector spinae and transversospinalis muscles are divided over the costotransverse junction. The rib is divided 6 to 8 cm lateral to the midline and disarticulated medially. The transverse process is removed. The pedicle, disc space, and foramen are identified. The disc is removed in a direction opposite the spinal cord. Part of the inferior pedicle can be removed to gain exposure. A cavity can be created in the vertebral bodies for the disc to be pushed into similar to that of a lateral transthoracic approach.

The lateral extracavitary approach for TDH begins by placing the patient in a prone position. A hockey-stick incision is made beginning three levels above the area to be approached and curving laterally two levels below. Alternatively, a curved longitudinal incision can be made with its apex 12 cm from the midline. Depending on the level, the trapezius, latissimus dorsi, or rhomboids are split or retracted. The rib is cut 8 to 10 cm lateral and disarticulated medially. The intercostal nerve is identified and cut 3 cm distal to the dorsal root ganglia. The parietal pleura is dissected off the vertebral bodies. The inferior portion of the cephalad pedicle and the superior portion of the caudal pedicle are removed. A cavity is created by removal of part of each adjacent vertebral body. The disc is pushed into this cavity. Removal of the articular facet may also be performed to increase exposure.

For the transpedicular approach, the patient is placed in the prone position. A midline incision is made down to the deep fascia. This is incised and muscle is dissected off to expose laterally out to the facet joint. A high-speed burr is used to remove the facet and pedicle on the symptomatic side caudal to the herniation. This is carried down to the posterior wall of the vertebral body. Lateral herniations can be directly removed, or if needed an anterior bony cavity can be created for the disc to be pushed into.

Thoracoscopic discectomy can also be performed. The patient is intubated with a double-lumen endotracheal tube for single lung ventilation. A lateral decubitus position is used. The spine is approached from the symptomatic side, although the right side is preferred. Three to four portals are established in the lateral chest wall. With the use of special endoscopic instruments, the rib head over the disc space is removed. Part of the pedicle caudal to the herniation is also resected for visualization. The disc is identified by tracing the pedicle to the body and removed with curettes.

Alternative Methods of Management

Type of Management	Disk Herniation	Advantages	Disadvantages
Costotransversectomy	Soft—Central Centrolateral Lateral Hard—Centrolateral Lateral	Extrapleural Avoid pulmonary complications	Difficult in scapular region Decreased visualization across midline Hard to remove calcified disc/osteophytes Difficult to repair dural tears
Lateral Extracavitary	Soft—Central Centrolateral Lateral Hard—Central Centrolateral Lateral	Extrapleural Better visualization across cord Multilevel potential Ability to graft No diaphragmatic takedown at T-L junction	Difficult in scapular region Total visualization across cord Difficult to repair dural tears Increased time/blood loss Large dissection/bone resection
Transpedicular	Soft—Lateral Hard—Lateral	Extrapleural Less extensive dissection Simple/familiar approach Decreased time/blood loss Good in scapular region (T2 to T4)	Limited central/centrolateral exposure Lack of direct visualization/decompression Hard to remove calcified disc Facet and pedicle removal with no ability to graft
Thoracoscopic	Soft—Lateral Small Focal	Good direct visualization Decreased pain/recovery Decreased blood loss Decreased rib distraction/resection	Technically demanding Trocar injuries Atelectasis/pulmonary complications Thoracic surgeon needed

Suggested Readings

Dietze DD, Fessler RG. Thoracic disc herniations. Neurosurg Clin North Am 1993; 4:75–90.

Mulier S, Debois V. Thoracic disc herniations: transthoracic, lateral, or posterolateral approach? A review. Surg Neurol 1998; 49:599–608.

Stillerman CB, Chen TC, Couldwell WT, et al. Experience in the surgical management of 82 symptomatic herniated thoracic discs and review of the literature. J Neurosurg 1998; 88:623–633.

Stillerman CB, Weiss MH. Management of thoracic disc disease. Clin Neurosurg 1992; 38:325–352.

Case 8

Thoracic Disc Herniation: Posterior Approach

Douglas M. Ehrler and Alexander R. Vaccaro

History and Physical Examination

A 34-year-old man presented with a chief complaint of back pain associated with anterior leg pain, numbness, and weakness. The pain is in his midback and had been present for almost 1 year and was increasing in intensity. It is now always present. It radiates to both thighs, knees, and lateral calves, with the left side affected more than the right. He also reports numbness primarily in the left leg down to the foot. Over the past 4 weeks he has been unable to run and has had increasing difficulty with balance. He has had difficulty initiating urination over the past 2 weeks but denies frank retention or incontinence. He denies fever, chills, weight loss, or any previous back/neck trauma. Past medical history is insignificant.

On physical exam the patient walks with a broad-based gait, and had moderate difficulty with balance especially while turning. He is able to toe walk but cannot heel walk. He lacks 24 inches with forward bending and has 10 degrees lateral bending. Motor testing reveals 5-/5 iliopsoas bilaterally; 5/5 hamstrings and quadriceps bilaterally; 3/5 foot dorsiflexors bilaterally; 3/5 right extensor hallucis longus (EHL)

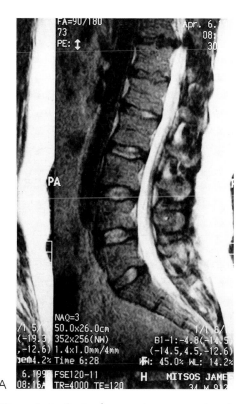
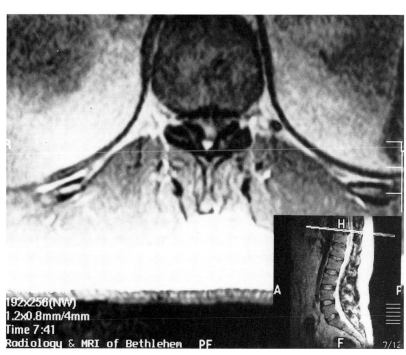

Figure 8–1. Sagittal magnetic resonance imaging (MRI) (A) of a thoracic disc herniation (TDH) at T11/T12. An axial MRI (B) of the same TDH with resultant spinal cord compression.

and 4+/5 EHL left; and 4+/5 plantar flexors bilaterally. There is decreased sensation in the L5 and S1 dermatomes bilaterally, left more than right. Straight leg raise (SLR) is negative. Deep tendon reflexes (DTRs) are bilateral patella 1/4 and bilateral Achilles 3/4. He has bilateral up-going Babinski's and sustained clonus. Vascular, rectal, and upper extremity exam is within normal limits.

Radiologic Findings

Plain radiographs of the entire spine demonstrate no abnormalities. Magnetic resonance imaging (MRI) demonstrates a left centrolateral thoracic disc herniation (TDH) at T11/T12 (Fig. 8–1). Due to the MRI findings and the progressive nature of his symptoms, no other studies were ordered.

Diagnosis

The patient was diagnosed with a soft centrolateral disc herniation at T11/T12 with resultant myelopathy. The disc herniation was suggested by the history of atraumatic midback pain radiating to his legs, associated numbness, and leg weakness. The presence of leg weakness, decreased sensation, hyperreflexia, and upper motor neuron (UMN) findings on physical exam supported the diagnosis of a TDH. Recent increase in weakness, loss of balance, and urinary retention suggested a progressive course. The TDH was confirmed by MRI. It was designated a soft herniation due to a lack of extravertebral calcification.

Surgical Management

After explanation to the patient of his diagnosis, prognosis, and treatment plan, the patient decided to proceed with surgical management. The patient was taken to the operating room and induction of anesthesia with a double-lumen endotracheal tube was performed. Spinal cord monitoring leads were attached to the patient. Pneumatic compression boots were applied to his calves. He was placed in a prone position with two chest rolls placed longitudinally, lateral enough to allow chest expansion. All pressure points were padded. The patient's back was prepared and draped. One gram of cefazolin was given intravenously. A radiograph was taken to identify the T11/T12 interspace and the T11 rib.

A curved incision was made from T9 to L2 with its apex centered at T11, 10 cm left of the midline. The subcutaneous tissue and deep fascia were incised in line with the skin incision. The trapezius and erector spinae muscles were split in line with the 11th rib. The intercostal neurovascular bundle was identified and separated from the inferior rib margin. The periosteum of the rib was incised and then stripped circumferentially. The rib was cut 5 cm from the costotransverse articulation. This articulation was then transected and the rib manipulated off. The medial edge of the rib was beveled to a smooth surface. The parietal pleura was dissected off the T10 and T12 rib above and below and depressed with a malleable retractor. The transverse process of T11 was then removed with a high-speed burr and rongeurs down to its junction with the superior facet and pedicle. The neurovascular bundle was traced back to identify the T11 pedicle and neuroforamen. The T11 vertebral body was followed inferiorly to identify the T11/T12 disc. A needle was placed in the disc space and confirmed with a radiograph. The parietal pleura was dissected off the posterior lateral portion of T11 and T12 to expose the T11/T12 disc space. The lateral margin of the T11/T12 disc was incised with a no. 15 blade well away from the spinal cord. Disc material was then removed with curettes and a pituitary rongeur. Disc material adjacent to the thecal sac was pushed back into the evacuated interspace in an atraumatic fashion. This was done until the cord was decompressed. There were no changes in the spinal cord monitoring throughout the case. Epidural bleeding was controlled with use of a bipolar electrocautery. Meticulous hemostasis was achieved.

Through positive pressure ventilation, the pleura was checked for any leaks. The wound was copiously irrigated. Deep fascia was closed with interrupted heavy absorbable suture. Subcutaneous tissue was closed with absorbable suture. The skin was closed with staples. A chest X-ray was taken in the recovery room to check for a pnuemothorax.

Postoperative Management

The patient was admitted to the neurosurgical intensive care unit (NICU) overnight. Morphine, administered by patient-controlled anesthesia (PCA), was used for pain. No postoperative immobilization or bracing was required. The patient ambulated on postoperative day 1. Prophylactic antibiotics were continued for 24 hours. Ambulation and incentive spirometry were encouraged. Pneumatic compression stockings were used while the patient was in bed. The patient was discharged on postoperative day 4.

The wound healed uneventfully. Skin staples were removed 15 days after surgery. The patient's midthoracic back and leg pain had resolved by $2\frac{1}{2}$ weeks postoperation. Lower extremity strength returned to between 4 and 5/5 strength for all roots by 9 weeks. A postoperative anteroposterior (A/P) radiograph was taken (Fig. 8–2).

Discussion

Eighty percent of patients with a symptomatic disc herniation present between their third and fifth decade of life. Male to female ratio is 1.5 : 1. Sixty-six percent occur between T8 and T11, with a peak at T9/T10 (26%). A history of torsional or twisting trauma is associated in 25% of cases. The low incidence is due to several anatomic factors. These include the limited mobility of the thoracic spine, small intervertebral discs, rib and sternal stability, and facet orientation. Asymptomatic subjects have a 37% incidence of a TDH on MRI. TDHs are classified by level, consistency (hard or soft), and location (central, centrolateral, lateral, or intradural). Seventy to ninety percent are central or central lateral.

The presenting symptoms of a TDH vary from patient to patient. Pain is the most common presenting symptom. It is present in 49 to 70% of patients. The pain can be localized to the axial thoracic spine or is radicular in nature. Sensory impairment ranges from 24 to 61%, and can vary from dysesthesias/paresthesias to complete loss in the chest, groin, or legs. Motor impairment ranges from 17 to 61%. Any one or a combination of these symptoms can be present. Physical exam may reveal deficits involving sensory and or motor function. Weakness, hyperreflexia, spasticity, clonus, or a Babinski sign may be present. These indicate upper motor neuron involvement. A TDH at C7/T1 or T1/T2 may produce a Horner's

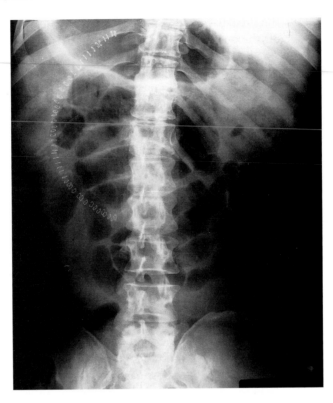

Figure 8–2. Postoperative plain film after T11/T12 discectomy via a costotransversectomy.

syndrome (miosis, ptosis, anhidrosis) due to preganglionic sympathetic fiber injury. A herniation at these levels may also mimic cervical degenerative disc disease. Midthoracic disc herniation can present as Brown-Séquard syndrome, whereas low TDHs can present as conus medullaris syndrome. A broad differential diagnosis must be considered. These include referred pain from myocardial infarction, cardiac angina pulmonary embolus, pulmonary infarction, hepatobiliary colic, colitis, pancreatitis, renal pathology, and retroperitoneal vascular abnormalities. Spinal pathology such as infection, neoplasm, arteriovenous malformations, deformity, degeneration, and occult trauma must be considered. Fibromyalgia, intercostal neuritis, costochondritis, muscle strain, or herpes zoster may cause chest wall pain. Demyelinating disease, primary motor neuron dysfunction, muscular dystrophy, and myopathies should also be considered especially in the absence of pain.

The diagnostic study of choice for a TDH is MRI. It has several advantages, including multiplanar imaging, identification of disc dehydration, lack of ionizing radiation, demonstration of marrow changes, and soft tissue definition, and it is non-invasive. Its disadvantages are difficulty distinguishing between hard and soft discs and detecting asymptomatic lesions, and it overestimates cord compression. Disc herniations are isointense or slightly hypointense on T1 images and hypointense on T2. A T2-weighted image produces a myelogram effect providing better contrast between structures. Any finding on MRI cannot be used to determine the need for surgical treatment.

Vascular occlusion or mechanical compression may produce the signs and symptoms associated with a TDH. The midthoracic region from T4 to T9 is termed the watershed zone due to its poor vascular supply. Any compression in that area can diminish an already tenuous blood supply. The thoracic spinal cord to canal area ratio is the largest of the entire spine. The spinal cord occupies 40% of the subarachnoid space in the thoracic area compared to 25% in the cervical spine. Even small amounts of compression may be clinically significant.

The most agreed upon absolute indication for surgical intervention is severe static or progressive myelopathy. The presence of either indicates a poor prognosis. Mild static or improving myelopathy may be treated conservatively. This may be considered an indication for operative treatment by some surgeons. Localized axial and radicular pain is treated conservatively. Radicular pain may be selected for surgical treatment if medical means fail. Mild and moderate motor dysfunction can be treated conservatively, but severe static or progressive deficits should be treated surgically. Conservative treatment consists of steroidal and nonsteroidal antiinflammatory drugs, steroid injections, and controlled physical therapy concentrating on stretching, strengthening, controlled hyperextension exercises, as well as education. The judicious use of narcotics is also acceptable.

A costotransversectomy can be used at any level of the thoracic spine. It can be especially useful in the upper thoracic spine (T2 to T4) where an anterior approach would necessitate a sternal splitting procedure. Likewise, if used at the Thoracolumbar (T-L) junction, a takedown of the diaphragm can be avoided. It allows the decompression of soft TDHs that are central, centrolateral, and lateral as well as a hard TDH that is centrolateral or lateral. Its advantages are that it is extrapleural, avoids potential pulmonary complications associated with an anterior approach, and does not require the addition of a second (thoracic) surgeon. Its disadvantages are the disruption of the paraspinal musculature, difficulty in repairing dural tears, and decreased access across the midline. It should not be used for large central calcified discs or when large osteophytes are present.

The patient was placed in a prone position. This facilitates taking a true lateral intraoperative radiograph. The patient could also have been placed in a lateral decubitus or a 15- to 30-degree semiprone position to facilitate exposure. A left-sided approach was chosen because of the patient's greater signs and symptoms on the left side, which correlated with the left-sided pathology found on MRI. The patient should be approached from the side of pathology. If there are no localizing signs or symptoms and a midline disc, a right-sided approach is chosen in the lower thoracic spine to avoid the artery of Adamkiewicz. A curved incision with its apex 10 cm lateral was chosen to facilitate dissection over the rib and transverse process and to allow a more horizontal angle of approach. The incision can be a straight paramedian or more or less curved depending on the number of levels and surgeon's preference. Dissection is carried down through the trapezius and rhomboids (for high approaches) or latissimus dorsi (for lower approaches). Dissection can be in line with their fibers if the plane permits or transversely if needed. The deep paraspinal muscles, erector spinae, and transversospinalis are dissected in line with the skin incision. These can be divided transversely if exposure is difficult, although this makes for a more difficult closure. In this case, dissection was carried down upon the 11th rib and traced to the transverse process and pedicle of the 11th vertebral body to access the anteriorly situated T11/T12 interspace. At higher levels in the spine (T2 to T8) and less so at T9/T10, the rib/vertebral body anatomy is more predictable. At these levels, the rib articulates with the superior aspect and transverse process of the similarly numbered vertebra and the inferior aspect of the cephalad vertebra. Thus, following the eighth rib will lead to the T7/T8 disc space. However, the T12 rib only articulates to the body of T12 and does not lead directly to the T11/T12 disc. Therefore, it was chosen to follow and subsequently resect the 11th rib, identify the 11th pedicle, and dissect inferiorly to the T11/T12 disc. The transverse process was removed with a burr, which is less traumatic than using an osteotome. Once the T11 pedicle is identified, it is traced to the posterolateral vertebral body. The parietal pleura is dissected off the vertebra in a caudal direction to find the disc space. Care should be taken not to damage the sympathetic chain while this is being done. A portion of the exposed or caudad pedicle can be resected with a burr or Kerrison if needed for exposure. The disc is incised well away from the cord and removed in the usual fashion. The herniated portion of the disc is then pushed away from the cord into this space. A cavity can be created by vertebral body resection on each side of the disc space if additional space is needed. It is important that the cord is not manipulated.

A thorough decompression should be achieved. Hemostasis is achieved to avoid hematoma formation, which could compress the cord. The lung is inflated to check for air leaks. A leak can be better appreciated if the wound is filled with saline. If a tear is present, it should be repaired and consideration given to placing a chest tube. The wound is closed as previously described.

Alternative Methods of Management

There is no single approach that is accepted for the removal of a TDH. In choosing an approach, one must consider the disc level, consistency, relation to the spinal cord, dural attachment, patient's medical condition, and surgeon's experience. Surgical principles common to any approach are, (1) minimal spinal cord manipulation, (2) preservation of bony architecture, and (3) a thorough decompression. Alternative approaches include transthoracic, lateral extracavitary, transpedicular, and thoroscopic.

The transthoracic approach for a TDH begins by placing the patient in a right lateral decubitus position (left side up). The table is flexed under the patient to aid in exposure. An incision is made over the rib to be resected. This rib in question corresponds in number to the inferior vertebral body. Dissection is carried down to the rib periosteum, which is stripped circumferentially. The rib is then resected. The pleura is incised in line with the skin incision and the lung deflated and retracted. The parietal pleura is reflected off the vertebral bodies, and the segmental vessels are ligated if necessary. A burr is used to remove the rib head, transverse process, and caudal pedicle. A cavity is created by resecting the inferior portion of the cephalad vertebra and the superior portion of the caudal vertebra. Disc material is then pushed away from the cord into this area. The resected rib is fashioned as a graft and inserted into the cavity.

The lateral extracavitary approach for TDH begins by placing the patient in a prone position. A hockey-stick incision is made beginning three levels above the area to be approached and curving laterally two levels below. Alternatively, a curved longitudinal incision can be made with its apex 12 cm from the midline. Depending on the level, the trapezius, latissimus dorsi, or rhomboids are split or retracted. The rib is cut 8 to 10 cm lateral and disarticulated medially. The intercostal nerve is identified and cut 3 cm distal to the dorsal root ganglia. The parietal pleura is dissected off the vertebral bodies. The inferior portion of the cephalad pedicle and the superior portion of the caudal pedicle are removed. A cavity is created by removal of part of each adjacent vertebral body. The disc is pushed into this cavity. Removal of the articular facet may also be performed to increase exposure.

For the transpedicular approach, the patient is placed in the prone position. A midline incision is made down to the deep fascia. This is incised and muscle is dissected off to expose laterally out to the facet joint. A high-speed burr is used to remove the facet and pedicle on the symptomatic side caudal to the herniation. This is carried down to the posterior wall of the vertebral body. Lateral herniations can be directly removed, or if needed an anterior bony cavity can be created for the disc to be pushed into.

Thoracoscopic discectomy can also be performed. The patient is intubated with a double-lumen endotracheal tube for single lung ventilation. A lateral decubitus position is used. The spine is approached from the symptomatic side, although the right side is preferred. Three to four portals are established in the lateral chest wall. With the use of special endoscopic instruments, the rib head over the disc space is removed. Part of the pedicle caudal to the herniation is also resected for visualization. The disc is identified by tracing the pedicle to the body and removed with curettes.

Type of Management	Disc Herniation	Advantages	Disadvantages
Transthoracic	Soft—Central Centrolateral Lateral Hard—Central Centrolateral Lateral	Excellent exposure Direct decompression Access across midline Ability to fuse	Pulmonary complications/chest tube Limited intradural access Diaphragmatic takedown at T-L junction Need for thoracic surgeon
Lateral Extracavitary	Soft—Central Centrolateral Lateral Hard—Central Centrolateral Lateral	Extrapleural Better visualization across cord Multilevel potential Ability to graft No diaphragmatic takedown at T-L junction	Difficult in scapular region Total visualization across cord Difficult to repair dural tears Increased time/blood loss Large dissection/blood loss
Transpedicular	Soft—Lateral Hard—Lateral	Extrapleural Less extensive dissection Simple/familiar approach Decreased time/blood loss Good in scapular region (T2 to T4)	Limited central/centrolateral exposure Lack of direct visualization/decompression Hard to remove calcified disc Facet and pedicle removal with no ability to graft
Thoracoscopic	Soft—Lateral Small Focal	Good direct visualization Decreased pain/recovery Decreased blood loss Decreased rib distraction/resection	Technically demanding Trocar injuries Atelectasis/pulmonary complications Thoracic surgeon needed

Suggested Readings

Dietze DD, Fessler RG. Thoracic disc herniations. Neurosurg Clin North Am 1993; 4:75–90.

Mulier S, Debois V. Thoracic disc herniations: transthoracic, lateral, or posterolateral approach? A review. Surg Neurol 1998; 49:599–608.

Stillerman CB, Chen TC, Couldwell WT, et al. Experience in the surgical management of 82 symptomatic herniated thoracic discs and review of the literature. J Neurosurg 1998; 88:623–633.

Simpson JM, Silveri CP, Simeone FA, et al. Thoracic disc herniation. Re-evaluation of the posterior approach using a modified costotransversectomy. Spine 1993; 18:1872–1877.

Case 9

Thoracic Disc Herniations: Minimally Invasive Approach

Srdjan Mirkovic

History and Physical Examination

A 35-year-old woman presented with a 9-month history of middle to low back pain. She states that her symptoms began acutely after she moved some furniture. In the preceding 9 months, she was treated by chiropractic manipulations and antiinflammatory medications, with some improvement. However, she experienced reexacerbation in her symptoms and was reevaluated and then referred to therapy.

On physical examination, her motor strength was 5/5 in the upper and lower extremities. The patient had no difficulty toe walking or squatting and the sensory examination to pinprick and light touch was normal in the upper and lower extremities, as well as in her back and along her chest. Reflexes were 1+ and equal bilaterally.

She presented without evidence of tension signs. She had a down-going Babinski's sign and no evidence of clonus. Her proprioception was intact. Waddell sign's were 0/5.

Radiologic Findings

Anteroposterior (AP) and lateral radiographs of the thoracic and lumbar spine demonstrated good alignment without suggestion of deformity. The disc spaces were well maintained without evidence of a destructive process or suggestion of endplate erosion consistent with infection. Sagittal and transverse magnetic resonance

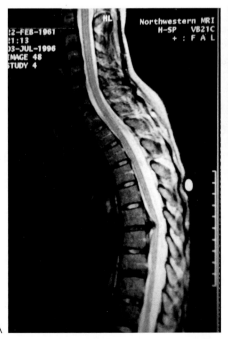

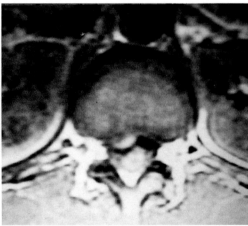

Figure 9–1. Sagittal (A) and axial (B) magnetic resonance imaging (MRI) of a T6/T7 thoracic disc herniation.

imaging (MRI) of the thoracic spine demonstrated a calcified herniated disc at T6/T7, with posterior compression of the thoracic cord. There was no abnormal signal intensity within the thoracic cord parenchyma. The thoracic spine was otherwise unremarkable (Fig. 9–1).

Diagnosis

Symptomatic degenerative disc herniation at T6/T7.

Surgical Management

The surgical procedure is performed under general anesthesia with the patient in the lateral decubitus position. A double-lumen endotracheal tube is preferred to allow unilateral lung ventilation; the lung is collapsed on the operative side, facilitating exposure. Two large-bore intravenous lines and/or a peripheral large-bore line with a central line are placed. In addition, we prefer an arterial line for close pressure monitoring. Somatosensory and motor evoked potential spinal cord monitoring is instituted throughout the procedure. The patient is approached from the side of the herniation, facilitating the thoracoscopic approach. The patient is positioned in the lateral decubitus position, using Stulberg hip positioners, which can also be placed at the chest level, securing the patient to the operative table. We have avoided the use of a beanbag, because of difficulty with secure patient positioning and occasional interference with the operative field. A Foley catheter is inserted and the lower extremities are placed in thromboembolic disease stockings (TEDS) and compression boots. Hips and knees are flexed and all extremities are carefully padded. An axillary roll is placed with the arm closest to the table extended on an arm board, whereas the arm on the side of the approach is placed in an airplane splint. The head is placed in neutral on pillows or blankets. The operative field extending anteriorly over the chest wall and posteriorly over the lateral back is prepped and draped. The operative field includes the left iliac crest in cases where iliac crest bone harvesting may be necessary. The surgeon and first assistant stand anterior to the patient. The surgeon holds working instruments and suction-irrigation, and the first assistant holds the fan retractor and the camera. If the surgeon needs to use both hands for manipulating sharp instruments, a second assistant can hold the suction-irrigation. The second assistant faces the camera and instrument and needs to adjust to the mirror imaging that occurs (Fig. 9–2).

The initial trocar is placed in the anterior axillary line at the level of the disc herniation. The appropriate surgical level is identified following placement of a metallic object over the thoracic spine and identification of this level through fluoroscopy or X-rays. Vertebrae are counted from the sacrum proximally and the appropriate level is thus identified, or it can be confirmed by counting ribs. Preoperatively, X-rays and MRIs are reviewed to ensure that no spinal anomalies are present, notably, the presence of a sixth lumbar vertebra. The initial trocar is placed in the T6/T7 intercostal space following a 2-cm incision. Trocar placement is performed without direct visualization of the cavity and is done bluntly with digital palpation to avoid injury to the lung parenchyma, which can occur in cases of pleural adhesions. The ipsilateral lung is then collapsed through resorptive atelectasis. A 30-degree angle rigid scope was then placed. If the lung cannot be collapsed sufficiently, a second portal is placed in the anterior axillary line at the T9 intercostal level. A fan retractor

PEARLS

The surgical approach should be determined by the disc consistency, location, level of herniation, and the surgeon's experience (see Table 9–1). The following technical surgical principles should be adhered to:

- Instrumentation crowding and the ensuing fencing can be avoided by spacing the portals.
- To avoid mirror imaging, the instrumentation and camera should be positioned in a 180-degree arc in the same direction.
- Avoid simultaneous movement of instrument and camera.
- Manipulation of instruments should proceed under direct thoracoscopic visualization.

PITFALLS

- Overtreatment, particularly in the presence of asymptomatic lesions, should be avoided.
- In the absence of neurologic involvement, conservative management is indicated.
- Thoracoscopic discectomy has a sharp learning curve.
- A laboratory setting is advisable to familiarize the surgeon with the instrumentation and thoracoscopic techniques.
- The development of tactile sensation when working with long instruments a significant distance from the pathology, as well as an appreciation for depth perception, will ensure intraoperative success and avoidance of disastrous neurologic complications.

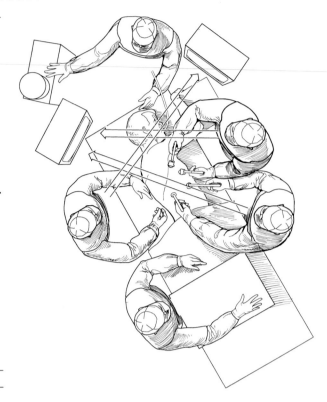

Figure 9–2. An illustration of patient positioning with surgeon location.

is placed through this portal, allowing the lung to be retracted, thus enhancing visualization of the thoracic spine. With the thoracic spine fully visualized, the correct level is identified by counting from the first rib distally to the T7 rib corresponding to the T6/T7 disc interspace. A 10-inch spinal needle is then placed cephalad to the presumed T7 rib head in the disc space to verify the appropriate level. AP and lateral X-rays are then obtained, verifying the appropriate disc level. Under endoscopic visualization, a third working portal is placed in the midaxillary line located at the T9/T10 intercostal space. The 30-degree scope is then switched from the T6/T7 portal to the T9/T10 midaxillary portal. A fourth working portal, under direct endoscopic visualization is then placed in the anterior axillary line at the T4/T5 intercostal space through which suction irrigation is inserted (Fig. 9–3).

Through the working T6/T7 midaxillary portal, insulated Bovie cautery is then inserted and the pleura over the T7 rib head extending from its most anterior border to 3 to 4 cm posteriorly is reflected and the costotransverse ligaments are transected with Bovie cautery. Using a 10-inch Cobb elevator and a 45-degree curbed dissector, the rib head is then freed from its cephalad attachment to the T7 vertebral body (Fig. 9–4). A $\frac{1}{4}$-inch osteotome is then used to osteotomize the most anterior 2 cm of the rib head. This allows complete visualization of the T6/T7 disc space. Intercostal vessels are coagulated with bipolar cautery. A long Penfield probe is then used to gently dissect through the foraminal soft tissues, allowing identification of the T7 pedicle. The T6/T7 trocar is removed, allowing evacuation of the rib head with a 10-inch pituitary through the T6/T7 working portal. The trocar is then replaced and bipolar cautery is inserted, permitting coagulation of the epidural and foraminal soft tissues and clear identification of the T7 pedicle. Intermittent suction irrigation through the T4/T5 portal facilitates exposure. Once the pedicle is fully visualized, a 45-degree Kerrison rongeur is used to resect the cephalad aspect of the

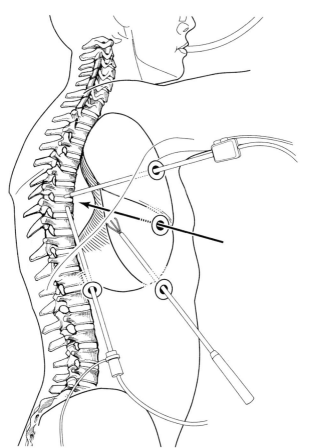

Figure 9–3. An illustration of thoracic instrument placement.

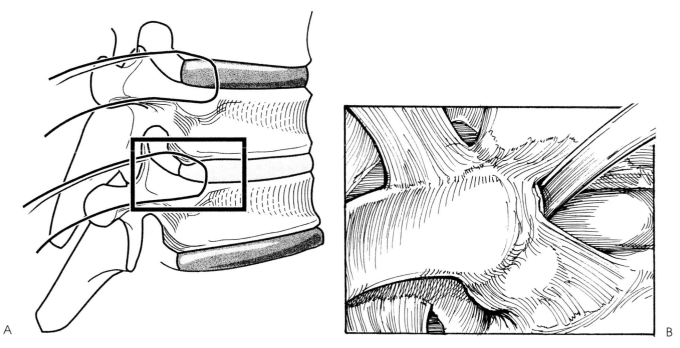

A

B

Figure 9–4. (A) An illustration of surgical field outlining area of anticipated decompression. (B) An illustration of subperiosteal rib exposure with ligamentous dissection with a cobb elevator.

pedicle (Fig. 9–5). This allows better visualization of the posterior aspect of the disc herniation. Intermittently, the 30-degree scope may need removal and cleansing with the defogging solution to allow consistent clear visualization.

The herniated calcified disc was found by tracing the pedicle back to the T7 vertebral body. A Penfield dissector and Bovie cauterization allows identification of the anterior aspect of the dura at this junction. The disc was incised with a no. 15 blade, angling the cutting edge of the blade away from the dura. A transverse cut is made in the sagittal plane, anteriorly freeing up the bulk of the disc. The disc must be incised sufficiently anteriorly to allow placement of pituitaries and curettes. The superior and inferior end plates are similarly incised with a no. 15 blade. Then 2-0 and 3-0 angled curettes are used to free up the bulk of the disc, angling the curettes away from the dura and pulling the disc material anteriorly (Fig. 9–6). A pituitary is used to remove the disc material in addition to the suction irrigation. Epidural bleeding is controlled with bipolar cautery, as well as Avitene plugs or Gelfoam impregnated in thrombin. Optimal visualization must be maintained at all times, allowing clear distinction between the dura and the disc material. Once sufficient soft disc material is removed, the most posterior aspect of the calcified disc herniation was approached with angled curettes. The calcified disc was adherent to the dura, requiring careful dissection. Commonly, however, the plane between the posterior annulus and the posterior longitudinal ligament is identified. The junction at the posterior longitudinal ligament was visualized. Angled curettes are then used to section the anterior longitudinal ligament, and epidural bleeding posterior to the ligament is controlled with bipolar cautery. A ball-ended probe or nerve hook is used to ensure that the anterior aspect of the dura remains free of all disc material. A ball-ended probe is placed into the discectomy defect, and AP and lateral X-rays obtained to ensure that the dissection has proceeded to the midline. The segmental vessels are spared.

In cases where the disc space is significantly collapsed, access with curettes and pituitaries is difficult, requiring resection of the posterior cephalad and caudal vertebral bodies with a burr. The dissection is then taken posteriorly until a thin eggshell of the posterior vertebral cortex remains, which is then removed with the angled

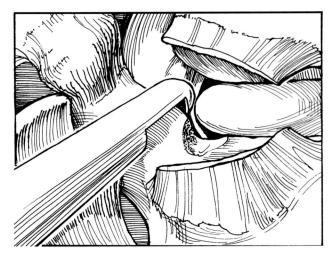

Figure 9–5. An illustration of Pedicle decompression with use of a Kerrison rongeur.

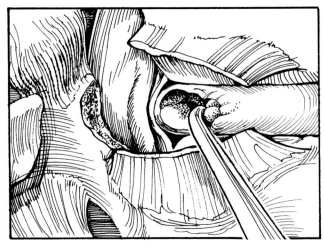

Figure 9–6. An illustration of partial disc removal with a curved currette.

Kerrisons or curettes prior to disc removal. A fusion at this junction may be necessary, which can be performed by morcelizing the rib head or harvesting the anterior iliac crest.

Gelfoam is placed over the anterior aspect of the dura and the graft is impacted with a bone tap. A Penfield probe is then placed posterior to the graft, ensuring ample space between the graft and the anterior aspect of the dura. A 24-French chest tube is inserted through one of the trocar sites prior to lung reexpansion and wound closure. Marcaine 0.75% is injected around the trocar sites to control postoperative pain.

Postoperative Management

The chest tube was removed on the second postoperative day when average drainage was less than 50 mL per shift. Postoperatively, the patient was fitted with a thoracolumbar spinal orthosis (TLSO) brace for postoperative comfort. An incentive spirometer was instituted immediately postoperatively and deep-breathing exercises were encouraged. A patient-controlled analgesia (PCA) pump was used by the patient for 48 hours, after which the patient was switched to oral medications. The patient was mobilized on the first postoperative day and discharged on day 4.

Discussion

Although a variety of techniques have been successful in removing thoracic disc herniations, these procedures oftentimes result in significant postoperative morbidity due to respiratory complications, incisional pain, and shoulder girdle dysfunction. The first report to address spinal disorders using video-assisted thoracoscopy was in 1991. Video-assisted thoracic spinal surgery (VAT) offers several advantages over conventional open procedures in the surgical treatment of thoracic disc herniations. Thoracoscopy allows greater visualization of the thoracic spine with the use of a 30-degree angled scope, beyond that seen with an open incision. The magnified visualization, despite small incisions, facilitates precise dissection, while minimizing surgical trauma. Standard open thoracotomy procedures involve either spreading of the ribs or rib resection to optimize visualization. This is avoided with thoracoscopic discectomy, resulting in less incisional pain and diminished postoperative chest tube drainage, reduced postoperative pain, and improved postoperative ventilation, which potentially decreases the need for intensive care and diminishes blood loss. Due to limited soft tissue trauma, postoperative hospitalization is shorter and oftentimes the need for postoperative rehabilitation is minimized. Consequently, the overall cost for medical care is lower. Proximal thoracotomy approaches can lead to shoulder girdle dysfunction, which is infrequently seen in thoracoscopic procedures. Less invasive dissection with VAT diminishes the potential for infection, in contrast to the long incisions used in the open procedure, requiring rib distraction and inherently more extreme soft tissue trauma.

Thoracoscopic discectomy is particularly indicated for treatment of disc herniations in the midthoracic spine, typically from T6 to T7. Because 75% of thoracic disc herniations occur between T8 and T12, VAT discectomy is an acceptable alternative in the treatment of these disorders.

Table 9–1
Surgical Approaches for Varying Pathologies

Levels	Disc Herniation	Approaches
Soft discs		
T1 to T4	Central, centrolateral	Transsternal
	Central, centrolateral	Medial clavisectomy
	Centrolateral, lateral	Costotransversectomy
T4 to T12	Central, centrolateral, lateral	Transthoracic
	Central, centrolateral, lateral	Thoracoscopy
	Centrolateral, lateral	Lateral
	Central, centrolateral, lateral	Costotransversectomy
	Lateral	Transpedicular
Calcified discs		
T1 to T4	Central, centrolateral	Transsternal
	Central, centrolateral	Medial clavisectomy
	Lateral	Costotransversectomy
T4 to T12	Central, centrolateral, lateral	Transthoracic
	Lateral	Lateral
	Lateral, centrolateral	Costotransversectomy

From Orthopaedic Knowledge Update. Spine. Mirkovic S, Cybulski G. Thoracic Disc Herniations. American Academy of Orthopaedic Surgeons. Garfin SR, Vaccaro AR, eds, North American Spine Society, pp. 91–96.

Thoracic disc herniations are a difficult diagnostic entity due to the variation in their clinical presentation. Symptoms are commonly exacerbated by sneezing, coughing, and increased activities, and improved with rest. Physicians must be aware of atypical radiating pain, occasionally in the groin and testicles, seen with T11/T12 disc herniations, simulating renal and degenerative hip disease. Midthoracic disc herniations may present with abdominal and chest pain. T1 or T2 disc herniation can elicit neck and upper extremity pain, which mistakenly can be associated with degenerative cervical disease.

Both spinal and nonspinal pain origin should be considered in the differential diagnosis. Neurologic disorders with similar symptomatology include multiple sclerosis, spinal cord tumors, amyotrophic lateral sclerosis, transverse myelitis, and arteriovenous malformations. Nonspinal disorders, which in the past have been mistaken for thoracic disc herniations, include cholecystitis, aneurysms, and retroperitoneal neoplasms.

For patients who present with myelopathy and those with relenting pain of greater than 6 months' duration who have failed a course of nonsurgical treatment, surgery should be considered. The most appropriate surgical approach is based on location (central, centrolateral, or lateral) relative to the spinal cord, the level of herniation, disc consistency, as well as the surgeon's familiarity with different approaches. Surgical approaches can either be posterior or anterior (Table 9–1).

Alternative Methods of Management

Surgical approaches to thoracic disc herniations involve both posterior and anterior approaches. The posterior treatment options include the lateral (extracavitary) approach, costotransversectomy, transpedicular approach, and laminectomy. An anterior transthoracic approach is currently the preferred approach for the majority of thoracic disc herniations. In addition, access to the upper thoracic spine (T2 to T4) can be gained through a transsternal or a medial claviclectomy approach.

The lateral extracavitary approach (Fig. 9–7) can be applicable to any level of the thoracic spine and is particularly suited for centrolateral and lateral soft disc herniations, as well as lateral calcified disc herniations.

Posterior access to the central and centrolateral canal can also be accomplished via costotransversectomy (Fig. 9–7). This is a posterolateral-extrapleural approach with resection of the medial portion of the rib, articulating with the transverse process.

The transpedicular approach (Fig. 9–8) involves resection of the facet joint and at least the medial portion of the pedicle, caudal to the disc. A trough can be created with a high-speed burr, facilitating removal of hard discs.

Laminectomy (Fig. 9–8) has fallen into disfavor due to the poor results and high rates of paraplegia. This approach should be avoided.

The transthoracic transpleural (Fig. 9–9) approach allows excellent visualization of the central and centrolateral canal from T3/T4 to the thoracolumbar junction. The approach can be performed on either side, depending on the level of pathology. The VAT thoracoscopic approach is essentially a magnification of the transthoracic approach.

Type of Management	Advantages	Disadvantages
Lateral extracavitary	Any level Centrolateral and lateral soft discs Lateral calcified discs	Paraspinal muscle disruption Dural tear repair Chest wall numbness
Costotransversectomy	Medically compromised patients in whom thoracotomy is contraindicated Centrolateral and lateral herniation Fusion	Central calcified discs Degenerative osteophytes Paraspinal dissection
Transpedicular	Soft lateral disc herniations Medically compromised patients	Limited visualization Calcified disc/osteophyte complex Possible instability
Laminectomy	None	Paraplegia Paraparesis
Transthoracic	Enhanced visualization Calcified discs Disc/osteophyte complex	Thoracotomy

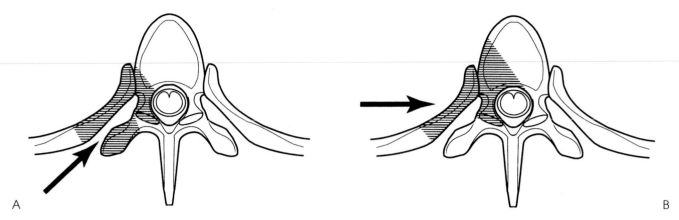

Figure 9–7. An illustration of various posterolateral decompressive procedures. The area of bony resection (cross hatch) and direction of approach (arrows) to the herniated disc is illustrated with the costotransversection approach (A) and lateral extracavitary approach (B).

Complications

Blind insertion of the first trocar in the presence of inadequate lung collapse can lead to injury of the lung parenchyma and bleeding. Injury to the lung parenchyma can also occur when pleural adhesions do not allow adequate lung collapse. Injuries to the hemidiaphragm during trocar insertion have also been reported. Placement of trocars in the intercostal space can injure the intercostal neurovascular bundle. This can be avoided by using blunt dissection during the initial incision, placement of soft rubber trocars, and gentle handling of instruments, avoiding levering against intercostal structures. Postthoracoscopy and intercostal neuralgia has been reported in up to 21% of cases. Direct injury to the lung by the instrument or scope can be avoided by ensuring that the lung has been collapsed fully and with the use of retractors. Wedging of the lung parenchyma between the fan blades of the retractor can be avoided by direct visualization during fan retraction opening and closing. Neurologic injury, including paraplegia, remains the most catastrophic complication. The

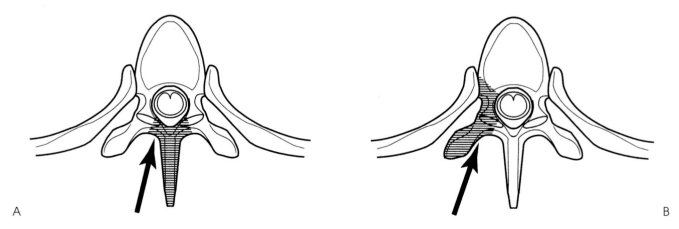

Figure 9–8. Extent of bony resection (cross-hatch) and angle of approach (arrows) to disc space with laminectomy (A) and facetectomy/transpedicular (B) procedures.

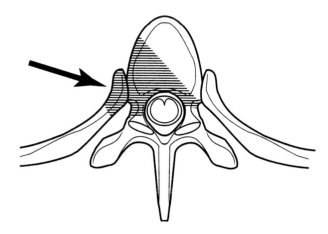

Figure 9–9. Extent of bony resection (cross-hatch) and angle of approach (arrow) to disc space with transthoracic approach.

proximity of the spinal cord requires careful instrument handling and familiarity with three-dimensional thoracoscopy and depth perception. A history of previous thoracotomy and/or tube thoracostomy, depending on the extent of pleural adhesions, is a relative contraindication to this procedure.

Suggested Readings

Ben-Ishy A, Regan JR, McAffee P. Early results of excision of herniated disc utilizing video-assisted thoracoscopy. Presented at the 29th annual meeting of the Scoliosis Research Society, Portland, Oregon, September 21, 1994.

Dickman CA, Karahalios DJ. Thoracoscopic spinal surgery. Clin Neurol Surg 1996; 43:392–422.

McAffee P, Regan JR, Zedblick T, et al. Complications in endoscopic anterior thoracolumbar spinal reconstructive surgery, prospective multi-center study comprising the first 100 consecutive cases. Spine 1995; 20:1624–1633.

Case 10

Axial Low Back Pain: Nonoperative Approach

Mitchell K. Freedman

History and Physical Examination

A 31-year-old man presents with generalized lower back pain that developed 1 year ago when picking up a 50-lb piece of equipment. He was treated with nonsteroidal antiinflammatories and physical therapy without much success. He had one epidural steroid injection under fluoroscopy, which gave him transient relief. He currently describes his back pain as achy. It radiates into the left buttock. He denies paresthesias, weakness, or bowel and bladder dysfunction. Pain is worse with sitting and bending and better in bed. He has become despondent. He is not sleeping well and has lost 10 pounds. He is a construction worker who has not worked since his

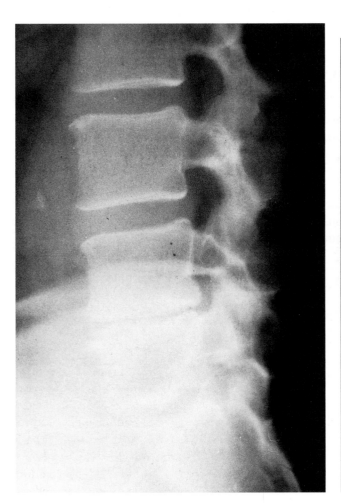

Figure 10–1. A lateral plain radiograph revealing marked narrowing of the lysis disc space.

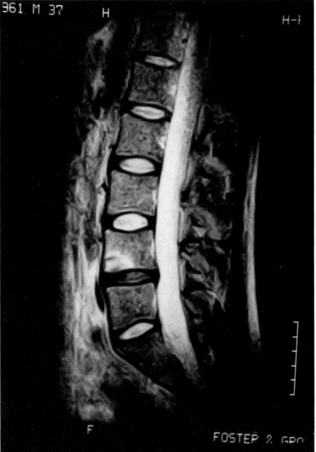

Figure 10–2. Sagittal magnetic resonance imaging (MRI) revealing decreased signal intensity at the L4/L5 disc space with evidence of disc bulging at this level.

injury. He has become depressed over his ongoing pain and inability to work. Marital strife has developed related to his irritability and ongoing pain.

Physical examination reveals a despondent male with a flat affect. He became teary-eyed throughout the evaluation. He was able to sit throughout the 30-minute evaluation. Lumbar flexion is limited to 60 degrees with poor reversal of the lumbar lordosis. Lumbar extension is present to 30 degrees. There is pain at the end-range of motion with both movements. There is tenderness in the left sacroiliac joint as well as over the lumbar paraspinal musculature on the left. There is palpable spasm into the thoracic paraspinal musculature. Straight leg raise causes pain into the back and buttock at 90 degrees. The hamstrings are tight bilaterally. Hip range of motion is full and there is pain in the low back at the end-range of motion. Peripheral pulses are intact. Abdominal examination is benign. Strength, sensation, and reflexes are intact. Ambulation reveals a flexed posture; he is antalgic on the left.

Radiologic Findings

X-rays of the lumbar spine reveal narrowing of the disc space at L4/L5 (Fig. 10–1). Magnetic resonance imaging (MRI) of the lumbar spine reveals a mild disc bulge at L4/L5 (Fig. 10–2). Mild disc desiccation is present at L4/L5. A bone scan is negative. Intraarticular blocks were performed to the facet joints under fluoroscopic guidance; 0.2 cc of nonionic contrast medium was used to confirm proper placement of the needle into the facet joints at L3/L4, L4/L5, and L5/S1 bilaterally. The joints were then injected with 0.5 cc of 2% lidocaine. The patient had 75% pain relief for 1 hour. One week later, he returned to the clinic and had repeat facet joint injections under fluoroscopy with 0.5 cc of 2% bupivacaine. The patient had nearly full resolution of his discomfort for 4 hours.

Diagnosis

This patient has a chronic pain syndrome. He has evidence of depression and functional deficits. His pain has been present for more than 6 months. Diagnostic blocks would indicate that there is evidence of facet joint dysfunction. A component of his pain may also be related to underlying lumbar disc pathology. Discography was not performed to ascertain this diagnosis, as the patient was not deemed to be an optimal surgical candidate for lumbar fusion.

Management

At the outset of the pain management program, the patient received therapeutic facet joint injections with 0.5 cc of 1% lidocaine and 0.5 cc of Celestone soluspan at L3/L4, L4/L5, and L5/S1 bilaterally. This was performed under fluoroscopic guidance. Daypro was discontinued; it was reinstituted when his pain flared. He was placed on nortriptyline 25 mg nightly, and this was gradually increased to 75 mg at night. He was able to utilize capsaicin 0.025% as needed to the lower back.

The patient entered a 6-week interdisciplinary pain management program. He was placed on a quota system of exercise. Initial levels of exercise were determined by having him perform a series of exercises to tolerance. He then was placed on an exercise program that was 80% of his initial exercise tolerance. Quotas were progressed every 3 to 5 days. Initial exercises included aerobic conditioning on the bicycle and an ambulation program. Abdominal strengthening and lumbar extension exercises short of pain were initiated. Stretching was performed to the tensor fasciae latae, hamstrings, and hip rotators. He reviewed good body mechanics with functional activities. Homemaking, activities of daily living (ADLs), and recreational, vocational, and sexual activities were addressed.

The patient received individual counseling to address his depression. His spouse came in for counseling for several sessions to address marital issues. Group counseling was performed once weekly; he met with other patients with long-term pain syndromes to discuss methods of pain management and developing coping skills for pain. The patient received a course of biofeedback and relaxation techniques to develop pain management strategies. During the second week of the program, the patient was placed on work tolerance. He progressively increased his activity throughout the 6 weeks in the program.

At the end of the program, the patient had significantly less lower back pain. The pain continued to radiate into the buttock on occasion. He felt that he was able to manage his discomfort with the strategies that he had learned. His depression was significantly diminished. He was sleeping well. He returned to work at a modified job as a machinist. He was not allowed to work with more than 30 pounds.

Discussion

A thorough history and physical is essential in all patients with lower back pain. Emergencies including cauda equina syndrome and spinal cord injury must be ruled out rapidly. Visceral pathology and malignancy, as well as metastatic bone disease must be considered.

The history reviews how the pain started as well as the location and severity of the pain. Positions that worsen or lessen the discomfort are identified. Pain that radiates below the knee is often indicative of a radiculopathy. However, radicular symptoms may also present with pain into the buttock or posterior thigh. Paresthesias may be present in the sensory distribution of the damaged nerve root. The patient must be questioned about weakness. With diffuse weakness, one must consider the possibility of a central nervous system lesion or cauda equina syndrome versus weakness associated with pain from movement.

The sleep/wake pattern may be disrupted in patients who are in pain. This is important to treat because patients who are sleep deprived may develop myofascial discomfort. A general medical history must be obtained to rule out visceral pathology and infection.

Social and functional history should guide goals and therapeutic strategies. Because patients may not be able to return to jobs that are physically demanding, it is important to get a history of previous vocation and education.

Physical examination begins when the patient enters the physician's office suite. Casual activities including sitting, ambulation, and undressing should be evaluated; these movements are compared to the rest of the formal examination. Sitting and standing posture should be observed. Spinal curvature should be evaluated. Lumbar mobility including flexion, extension, rotation, and lateral bending should be observed. The paraspinal musculature, vertebral spinous processes, sacroiliac joint, and greater trochanter must be palpated. Motion should be evaluated in the hip joints as well as the knees and ankles. Hamstring, tensor fasciae latae, rectus femoris, and gastroc-soleus flexibility should be evaluated. Straight leg raise should be performed actively and passively. Straight leg raise maneuver is generally compatible with radicular symptomatology when pain radiates below the knee at 30 degrees of hip flexion. Patients with bowel and bladder complaints should have an evaluation of their perirectal sensation, rectal contraction, and anocutaneous and bulbocavernosus reflexes. The abdominal aorta and the peripheral pulses should also be evaluated.

Discography is arguably considered to be the best test to evaluate whether or not a given lumbar disc is painful. It is indicated when a patient has unremitting spinal pain, with or without extremity pain, of greater than 4 months of duration and when pain has been unresponsive to all appropriate methods of conservative therapy.

The current method to diagnose a pain generator in the facet or sacroiliac joint is based on the resolution of pain following anesthetic injections. Relief with anesthetic injections in the facet joint or to the medial branch of the dorsal roots that innervate the facet joint are used to diagnose facet dysfunction. Anesthetic injection directly into the sacroiliac joint is utilized to diagnose sacroiliac joint pathology. Double- or triple-block paradigms minimize false-positive findings. A short-acting agent such as lidocaine should provide relief of at least 50% of the patient's discomfort. If the patient responds to the first injection, then injection with a long-acting agent such as bupivacaine is carried out to the target site. The patient should have at least 50% relief of pain for a duration appropriate to the physiologic effect of the longer-acting anesthetic agent. On occasion, a third block is performed with saline, which should not provide any relief.

Exercise is the core of the treatment program in patients with axial back pain. Following acute injury, patients should not be at bed rest for more than 2 to 7 days. Exercise should be targeted to stretching tight musculoskeletal structures and strengthening weak musculature.

Medication options include nonsteroidal antiinflammatories, nonnarcotic analgesics, counterirritant creams, opioid analgesics, muscle relaxants, and antidepressants. The antiinflammatories provide analgesia and help to decrease inflammation. Patients must be monitored carefully for gastrointestinal side effects. Muscle relaxers are centrally acting agents that have uncertain rationale and efficacy in the treatment of pain syndromes. They may help patients to sleep during the acute phases of their injury. Benzodiazepines are used as a sedative and muscle relaxant. They are potentially addictive medications. There is some evidence that benzodiazepines increase sensitivity to pain. In general, the use of these agents should be avoided. The one benzodiazepine that has been used with some success in pain management is clonazepam. Opioid analgesics are used for the treatment of acute pain. On occasion, a patient with chronic unremitting pain may utilize long-acting narcotics to allow some degree of pain relief and promote an increase in function. Antidepressant medications can be utilized to treat depression in patients who become depressed from their pain syndrome. The tricyclic antidepressants are also excellent sedative agents, and can provide pain relief in patients with neuropathic pain. Side effects may be considerable and include anticholinergic sequelae with urinary retention, constipation, cardiac arrhythmias, and weight gain.

Spinal injections provide analgesia that allows the patient to participate in an exercise program. Lumbar epidural steroid injections via an interlaminar or a transforaminal route are most useful for radiculopathy but often provide relief for axial pain of discogenic origin as well. Intraarticular steroid injections have been used with varying degrees of success in the facet and sacroiliac joints. Trigger-point injections may be useful in patients with focal muscular tenderness.

Psychological management is important in patients who become depressed or have adverse psychological responses to their injury. Inappropriate illness behaviors and functional deficits beyond what is expected for a given pain syndrome may develop.

Interdisciplinary pain management programs are indicated in patients with chronic low back pain who have significant functional deficits. These programs focus on pain management and pain reduction.

Alternative Methods of Management

Treatment with pulsed electromagnetic fields has become popular. There have been two double-blind randomized treatment trials in patients with osteoarthritis. The conclusion of these studies was that magnets were useful for pain control.

Manipulation is a mobilization technique that attempts to remove restrictions in range of motion. Soft tissue techniques stretch out tight musculature. Long-lever techniques involve gross rotational movements to the lumbar spine. Efficacy is uncertain.

Prolotherapy is intraligamentous and intratendinous injection of solutions that induce proliferation of new cells. The new cells strengthen lax soft tissue structures and promote stability, which decreases pain. Proliferating solutions may include dextrose, which is injected into the soft tissue every 6 to 12 weeks. The alternative method is to inject preparations containing phenol or sodium morrhuate into the soft tissue structures weekly. Injection targets are lax musculotendinous and ligamentous areas. Efficacy is unclear.

Acupuncture was recently endorsed by the National Institutes of Health as a promising modality in the treatment of low back pain (as well as other painful syndromes). Acupuncture involves the insertion of small gauge needles into strategic points of the body. It is based on a theory that there are disruptions in patterns of energy flow (*Qi*) through the body that are essential for health. Proposed mechanisms include stimulation of small myelinated afferent fibers of peripheral nerves to transmit an analgesic effect. Other possibilities include the release of endogenous opioids.

Type of Management	Advantages	Disadvantages	Comments
Magnets	Possible pain relief No known side effects		Efficacy uncertain
Manipulation	Possible pain relief Improves range of motion	Rare but potential complications: fractures, spinal cord injury Potential dependency on medical practitioner	Useful for subacute pain Should be used in conjunction with an exercise program Contraindicated with fracture, metastasis to bone, spinal stenosis
Prolotherapy	Possible pain relief	Potential complications: pneumothorax, neurologic impairment, pigmentation from anesthetic gun	Efficacy uncertain
Acupuncture	Possible pain relief	Potential (rare) complications: pneumothorax, hepatitis, local infection	Endorsed by the National Institutes of Health as a promising modality for the treatment of low back pain

Suggested Readings

Deyo RA, Diehl AK, Rosenthal M. How many days of bed rest for acute low back pain? N Engl J Med 1986; 315:1064–1070.

Lee MHM, Liao SJ. Acupuncture for pain management. In: Lennard TA, ed. Physiatric Procedures in Clinical Practice, pp. 49–56. Philadelphia: Hanley and Belfus, 1995.

MacDonald RS, Bell CM, Janine Bell CM. An open controlled assessment of osteopathic manipulation in nonspecific low back pain. Spine 1990; 15:364–370.

Saal JA, Saal JS. Initial stage management of lumbar spine problems. Phys Med Rehabil Clin North Am 1991; 2:187–204.

Trock DH, Bollet AJ, Dyer RH, et al. A double-blind trial of the clinical effects of pulsed electromagnetic fields in osteoarthritis. J Rheumatol 1993; 20:456–460.

Trock DH, Bollet AJ, Markoll R. The effect of pulsed electromagnetic fields in the treatment of osteoarthritis of the knee and cervical spine. Report of randomized double blind placebo controlled trials. J Rheumatol 1994; 21:1903–1911.

Vallbona C, Hazlewood CF, Jurida G. Response of pain to static magnetic fields in postpolio patients: a double blind pilot study. Arch Phys Med Rehabil 1997; 78:1200–1203.

Case 11

Lumbar Degenerative Disc Disease—Axial Back Pain: Anterior Approach

Stephen D. Kuslich

History and Physical Examination

A 40-year-old woman presented with a 10-year history of low back pain. She had undergone three previous decompression operations at L4/L5. She complained mainly of low back pain, but also admitted to an intermittent history of leg pains and numbness. Twelve years ago she developed a large herniated disc at L4/L5 with compression of the left L5 nerve root dysfunction. A new imaging study, myelogram,

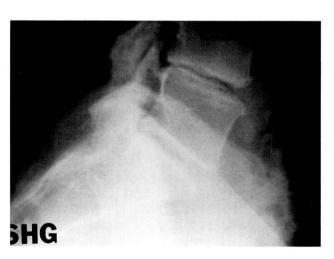

Figure 11–1. Lateral preoperative X-ray showing narrowing of L4/L5 disc space, marginal osteophytes and mild retrolisthesis of the L4 vertebral body. None of these changes is diagnostic in and of itself, but when considered along with the magnetic resonance imaging (MRI) and history, we can conclude that the L4/L5 disc is probably the source of chronic mechanical back pain.

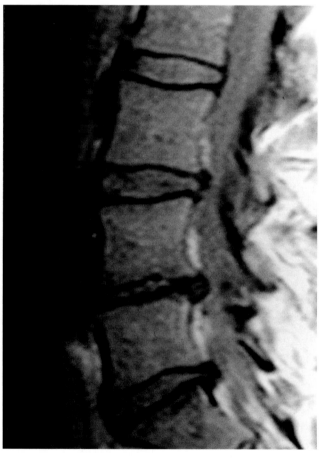

Figure 11–2. MRI reveals low discal signal intensity, annular delaminations, and an insignificant bulge of the disc at L4/L5. Other levels are normal. Discography is not needed in such cases because the painful level is obvious from the history and MRI findings.

computed tomography (CT) confirmed the diagnosis of large recurrent herniated nucleus pulposus (HNP).

Exploration at the time of a second decompression revealed that the recurrent disc had actually passed into and through the adherent nerve root, producing severe damage to the nerve. A durotomy of the nerve root sleeve, followed by removal of the recurrent fragment, resulted in moderate improvement in the sciatic pain, but the patient continued to experience mechanical low back pain and dysesthesias in the distribution of the left L5. About 2 years later, she consented to a third exploration and decompression, but no relief resulted from that operation. She refused additional surgical treatment during the ensuing 9-year period, and required codeine-level oral analgesics on a regular basis. Persistent pain and child care responsibilities precluded gainful employment for 3 years, but a divorce, with loss of spousal support, necessitated a return to work. Her sciatic pain gradually abated but the mechanical low back pain increased in frequency and severity. The remainder of her past history was not significant. She had no diseases or conditions that would contraindicate further surgical treatment. She was intelligent, self-supporting, nonlitigious, and emotionally stable.

The patient had tried many nonsurgical treatments over the years, including chiropractic manipulations, physical therapy, exercise programs, antiinflammatory medications, steroid injections, and braces, without any significant or long-lasting relief.

The physical examination revealed a well-healed posterior lumbar surgical incision, moderate restriction of lumbar range of motion, some restriction in left-sided straight leg raising, and a decrease in L5 dermatomal sensation. Abdominal palpation and gynecologic evaluations were negative.

Radiologic Findings

Routine anteroposterior (AP) and lateral X-rays of the lumbar spine revealed only narrowing of the L4/L5 disc space with slight marginal osteophytes (Fig.11–1). Lumbar magnetic resonance imaging (MRI) demonstrated advanced degenerative disc disease at L4/L5 with low signal intensity in the disc (Fig.11–2). There was a posterior bulge at the left side of the L4/L5 disc, and some loss of normal epidural fat around the L5 nerve behind the disc, but no significant nerve compression. Other levels were unremarkable.

Diagnosis

Chronic mechanical low back pain secondary to advanced degenerative disc disease at L4/L5. Old, quiescent, L5 nerve neuropathy.

Surgical Management

After a thorough discussion of the risks, benefits, and alternative treatments, the patient consented to an anterior interbody fusion using BAK (Bagby and Kuslich) hollow titanium cylinders filled with autogenous bone graft. We used a left-sided open, anterior, retroperitoneal exposure, and obtained bone graft from the left anterior·superior iliac crest. Figure 11–3A demonstrates the skin and subcutaneous

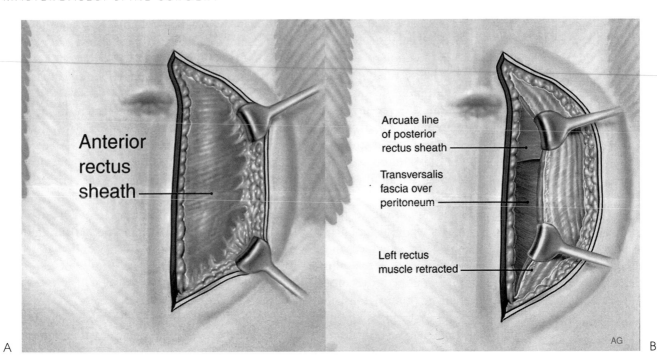

Figure 11–3. (A) The anterior retroperitoneal exposure begins with either a longitudinal or transverse incision through the skin and sub-cutaneous tissue. L4/L5 is normally located about 4 cm below the umbilicus. The anterior rectus sheath is split longitudinally just lateral to the midline. The rectus muscle is reflected laterally, exposing the arcuate line with the posterior rectus sheath above and the transversalis fascia and peritoneum below. (B) Lateral retraction of the rectus preserves its blood and nervous supply and allows direct anterior access to the spine.

incision down to the level of the anterior rectus sheath. We retracted the left rectus abdominus muscle to the left (Fig. 11–3B) and developed the retroperitoneal plane by bluntly mobilizing the peritoneal cavity toward the right side of midline (Fig. 11–4), exposing the L4/L5 space above the bifurcation of the great vessels (Fig. 11–5 and Fig. 11–6). We used stationary retractors to retract the peritoneal contents, and hand-held Wiley retractors to mobilize and protect the ureter and the great vessels (Fig. 11–7). We distracted the disc space using a 12-mm BAK re-traction plug, after which we drilled, debrided, and tapped the opposite-side hole, and then placed a 15-mm by 20-mm BAK implant deeply into the hole. After re-moving the distraction plug, we debrided the disc and prepared the second cylin-drical hole, into which we inserted the second implant (Fig. 11–8). We filled each implant with about 7 cc of morselized cancelleus autogenous bone graft. We closed the anterior rectus sheath and subcutaneous and cutaneous tissues using resorbable sutures. We placed no drains or nasogastric tubes, but did insert a Foley catheter before the operation.

Postoperative Management

The patient received routine antibiotic prophylaxis preoperatively and postopera-tively for 48 hours. Nurses removed the Foley catheter on the first postoperative day. We did not order a postoperative brace, but did provide he patient with an ab-dominal corset to support the abdominal incision. Postoperatively, she used a pa-tient-controlled analgesic device delivering morphine in small doses intravenously

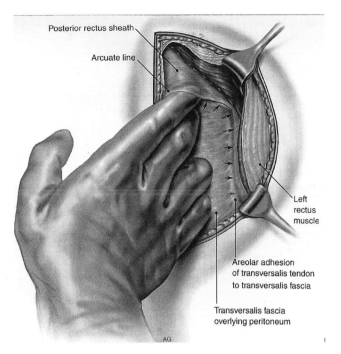

Posterior rectus sheath

Arcuate line

Left rectus muscle

Areolar adhesion of transversalis tendon to transversalis fascia

Transversalis fascia overlying peritoneum

AG

Figure 11–4. The surgeon uses blunt dissection to separate the peritoneum from the lateral abdominal wall and the undersurface of the posterior rectus sheath along the line of arrows.

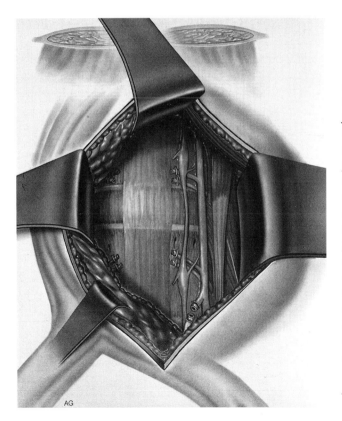

AG

Figure 11–5. As the peritoneal membrane is stripped from the psoas medially, the deep structures of the retroperitoneal space are exposed. Any nerves lying on the surface of the psoas must be carefully protected. The left sympathetic chain is identified and left in its place. The segmental vessels above and below the disc space must be cut and tied or clipped. The ascending lumbar vein, seen at the bottom right of the exposure, might need to be tied and sectioned if its tightness restricts the vena cava or left iliac vein from being mobilized to the right side of the spine.

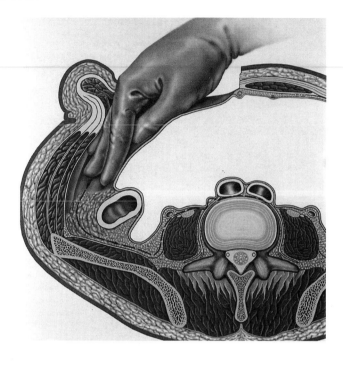

Figure 11–6. The path of the blunt dissection through the left side of the retroperitoneal space. The left ureter and all intraperitoneal contents are mobilized to the right side of the spine.

for 2 days. Thereafter, acetaminophen with codeine, orally, was sufficient. She began eating solid food on the second day.

The patient stood and sat on the first postoperative day, walked on the second day, and was ready for discharge on the third day. After a clinic visit at 2 weeks, and gradual recuperation at home, she returned to her office-based employment at 6 weeks.

Her low back pain improved dramatically, and continued to be relieved at 2-year follow-up, although her L5 parasthesias persisted, but in diminished form. X-rays at 2 years postoperation showed solid fixation with no radiolucencies and no motion of flexion-extension bending (Fig. 11–9 and 11–10). She currently takes no analgesic

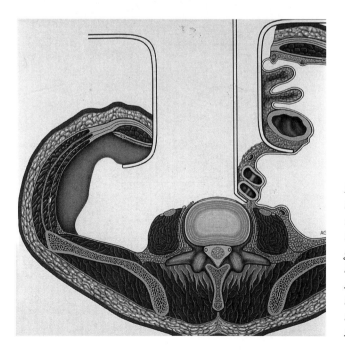

Figure 11–7. Stationary retractors may be used on the muscles and visceral layers, but the author strongly suggests that the great vessels be held in place by deep, blunt smooth, hand-held retractors, such as Wiley retractors, to prevent damage to these structures.

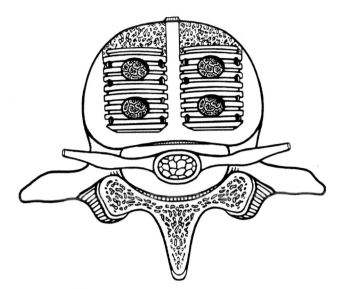

Figure 11–8. After placement of the appropriately sized distraction plug on the left side, the right side is drilled and tapped, and an implant is screwed into a position deep in the disc, guided by preoperative templates and intraoperative fluoroscopy. The resulting cavity anterior to the implants will be filled with additional bone graft. Not noted here is the fact that disc tissue should be curetted from the middle of the disc before the second implant is installed.

medication. She works full time, cares for her children without assistance, and engages in recreational sports without limitation.

Discussion

The diagnosis and treatment of chronic low back pain continues to be a difficult medical challenge. Patients who have had previous unsuccessful laminectomies are particularly frustrating to manage. Some experts believe that surgical treatment of such cases is futile. Others recommend surgical treatment only when there are

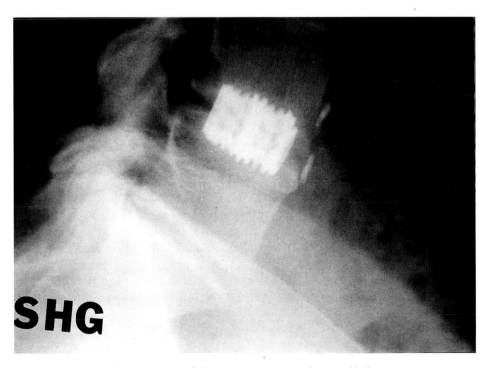

Figure 11–9. Lateral X-ray 2 years following surgery. Note absence of halos, migration, or rotation of the implants. Flexion-extension views showed no motion—all signs of solid fixation and probably bony union. By this time, the patient is pain free and fully active without restrictions.

PEARLS

Interbody cage stabilization is now a proven method of spinal arthrodesis. Almost all cases eventually fuse. However, faster fusion and better results are obtained if certain details are known and practiced:

- Choose the largest possible diameter of cage.
- Drill long and place the cage deep into the cavity.
- Place additional bone graft in front of and beside the cages.
- Debride the space of loose material prior to cage placement.
- Utilize a vascular surgeon to assist in the anterior exposure.
- Take specialized training before attempting these procedures.
- Don't operate on patients with significant psychosocial pathology.

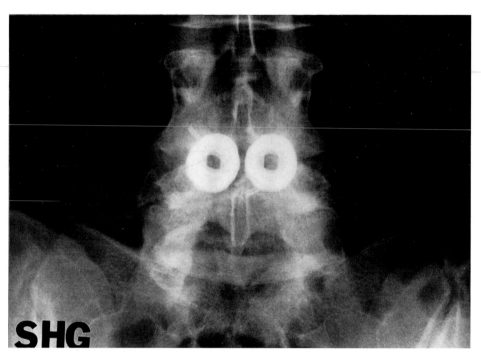

Figure 11–10. Anteroposterior (AP) X-ray showing perfect position of the implants. We have never observed a late nonunion or change in implant position when the X-ray looks this good, this late into follow-up.

obvious signs of new nerve root compression or gross instability of the motion segment. Most authorities recommend conservative rather than operative treatment for back pain, regardless of cause.

I chose interbody fusion in this case because I felt very confident that the pain was mechanical and discogenic. The patient was emotionally intact, otherwise healthy, middle-aged, working, and nonlitigious, with single-level, obvious degenerative disc disease. She represents one subgroup of patients that can benefit from fusion. The other group consists of spondylolisthesis patients with mechanical low back pain.

In spite of the advances of technology during the past two decades, including CT, MRI, pain drawings, discography, microsurgery, and an array of spinal surgical tools and implants, back pain patients remain our most difficult and challenging cases. A certain percentage of these patients cannot be diagnosed with certainty (my estimate is about 10 to 15%). I recommend conservative measures such as steroid injections into the facet and sacroiliac (SI) joints in such cases. Others can be diagnosed, but they exhibit more than two levels of disease, or they have other serious organic, psychiatric, or sociologic disorders that adversely affect outcome. The wise and successful surgeon learns to offer fusion only to those rare patients who exhibit certain features that correlate with good results.

1. A high ratio of organic to functional signs and symptoms
2. No personal injury, product liability, or malpractice litigation pending
3. Workers' compensation insurance issues are settled
4. MRI scan showing one- or two-level moderate to severe degenerative disc disease, other levels normal
5. Otherwise healthy patient with strong motivation to get well

PITFALLS

Retrograde ejaculation is a risk when the anterior approach is used. Knowledge of the following technical considerations can reduce the risk to a minimum:

- The nerves involved are the fine, filmy strands of the parasympathetic nerves contained in the periaortic fat and prevertebral tissues.
- Use blunt dissection from the midline laterally, splitting the tissue longitudinally, not transversely.
- Do not use high power cautery on the prevertebral tissues.
- Do not use heavy packing in the presacral area.
- Warn young and middle-aged male patients of the possible complication.
- Most cases self-resolve, but resolution may take a year or more.

Delayed union can occur when less than perfect technique is utilized.

- Do not remove cages unless they are migrating into dangerous areas (very rare).
- Most cases will eventually fuse after 12 to 24 months.
- If nonunion is proven by flexion-extension films and thin-cut CT scanning, augment the cage fusion with posterolateral graft, translaminar facet screws, or pedicle fixation systems. Cage removal is almost never necessary.

Do not use electrocautery on the skin. It is the most common cause of superficial infection.

At this time, anterior interbody fusion with hollow titanium cylinders containing autogenous bone graft appears to be the best choice of treatment for most cases of one- and two-level lumbar degenerative disc disease. Whether the cages are installed using open, mini-open, or laparoscopic technique does not seem to matter in terms of safety or efficacy. Cage-type fusions appear to be superior to other surgical methods when one compares surgical time, operative bleeding, reoperation rates, return to work rates, infection rates, overall complications, and degree and duration of pain relief. Since 1996, the year of Food and Drug Administration (FDA) approval of the BAK and Ray devices, surgeons have performed more than 40,000 procedures. There is a learning curve involved, but experience has shown that skilled surgeons can become facile with the cage fusion technique in 10 to 20 cases. The main obstacle is case selection. That skill is more difficult for some surgeons to master.

Alternative Methods of Management

Posterior interbody fusion using bone dowels, autogenous rectangular grafts (Cloward type procedures), or posterior lumbar interbody fusion (PLIF) with cages can also be effective. However, PLIF procedures require significant removal of posterior stabilizers, making them less stable than anterior lumbar interbody fusion (ALIF) procedures. Allografts do not incorporate as swiftly as autografts. Iliac autografts are not as stable as cages filled with bone. PLIF always involves an invasion of the epidural space with the possible production of dural tears, nerve root trauma, epidural scarring, and arachnoiditis. Posterior procedures, however, have one advantage over ALIF: they allow direct decompression of compressed nerve roots at the time of fusion operation.

ALIF using allograft bone dowels is popular and may be as effective as cage fusion. Allografts, however, take longer to incorporate and there will always be a small risk of disease transmission.

Posterolateral fusion with and without pedicle or other fixation methods is still the standard operation for some surgeons, but surgical time, bleeding, reoperation rates, and overall complications are higher with the cage fusion procedures. The latest research indicates that the pain of degenerative disc disease is derived mainly from the anulus of the disc. If only the posterior portion of the motion segment is fused, the disc continues to be loaded during the activities of daily living. Therefore, pain can continue in spite of a solid posterior or posterolateral fusion.

Circumferential fusion with bone graft in the disc space and pedicle fixation posteriorly is very effective in achieving a fusion. However, the procedure is lengthy and bloody, and the reoperation rates for metal removal and other reasons are high. The overall complication rates appear excessive when compared to those of fusion cage procedures.

Finally, we must always remember that chronic low back pain is not a fatal disease, and, in the absence of societal programs that reward illness behavior, it is not ordinarily a debilitating condition. Therefore, the physician must always consider nontreatment or simple conservative management as an option. Do not fuse in the following situations:

Type of Management	Advantages	Disadvantages	Comments
ALIF with cages	Fast surgery, low blood loss, no epidural complications, highly effective	Less traditional, risk of great vessel injury, risk of retrograde ejaculation	Author's preferred method, simple once learning curve is mastered
PLIF with bone dowels, rectangular grafts (Cloward) or PLIF with cages	Allows concomitant decompression	Dural and nerve damage, bleeding, less stable	Most experienced cage surgeons eventually abandon this for anterior approach
ALIF with allograft dowels	Fast surgery, low blood loss, no graft site morbidity, no epidural complications	Longer time to graft incorporation, risk of disease transmission	Not proven in large multicenter trials, older studies had 20 to 30% nonunion rates
Posterolateral fusion with and without pedicle fixation	Traditional approach	Does not completely immobilize disc, damage to musculature	Higher morbidity, less complete pain relief than interbody methods
Circumferential fusion with anterior graft and fixation posteriorly	High fusion rate	Long, bloody procedure, high reoperation rates, high complication rates	Becoming less popular since advent of cage fusion technology. Morbidity is greatest negative feature
Conservative management	Safest form of treatment	Not very effective for chronic back pain	Always try first, may be the only feasible alternative in certain patients

ALIF, anterior lumbar interbody fusion; PLIF, posterior lumbar interbody fusion.

- Contraindications are present
- The disease is only mild or moderate
- The disease extends over more than two segments
- The patient exhibits behavioral patterns that are pathologic
- The pain, however severe, is of short duration

Acute low back pain self-resolves in about 85% of cases, with or without treatment!

Suggested Readings

Kuslich SD. Lumbar interbody cage fusion for back pain: an update on the BAK (Bagby and Kuslich) system. In: Erroco T, ed. Spine: State of the Art Reviews, Spinal Instrumentation. Philadelphia: Hanley and Belfus, 1999.

Kuslich SD, Ulstrom CL, Griffith SL, Ahern JW, Dowdle JD. The Bagby and Kuslich method of lumbar interbody fusion. Spine 1998; 23:1267–1278.

Kuslich SD, Ulstrom CL, Michael CJ. The tissue origin of low back pain and sciatica. Orthop Clin North Am 1995; 22:1020–1027.

Weinstein JN, Gordon SL, eds. Low Back Pain—A Scientific and Clinical Overview. Rosemont, IL: American Academy of Orthopedic Surgeons, 1996.

Case 12

Lumbar Degenerative Disc Disease—Axial Back Pain: Posterior Approach

Stephen D. Kuslich

History and Physical Examination

A 38-year-old man who works as an airline baggage handler described an 8-year history of intermittent mechanical low back pain and 1 year of constant low back pain and leg pains. The problems began following an incident in which a baggage cart struck him. Conversion to light duty work decreased the pain, but he intensely disliked the work and was unwilling to accept the limitations on his sporting activities. Multiple trials of conservative treatments including chiropractic manipulations, physical therapy, and antiinflammatory medications failed to change the nature or intensity of the pain. Multiple attempts to return the patient to his baggage-handling duties resulted in frustration because of increased pain.

Before his injury, the patient had been a highly valued employee with a good work history. He was known to be an honest, hard-working individual who was well liked by his supervisors and coworkers. His pain drawing revealed no signs of symptom exaggeration. Waddell testing revealed no signs of functional overlay, and his family and social situations were stable and supportive. The physical examination revealed a 6'5", athletic-appearing male, weighing 225 lbs. We recorded a 30%

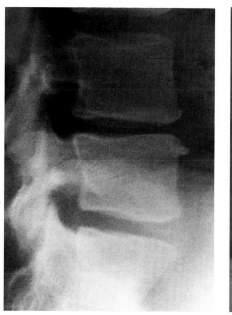
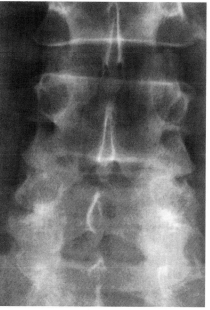

A   B

Figure 12–1. Anteroposterior (AP) (A) and lateral (B) X-ray of the lumbar spine showing some narrowing of the disc spaces at L4/L5 and L5/S1.

Posterior lumbar interbody fusion (PLIF) using bone-filled cages is most appropriately performed when the following circumstances are present:

- At L5/S1 there exists a large interlaminar window, so that exposure can be accomplished without total removal of the laminae and facet joint.
- The surgeon is able to retract the dural sac to the midline without excessive stretch.
- A younger male patient requires interbody stabilization and he is unwilling to accept a 2 to 4% chance of retrograde ejaculation as a possible complication.
- An extensive decompression is necessary, and the resulting exposure allows for disc debridement and cage placement.

reduction in lumbar spinal motion. There was flattening of the lumbar lordosis. His neurologic examination was unremarkable.

Radiologic Findings

Routine X-rays of the lumbar spine showed only slight loss of disc height at L4/L5 and L5/S1 (Fig. 12–1). Magnetic resonance imaging (MRI) revealed degenerative changes at the lower two lumbar discs with dehydration of the nucleus, posterior annual tears, and posterior protrusions of the discs, causing mild subarticular zone stenosis at both levels (Fig. 12–2).

Diagnosis

Chronic mechanical low back pain and leg pain secondary to degenerative disc disease and subarticular zone nerve root irritation at L4/L5 and L5/S1.

Surgical Management

Decompression alone might have helped the leg pain, but the mechanical backache required stabilization. Because our goal was to return the patient to full activities including occupational lifting and active sports participation, we needed to choose a procedure that would be stable and permanent. We informed the patient of all of

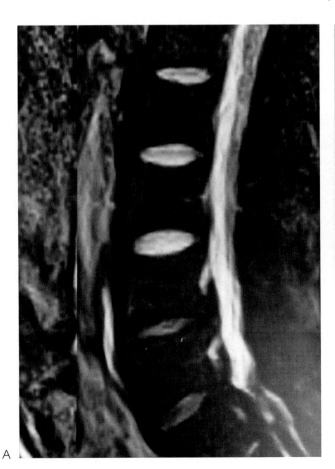

A

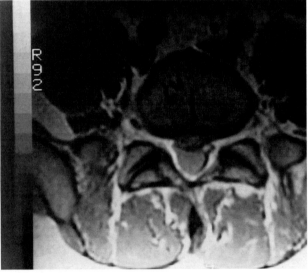

B

Figure 12–2. Magnetic resonance imaging (MRI) demonstrating advanced degenerative disc disease at L4/L5 (A) and L5/S1 (B). Minimal disc protrusions are not causing significant nerve root compression. Mild subarticular zone stenosis is present.

Most experienced cage surgeons eventually prefer the anterior retroperitoneal route for interbody stabilization. Reasons for avoiding the PLIF approach are the following:
- PLIF operations are more difficult, more bloody, and take longer to perform than anterior lumbar interbody fusion (ALIF) operations.
- PLIF operations require the removal of several posterior stabilizers, leading to a less stable construct.
- Invasion of the epidural space increases the risks of spinal fluid leaks, arachnoiditis, nerve root trauma, and epidural fibrosis.
- PLIF patients seem to take longer to recuperate, have more postoperative leg pain symptoms, and require longer periods off of work before recovery.

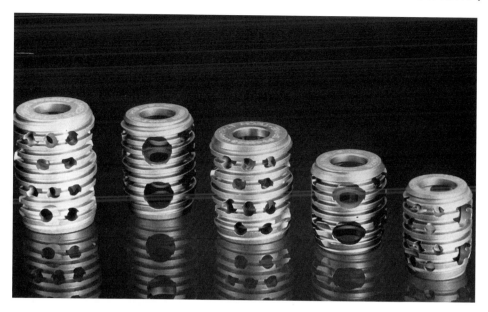

Figure 12–3. The BAK device in a titanium hollow cylinder with multiple perforations to allow bone ingrowth. The leading edge is beveled into a slight bullet shape to facilitate insertion. Square threads that feed into a triangular cut bed to remove some bone during screw-in, partially filling the perforations and the internal cavity. Three internal ribs provide the strength needed to withstand the compression forces on the implant.

the available surgical treatment options. In general, and especially in cases of two-level disease, I prefer the anterior approach. However, after the patient considered the slight risk of retrograde ejaculation with the anterior approach, he opted for a posterior interbody fusion using bone-filed titanium BAK (Bagly and Kuslich) cages (Fig. 12–3).

The operation consisted of a wide central subarticular decompression and exposure of the L5/S1 and L4/L5 disc spaces posteriorly (Fig. 12–4) followed by the placement of two BAK titanium cylinders at each level (Fig. 12–5). Postoperative X-rays showed good alignment and depth of the implants (Fig 12–6). The operation lasted 4 hours and the patient was hospitalized for 4 days following surgery. Blood loss was about 550 cc. We used no braces or additional fixation. We derived bone graft by processing the resected spinous processes and laminae in a bone mill.

Postoperative Management

The patient walked on the first postoperative day and we discharged him on the fourth day. His back pain improved immediately but he experienced leg pains during the first few weeks following the operation, probably as a result of the nerve root retraction necessary to obtain exposure of the disc for the posterior lumbar interbody fusion (PLIF) procedure. After about 6 weeks the leg pain subsided.

The patient gradually increased his activities during the first 3 months following the operation. When he became more active, he noted some recurrence of back pain. We treated the pains with oral medication and sacroiliac (SI) joint injections on two occasions. He returned to part-time light-duty work at 4 months and by 7 months he was back to heavy-duty lifting 4 to 6 hours per day. At 1 year following

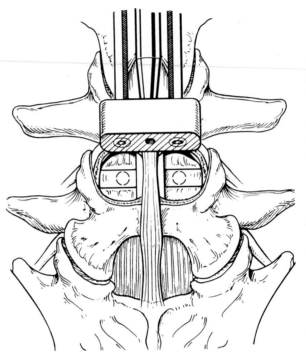

Figure 12–4. The minimum posterior exposure needed to insert two BAK implants from the posterior approach. At L5/S1, it is usually possible to preserve at least half of the facet joint, but at L4/L5 or above, total facetectomy is usually necessary. The surgeon must be able to retract the dural sac to midline to safely perform the procedure. Marginal osteophytes should be removed prior to placement of the distraction plug to establish normal lordosis. The exiting nerve root must be identified and protected from injury during the drilling and implantation.

the operation, he was working full time and lifting 10,000 to 15,000 lbs of luggage per day with only occasional tolerable discomfort in the back. His last follow-up examination took place 4 years following the operation. X-rays revealed no motion on flexion-extension and there were no radiolucencies above or below the implants. Normal lordosis was maintained (Fig. 12–7). He works full-time (with some overtime) as a baggage handler and participates in several sports activities without

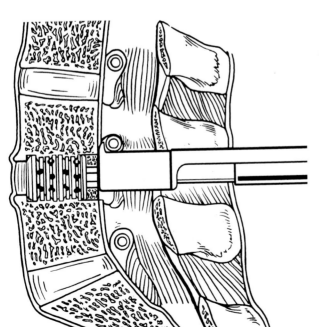

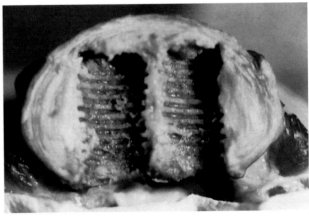

Figure 12–5. (A and B) The implant should be placed deep within the disc space and parallel to each other. The implants are separated from one another by 4–6 mm. The space in between should be curetted to remove disc material. The implants are filled with morcelized bone graft.

A

B

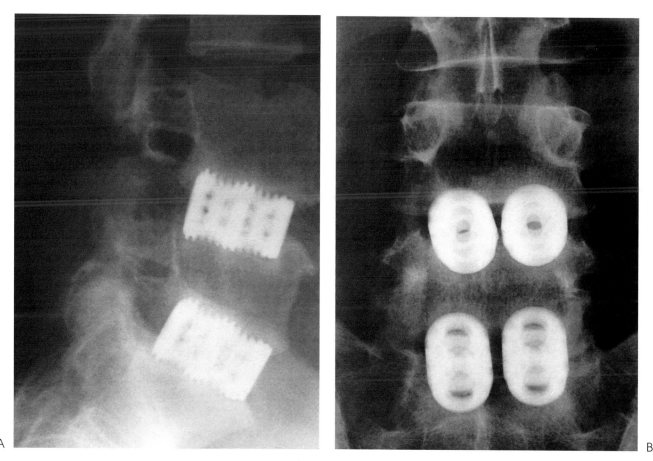

Figure 12–6. Postoperative AP (A) and lateral (B) X-rays show good position of implants.

limitation. He requires no medication or treatments for back pain. The patient, his employer, and his insurance company are very satisfied with the result.

Discussion

The management of chronic mechanical low back pain can be a frustrating and unrewarding experience for the physician and therapist. Although acute cases usually resolve without any therapy (and sometimes in spite of therapy!), back pain lasting more than 6 months is remarkably resistant to conservative measures. Often, employers and health care workers believe that the patient is a malingerer primarily motivated by secondary gain. Chronic pain can generate anxiety and depression, and the physician may then confuse cause with effect.

Although inflammatory conditions of the facet and/or sacroiliac joints may be implicated as the cause of pain in 20 to 30% of new patients, degenerative changes in the disc are the most common etiology. My 20-year experience with tissue sensitivity testing during the course of operations using local anesthesia has taught me that the disc is the only tissue capable of causing the deep, nauseating, dull pain of lumbago.

Before the advent of modern diagnostic technology (MRI and discography) and effective interbody stabilization methods (interbody cages and 360-degree fusions

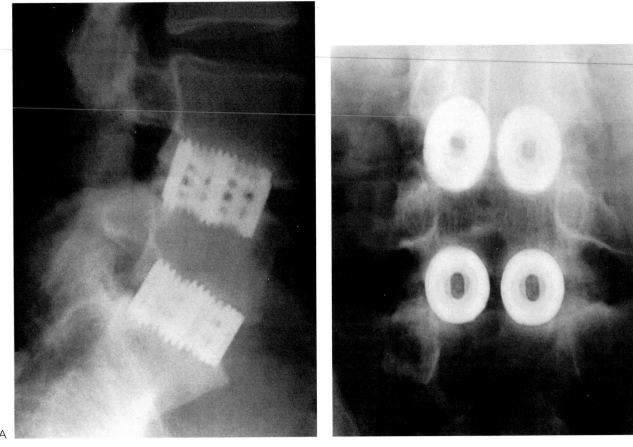

A

B

Figure 12–7. AP (A) and lateral (B) X-rays at 4 years postoperation. Some settling has taken place. No radiolucencies are present. Lordosis is maintained. The patient is stable and pain free.

with interbody graft), many patients suffered in silence. Others chose to "fight the system," so to speak, because of the inability of their physicians to make a tissue-specific diagnosis and offer effective treatment. Although it is still true that some patients cannot be specifically diagnosed and effectively treated, modern methods do provide accurate diagnoses and definitive treatment options to a majority of patients with organically caused chronic mechanical low back pain.

The greatest remaining challenges are (1) learning how to select appropriate candidates for surgery, and (2) learning how to perform disc debridement and stabilization with the least possible collateral damage. Case selection requires knowledge, logic, and the establishment of a personal relationship with the patient. To make decisions about where, when, and how to operate, the surgeon must understand the physical, mental, and emotional state of the patient. Interbody fusion using bone-filled cages provides one more option for effective stabilization. This method is not ideal (complications and failures do occur), but currently it is the best we have. Large multicenter studies conclusively demonstrate that properly selected cases can be treated successfully and safely with cage technology.

Alternative Methods of Management

The alternative methods are the same as those discussed in Case 11.

Type of Management	Advantages	Disadvantages	Comments
ALIF with cages	Fast surgery, low blood loss, no epidural complications, highly effective	Less traditional, risk of great vessel injury, risk of retrograde ejaculation	Author's preferred method, simple once learning curve is mastered
PLIF with bone dowels, rectangular grafts (Cloward) or PLIF with cages	Allows concomitant decompression	Dural and nerve damage, bleeding, less stable	Most experienced cage surgeons eventually abandon this for anterior approach
ALIF with allograft dowels	Fast surgery, low blood loss, no graft site morbidity, no epidural complications	Longer time to graft incorporation, risk of disease transmission	Not proven in large multicenter trials, older studies had 20 to 30% nonunion rates
Posterolateral fusion with and without pedicle fixation	Traditional approach	Does not completely immobilize disc, damage to musculature	Higher morbidity, less complete pain relief than interbody methods
Circumferential fusion with anterior graft and fixation posteriorly	High fusion rate	Long, bloody procedure, high reoperation rates, high complication rates	Becoming less popular since advent of cage fusion technology. Morbidity is greatest negative feature
Conservative management	Safest form of treatment	Not very effective for chronic back pain	Always try first, may be the only feasible alternative in certain patients

ALIF, anterior lumbar interbody fusion; PLIF, posterior lumbar interbody fusion.

Suggested Readings

Kuslich SD. Lumbar interbody cage fusion for back pain: an update on the BAK (Bagby and Kuslich) system. In: Errico T, ed. Spine: State of the Art Reviews, Spinal Instrumentation. Philadelpia: Hanley and Belfus, 1999.

Kuslich SD, Ulstrom CL, Griffith SL, Ahern JW, Dowdle JD. The Bagby and Kuslich method of lumbar interbody fusion. Spine 1998; 23:1267–1278.

Kuslich SD, Ulstrom CD, Michael CJ. The tissue origin of low back pain and sciatica. Orthop Clin North Am 1995; 22:1020–1027.

Weinstein JD, Gordon SL, eds. Low Back Pain—A Scientific and Clinical Overview. Rosemont, IL: American Academy of Orthopaedic Surgeons, 1996.

Case 13

Lumbar Spinal Stenosis
without Instability

John A. McCulloch

History and Physical Examination

An 82-year-old healthy man presented with a long history (years) of back pain and a more recent (2-year) gradual onset of bilateral claudicant leg pain. He described his leg symptoms as somewhat radicular in nature, but more so a sensation of tiredness, heaviness, and some numbness. The right leg was a little more symptomatic than his left. His leg symptoms had become more of a problem than his back pain because they limited his ability to walk more than three or four blocks, or stand more than 5 to 10 minutes. He could not relieve his symptoms by standing, but rather had to sit down for a few minutes before he could start walking again.

Although he was 82 years of age, he was very healthy, driving his car back and forth between Ohio and Florida each year. Also, he did not wish to give up his "boat-centered" lifestyle that required a lot of standing and walking.

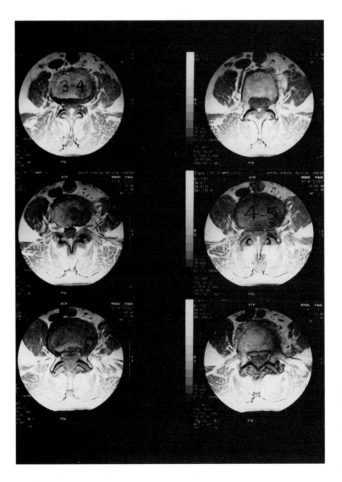

Figure 13–1. Assembled T1 axial magnetic resonance imaging (MRI) images showing spinal canal stenosis (SCS) L3-4 (top left) and L4-5 (middle right).

On physical examination he stood in a slightly forward flexed position. He had mild reduction in straight leg raising with average knee reflexes and reduced ankle reflexes. He had good strength on testing individual muscle groups. He had booming ankle and foot pulses and a full range of movement in his hips.

Radiologic Findings

Magnetic resonance imaging (MRI) of the patient's lumbar spine (transaxial views) revealed significant tricompartmental stenosis at the L3/L4 and L4/L5 levels (Fig. 13–1).

Diagnosis

Patients with symptomatic lumbar stenosis often present with significant limitations in their ability to stand and walk, yet there is little to find on physical examination. Rather, the physical examination is important in ruling out other conditions that limit one's ability to walk, such as vascular claudication. Patients with ischemic claudicant leg pain have absent pulses and have a sharper pain that is more distally located, rarely associated with neurologic symptoms, and the pain can be relieved very quickly simply by stopping the activity, even in the standing position. Another differential diagnostic possibility is bilateral hip disease, which is easy to determine through loss of range of movement in the hip joints and flexion deformities. A further diagnostic conundrum is peripheral neuropathy, which is a less painful, more sensory, and weakness-oriented collection of symptoms. Finally, spinal canal stenosis can be combined with any of the above conditions and cause considerable consternation in arriving at a suitable diagnosis.

As long as there is no structural deformity such as scoliosis or a severe degenerative spondylolisthesis, then surgical game planning can be done entirely on the basis of an MRI and plain radiographs. MRI, although twice as expensive as computed tomography (CT) scanning, delivers at least twice as much information as the CT scan. Most importantly, it distinguishes congenital from acquired stenosis (Fig. 13–2). It shows the exact localization of the lesion within the anatomic segment so that limited surgery can be planned (Fig. 13–3).

When looking at an MRI, remember that over 60% of patients 60 years of age or over have degenerative changes and even spinal canal stenosis with no symptoms at all. In addition, it's important to remember that someone who is significantly disabled in terms of lower extremity symptoms needs to have a significant MRI defect or the physician is missing some other condition causing the leg symptoms.

Conservative Management

Providing that there are no bladder or bowel symptoms and no specific weakness on physical examination, it is okay to wait out the patient's symptoms until the patient decides he has reached a stage of functional limitation that he can no longer tolerate. It is at that stage that one intervenes with radiographic investigation, possibly leading to decompressive surgery.

Once patients reach a threshold of walking limitation of three to four blocks, or standing limitation of 5 to 10 minutes, then probably conservative management will be of little long-term benefit. There may be temporary relief through

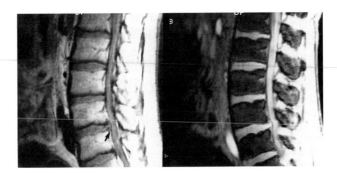

Figure 13–2. Congenital (developmental) SCS. Note the global nature of the stenosis.

conservative treatment efforts such as physical therapy and epidural cortisone. If patients reach the thresholds mentioned above, then surgical intervention should be considered. Patients should clearly understand that the condition is not a dangerous problem and they can afford to live with their stenosis if they wish to limit their standing and walking times. If a patient is medically unfit for surgery, then conservative management in the form of epidural cortisone may be useful. For the early stages of spinal canal stenosis with limited symptoms and a good ability to stand and walk, epidural cortisone, nonsteroidal antiinflammatory drugs (NSAIDs), and physical therapy are indicated.

Surgical Management

Indications

Bladder and bowel symptoms and actual measurable weakness on specific muscle group testing are unusual but absolute indications for surgical intervention. Ninety-nine percent of the patients will have the surgical indication of significant limitation in the ability to walk and stand. In addition, surgery should be proposed *only* to those patients who have significant limitation in walking and standing time due to their claudicant leg pain. Surgery is not a good treatment for the back pain associated with spinal canal stenosis.

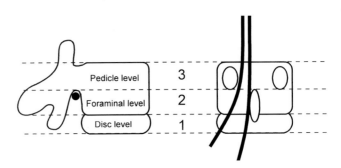

Figure 13–3. The three-storied anatomic segment. The stenotic lesion in Figure 13–1 is predominantly in the first story of the L3 and L4 segments, whereas adjacent axial cuts (top right, middle left, bottom right) show a canal of normal dimensions. Every story in Figure 13–2 (1st, 2nd, and 3rd) of each anatomic segment L2 to L5 is narrowed. This is the difference between acquired (degenerative) SCS (Figure 13–1) and congenital (developmental) SCS (Figure 13–2).

Diagnosis

It is important to be sure that the patient has a clear-cut case of spinal canal stenosis. It is also important to ascertain the general medical state of these patients, as they often have comorbid conditions. Patients who have limited ability to walk can easily develop severe heart disease without angina because their limited ability to walk means they are not pushing their heart to any great extent. Finally, it is important to separate congenital (developmental) from acquired stenosis (Fig. 13–2). The former requires a more aggressive open procedure, and the latter can be treated with limited surgical intervention.

How Many Levels to Decompress

It is wise to decompress all stenotic levels but to do so in a limited fashion. Even though this patient had pain down the back of his legs, the L3/L4 stenosis was significant enough that it was also decompressed at the time of surgery. The decompression that the patient underwent was limited in that it was a laminoplasty type of decompression of the spinal canal and the subarticular recess at the L3/L4 and L4/L5 levels (Fig. 13–4). He had no foraminal stenosis.

Foraminal stenosis is probably overreported by radiologists and underoperated by surgeons (Fig. 13–5). It is an associated stenotic lesion that can only be seen on sagittal X-ray. If it is present, it is best to decompress the foraminal component of the stenosis through a lateral approach to the pars (Fig. 13–5).

Surgery in This Patient

The patient underwent a bilateral laminoplasty-type decompression at L3/L4 and L4/L5 from his right side because he was more symptomatic on the right. No elevation of the paraspinal muscles was done on the left side. This approach allows the surgeon to save the spinous process and the interspinous-supraspinous ligament complex. The anterior surface of the lamina is also removed to enlarge the spinal canal. There was no role for fusion in this patient or any other patient that has spinal canal stenosis without instability.

Postoperatively, this age group warrants special attention to prophylaxis for pulmonary problems, deep venous thrombosis (DVT), and pulmonary embolus. This limited surgical intervention allows for quick ambulation of the patient in a simple canvas corset.

Discussion

Spinal canal stenosis is defined as narrowing of the central spinal canal or lateral zone of the spinal canal (Fig. 13–6). With our increasing aging population, more and more patients with this condition are showing up in spine surgeons' offices. With a better understanding of the actual structural lesion, better anesthesia, and better surgical techniques, it is possible to perform very limited surgical intervention for pure acquired spinal canal stenosis. Laminoplasty with quick ambulation is the procedure of choice in these patients. Each level of stenosis seen on MRI, unless it is a minor degree of stenosis, warrants surgical attention. The objective of the surgery is to increase the patient's walking distance and standing time.

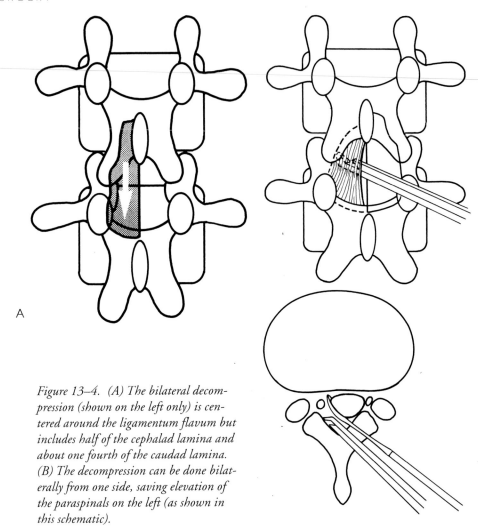

Figure 13–4. (A) The bilateral decompression (shown on the left only) is centered around the ligamentum flavum but includes half of the cephalad lamina and about one fourth of the caudad lamina. (B) The decompression can be done bilaterally from one side, saving elevation of the paraspinals on the left (as shown in this schematic).

It is prudent to differentiate patients with cauda equina–type stenosis from those with radicular stenosis (Fig. 13–6). Cauda equina stenosis patients have a more diffuse type of leg syndrome with less radicular pain. These patients are thought to have central canal stenosis. Patients with a radicular type of stenosis have very definite radicular pain, usually due to stenosis in the lateral zone, such as subarticular or foraminal stenosis. Many patients present with combined cauda equina and radicular pain.

The structural cause of the stenosis is predominantly infolding of the ligamentum flavum. In addition, a bulging annulus, hypertrophied facet joints, and hypertrophied facet capsule contribute to the stenosis. The stenotic lesion occurs predominantly in the first story of the anatomic segment and extends a little bit up into the second story of the anatomic segment, and a little bit down into the third story of the anatomic segment below (Figs. 13–1 and 13–3). Recognizing this isolated intrasegmental lesion allows one to plan a very limited laminoplasty type decompression (Fig. 13–7).

The pathophysiology of the stenotic symptoms obviously has to be something more than mechanical. Supporting this argument is the fact that when the patients are at rest, they are symptom-free, yet the stenotic lesion is still present. It is only when the patient is walking or standing that symptoms appear, and this indicates a dynamic component. The dynamic component is thought by various experts to be due to venous stasis, nerve root ischemia, or decreased nutrition to the nerve roots brought on by activity.

Acquired spinal canal stenosis is a manifestation of the aging process. As such it should not be conveyed to patients as anything serious, or as due to any misadventure in their past life. As mentioned above, it is important to distinguish intersegmental acquired spinal canal stenosis (SCS) from congenital or developmental SCS (Fig. 13–2).

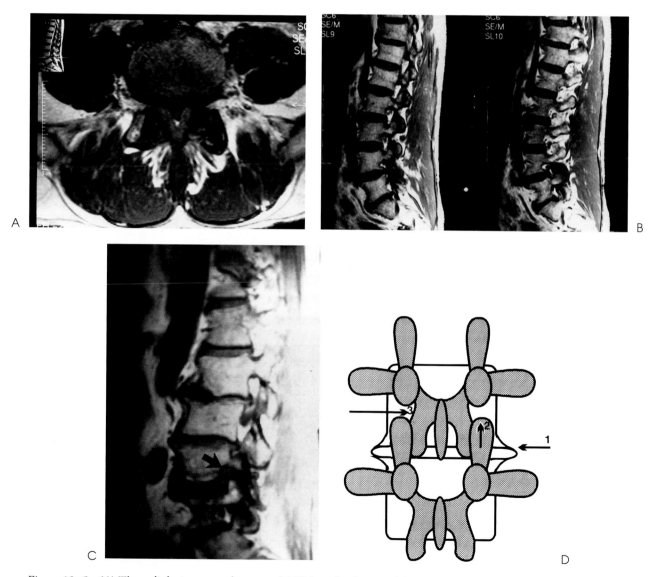

Figure 13–5. (A) The radiologists correctly reported SCS but also diagnosed foraminal stenosis on this axial. (B) The foramen can only be accurately read on (para)sagittal cuts, which for the patient in part A shows all the foramina wide open. (C) This (para)sagittal T1 MRI shows a stenosed L4 foramen (arrow). (D) With disc space narrowing comes (1) facet subluxation with or without (2) facet hypertrophy. Decompression is best accomplished from "outside-in" (3).

PEARL
• Spinal stenosis is a diagnosis made on history, with usually little in the way of supportive physical findings.

PITFALLS
• Be wary of proposing surgery in a patient with spinal stenosis (claudicant leg pain) who has a minor encroachment lesion on investigation.
• Aggressive decompressive surgery may adversely impact the cascading events of degenerative spinal canal stenosis. By carefully studying the sagittal and axial MRI images, it is possible to rethink the three-dimensional constricting lesion of acquired SCS. With an understanding of the three-storied anatomic house of each anatomic segment, along with the posterior interlaminar window of decompression, it is possible to do a limited microsurgical decompression of acquired SCS, save many of the soft tissue supporting structures (such as interspinous/supraspinous ligaments), and have a less detrimental impact on the degenerative cascade.

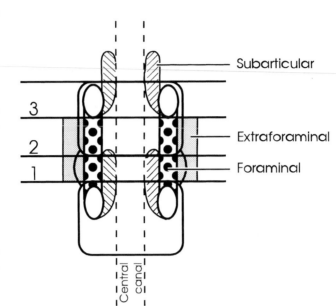

Figure 13–6. The spinal canal is divided into a central zone (spinal canal) and lateral zone. The subdivisions of the lateral zone are (a) subarticular, (b) foraminal, (c) extraforaminal.

The surgical procedure of choice for SCS of an acquired nature, without instability, is the laminotomy or laminoplasty procedure (Fig. 13–7), which saves the supraspinous and the interspinous ligaments, and saves the facet joints and the disc spaces.

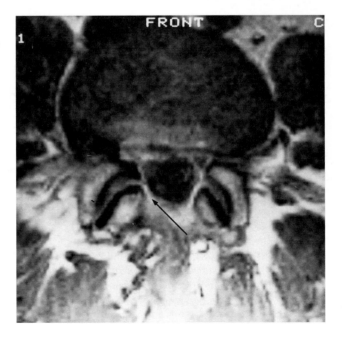

Figure 13–7. A postoperative SCS bilateral decompression from the left. The arrow points to the right-sided decompression from the left.

Alternative Methods of Management

Conservative care is indicated in those patients who have minor claudicant leg pain. Physical therapy, NSAIDs, and epidural cortisones are useful. Chiropractic adjustments may be useful for the management of the patient's back pain.

Once a patient reaches the threshold of walking ability limited to three or four blocks and standing ability limited to 5 or 10 minutes, then conservative treatment efforts are going to be of limited and temporary benefit.

Type of Management	Advantages	Disadvantages	Comments
Conservative	Simple	Fails routinely when patient significantly limited in walking distance and standing time	First line of treatment
Midline decompression	Standard procedure	Removes supporting bone and ligaments that do not have to be removed	Will be replaced by laminoplasty
Microdecompression (laminoplasty)	Simple and minor surgery in this age group	Longer learning curve than for microdiscectomy	Will replace midline decompression in acquired spinal cord stenosis (SCS)
Percutaneous procedures	None	No indication for their use	Just another example of how limited percutaneous surgery is for degenerative spine conditions

Complications

Following surgery there are many general complications to deal with that largely center around the pulmonary tree, the venous system in the lower extremities, and the bladder. It is important to stay on top of these systems in the first 24 hours. With the limited laminoplasty-type decompression, blood loss is very limited and a transfusion is usually not required.

Specific complications center around dural tears and root injuries due to the fact that synovial tissue in the spinal canal is often part of the spinal stenotic lesion. Once synovial tissue gets into the spinal canal, it usually scars itself to the dura, and aggressive surgery may open a rent in the dura that requires repair. One should always be aware of the potential for a postoperative hematoma causing thecal sac compression and the so-called cauda equina syndrome. With the frequency of postoperative bladder problems in this patient population, it is very easy, especially in the catheterized patient, to miss a cauda equina syndrome that develops as the hematoma forms over the first few postoperative days.

Suggested Readings

Arnold CC, Brodsky AE, Cauchoix J, et al. Lumbar spine stenosis and nerve root entrapment syndromes: definition and classification. Clin Orthop Rel Res 1976; 115: 4–5.

Boden SD, David DO, Dina TS, Patronas NJ, Wiesel SW. Abnormal magnetic resonance scans of the lumbar spine, asymptomatic subjects. J Bone Joint Surg 1990; 72A:403–408.

Ciol M, Deyo R, Howell E, Krief S. An assessment of surgery for spinal stenosis: time trends, geographic variations, complications and reoperations. J Am Geriatric Soc 1996; 44:285–290.

Deyo R, Cherkin DC, Loeser JD, et al. Morbidity and mortality in association with operations on the lumbar spine. J Bone Joint Surg 1992; 74:536–543.

Johnsson KE, Rosen I, Uden A. The natural course of spinal stenosis. Clin Orthop 1992; 279:82–86.

Katz J, Lipson S, Chang L, Levine S, Fossel A, Liang M. Seven to ten year outcome of decompressive surgery for degenerative lumbar spinal stenosis. Spine 1996; 21:92–98.

Verbiest H. Results of surgical treatment of idiopathic developmental stenosis of the lumbar vertebral canal. J Bone Joint Surg 1977; 59B:181–188.

Case 14

Lumbar Degenerative Spondylolisthesis

Eeric Truumees and Harry N. Herkowitz

History and Physical Examination

A 70-year-old woman with a medical history of hypertension and asthma presented with complaints of bilateral buttock, posterior thigh, and lateral calf pain of 2 years' duration. Her pain increased with activity and was relieved by periods of rest. Further, forward flexion with sitting, cycling, or shopping-cart use decreased her pain. She noted mild weakness that worsened after walking. She denied bowel or bladder complaints. She had no history of cancer or trauma and denied fever, chills, night pain, or other systemic complaints. On physical examination, this well-nourished, pleasant female demonstrated a normal gait. Her back was nontender, but an L4/L5 step-off was palpated. Clinically she was in coronal and sagittal spinal balance. Although she had normal forward flexion, extension maneuvers increased her pain.

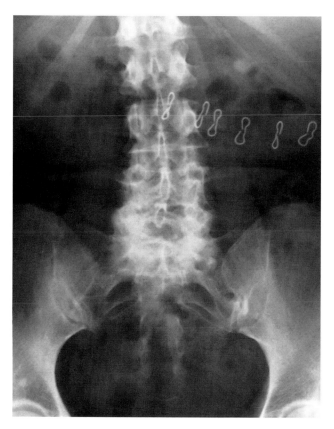

Figure 14–1. Anteroposterior (AP) radiograph of the lumbosacral spine demonstrating degenerative changes.

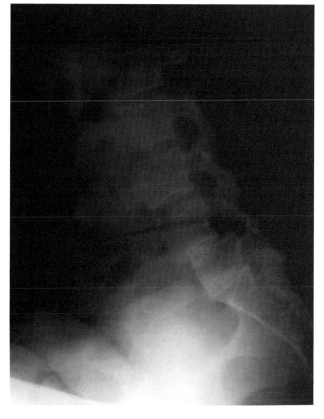

Figure 14–2. Flexion lateral projection of the lumbosacral spine demonstrating 25% spondylolisthesis of the L4/L5 level. The extension film demonstrated correction of approximately 50% of the deformity.

Her hip and extremity exams were within normal limits. She exhibited normal capillary refill and pulses in the distal lower extremities. Abdominal examination was negative for masses, pain, or bruits. Sensory exam was grossly normal, including position and vibratory sense. She had no tension signs.

Radiologic Findings

Radiographic evaluation began with anteroposterior (AP) and lateral projections of the lumbosacral spine (Figs. 14–1 and 14–2) as well as an L4/S1 cone-down view. These studies demonstrated degenerative changes of the spine with loss of disc height at L4/L5 and L5/S1. Further, a 25% anterolisthesis of L4 was noted on L5. The posterior elements appeared intact. Normal psoas shadows and intact pedicular anatomy were noted.

After initial plain radiographic evaluation, a period of nonoperative management was undertaken. The patient noted some functional improvement, but her leg pain continued to interfere with her normal daily activities. Therefore, further imaging studies were requested. Included among these were flexion and extension lateral radiographs of the lumbosacral spine. Although partial correction of her spondylolisthesis was noted, no evidence of instability of adjacent segments was appreciated. Magnetic resonance imaging (MRI) scan of her lumbosacral spine was obtained, including T1 and T2 parasagittal images (Fig. 14–3) and disc level axial images from L1/L2 to L5/S1. This study demonstrated diffuse degenerative changes, the L4/L5 spondylolisthesis, as well as central canal and foraminal stenosis of the L4/L5 level (Fig. 14–4). No evidence of posterior element defects, foraminal stenosis, or involvement of other levels was noted.

Diagnosis

This generally healthy 70-year-old woman had lumbar spinal stenosis in conjunction with a mobile spondylolisthesis at the L4/L5 level. Her symptoms of pseudoclaudication and L5 radiculopathy are consistent with physical and imaging findings. These symptoms had not been responsive to nonoperative treatment. For this reason, the risks, benefits, and alternatives of surgical intervention were discussed with the patient. Because of the significant limitations imposed on her lifestyle by her stenosis, she agreed to proceed. Preoperative imaging tests were then ordered to confirm the diagnosis, provide a surgical roadmap, and exclude subtle pathology elsewhere. Surgical planning included a lumbar laminectomy of the stenotic level. A posterolateral fusion of this segment was recommended because of the presence of degenerative spondylolisthesis. Instrumentation was elected in this patient to improve fusion rates and because of the mobility of the slip. Careful measurement of pedicular size and orientation was carried out preoperatively as well. Pedicular fill was maximized. Screw length was based on penetration of 75% of the vertebral body. A triangulated screw configuration was planned to increase pull-out strength and decrease the injury to the L3/L4 facet.

Surgical Management

Further preoperative planning included standard preanesthesia laboratory studies, EKG, and chest radiographs. Dual energy x-ray absorptiometry (DEXA) scanning is

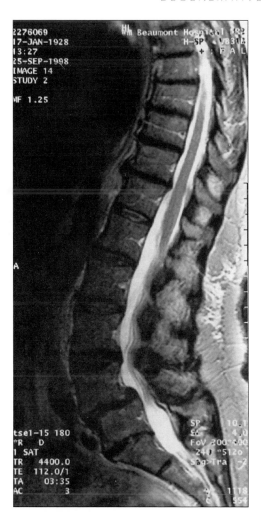

Figure 14–3. Sagittal T2-weighted magnetic resonance imaging (MRI) demonstrating spondy-lolisthesis with spinal stenosis at L4/L5.

recommended in patients with osteopenic bone should instrumentation be contemplated. Preoperatively, two units of autologous blood were obtained.

The patient was given a dose of antibiotics prior to skin incision. To decrease bleeding during decompression by decreasing venous tension, she was positioned without pressure on her abdomen. Further, because a concomitant fusion was planned, maintenance of lumbar lordosis was important. This lordosis further ensured a complete decompression would be performed by placing the spine into a simulated erect posture. A Jackson or other four-poster frame allows both abdominal decompression and, as the hips may be extended, maintenance of lordosis. All bony prominences were carefully padded. Careful attention was paid to pressure on the eyes. A general endotracheal anesthetic was used. However, for short-segment fusions, occasionally spinal or epidural anesthesia may be employed. If the patient's general condition allows, mean arterial pressure is maintained at 70 mm Hg to decrease intraoperative blood loss.

Standard skin preparation and draping, including the iliac crest, were undertaken. For this patient's one-level disease, a 5-cm incision was made centering over

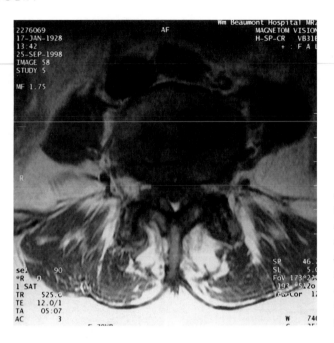

Figure 14–4. Axial T1-weighted MRI image at L4/L5 demonstrating central and lateral recess spinal stenosis, facet and ligamentum flavum hypertrophy. Images at L3/L4 and other neighboring levels did not demonstrate stenosis.

the involved disc space. The subperiosteal dissection was carried to the facets of the level above and below the subject level. This additional dissection allowed adequate retraction of the erector muscles to facilitate exposure to the tips of the transverse processes of L4 and L5. Care was taken not to fracture the transverse processes. Careful preservation of the facet capsules was maintained until local bony anatomy or radiographic confirmation of the level had been achieved. At this point, the facet capsule of the level to be fused was stripped and complete exposure of the lateral pars was undertaken.

Decompression began by removal of the inferior half of the superior and the superior half of the inferior spinous process with a double-action rongeur. A Leksell rongeur was used to thin the laminae at the level of the disc space. A burr may also be used for this purpose. The ligamentum flavum was dissected from the inferior aspect of the superior level lamina with a 3-0 curette. This allowed introduction of a 3-mm Kerrison punch. A midline decompression was performed to the level of the superior border of the facet. Next, the decompression was carried inferiorly through the superior aspect of the inferior lamina and continued to the inferior border of the facet. Occasionally an angled dural elevator was used to lift the intervening ligamentum flavum, which was then cut with a no. 15 blade. With a midline decompression completed, the lateral recess decompression began with a partial medial facetectomy. In the presence of severe facet hypertrophy, this lateral decompression could be started with a 5-mm burr to thin the lateral bone. A straight half-inch osteotome may also be used for this purpose. A 2-mm Kerrison punch was introduced and the decompression was carried laterally to the level of the pedicles. A Penfield no. 4 dural separator is helpful to dissect any dural adhesions from the bony lamina. The extent of decompression was then assessed with a probe. Evidence of foraminal stenosis of both the traversing and exiting nerve roots was sought. In this case, the L5 foramina did not allow easy passage of the 3-mm probe.

Further facet undercutting at the foraminal level was performed using angled Kerrisons. Then, the Kerrison was placed superficial to the root and hypertrophied ligamentum flavum and more lateral facet osteophytes were removed. Had such undercutting not been possible, further lateral resection of the facets would have been undertaken. Then, the planned fusion would have been mandatory. Finally, the superior and inferior extent of the decompression is assessed and may be carried cephalad or caudad as needed.

At the conclusion of the lateral and foraminal decompression, the roots displaced 1 cm medially without undue tension. At the time of this testing, the absence of soft disc pathology was confirmed. Hard posterior vertebral body osteophytes were left in place. With an adequate decompression completed, transpedicular hardware was inserted. The medial, superior, and inferior pedicular borders were directly palpated with the Woodson from inside the canal. External bony landmarks included the lateral pars, the lateral facet, and the transverse process. Axial MRI or computed tomography (CT) cuts were used to confirm pedicular angulation. General landmarks used included the lateral pars and the outer border of the facet in the mediolateral plane. The pedicle screw entry site was selected 2 to 3 mm lateral to the pars in a vertical line connecting the lateral pars with the inferior border of the superior facet at each level. This insertion point was slightly lateral to the direct center of the pedicle to afford triangulation of the screw. In the superoinferior plane, the line bisecting the transverse processes was used to identify the level of the pedicle. This level was 1 to 2 mm below the inferior border of the facet. In this patient, an accessory process was noted at L4 and provided an excellent entry point for screw insertion. A 4-mm burr was used to enter the cortex of the pedicle entry site. A pedicle probe or 3-0 curette was used to sound the pedicle. Superoinferior inclination of the pedicle was ascertained from the lateral intraoperative localization radiograph. A 15-degree medial-lateral inclination was chosen at L4 with approximately 30 degrees of inclination at L5.

Next a thin probe was inserted into the pedicle to ensure cortical continuity. The Woodson may be used to assess the outer pedicular cortex. As the pedicles were intact, a 5.5-mm tap was used to prepare the pedicle tract. A marker and intraoperative fluoroscopy was employed to confirm localization. Once tapped, the tract was again probed and the screw was inserted. At this point, and intermittently throughout the procedure, the wound was copiously irrigated.

Next, attention was paid to complete decortication of the transverse processes, facets, and lateral pars. A combination of burr, gouges, and rat-tooth rongeurs were be used for this purpose. Autogenous bone graft was obtained from the posterior iliac crest and packed into the posterolateral gutters. Next, the longitudinal member of the instrumentation system was placed. In this single-level fusion we used plates, which confer more rigidity at the plate-screw interface than rods and further assist in compressing the bone graft in place. Careful attention was paid to the height and angulation of the screws. If necessary, straight and angled washers are used to equalize screw-plate geometry of both levels. After the completion of instrumentation, the decompression is reassessed with a Woodson. Occasionally, inadvertent compression through the transpedicular instrumentation results in foraminal stenosis. No such stenosis or misplaced bone graft was noted in this patient. Therefore, a watertight fascial closure was completed over suction drains at both the iliac crest and midline sites. Cutaneous sutures were followed by staples. A sterile, bulky postsurgical bandage was applied.

Postoperative Management

The patient was taken from the operating room to the recovery room. Once vital signs had been stabilized, she was transported to the regular nursing floor. Postoperative braces and corsets are generally not employed. The patient was mobilized to a chair the evening of surgery. Drains were removed, and diet and pain medications were advanced on the first day after surgery. Antibiotics were continued for 24 hours. Ambulation was progressed with physical therapy over the next several days. Initial activity restrictions include avoidance of bending, lifting, and twisting. Most patients are able to return home within 3 to 5 days.

Office follow-up began with a wound check and staple removal at 10 days; 15 to 30 minutes of walking twice a day were encouraged at this point. Stationary bicycling and swimming were resumed at 4 to 6 weeks. Further follow-up was planned at the 6-week, 3-month, 6-month, and 1-year mark. Instrumented spinal fusion patients warrant long-term follow-up because of the possibility of adjacent segment degeneration. This may be carried out at a yearly interval. Radiographs are obtained intermittently to assess progression of fusion, bony alignment and hardware positioning (Figs. 14–5, 14–6, and 14–7). Instrumentation is generally not removed.

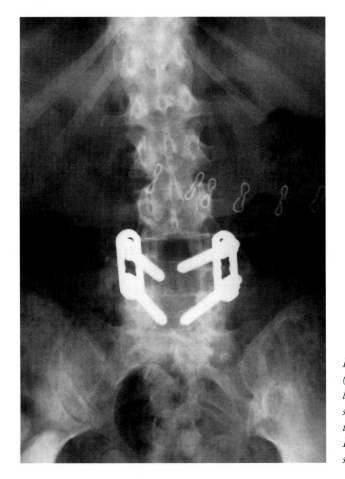

Figure 14–5. Postoperative (6 months) AP view of the lumbosacral spine demonstrating an instrumented posterolateral spinal fusion. Early consolidation of the fusion mass is evident.

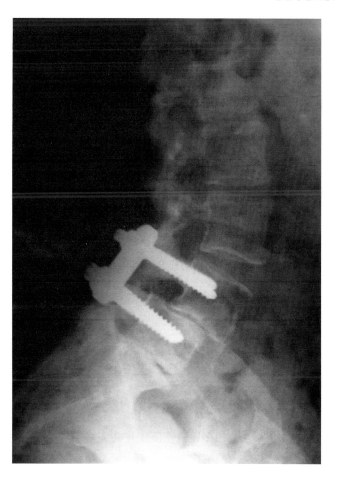

Figure 14–6. Postoperative (6 months) lateral view demonstrating instrumented posterolateral spinal fusion. Note the overall maintenance of lumbar lordosis. Only minimal correction of the slip was achieved.

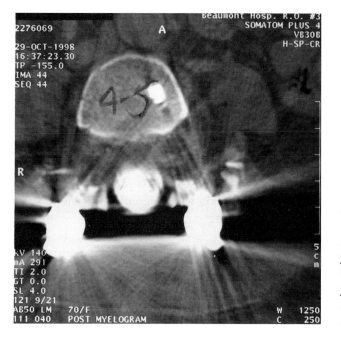

Figure 14–7. Postoperative CT image at the level of decompression demonstrating presence of posterior instrumentation. A wide decompression with complete filling of the thecal sac is appreciated.

- As back pain and degenerative changes (including stenosis and spondylolisthesis) are common in both the symptomatic and asymptomatic population, it is a mistake to assume that the spondylosis and slip identified on plain radiography account for the patient's symptoms, particularly when limited to back pain. A Venn diagram approach, with overlapping and consistent historical, examination, and radiographic findings, will more clearly identify patients likely to obtain relief with surgical intervention.
- Nonoperative measures are often sufficient to control symptoms. Further, symptoms rarely progress rapidly. Therefore, disease education, activity modification, and therapeutic exercises are the mainstays of treatment. Nonsteroidal and other medications may be added. Smoking cessation and weight loss should be encouraged.
- Because of increases in stenosis with extension, McKenzie-type exercises are not recommended in this patient group. Rather, flexion exercises are ordered.
- The iliac crest is prepared in all decompression patients as iatrogenic destabilization may necessitate fusion, even if fusion is not initially intended.
- Epidural steroid injections may offer transient relief in some patients.

Discussion

Spinal stenosis and degenerative spondylolisthesis are rare in patients under 40 years of age. Yet, 10% of women above the age of 60 have evidence of a degenerative slip, most commonly at L4/L5. Such slips are more common in diabetics and in women status postoophorectomy and may be related to hormonally derived alterations in ligamentous laxity and arthritis of the facet joints. Also, biomechanical factors such as hemisacralization of the L5 body, sagittal orientation of the facets, and lowered intercrestal line (passing through L5 instead of L4) are more common in spondylolisthesis patients than in the population at large. The restraining effect of the iliolumbar ligament on L5 keeps it in place while L4 slides over it anteriorly. Unlike isthmic spondylolisthesis, the posterior arch is intact and may contribute to stenosis in these patients. The intact posterior elements also restrict the degree of slippage, however. Most cases have less than 30% sagittal width slip.

Three distinct pain syndromes are encountered in patients with degenerative spondylolisthesis. The first is that of mechanical back pain. Next, the slip may accentuate central canal stenosis, and symptoms of central thecal sac compression may exist. Finally, the L5 root may become entrapped between the upper edge of the L5 body and the superior facet. With more severe slips and stenosis, the L4 root may become compressed in its foramen.

Regardless of the symptoms, the majority of patients respond to nonoperative treatment. Therefore, except in the rare cases of rapidly progressive neurologic deficits, at least a 3-month trial of nonoperative measures is attempted prior to consideration of surgery. Indications for surgery include increasing neurologic deficits, intractable pain, and persistent functional limitations. As back pain is not reliably relieved with surgery, surgery is not recommended for patients with axial complaints only. The primary goal of treatment in this patient with refractory spinal stenosis is adequate decompression of the neural elements. Secondarily, concomitant arthrodesis is associated with decreased rates of postoperative slip progression. Further, it appears that concomitant fusion improves clinical outcome. The use of instrumentation is recommended by some as a means to increase the fusion rate. However, the relationship between fusion status and continued symptoms is debated.

Alternative Methods of Management

Traditionally, degenerative spondylolisthesis has been treated with decompression alone. Yet, significant postoperative slip progression and inferior outcomes were reported. Routine addition of fusion was recommended as a means to halt this progression and diminish the rate of laminar regrowth in these patients. Some authors recommended fusion based on certain identified risk factors for progression, such as female gender and disc space penetration.

The use of instrumentation is more controversial still. Clearly, fusion and instrumentation add to the potential morbidity and cost of surgical treatment. Although we fuse most patients undergoing decompression for stenosis in association with degenerative spondylolisthesis, there are no hard-and-fast rules for the addition of instrumentation. Some authors use instrumentation only in those cases in which significant risk of early postoperative progression is present, such as >50% or 3.5-mm slip, >6-mm disc height, or >10-degree angular motion on flexion-extension radiographs. However, there are no prospective data to support such risk stratification in these patients. Further, although some authors fuse all segments decompressed, we fuse only the listhetic segment.

Another option is posterior element preserving decompression. Microsurgical decompression techniques and laminotomy techniques have been described. Their exact indications and associated outcomes are not well known, however. Use of bilateral laminotomy or fenestration procedures seems to be increasing as a means of removing only that bone and soft tissue responsible for neural element compression. Although appealing in concept as a means of obviating fusion, early reports suggest that the risk of iatrogenic neurologic injury increases with these procedures.

Reduction maneuvers have been recommended by some authors as means to improve cosmesis, sagittal contour, and tension on the bone graft. Further normal alignment relaxes involved nerve roots by shortening their course. Presently, methods have included preoperative casting and halo-femoral traction; however, more commonly, an active intraoperative maneuver through the instrumentation is reported. Often, additional levels of cephalad and caudal fixation are required to increase the stability of the construct during these maneuvers.

Type of Management	Advantages	Disadvantages	Comments
Nonoperative management	Least costly Least morbid	Some patients will fail	A trial of nonoperative management is attempted in all patients
Decompression alone	Least surgical morbidity	May allow progression of deformity May be associated with laminar regrowth	Appropriate in hyperstable segments with significant disc height collapse and anterior osteophyte formation
Laminotomy	May preserve stability May obviate need for fusion	Greater chance of injury to neural elements Benefits regarding fusion avoidance unproven Increased time and skill required	May be an excellent alternative in the future
Laminectomy	Technically easier	Further destabilizes an unstable spine	Standard for decompression presently
Decompression and fusion	May decrease axial pain Prevents progression	Increased surgical morbidity	Appropriate in most cases to fuse the slip level
Uninstrumented	Less morbidity and cost than instrumented	Increased surgical morbidity Some early postoperative progression possible	Appropriate in most cases
Instrumented	Ability to obtain correction May allow higher fusion rates	Increased surgical morbidity Increased costs Increased early stability Failure in osteopenic bone	Appropriate for grossly unstable segments; increased fusion rates may or may not be related to improved outcomes

Complications

Rates of morbidity and mortality increase proportionally with age and the lengths and complexity of the procedure. Complications increase twofold, and overall outcomes decrease in patients with three or more medical comorbidities. The most serious potential complications are hardware-related injury of neural, vascular, or enteric structures. Vascular injury rates are low with laminectomy alone, but increase with the addition of bone graft harvest and instrumentation. A careful appreciation of the anatomy and stepwise palpation of the screw tract should minimize this complication. Neurologic injury may stem from instrumentation, mishandling of the roots (battered root syndrome), or postoperative arachnoiditis. An overall 4% rate of durotomy is reported; however, if primarily repaired in a watertight fashion, outcomes are not significantly affected. More likely problems include pseudarthrosis and wound infection.

Suggested Readings

Fischgrund J, Kurz LT. The radiographic assessment of spondylolisthesis. Semin Spine Surg 1993; 5:301–307.

Fischgrund J, MacKay M, Herkowitz HN, et al. Degenerative lumbar spondylolisthesis with spinal stenosis. A prospective randomized study comparing decompressive laminectomy and arthrodesis with and without spinal instrumentation. Spine 1997; 22:2807–2812.

Herkowitz HN, Kurz LT. Degenerative lumbar spondylolisthesis with spinal stenosis. A prospective study comparing decompression with decompression and intertransverse process arthrodesis. J Bone Joint Surg 1991; 73(A):802–808.

Hu SS. Internal fixation in the osteoporotic spine. Spine 1997; 22:43S–48S.

Katz J, Lipson S, Lew R, et al. Lumbar laminectomy alone or with instrumented or noninstrumented arthrodesis in degenerative lumbar spinal stenosis. Patient selection, costs, and surgical outcome. Spine 1997; 22:1123–1131.

Matsunaga S, Sahou T. Natural history of degenerative spondylolisthesis. Pathogenesis and natural course of the slippage. Spine 1990; 15:1204–1214.

Postacchini F, Cinotti G, Perugia D, Gumina S. The surgical treatment of central lumbar stenosis. Multiple laminotomy compared with total laminectomy. J Bone Joint Surg 1993; 75(B):386–392.

Spivak J. Degenerative lumbar spinal stenosis. Current Concepts Review. J Bone Joint Surg 1998; 80(A):1053–1066.

Case 15
Lumbar Degenerative Scoliosis with Spinal Stenosis
Eeric Truumees and Harry N. Herkowitz

History and Physical Examination

A 65-year-old woman with a medical history of diabetes presented with complaints of left greater than right leg pain as well as back pain of 6 years' duration. The pain proceeded from the back, around the buttock, and into the anterior-lateral thigh. The pain increased with increasing activity and was relieved by periods of rest. She noted a change in her waistline over the past several years as well. She denied bowel or bladder complaints or a history of cancer or trauma. She denied fever, chills, night pain, or other systemic complaints.

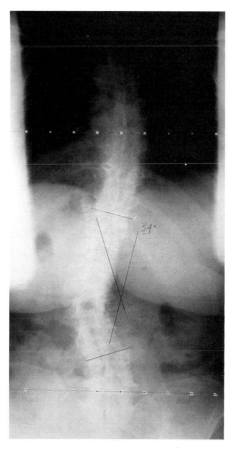 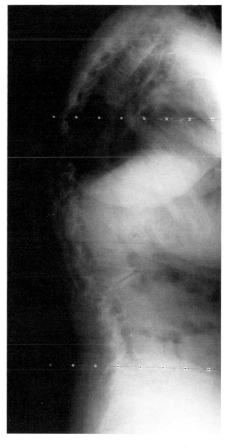

Figure 15–1. Anteroposterior (AP) long-cassette view of the thoracolumbar spine demonstrating a 34-degree lumbar scoliosis with lumbosacral and thoracic compensation. The spine is balanced in the coronal plane.

Figure 15–2. Lateral long-cassette view of the thoracolumbar spine demonstrating hypolordosis of the lumbar spine with increased thoracic kyphosis. Overall sagittal balance is forward 2 to 3 cm.

On physical examination, this well-nourished, pleasant female demonstrated a normal gait. She had mild tenderness in her midlumbar spine in both the midline and in the paravertebral muscles. She exhibited no unusual cutaneous findings in her back or lower extremities. On forward flexion, prominence of the left side ("lumbar hump") was noted. Leg lengths were equal, and coronal balance was maintained with symmetric shoulder heights. Clinically, sagittal balance was acceptable. A plumbline dropped from C7 passed along the gluteal cleft. The patient exhibited limitation of spinal range of motion (ROM) in all planes. Examination of the patient's hips failed to elicit pain or restriction in ROM. The remainder of her extremity and vascular exams were within normal limits. Abdominal examination was negative for masses, pain, or bruits. Neurologic exam was grossly normal with full strength and sensation. She had no tension signs.

Radiologic Findings

Radiographic evaluation began with anteroposterior (AP) and lateral projections of the lumbosacral spine as well as L5/S1 cone-down views. Incidental note of a lumbarized first sacral segment was made. This mobile segment will referred to as L6 for the purposes of the present evaluation. These studies also demonstrated degenerative changes of the spine with loss of disc height at L4/L5 and L5/S1. Further, a 34-degree curve of the lumbar spine with an apex at L3 was noted. The involved levels demonstrated little rotation; however, lateral and anterior olistheses are noted at the periapical segments. The posterior elements appeared intact. Normal psoas shadows, mild osteopenia, and intact pedicular anatomy were noted. As clinical evaluation of spinal balance was acceptable, 36-inch-long views were not obtained initially.

After initial plain radiographic evaluation, a period of nonoperative management was undertaken. The patient noted some improvement, but her leg pain continued to interfere with her daily activities. Therefore, further investigations were obtained, including long-cassette standing views of the thoracolumbar spine. A plumbline dropped from C7 fell to the middle of the sacrum, demonstrating good coronal balance (Fig. 15–1). On the lateral projection, a plumbline dropped from the anterior aspect of the C7 body fell 2 to 3 cm anterior to the L5/S1 disc, demonstrating slight forward sagittal balance (Fig. 15–2). Side-bending supine films were also obtained and demonstrated partial correction of her scoliosis to 12 degrees on right-side bend (Fig. 15–3). On left side-bending, an increase in the curve to 43 degrees was appreciated (Fig. 15–4). Flexion and extension lateral views were also obtained to exclude subtle instability patterns outside the curve. Magnetic resonance imaging (MRI) scan of the lumbosacral spine was obtained, including T1 and T2 parasagittal images and disc level axial images from L1/L2 to L6/S1. This study demonstrated diffuse degenerative changes, the lumbar scoliosis, as well as central canal and foraminal stenosis from L2/L3 to L5/L6 (Fig. 15–5). Parasagittal images demonstrated decreased interpedicular height with foraminal stenosis on the left at the L3/L4 and L4/L5 levels. Although invasive, computed tomography (CT) myelography is another option for imaging and may be preferable in certain difficult-deformity patients. The myelogram typically demonstrates indentation of the dye column at the apex of the curve.

Diagnosis

This generally healthy 65-year-old woman has lumbar spinal stenosis in conjunction with a nonrigid scoliosis. Her symptoms include diffuse pseudoclaudication as well as radiculitis from left-sided foraminal compression at the L3/L4 and L4/L5

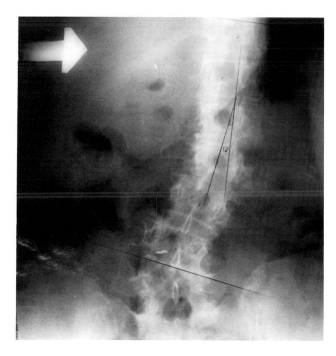

Figure 15–3. Right supine side-bending AP demonstrating correction of the deformity to 12 degrees. Note the overall lack of rotation of the involved vertebral segments.

segments. These symptoms have not been responsive to nonoperative treatment. Further, although no definitive evidence of interval progression was available, the patient's report of a sense of waistline symmetry changes suggests curve progression. For this reason, the risks, benefits, and alternatives of surgical intervention including laminectomy and instrumented spinal fusion were discussed with the patient.

Surgical Management

Further preoperative planning included standard preanesthesia laboratory studies, EKG, and chest radiographs. Dual energy x-ray absorptiometry (DEXA) scanning is

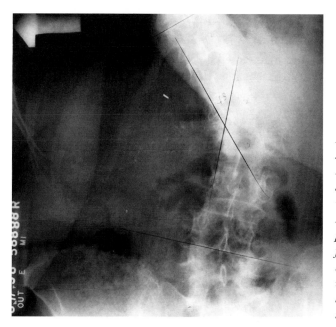

Figure 15–4. Left supine side-bending AP view of the lumbar spine demonstrating accentuation of the deformity with 43 degrees of scoliosis. Note the lateral listhesis of the periapical segments and the failure of the L5/L6 disc space to become parallel. Thoracic views on side bending similarly demonstrated failure of the secondary curve to correct.

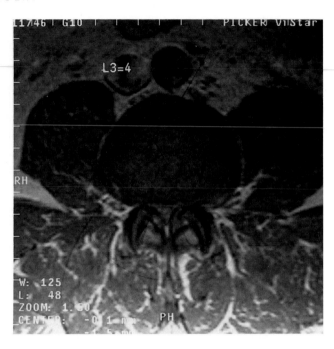

Figure 15–5. Sample T1-weighted axial MRI image at the L3/L4 interspace demonstrating severe stenosis with facet and ligamentum flavum hypertrophy.

recommended in patients with osteopenic bone should instrumentation be contemplated. As in all patients undergoing multilevel fusions, preoperative donation of three units of blood was recommended. Cell saver was also used. Electrodiagnostic monitoring was requested in this case because of anticipated conus level manipulations and instrumentation. A combination of sensory and motor evoked potentials along with electromyogram (EMG) testing of individual pedicle screws was obtained.

The patient was given a dose of antibiotics prior to skin incision. A generous skin preparation and draping were undertaken. Even if only a lumbar instrumentation is to be undertaken, the ability to inspect and palpate the entire spine is helpful in assessing coronal balance. A straight incision was marked using a long ruler or Bovie cord from the top of the intended fusion to the bottom. Alternatively, a straight line from the C7 spinous process to the sacral spine can be used. A generous incision is then made along this mark to facilitate exposure to the tips of the transverse processes. Careful preservation of the cranial and caudal-most facet capsules was maintained until local bony anatomy or radiographic confirmation of the level had been achieved. At this point, the capsules of the levels to be fused were excised and complete exposure of the lateral pars of each level was undertaken.

Decompression began with the removal of spinous processes with a double-action rongeur. The superior half of the superior process and the inferior half of the inferior process were preserved to maintain interspinous ligament integrity of neighboring levels. A Leksell rongeur was used to thin the laminae. A burr may also be used for this purpose. The ligamentum flavum was dissected from the inferior aspect of the superior level lamina of the inferior-most level with a 3-0 curette. This allowed introduction of a 3-mm Kerrison punch. A midline decompression was performed to the level of the superior border of the facet of the superior-most level. Next, the decompression was carried inferiorly through the superior aspect of the inferior lamina and then carried caudally to the inferior border of the inferior-most facet. With a midline decompression completed, attention was paid to the lateral recesses. A Penfield no. 4 dural separator was helpful to dissect any dural adhesions from the bony lamina. A 2-mm Kerrison punch was introduced and the decompression was carried laterally to the level of the pedicles. The extent of decompression was then assessed with the Woodson, or similar probe. Ample room for the thecal sac was present throughout. Evidence of foraminal stenosis was sought, particularly in the curve concavity. In the convexity, the Woodson passed freely out laterally. In this case, the concave side foramina of the periapical segments restricted passage of the probe. Therefore, further lateral decompression was attempted with an angled Kerrison punch in an effort to undercut the facets and prevent further destabilization. Had this not been possible, resection of the facets or pars would have been undertaken. Finally, the superior and inferior extents of the decompression were assessed. Had stenosis been encountered, the decompression would have been carried cephalad or caudad as needed.

With an adequate decompression completed, transpedicular hardware was inserted. In this patient with scoliosis, identification of appropriate entry sides and angles of approach was more difficult. An appreciation of the degree of rotation and translation of each involved segment was mandatory. The medial, superior, and inferior pedicular borders may be directly palpated with the Woodson from inside the canal. External bony landmarks include the lateral pars, the lateral facet, and the transverse process. In the medial-lateral plane, the pedicle usually lies between the pars and the outer border of the facet. Further, a line transecting the point of facet confluence with the lateral pars should accurately predict the dorsal-most aspect of the pedicle. In the superoinferior plane, the pedicles are bisected by the midline of the transverse process. This line should be 2 to 3 mm inferior to the midpoint of the facet joint. A 4-mm burr was used to enter the cortex of the pedicle entry site. A pedicle probe or 3-0 curette was used to sound the pedicle. Next, a thin probe was inserted into the pedicle to ensure cortical continuity. The Woodson was used to assess the outer pedicular cortex. A marker was then inserted and intraoperative fluoroscopy was employed to confirm localization. As the cortices were intact and imaging confirmed localization, a 5.5-mm tap was used to prepare the pedicle tract. Once tapped, the tract was again probed and the screw was inserted. Standard values of pedicle inclination, declination, or medial-lateral angulation are of little use in deformity cases. Some authors recommend intraoperative three-dimensional localization, such as the Stealth Station, in complex deformity cases. In most cases, however, careful assessment of the deformity and bony landmarks both in and outside the canal allows accurate pedicle identification.

As in all long spinal fusions, the retractor system was relaxed intermittently to allow vascularity to return to the paraspinal muscles. Further, the wound was copiously irrigated. Next, a complete decortication of the transverse processes, facet, and lateral pars was undertaken. A burr, rat-tooth rongeur, and gouges were used for this purpose. Autogenous bone graft was obtained from the posterior iliac crest and packed into the posterolateral gutters. In this patient, as in many older patients with multilevel fusions, augmentation of available iliac crest bone was required. Allograft croutons or demineralized bone matrix or both are acceptable in this context. With copious bone graft tamped into place, the longitudinal member of the instrumentation system was placed. Rods, rather than plates, were placed because of the greater ease of application in long deformity fusions and the room spared for bone graft.

Careful attention to maintenance of lumbar lordosis is critical in long lumbar fusions, particularly in this patient with slight positive sagittal balance preoperatively. The rod was precontoured. Then, the convex side was tightened first with only mild compression on the screws while the rod-screw connectors were tightened. Next,

- Other dynamic studies that may be employed in evaluating the adult deformity patient include standing side-bending and axial traction films, which are particularly helpful in severe deformities or when significant sagittal plane abnormalities are present.
- Curve characteristics that suggest progression or the need for fusion:
  - An intercrestal line through L5, not L4
  - Flexibility, as evidenced by greater than 50% correction on side bending
  - Loss of lordosis to the extent that sagittal balance is lost
  - Asymmetric tilt of a single interspace
  - Lateral spondylolisthesis or multiplanar instability (especially if >6 mm)
  - Documented curve progression
- If a fusion is required, include levels with
  - Subluxations
  - Stenosis
  - Posterior element deficiencies
- Careful preoperative planning will significantly increase operating-room efficiency. A surgical plan with estimated screw and hook types and sizes both encourages careful evaluation and measurement of the bony anatomy by the surgeon and allows the scrub personnel to anticipate hardware requests during the case.

the concave side was tightened with only a minimal amount of distraction. No rod rotation maneuvers were attempted. An intraoperative X-ray to further assess coronal balance was obtained. Watertight fascial closure was completed over suction drains at both the iliac crest and midline sites. Cutaneous sutures were followed by skin staples. A sterile, bulky postsurgical bandage was applied.

Postoperative Management

The patient was taken from the operating room to the recovery room. Once vital signs stabilized, she was transported to the regular nursing floor. If significant fluid shifts had occurred, especially in patients with limited cardiopulmonary reserve, a period of observation in the surgical intensive care unit would have been warranted. In this case, no bracing was required. However, postoperative use of a Thoracolumbosacral orthosis (TLSO) may be necessary in osteopenic patients with tenuous screw purchase. Protection of the low lumbar segments may require a pantaloon extension. The patient was mobilized to a chair the evening of surgery. Ambulation was progressed with physical therapy over the next several days. The drains were removed, and diet and pain medications were advanced on the second day after surgery. Antibiotics were continued for 48 hours. This patient was able to return home after 6 postoperative days in the hospital (Figs. 15–6 and 15–7).

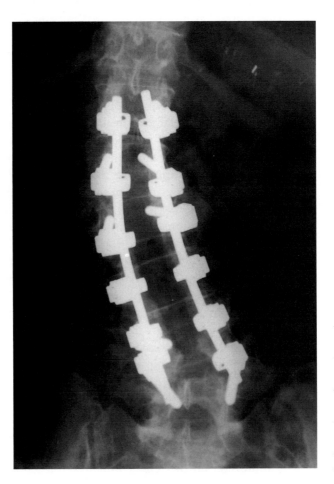

Figure 15–6. Postoperative (6 months) AP view of the lumbar spine demonstrating a multiple level posterolateral spinal fusion with transpedicular instrumentation (L1 to L6). A wide decompression of the spinal canal is demonstrated. Overall coronal balance has been maintained.

PITFALLS

- In patients with significant deformity, axial MRI scanning may give the appearance of displaced disc material. Most often this appearance is due to a nonorthogonal slice through the disc space.
- In patients with degenerative scoliosis and stenosis, decompression, spinal balance, and curve stabilization, not correction, are the critical surgical goals. Major curve correction at the level of primary curve may leave the spine unbalanced as compensatory curves are likely to be rigid.
- Hip pain may mimic an L4 radiculopathy and hip flexion contractures may cause or contribute to positive sagittal imbalance. Therefore, careful examination of the hips is crucial.
- Do not end fusions
  - At the apex of secondary deformities.
  - At kyphotic segments.
  - At segments with significant rotational deformity.

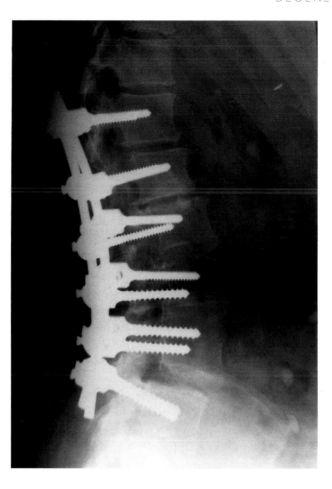

Figure 15–7. Postoperative (6 months) lateral view of the lumbar spine demonstrating instrumented spinal fusion with maintenance of lumbar lordosis.

Discussion

There is a 6 to 10% incidence of scoliosis in the older adult population. Approximately half represent de novo curve formation in association with degenerative destabilization of the spine in later life. The mean age for such curves is 60 years. Males and females are equally involved. These curves, overall, are smaller than residual idiopathic curves, and they exhibit less rotation and more segmental translation and instability. Progression of up to 3.3 degrees per year has been reported. Although Kostuik and Bontiviglio found the incidence of back pain in patients with adult scoliosis to be the same as that of the population at large, they did note an increase in incapacitating pain in those with curves greater than 45 degrees. Spinal fatigue, pain over the scoliotic prominence, and rib on iliac crest abutment pain are often reported. Other common symptoms involve those of compression of the central canal and the roots of L3/L4/L5 on the concave side.

Operative indications vary in the literature. In the absence of pain, the risk of progression might necessitate fusion. As younger and healthy patients have a longer life expectancy in which to progress, many authors recommend fusion for curves greater than 50 degrees. Fusion might be delayed in older patients until the curve exceeds 90 degrees. Other writers recommend fusion for all patients at 60 degrees because of the risk of progression and the high incidence of mechanical pain. More commonly, however, surgery is recommended for symptoms of neurologic compression.

In the absence of sagittal or coronal imbalance, reduction maneuvers are not indicated in these patients. If prestressed, older and osteopenic patients may experience screw failure.

If a fusion is to be undertaken, levels with rotatory or multiplanar subluxation should be included as should those that are stenotic or have posterior column deficiencies (prior laminectomy or spondylolysis, for example). The fusion should be extended cranially and caudally into an area of lordosis to prevent junctional kyphosis. In the coronal plane, the top and bottom of the instrumentation should pass through the central sacral line. The fusion should not end at the apex of any secondary deformity. If there is a major rotatory component, end the fusion at neutral vertebrae cranially and caudally. Whenever possible, the lumbosacral motion segment (L6/S1 in this case) should be excluded from the fusion.

Alternative Methods of Management

There is no universal approach to adult scoliosis. Further, careful distinction must be drawn between those cases of holdover patterns of idiopathic scoliosis and de novo patterns of spinal curvature stemming from degenerative destabilization. Some authors recommend decompression without fusion. The use of instrumentation is more controversial still. Clearly, fusion and instrumentation add to the potential morbidity and cost of surgical treatment.

Another option is posterior element preserving decompression. Microsurgical decompression techniques and laminotomy techniques have been described. Their exact indications and associated outcomes are not entirely established, however.

The anterior approach alone may be considered in patients undergoing fusion for curve progression in the absence of significant neural compression. This is particularly appropriate in younger patients. In older patients, osteopenia limits the usefulness of anterior instrumentation and hypertrophied facets are obstacles to correction from an anterior approach.

However, certain curves require even more challenging surgical intervention. Triplane osteotomies are recommended for severe, out of balance, and highly inflexible curves. Circumferential release and fusion procedures, or posterior lumbar interbody fusion (PLIF) procedures, may allow for greater correction and increased fusion rates, and are often recommended in curves greater than 70 degrees with rigid, unbalanced segments.

Type of Management	Advantages	Disadvantages	Comments
Nonoperative measures	Least morbid Least costly	Curve may progress Patient may not respond	Most cases are initially managed nonoperatively
Decompression alone	Least surgical morbidity	May allow progression of deformity	Appropriate in single root involvement when facets are preserved and in patients with hyperstable spines

Continued on next page

Continued

Type of Management	Advantages	Disadvantages	Comments
Laminotomy	May preserve stability May obviate need for fusion	Greater chance of injury to neural elements Benefits regarding fusion avoidance unproven Increased time and skill required	May be an excellent alternative in the future
Laminectomy	Technically easier May provide wider decompression in deformity patients	Further destabilizes an unstable spine	Standard for decompression presently
Fusion alone	May decrease axial pain Prevents progression	Increased surgical morbidity Will not relieve extremity pain	Appropriate when axial pain and fusion progression are the main considerations
Anterior	May preserve fusion segments May improve fusion rates	Decompression not possible Instrumentation fails in osteopenic bone Difficult to achieve lordosis	Rarely indicated in degenerative curves
Posterior	Allows decompression Allows restoration of lordosis	Extensor muscle disruption Increased blood loss Fusion rate may be lower	Primary means of fusion in degenerative scoliosis
Uninstrumented	Less morbidity and cost than instrumented	Increased surgical morbidity Some early postoperative progression possible	Appropriate in mild curves and 1–2 level fusions when foraminal stenosis from collapsed interpedicular height not present
Instrumented	Ability to obtain correction May allow higher fusion rates Increased early stability	Increased surgical morbidity Increased costs Failure in osteopenic bone Technically difficult in curve	Appropriate for most long decompressions, around apical segments, wide decompressions
Decompression and fusion	Single-stage procedure to address entire problem See individual advantages above	Compounds surgical time, cost, and morbidity	Procedure of choice in most cases of degenerative scoliosis
Posterior lumbar interbody fusion (PLIF)	Also a single-stage procedure to address entire problem May increase fusion rate May allow increased correction due to indirect anterior release	Additional morbidity Nerve root injury from traction Technically more difficult	Rarely needed as a primary procedure; useful in revisions in which anterior approach technically difficult
Osteotomy	Allows correction in stiff spines	Most surgical morbidity	Often performed as a 360-degree procedure in severe, out of balance curves

Complications

Overall, the long, instrumented fusions required in reconstruction of adult deformity patients are associated with much higher rates of morbidity and mortality than other procedures for degenerative diseases of the spine. Nelson and Trummel found an 80% rate of at least one complication, although only 23% were considered major. The most common complications included urinary retention and urinary tract infection. Pneumonia and other cardiopulmonary problems were not uncommon.

The most serious potential complications are hardware-related injury to neural, vascular, or enteric structures. A careful appreciation of the anatomy and stepwise palpation of the screw tract should minimize the risks of such injuries. In one series, a 3% rate of hardware-related root injury was reported in deformity patients.

Clinically apparent pseudarthroses are seen in 15 to 60% of patients undergoing multilevel posterior spinal fusion. Degeneration of adjacent segments may require further surgery in up to 25% of patients undergoing long spinal fusions. Another major problem in long lumbar fusions in elderly patients involves compression fractures at adjacent segments.

Finally, a syndrome of inappropriate release of the pituitary antidiuretic hormone (SIADH) is occasionally noted in spinal fusion patients. ADH release begins during surgery and usually resolves by the third postoperative day. It is important that electrolytes be monitored so that a rational volume management program is maintained and overhydration, in an effort to increase urine output, is avoided.

Suggested Readings

Bradford DS, Tribus CB. Current concepts and management of patients with fixed decompensation spinal deformity. Clin Orthop 1994; 306:64–72.

Dawson EG, Moe JH, Caron A. Surgical management of scoliosis in the adult. J Bone Joint Surg 1973; 55(A):437–441.

Hu SS. Internal fixation in the osteoporotic spine. Spine 1997; 22:43S–48S.

Kostuik JP. Recent advances in the treatment of painful adult scoliosis. Clin Orthop 1980; 147:238–252.

Marchesi DG, Aebi M. Pedicle fixation devices in the treatment of adult lumbar scoliosis. Spine 1992; 17(S):235–243.

Simmons EH, Jackson RP. The management of nerve root entrapment syndromes associated with the collapsing scoliosis of idiopathic lumbar and thoracolumbar curves. Spine 1979; 4:533–541.

Case 16
Microdiscectomy, Arthroscopic Discectomy, Chymopapain Injection
John A. McCulloch

History and Physical Examination

A 40-year-old man who worked as an executive presented with a 3-month history of spontaneous left-sided back pain. He had been working in the garden a few days before but had no specific injury. He noticed the back pain on arising one morning, and within a few days developed radiating left leg pain in a radicular distribution. He also noticed paresthetic symptoms over the dorsum of his left foot and when walking experienced a mild floppy foot left. When seen by his primary care doctor 3 weeks into symptoms, plain X-rays of the lumbar spine were ordered and reported as normal. Because of the severity of the sciatic discomfort, his primary care physician treated him with 7 days of bed rest, antiinflammatories, muscle relaxants, and pain medication. He did not improve and was referred to a spine surgeon. Three months into symptoms he described exclusively left leg pain in a typical radicular distribution down the back of his leg. He had 30 degrees of straight leg raising, crossover, and bowstring discomfort. He had 4+

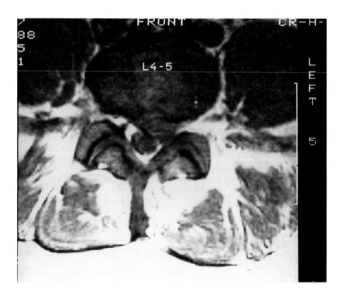

Figure 16–1. T1-weighted axial magnetic resonance imaging (MRI) showing a lumbar disc herniation (LDH) L4/L5 left. One should try to identify the nerve root.

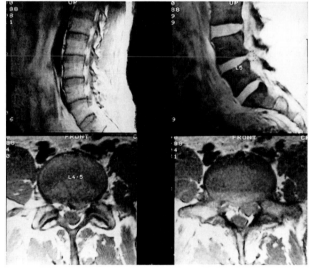

Figure 16–2. Top left: T1-weighted sagittal MRI showing a fragment not only opposite the disc space but also down behind the vertebral body of L5. Top right: Gradient echo sagittal MRI showing outline of disc herniation L4/L5. Bottom left: A T1-weighted axial showing the LDH opposite the disc space. Bottom right: A T1-weighted axial slice at the pedicle level showing a disc extrusion down behind the vertebral body of L5 and medial to the L5 root (an axillary disc herniation). There is much more operative information on these MRI cuts than on a computed tomography (CT) scan.

weakness in the L5 root distribution and had a sensory loss over the dorsum of his left foot. His reflexes were intact.

Radiologic Findings

Magnetic resonance imaging (MRI) of the lumbar spine revealed a left-sided paracentral L4/L5 disc herniation (Fig. 16–1). MRI alone is the preferred investigation for most surgeons treating soft tissue lesions in the lumbar spine. Although computed tomography (CT) scanning is half the cost, MRI delivers more than twice the surgical planning information than CT (Fig. 16–2). The exception to this is a poor MRI, which is worse than nothing. The open MRIs, which are designed to appeal to claustrophobic patients, are particularly prone to produce poor images. Because an MRI is ordered for surgical planning, the surgeon should review it to glean such information as where in the anatomic segment the lumbar disc herniation lies (Fig. 16–3), and where it lies relative to the nerve root, for example, central, axillary, anterior, lateral, or down beside the pedicle (Fig. 16–4). This is information that cannot be obtained from a CT scan. In reviewing the MRI, one must remember that 60% of patients aged 60 years or older have false-positive MRIs. If the physician believes that a patient has a disc herniation and it is not evident on MRI (a very unusual event), then a CT/myelogram is indicated. Electromyogram (EMG) and discography are of no use in the evaluation of a patient with an acute radicular syndrome (sciatica) due to a lumbar disc herniation (LDH).

Diagnosis

Hearing the report of dominant buttock and leg pain in the absence of back pain, the examiner should immediately think of the acute radicular syndrome due to an LDH. By getting the patient to place his leg on a stool and draw a map of the radicular distribution of the pain, the examiner can very quickly arrive at not only the diagnosis of sciatica likely due to a lumbar disc herniation, but also at an anatomic level. The more distal the symptoms are in the leg, the more valuable they are in lo-

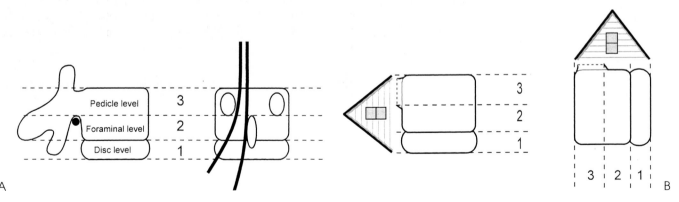

Figure 16–3. (A) The three stories (levels) of the anatomic "house" of each lumbar segment. The L5/L5 disc herniation in Figure 16–2 is not only in the first story of the fourth anatomic segment, it has migrated inferiorly into the third story of the fifth anatomic segment. (B) The three-storied house has a root of posterior elements, specifically the lamina (left). When the three-storied house is turned into the operative position (right), it is wise to know in which story the disc herniation lies so that appropriate but limited portions of the lamina can be removed to excise the LDH.

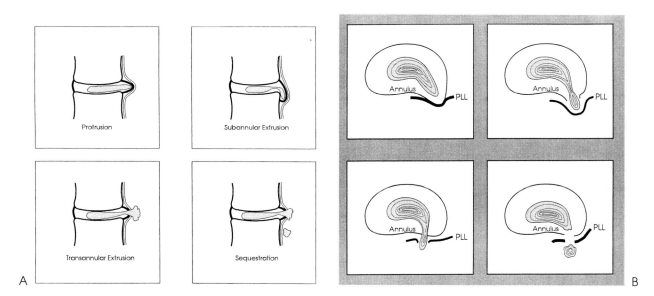

Figure 16–4. (A) Sagittal schematics of types of LDH. (B) Axial schematics of types of LDH. PLL, posterior longitudinal ligament.

calizing the anatomic level. With paresthesia over the dorsum of the foot, one should immediately suspect a fifth root involvement, and finding dorsiflexion weakness and an intact ankle reflex on examination supports this conclusion.

Surgical Management

In deciding on surgical management for such a patient, it is most important to keep in mind that one is performing nerve root surgery, not disc surgery. It is important to have a direct view of the nerve root intraoperatively so that it can be protected, retracted, and the encroachment pathology removed. Those procedures that primarily view the disc rather than the nerve root are doomed to failure. This would include automated percutaneous discectomy. Although these procedures do no harm, there are no randomized controlled trials showing they do some good. Procedures that forfeit clear three-dimensional viewing of the nerve root, such as microendoscopic discectomy (MED), have the potential of harming the nerve root and will eventually be discredited.

Today's gold standard for surgical management of a patient with an LDH is an open discectomy. This patient was taken to the operating room for a microdiscectomy, which was done on an outpatient basis. He received a single dose of Ancef 1 hour prior to surgery. If the patient had been allergic to penicillin we would have used clindamycin. The procedure was done in the kneeling (belly free) position under hypotensive anesthesia. Image intensifier localization of the surgical level was carried out prior to the skin incision. A 1- to $1\frac{1}{2}$-inch incision, centered over the skin marking line, was made. Single-segment paraspinal muscle elevation on the symptomatic left side over the L4/L5 disc space was completed. The wound was held open with a frame retractor. After exposing the interlaminar interval, the microscope was moved into position. The ligamentum flavum was not removed, but through peripheral dissection a flavum flap was designed, which in turn was used to reflect the fifth root medially. When in the spinal canal it is very important to first identify the

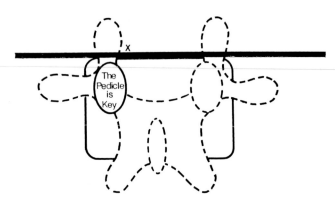

Figure 16–5. The pedicle is the key to nerve root anatomy. The heavy dark line (X) is the skin marking line the author places (with image-intensifier guidance) at the beginning of every microsurgical case. It is at the junction between the first story of one anatomic segment and the third story of the caudad anatomic segment. It marks the top edge of the pedicle. To prevent wrong-site spine surgery, extra special precautions such as the skin marking line are important when using small (microsurgical) incisions.

pedical (medial border) before identifying the lateral border of the nerve root (Fig. 16–5). It is always wise to know where the disc herniation lies relative to the nerve root by carefully reviewing the MRI (Fig. 16–2). An extruded or sequestered LDH may come to lie in the axilla of the nerve root (Fig. 16–2), displacing the root laterally where it can be damaged by the surgeon who does not first identify the pedicle. This exposure revealed a transligamentous disc extrusion (Fig. 16–1), which was removed; limited removal of intradiscal material was then carried out.

The patient was in the operating room for 1 hour; the blood loss was 25 cc. Within 3 hours of the operative procedure, the patient was discharged. No drain was placed.

Postoperative Management

The patient was given printed instructions that prescribed an immediate walking program and abstinence from bending and lifting. He was advised not to sit for prolonged periods of time, such as a for 2 or 3 hours, during the first two weeks. Within a week of the surgery he was allowed to take short drives and to return to work. In contrast, patients who work as laborers are prescribed work reconditioning for 6 weeks postoperatively, and do not return to work for 3 to 4 months after surgery. But this patient, an executive, was allowed to return to work 1 week postoperatively.

Discussion

Conservative Care

Ninety percent of patients who experience a lumbar disc herniation and sciatica will improve with conservative care. Only 10% of patients who experience their first-time LDH (causing the acute radicular syndrome) will require surgical intervention.

Adequate conservative care includes 3 days of rest off one's feet. This rest can be in bed, on the floor, on the sofa, or even in a recliner chair, provided that pressure is removed from the disc. The strongest antiinflammatory that is available is an oral steroid such as prednisone. It is probably just as effective as epidural cortisone, but research needs to be done to support this assertion. The severity of the pain dictates the analgesic medication that needs to be provided. In the acute radicular syndrome there is a limited role for exercise. Once the sciatica starts to settle in those 90% of patients who improve with conservative care, then the McKenzie exercise program is useful. Of limited use in the management of a patient with sciatica due to an LDH are muscle relaxants, root blocks, and chiropractic adjustments.

Conservative care should be provided for a minimum of 6 weeks and a maximum of 3 months. Lack of improvement in the sciatic discomfort and in the straight leg raising ability within 3 months is commonest indication for surgical intervention in an LDH.

If the patient presents with a cauda equina syndrome, progressive neurologic deficit, or a severe neurologic deficit such as a drop foot, then no time should be wasted on conservative care. Rather, the patient should undergo immediate investigation and surgical intervention. One must never let the sun set on a suspected cauda equina syndrome—it is a true spine surgical emergency. Other indications for surgical intervention besides the common failure of conservative care are recurrent history of sciatica and LDHs in special situations such as spinal canal stenosis and lytic spondylolisthesis.

Before proposing discectomy, one must be sure that one is dealing with an obvious radicular syndrome. It is also important to ascertain the anatomic level and to have a positive MRI that fits with the anatomic level. Also, it is best to have a motivated patient. Even Workers' Compensation patients with obvious disc herniations have a lower success rate than non-Compensation patients, and it is well to keep that in mind when proposing surgical intervention.

Surgery

In discussing surgical intervention with a patient, one should emphasize that the standard of care for an LDH causing sciatica that fails to respond to conservative care is open discectomy. All other techniques are unproven in scientific studies. A discectomy alters the short-term outcome by quickly relieving the patient's sciatica. However, in the long-term, a few years after the onset of acute sciatica due to an LDH, there is no difference between patients that have had surgery and patients that have followed a prolonged route of conservative care. Thus, the proposed surgical procedure should carry with it an effective outcome (90% success rate), should do no harm, and should cost as little to the system as possible. Microdiscectomy on an outpatient basis meets these requirements.

In discussing the risks, alternatives, and benefits with the patient, the surgeon should emphasize that the risks of a very limited skin and wound incision include (1) operating on the wrong level, which the surgeon is careful to avoid by doing pre-operative and intraoperative X-rays; (2) a dural tear; (3) nerve root injury; (4) retained pathology; and (5) a postoperative disc space infection, which is an extremely low risk (0.2%). Blood loss for a microdiscectomy is usually under 50 cc and averages about 25 cc. For this reason the risk of transfusion is low and the risk of a postoperative hematoma causing the cauda equina syndrome is low.

Lumbar Disc Herniations in Special Situations

There are many acute radicular syndromes due to an LDH that have, in addition, associated pathology. Such conditions as spinal canal stenosis and lateral zone stenosis can be compromised by an LDH. Disc herniations also occur in unusual locations, such as in the foramen and at higher lumbar levels such as L2/L3 and L3/L4. Disc herniations can be midline and cause bilateral leg pain, but they are very unusual and should constitute a very low percentage of surgeries. Equally unusual are multilevel LDHs and bilateral LDHs, which should constitute less than 1% of the indications for disc surgery. Even rarer still is the conjoint nerve root compromised by LDH.

Lumbar disc herniations also occur in instability syndromes such as degenerative spondylolisthesis and lytic spondylolisthesis, and in patients with a long history of significant back pain. In these three groups of patients, one needs to consider whether or not a lumbar fusion is required. Other than these three situations, there is no indication to consider a lumbar fusion in a patient with an acute radicular syndrome who is going to have a simple discectomy.

Alternative Methods of Management

The only other alternative method of treatment that has been proven in randomized control trials (RCTs) is chemonucleolysis. I reserve this technique for young patients because they usually have a wide disc space full of proteoglycan, which can be effectively hydrolyzed by the chymopapain. Also, patients below the age of 25 tend to have contained disc herniations rather than noncontained LDHs. Surgery in this young age group exposes the patient to a significant risk of recurrent symptoms and future surgery.

Other alternative methods of management have been unproven in randomized control trials. The automated percutaneous lumbar discectomy has been thoroughly discredited through a number of prospective randomized control trials.

The manual percutaneous lumbar discectomy procedure also has its problems. There are no published randomized control trials to support its efficacy. Kambin has completed a randomized control trial that is to be published in the near future. He has published a prospective paper on arthroscopic microdiscectomy, but with changing technology in his study period from 1988 to 1998, one has to wonder how prospective the trial was. As well, Kambin's technology has been changing over the years, but his results have not changed. In addition, these uniportal or biportal manual techniques are technically demanding and require a lot of time to complete the procedure, exposing the surgeon to excessive radiation. The instrumentation is necessarily small and less effective than instruments used in open discectomy. The main reason for questioning the efficacy of manual percutaneous lumbar discectomy is that is precludes three-dimensional visualization and the excellent illumination that is inherent in the microscope.

Adding a laser to the manual percutaneous lumbar discectomy has failed to live up to its expectations. The costs are high, it is difficult to control the laser and to avoid complications, and thermal endplate injuries, common dural sac injuries, and root injuries have occurred with too great a frequency.

The newest procedure available to remove an LDH is microendoscopic discectomy (MED). It is also experimental and unproven in clinical trials. It was born out of one neurosurgeon's frustration with the manual percutaneous discectomy techniques. It is being popularized in the spine surgery community, but with the high incidence of dural tears and root injuries due to the reduced visualization and the handcuff of the tubular retractor, it is likely going to be discredited in the near future.

Type of Management	Advantages	Disadvantages	Comments
Open discectomy	Simple, proven procedure	Bigger wound Poor visualization compared to microscope	Being superseded by microdiscectomy
Microdiscectomy	Equal to open discectomy results Better visualization	Minor learning curve	Microscope useful for many other conditions in spine
Automated percutaneous discectomy	Simple RCTs show it not to be effective	Simple RCTs show it not to be effective	Should not be used
Manual percutaneous discectomy	Less invasive	Poor visualization Technically demanding, labor intensive Unproven in RCTs	Desperately in need of RCTs
Chemonucleolysis	Needle procedure Proven efficacious in RCTs	High complications rate Increased back pain after injection Failure rate of 30%	Use should be confined to young patients
Conservative treatment	Works in at least 90% of patients	Fails in 10% of patients	The first line of treatment

RCTs, randomized controlled trials.

Summary

In dealing with the simple problem of a lumbar disc herniation that fails to respond to conservative care, "first do no harm." To avoid harm, the surgeon should not give up visualization and illumination, which is the strength of the microscope. Randomized controlled trials and multiple retrospective trials have clearly indicated that the gold standard for surgical intervention is an open discectomy. I believe that the microscope facilitates this surgical effort.

Suggested Readings

Delamarter RB, McCulloch JA. Microdiscectomy and microsurgical laminotomies. In: Frymoyer JW, ed. The Adult Spine, pp. 1961–1988. Philadelphia: Lippincott-Raven, 1997.

Kambin P, O'Brien E, Zhou L, Schaeffer J. Arthroscopic microdiscectomy and selected fragmentectomy. Clin Orthop 1998; 347:150–167.

Multiple authors. Focus issue on disc herniation. Spine 1996; 21:1S–78S.

Tullbert T, Isacson J, Weidenhielm L. Does microscopic removal of lumbar disc herniation lead to better results than the standard procedure? Spine 1993; 18:24–27.

Case 17

Lumbar Degenerative Disc Disease— Axial Low Back Pain: Minimally Invasive Laparoscopic Approach

John D. Tydings, Alexander R. Vaccaro, and Philip Minotti

History and Physical Examination

A 28-year-old white woman presented with a 3-year history of unrelenting low back pain without leg pain, as a result of a motor vehicle accident. This was unresponsive to conservative treatment. Her low back pain was primarily activity related and severely restricted her activities of daily living.

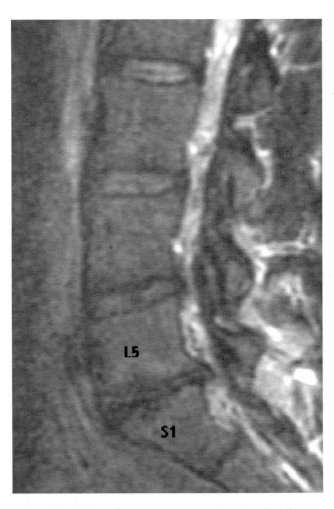

Figure 17–1. Lateral magnetic resonance imaging (MRI) showing disc degeneration with a herniation at the L5/S1 level.

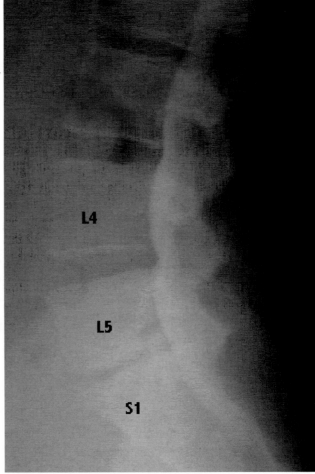

Figure 17–2. Lateral myelogram showing mild spinal stenosis at the L4/L5 level.

- In the setting of supporting radiographic studies, the key to deciding whether a decompression and/or a stabilization surgery is necessary is the proportion of leg pain to back pain. When back pain is overwhelming and predominant, a decompression alone will usually be ineffective for long-term pain relief.

- Discography is very user dependent. The skill, expertise, and experience of the discographer can be as important as that of the surgeon. Thus, the discographer should be experienced with the technique, familiar with the concept of pain provocation, and able to establish good rapport with the patient. The patient should understand the difference between simple pain production and typical pain reproduction.

Radiologic Findings

Plain anteroposterior (AP), lateral, and flexion extension radiographs revealed decrease in height of the L5/S1 disc space without translational instability. Magnetic resonance imaging (MRI) revealed multilevel lumbar disc degeneration with a left paracentral herniated disc at L5/S1 with a disc protrusion at the L4/L5 level (Fig. 17–1). A myelogram demonstrated tricompartmental stenosis left greater than right at the L4/L5 level as well as a left-sided disc herniation at L5/S1 (Fig. 17–2). Due to the patient's overwhelming back pain with minimal leg discomfort, the patient underwent provocative discography. The L3/L4 and L4/L5 levels produced no pain whatsoever (Fig 17–3). L5/S1 caused concordant provocation of the patient's typical pain complex of low back pain (Fig. 17–4).

Diagnosis

Symptomatic degenerative disc disease L5/S1.

Surgical Management

The patient was brought to the operating room where she underwent an anterior lumbar interbody fusion of L5/S1 with BAK (Bagby and Kuslich) cages and autologous right iliac crest bone graft via a laparoscopic approach. The laparoscopic approach was performed by a vascular surgeon with specialization in laparoscopy (Figs. 17–5 and 17–6). The interbody fusion was performed by the orthopaedic spine service (J.T.). The surgery took approximately $3\frac{1}{2}$ hours. The right anterior iliac crest bone graft was obtained first. Once this wound was closed, the surgical approach to the spine was commenced.

The laparoscopic portals were placed according to preincision radiographic assessment with fluoroscopy. A visualization portal was placed cephalad at about the

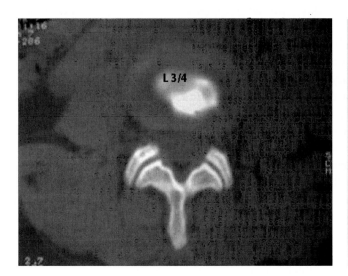

Figure 17–3. Axial postdiscogram CT of L4/L5 showing normal disc appearance.

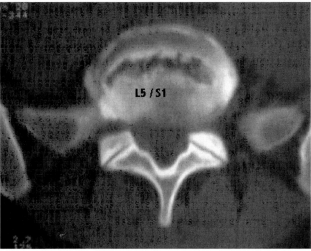

Figure 17–4. Axial postdiscogram CT of L5/S1 showing severe disc degeneration.

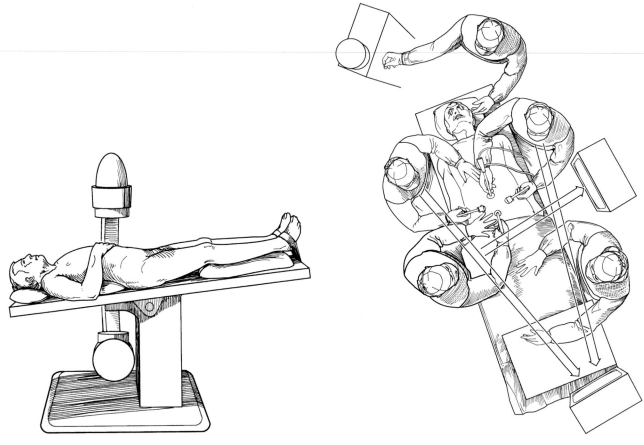

Figure 17–5. The patient is positioned in a slight Trendelenburg position to allow the abdominal contents to displace cephalad out of the surgical field.

Figure 17–6. An illustration of physician and monitor placement.

PITFALLS

- It is important to avoid the use of analgesics during discography as they can mask the pain response. Mild intravenous sedation is appropriate and often necessary during this procedure.
- It is important that a control level be present. If every disc that is injected produces severe unrelenting pain, surgery is to be avoided.
- The success rate for spinal fusion surgery is significantly lower in patients who have three or more positive levels.

umbilical area. Two working portals were placed on the right and left side. A standard laparoscopic setup was used, with insufflation with carbon dioxide. Visualization was with multiple TV monitors at both ends of the patient. The C-arm monitor was placed on the patient's left.

The abdominal surgeons took great care to mobilize the sigmoid colon and identify and protect all vascular structures. Once the L5/S1 disc space was identified, all soft tissues including fibers of the hypogastric nervous plexus were blunted and cleared to allow placement of the interbody cages. The alignment guide was placed under laparoscopic vision as well as fluoroscopic guidance. The appropriate entrance sites were marked with the alignment guide and again checked fluoroscopically. The 8-mm drill was placed through the suprapubic port. Long pituitary rongeurs were used to remove nuclear material at this time. Distraction plugs were placed. A 9-mm plug was placed on the patient's left. A 10-mm plug was placed on her right. This provided excellent distraction and an extremely tight fit. The position and orientation of the plugs were also confirmed fluoroscopically. The protective sheath from the instrumentation set was placed through the incision after the TEK-18 port was removed. Using the supplied tools, the protective sheath for cage insertion was placed through this wound.

PEARLS

- During surgery the patient must be placed in a steep Trendelenburg position. Use of a foam headrest and large IV bags under the shoulders may be useful to prevent pressure injury during this often long surgical procedure. Taping the ankles or using some type of harness such as Buck's traction boots is also appropriate to avoid patient movement during the surgical procedure.
- It is important to remember that the video camera is usually positioned in a cephalad to caudal direction. This will provide an image that is opposite to what the spinal surgeon is accustomed to viewing. It is sometimes easier to work fluoroscopically and use the video image to confirm safety when necessary.

The first step of the actual cage insertion was to place the primary reamer to establish the channel. The second step was to place the secondary reamer to complete the channel. After this was removed, another long pituitary rongeur was used to remove extra disc material, all the way back to the annulus. This was checked several times fluoroscopically. The channel was then tapped with the supplied bone tap. A 13- $\times$ 20-mm cage was placed on the insertion device. The leading edge was packed with the previously harvested cancellous bone graft. This was then driven into the channel until it was slightly recessed below the surface of the anterior longitudinal ligament. After this was completed, in the exact same manner, the left-side cage was then inserted (Fig. 17–7). Using the supplied bone tamp, the trailing edges of both cages were packed with additional cancellous bone. Visualization demonstrated that the cages were recessed below the level of the anterior surface of the spine and the bone graft was packed accordingly. All anatomic structures were safely identified and found to be in excellent condition. At this time, the wounds were closed. General anesthesia was reversed. The patient was then transported to the recovery room in stable condition (Fig. 17–8).

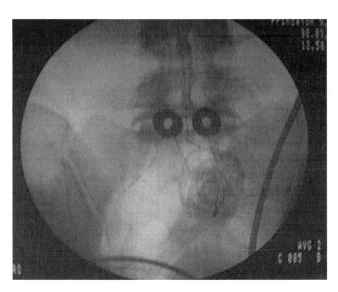

Figure 17–7. Intraoperative fluoroscopy showing final position of the cages.

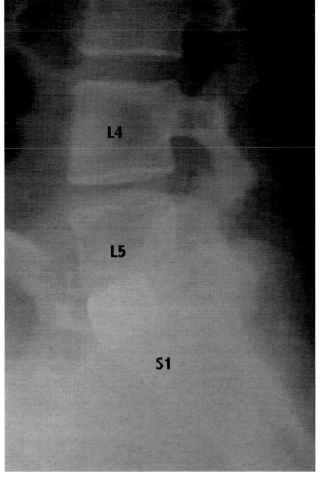

Figure 17–8. Postoperative lateral X-ray showing position of the cages.

- Placing a sponge into the abdomen is useful for dabbing small bleeders and maintaining a clear visualized field. Be sure its presence is accounted for at all times and that it is removed prior to closure.
- It is very important, especially at L5/S1, that the angle of approach be consistent with the most caudal portal, as this will determine the placement of the cages and the ease with which this can be accomplished.
- At all times surgical instrumentation must be checked both visually with laparoscopic video and radiographically with C-arm fluoroscopy.
- Postoperative mobilization should be swift. The sooner the patient is returned to normal activities, the better the rehabilitation process. The use of an abdominal binder or brace is not necessary but often provides an extra measure of comfort that allows these patients to be mobilized sooner and more aggressively. Extensive rigid bracing is neither necessary nor appropriate.

PITFALLS
- Contraindications to a laparoscopic approach include the presence of a peritoneal or pelvic infection or a history of a previous open anterior surgery of the lumbar spine.
- Relative contraindications include gross obesity, previous lower abdominal surgeries, previous laparotomy, endometriosis, and severe atherosclerosis.

Postoperative Management

The patient was supplied with a Warm and Forme type of abdominal binder/brace. She was started on ambulation as soon as she was awake. Later that night, she was independently walking around her room as well as up and down the hospital floor. Clear liquids were started that night. By the following morning, she was tolerating a general liquid diet without any signs of an ileus. She was discharged that morning, with appropriate follow-up appointments scheduled. Oral analgesics were necessary.

At follow-up, the patient has had an outstanding result. She has had no residual back discomfort as of her 1-year follow-up.

Discussion

Currently, the topic of degenerative disc disease as a pain generator is controversial. Many spine surgeons continue to feel that fusion surgery for back pain is to be condemned. However, recent controlled prospective studies have supported surgical intervention for the treatment of symptomatic degenerative disc disease in appropriately selected patients who have failed to improve with an extended period (greater than 6 months) of conservative therapy. With the advent of interbody lumbar cages, the success rate for this type of surgery has risen dramatically in terms of functional improvement. Additionally, the laparoscopic insertion of these cages has decreased the surgical morbidity of these procedures, allowing earlier patient mobilization and return to normal activities.

Surgery for lumbar degenerative disc disease is intended for patients with severe, unrelenting back pain of at least 6 months' duration, and who have undergone appropriate conservative modalities without any significant pain relief. The pain must be at a level where it is interfering not only with their occupational demands, but also with their activities of daily living and normal lifestyle. Conservative treatment at the least should include antiinflammatory medication, physical therapy with an appropriate exercise program, and the use of other modalities as determined by the treating physician. Because the natural history of low back pain for the majority of patients involves pain resolution without surgery, an ample time period must be provided to allow this to occur. Surgery for lumbar degenerative disc disease is an elective procedure, as bowel and/or bladder dysfunction or progressive paralysis are not associated with this spinal disorder in the absence of significant neural compression.

A vital diagnostic test to help identify patients' pain generator is lumbar discography. This test is still considered controversial as many surgeons feel that the false-positive rate, which varies depending on the spinal diagnostician's experience, is unacceptably high due to the subjective nature of a patient's pain response. Certainly, plain radiographic analysis alone in determining the cause of lower back pain has been shown to have no correlation with eventual surgical outcome. The key to discographic analysis of patients with back pain is not the objective radiographic data, but the pain response provided by the patient in reaction to pressurization of the disc. This is useful not only diagnostically but also for prognostication therapeutically. Due to the subjective nature of this diagnostic modality, it is appropriate that this testing be done by an independent physician well trained in this technique. In this patient's case, several other abnormal radiographic lesions were identified on computed tomography (CT) myelography and MRI, all of which were felt not to contribute significantly to her pain complaints. The discography showed that L5/S1 alone was responsible for generating her pain. For this reason, this isolated level was selected for surgical intervention.

Interbody fusions with cages have been Food and Drug Administration (FDA) approved since 1996. The laparoscopic approach for this procedure was approved by the FDA in July 1997. The patient presented here selected this technique after its decreased morbidity was explained to her. She had previously rejected an open posterior surgical approach due to the magnitude of the procedure and duration of expected rehabilitation.

L5/S1 is the easiest level to address laparoscopically due to its location below the bifurcation of the iliac vessels. More cephalad or multiple levels require significant manipulation of the great vessels and abdominal organs as well. A significant complication of both the anterior open and laparoscopic approaches is the risk of retrograde ejaculation in male patients. There appears to be an increased risk of developing retrograde ejaculation with laparoscopic approaches as compared to standard retroperitoneal approaches.

Alternative Methods of Management

A time-honored alternative method of management for this patient is continued physical therapy, activity modification, and antiinflammatory medication. Long-term narcotic usage should be discouraged with this spinal disorder due to the chronicity of symptom complaints and the potential for drug addiction. Many surgeons feel that a stand-alone anterior or posterior interbody fusion is inadequate biomechanically and have suggested the addition of adjunctive posterior instrumentation acting as a tension band for improved flexion and rotational stability. Less successful surgical interventions have included discectomy alone via open or fluoroscopically guided, minimally invasive techniques. The results of decompressive

Type of Management	Advantages	Disadvantages	Comments
Physical therapy Antiinflammatory medication Spinal injections	60 to 70% of patients report some degree of pain relief Minimal adverse side effects	A small percentage of patients are unresponsive to these treatment modalities	Time-honored treatment protocol for low back pain due to degenerative disc disease
Posterior lateral instrumented fusion (pedicle screws)	Avoids the anterior approach No risk of retrograde ejaculation	Does not surgically address the proposed pain generation—i.e., intervertebral disc and annulus fibrosus	Often results in immediate relief of pain but not to the degree of an anterior interbody fusion Greater soft tissue morbidity and longer rehabilitation period than anterior surgery
Anterior and posterior circumferential fusion	Rigid stabilization directly addressing the pain generator Improved flexion and rotational stability as compared to anterior alone procedure	Extended surgical time Increased soft tissue morbidity and prolonged rehabilitation period	Improved fusion rate and improved stability over anterior stand alone procedures

surgery alone for axial low back pain are universally poor. Alternative fusion procedures include an in situ posterolateral arthrodesis, posterior segmental instrumentation with a posterolateral arthrodesis, and reconstruction of the anterior and posterior spinal columns.

Complications

The majority of complications of this surgical technique are related to the approach and exposure. These include, but are not limited to, abdominal organ injury, vascular compromise, retrograde ejaculation, pelvic organ injury, and superficial or deep infection.

Suggested Readings

Hacker RJ. Comparison of interbody fusion approaches for disabling low back pain. Spine 1997; 22(6):660–666.

McAfee PC, Regan JJ, Geis WP, Fedder IL. Minimally invasive anterior retroperitoneal approach to the lumbar spine. Emphasis on the lateral BAK. Spine 1998; 23(13):1476–1484.

Obenchain TG, Cloyd D. Laparoscopic lumbar discectomy: description of transperitoneal and retroperitoneal techniques. Neurol Clin North Am 1996; 7(1): 77–85.

Zdeblick TA. Laparoscopic spinal fusion. Orthop Clin North Am 1998; 29(4): 635–645.

Case 18
Recurrent Lumbar Disc Herniation
R. Scott Meyer and Steven R. Garfin

History and Physical Examination

A 38-year-old woman presented with moderate low back pain and severe radiating right leg pain that had persisted for several weeks. A presumptive diagnosis of herniated lumbar disc was made and the patient was begun on a course of nonoperative treatment including activity modification, physical therapy, nonsteroidal antiinflammatory drugs, and a course of epidural steroid injections. After 3 months of nonoperative treatment she was still experiencing severe radiating right leg pain. Plain radiographs were normal (Fig. 18–1) and magnetic resonance imaging (MRI) of the lumbar spine confirmed a paracentral herniated disc at L5/S1 (Fig. 18–2).

The patient underwent a right L5/S1 laminotomy and discectomy without complication. Postoperatively she experienced immediate relief of her radiating right leg pain and after several weeks had returned to work and her usual activities. She continued to have mild low back pain.

Approximately 9 months following her surgery, the patient returned with increasing low back pain and an acute recurrence of right leg pain. Her pain was similar to the previous episode, radiating down the posterior thigh and into the lateral border of the foot. She had numbness in the same distribution but denied any leg weakness. She did not have any fevers, chills, recent weight loss, or any bowel or bladder dysfunction.

On physical examination the patient had a well-healed lumbar midline scar. She had palpable muscle spasm on the right in the lower lumbar spine. Range of motion of the lumber spine was approximately 50% of normal in both flexion and exten-

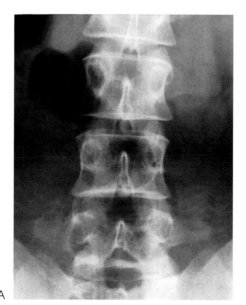
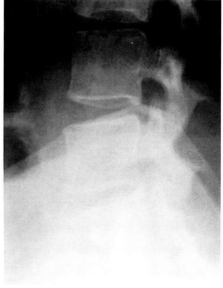

A   B

Figure 18–1. Anteroposterior (A) and lateral (B) radiographs of the lumbar spine.

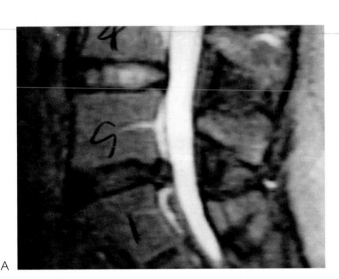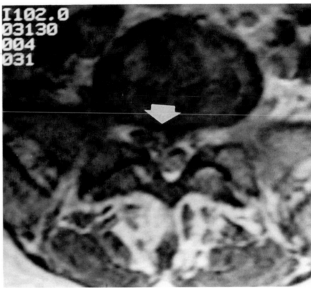

A   B

Figure 18–2. Magnetic resonance imaging (MRI) of the lumbar spine. Sagittal T2-weighted (A) and axial proton density (B) images show a herniated disc to the right at L5/S1.

sion. Motor strength in the lower extremities was normal throughout. Sensory examination revealed subjective diminished sensation in the lateral border and plantar aspect of the foot. Deep tendon reflexes were normal at the knees and left ankle, but the right ankle reflex was diminished. Straight leg raising reproduced her pain in the right foot. Vascular examination of the lower extremities was normal.

Radiologic Findings

Plain radiographs of the lumbar spine revealed slight disc space narrowing at L5/S1. Flexion-extension lateral radiographs of the lumbar spine did not reveal any instability. MRI with gadolinium showed a mass in the right lateral recess at L5/S1 with central low signal intensity on T1- and T2-weighted sequences. On the T1-weighted postgadolinium images, the mass was surrounded by a margin of enhancement (Fig. 18–3).

Diagnosis

Recurrent right L5/S1 herniated disc.

Surgical Management

Initially the patient was begun on a course of nonoperative treatment including activity modification, physical therapy, nonsteroidal antiinflammatory drugs, and a course of epidural steroid injections. She again failed this course of treatment and approximately 12 weeks later consented to a repeat right L5/S1 laminotomy and discectomy.

The patient was placed in the kneeling position, with the abdomen free, thus reducing intraabdominal pressure and minimizing epidural venous bleeding. One gram of intravenous cefazolin was used for antibiotic prophylaxis. The operation was performed under loupe magnification with a head light. An incision along the patient's previous scar was made. Dissection was then carried down to the lumbodorsal fascia, which was then incised off the midline to the right from L5 to S1. The right paraspinous musculature was stripped subperiosteally from the spinous processes and laminae of L5 and S1 and carried out to the facet joint of L5/S1. The presence of scar and palpation of the sacrum ensured dissection to the appropriate level. Prior to removing epidural scar, the previous laminotomy of both L5 and S1 were extended to find more normal anatomy. Using a combination of Penfield elevators, small curettes, and a dental pick, the epidural scar was carefully elevated from the previous laminotomy site. Working proximally and distally from normal to abnormal scarred anatomy, the lateral border of the nerve root was identified. A partial facetectomy was performed to safely stay lateral to the nerve root.

After exposure of the lateral border of the S1 nerve root, coursing medial to the pedicle wall, care was taken to dissect the root from the underlying disc. This was done using a combination of bipolar electrocautery and dissection with a small Penfield elevator and dental pick. A root retractor was placed and a knife used to cut a window in the

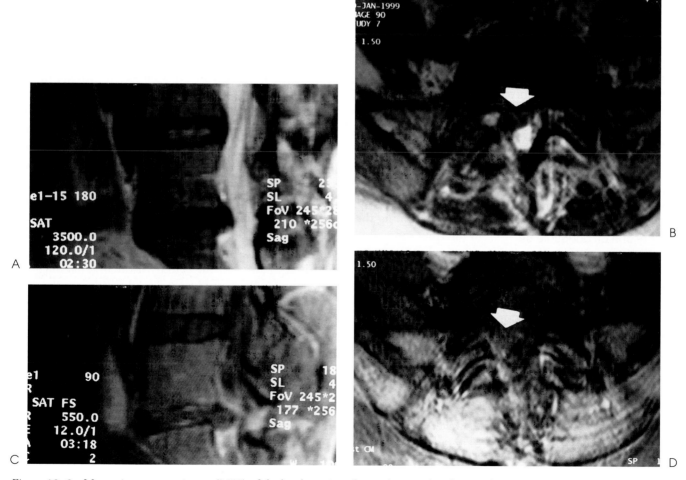

Figure 18–3. Magnetic resonance image (MRI) of the lumbar spine obtained 9 months after a right L5/S1 laminotomy and discectomy. Sagittal T2-weighted (A) and axial T2-weighted (B) images show a large mass in the right lateral recess (white arrow) with low signal intensity. After administration of intravenous gadolinium, sagittal T1-weighted (C) and axial T1-weighted (D) images show the mass continues to have low central signal intensity and is surrounded by a margin of enhancing material (white arrow). These imaging characteristics are consistent with a recurrent disc herniation to the right at L5/S1.

scar, posterior longitudinal ligament, and annulus overlying the disc space. A large amount of disc material was then removed using a combination of straight and angled pituitary rongeurs. A Scoville curette was used to impact any remaining disc material into the disc space, both medially and laterally, and this was removed. The disc space was then irrigated through a small catheter. No further free disc material was identified. A foraminotomy was performed to ensure that the S1 nerve root was completely free. A Frazier elevator could then be passed medially, anterior to the dura, and out the foramen anterior and posterior to the root, confirming that the nerve root was free in both tension and compression. The wound was closed in layers and a sterile dressing applied.

Postoperative Management

The patient experienced immediate partial relief of her leg pain. She was mobilized out of bed on the evening of surgery. She was given 24 hours of intravenous cefazolin and was discharged the next day after being cleared by the physical therapist. Her right leg pain continued to improve over a period of several weeks. At 1-year follow-up she had mild low back pain, but no radiating leg pain.

Discussion

Most patients undergoing laminotomy and excision of a herniated disc will experience immediate, or at least rapid, relief of leg pain. If the patient's postoperative pain persists beyond several weeks, or if the patient experiences a recurrence of similar pain shortly after the operation, the surgeon must consider that adequate decompression of the nerve root was not achieved. One reason for this may be disc excision at the wrong level. New lumbar spine radiographs should be obtained and the correct level of surgery confirmed with the preoperative imaging studies. If surgery at the wrong level is confirmed, this should be discussed with the patient and repeat surgery at the correct level should yield the expected good results.

A repeat imaging study, such as MRI with gadolinium enhancement, may be useful in determining the existence of a retained disc fragment, but it may be difficult to interpret soon after surgery because of hemorrhage and/or postoperative inflammatory changes.

A patient can also have persistent pain after discectomy if the original diagnosis was incorrect. The original imaging studies should be reviewed to confirm the diagnosis, and if there is any question as to its correctness, further workup should begin.

Patients following laminotomy and discectomy may initially have good relief of leg pain and a satisfactory clinical result, but experience recurrence of radicular pain over the next several weeks or months. Although a recurrent herniated disc may be responsible for a short-term failure, this is much more common in patients who have a pain-free interval greater than 6 months. More common causes of early recurrence of leg pain include infection, including discitis, vertebral osteomyelitis, and epidural abscess; meningeal cyst from inadvertent durotomy; and battered root syndrome. The latter may be associated with persistent leg pain following surgery, but may also be a reason for early recurrence of pain that was initially relieved. These patients may also have new neurologic findings such as numbness and weakness. Factors predisposing to the battered root syndrome include prolonged and aggressive root retraction, excessive bleeding, and the presence of a conjoined nerve root.

In patients such as the one presented above, an initial discectomy may be successful, but provide relief only for several months or years. In these cases a recurrent herniated disc should be suspected. The recurrent herniation can occur at the same level on the same side, the same level on the opposite side, or at a different level. The reported incidence of recurrent disc herniation following laminotomy and discectomy is variable. Within the first 6 weeks, the recurrence rate on the same side and level is rare. Recurrence at any level at any time after the original procedure has been reported to be from 1 to 19%.

Recurrent disc herniations usually have a rim enhancement pattern on T1 imaging shortly following the administration of intravenous gadolinium, whereas epidural scar uniformly enhances throughout the mass in question. Care must be taken in interpreting these images within the first few months following surgery, when the epidural space is filled with blood and early scar. Boden and colleagues have shown that a mass, similar in appearance to the original herniation, can be seen immediately following nearly all successful lumbar discectomies. In addition, 40% of the patients studied had gadolinium enhancement of the rim only, the classic finding of a recurrent disc herniation.

Patients who present with a recurrent lumbar disc herniation should initially be treated with a similar approach to a patient with a primary disc herniation. Only patients who fail an adequate trial of nonoperative treatment should be considered for repeat laminotomy and discectomy. Indications for more urgent surgical treatment, similar to cases of primary disc herniation, include cauda equina syndrome, a progressive neurologic deficit, a severe static neurologic deficit, and severe intractable radicular pain.

Reoperation for a different level recurrent disc herniation is no different than for a primary disc herniation. Reoperation for a same-site herniated lumbar disc, however, is technically more demanding than the primary operation. The risk of iatrogenic nerve root injury and/or dural tear is significantly reduced when dissection is begun in an area of normal anatomy. This is accomplished by enlarging the previous laminotomy, and may include partial facetectomy to adequately visualize the lateral border of the nerve root.

The results of reoperation after lumbar disc surgery are variable. Good to excellent results are reported in 28 to 100% of patients. The literature must be reviewed carefully, however, as these studies frequently include many diagnoses. The results following repeat laminotomy and discectomy for recurrent lumbar disc herniation are generally favorable. Results equal to primary surgery can be expected in many cases, particularly those with recurrent herniations at another level.

Alternative Methods of Management

Alternative surgical treatments to repeat laminotomy and discectomy include minimally invasive techniques such as chemonucleolysis, percutaneous lumbar discectomy (PLD), and arthroscopic microdiscectomy (AMD). Other alternatives include laminotomy and discectomy with posterolateral fusion, anterior lumbar interbody fusion (ALIF), posterior lumbar interbody fusion (PLIF), and front/back or 360-degree fusion.

Minimally invasive approaches to the lumbar spine are continuing to evolve and show significant promise as alternative techniques to open surgery. Several well-designed studies have proven the efficacy of chemonucleolysis with chymopapain compared with placebo. Although used infrequently in North America, chemonucleolysis continues to be widely used in Europe with reported good to excellent results in 75 to 80% of properly selected patients.

Percutaneous discectomy was independently developed by Hijikata and Kambin in the 1970s. This technique involves a posterolateral percutaneous approach to the lumbar disc followed by manual or automated retrieval of disc material. The published clinical success rates of automated percutaneous lumbar discectomy (APLD) are variable. Generally, good to excellent results can be expected in approximately 50 to 75% of patients. Complications occur in less than 1% of patients.

Frequently, the addition of a lumbar fusion is indicated in the treatment of recurrent disc herniation. We routinely add a posterolateral fusion to the repeat laminotomy and discectomy in cases of a second recurrence at the same level. Other indications for fusion include discectomy with facetectomy, such as in cases of foraminal or extraforaminal herniations approached from the midline, particularly at the L4/L5 level, where biomechanical stresses are high. Fusion should also be

Type of Management	Advantages	Disadvantages	Comments
Chemonucleolysis	Minimally invasive	Not useful in sequestered fragments Not as efficacious as laminotomy and discectomy	Contraindicated in same-site recurrences Complications rare if correctly used Still widely used in Europe
Percutaneous lumbar discectomy (PLD)	Minimally invasive	Blind technique Not as efficacious as laminotomy and discectomy	Used infrequently today
Arthroscopic microdiscectomy (AMD)	Minimally invasive Visualized technique Spinal canal is not violated	Migrated, sequestered fragment is relative contraindication Indirectly approaches the pathology	Appealing in same site recurrent herniation as reoperation through epidural scar is avoided More outcome studies needed
Laminotomy/discectomy with posterolateral lumbar fusion	Addresses back pain Prevents iatrogenic instability in some cases Decreases risk of recurrent herniation	More extensive surgery Longer recovery time Donor-site morbidity	Indications for fusion include 3rd recurrence, instability, discogenic back pain Consider instrumentation
Anterior lumbar interbody fusion (ALIF)	Directly addresses discogenic back pain Indirect foraminal decompression	? More extensive surgery Disc hernation often not directly visualized	Minimally invasive laparoscopic technique showing promise Cage techniques popular
Posterior lumbar interbody fusion (PLIF)	Direct approach for discectomy Indirect foraminal decompression Can easily add posterolateral fusion	Higher risk for neural injury at previously operated level	Technically difficult
Front/back (360-degree) fusion	Highest chance for fusion	Much more extensive surgery	Exact role is yet to be defined

considered in cases of recurrent disc herniation when low back pain is a major component of the patient's presentation. In these cases, flexion/extension radiographs should be evaluated for evidence of instability. Provocative tests such as discography may also be useful in the evaluation of discogenic low back pain.

In cases of recurrent disc herniation at the same level, the involved disc space may be significantly narrowed. These patients may have significant discogenic low back pain, but may also have radicular pain from secondary foraminal stenosis. When considering a fusion in such cases, some authors prefer an interbody fusion technique. This allows distraction of the disc space to its original height and indirectly decompresses the neural foramen. Approaches for interbody fusion include anterior (ALIF) and posterior (PLIF). In addition, some surgeons prefer combined anterior and posterior, or 360-degree, fusions. The role for these more extensive procedures remains to be defined.

Suggested Readings

Boden SD, Davis DO, Dina TS, et al. Contrast-enhanced MR imaging performed after successful lumbar disk surgery: prospective study. Radiology 1992; 182: 59–64.

Bundschuh CV, Stein L, Slusser JH, et al. Distinguishing between scar and recurrent herniated disk in postoperative patients: value of contrast-enhanced CT and MR imaging. AJNR 1990; 11(5):949–958.

Cinotti G, Roysam GS, Eisenstein SM, Postacchini F. Ipsilateral recurrent lumbar disc herniation. A prospective, controlled study. J Bone Joint Surg 1998; 80B(5):825–832.

Connolly ES. Surgery for recurrent lumbar disc herniation. Clin Neurosurg 1992; 39:211–216.

Ebeling U, Reichenberg W, Reulen HJ. Microsurgical reoperation following lumbar disc surgery. J Neurosurg 1989; 70:397–404.

Epstein JA, Lavine LS, Epstein BS. Recurrent herniation of the lumbar intervertebral disc. Clin Orthop 1967; 52:169–178.

Herron L. Recurrent lumbar disc herniation: results of repeat laminectomy and discectomy. J Spinal Disord 1994; 7(2):161–166.

Kambin P. Arthroscopic microdiscectomy. In: Frymoyer JW, ed. The Adult Spine: Principles and Practice, 2d ed., pp. 2023–2036. Philadelphia: Lippincott-Raven, 1997.

Nordby EJ, Wright PH. Efficacy of chymopapain in chemonucleolysis. A review. Spine 1994; 19(22):2578–2583.

Ross JS, Robertson JT, Frederickson RCA, et al. Association between peridural scar and recurrent radicular pain after lumbar discectomy: magnetic resonance evaluation. Neurosurgery 1996; 38(4):855–863.

Silvers HR, Lewis PJ, Asch HL, Clabeaux DE. Lumbar diskectomy for recurrent disk herniation. J Spinal Disord 1994; 7(5):408–419.

Sotiropoulos S, Chafetz NI, Lang P, et al. Differentiation between postoperative scar and recurrent disk herniation: prospective comparisons of MR, CT, and contrast-enhanced CT. AJNR 1989; 10:639–643.

Case 19

Intradural Disc Herniation—Lumbar Spine

Kush Singh and Alexander R. Vaccaro

History and Physical Examination

A 56-year-old woman presented with a 5-year history of low back pain that began abruptly after lifting a heavy object. She stated the pain had been increasing in intensity over the last 10 months. The pain radiated into both posterior thighs, posterolateral calves, and dorsum of both feet primarily involving the great toes. She has also experienced increasing weakness of both legs over the last 2 to 3 years. Three days prior to hospitalization, the pain in her back and legs intensified and was accompanied by urinary and fecal incontinence. Neurologic examination revealed hypesthesia and hyperalgesia of L5 and S1 bilaterally, with severe weakness (2–3/5) of her anterior tibialis, extensor hallucis longus, and gastrocnemius muscle groups. Achilles tendon reflexes were absent bilaterally. Straight leg raising was positive to 40-degrees bilaterally. Babinski's sign was negative bilaterally.

Radiologic Findings

Plain radiographs of the lumbar spine revealed disc space narrowing and posterior osteophyte formation at the L4/L5 level. Anteroposterior (AP) myelography demonstrated a near-complete filling defect in the dye column at the L4/L5 level (Fig. 19–1). Transaxial computed tomography (CT) confirmed lack of dye flow at this level (Fig. 19–2). Sagittal and transaxial magnetic resonance imaging (MRI) identified a large intracanal space-occupying lesion that was suspected to be an intradural disc herniation (Fig. 19–3).

Diagnosis

Intradural lumbar disc herniation.

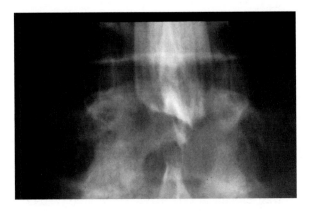

Figure 19–1. Anteroposterior (AP) myelogram demonstrating a near-complete filling defect in the dye column at the L4/L5 level.

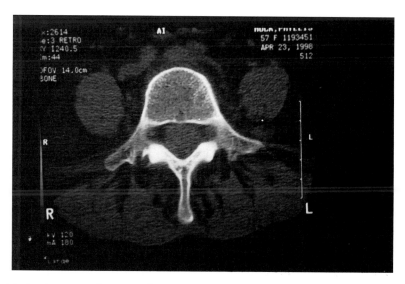

Figure 19–2. A transaxial computed tomography (CT) illustrating lack of dye flow at the L4/L5 level.

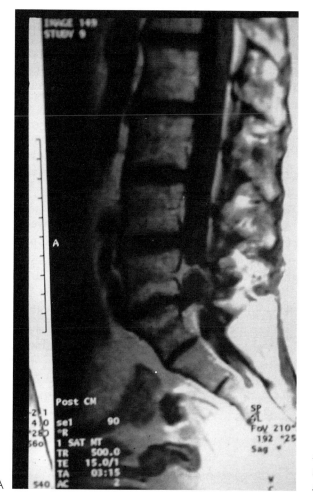

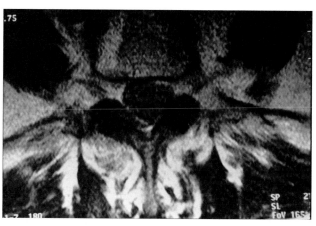

Figure 19–3. Sagittal (A) and transaxial (B) magnetic resonance imaging (MRI) revealing a large intracanal space-occupying lesion that was confirmed to be an intradural disc herniation.

Discussion

The primary diagnosis in the differential for an intracanal mass causing thecal sac compression in the lumbar spine is an intervertebral extradural disc herniation. The differential diagnosis of an intradural mass in the lumbar area includes an intradural disc herniation, neurofibroma, ependymoma, meningioma, neurilemoma, epidermoid tumor, arachnoid cyst, and an inflammatory mass such as may be seen with adhesive arachnoiditis.

A characteristic of an intradural lumbar disc herniation is the irregular border of the disc fragment, although irregular margins may also be seen with arachnoiditis and an associated inflammatory mass. The other pathologic entities in the differential tend to have a smooth contour to their external bodies. The identification of an intradural process is often appreciated on myelography or postmyelogram CT, but in most cases an MRI analysis is the most revealing imaging study. However, often the intradural status of the disc fragment is underappreciated in the preoperative period and is usually discovered at the time of surgery.

This rare occurrence has been reported to have an incidence of between 0.04 and 0.33% for all lumbar disc protrusions. Less than 100 cases of intradural lumbar disc rupture have been reported in the literature. The mechanism of intradural penetration of a lumbar disc herniation remains uncertain. Blikra (1969) reported on his morphologic evaluation of intradural disc herniations involving 40 cadavers. In affected patients, the author reported the presence of adhesions in close proximity to the posterior longitudinal ligament along the ventral aspect of the spinal dural sac. These adhesions, particularly at the L4/L5 level, are thought to be due to repeated minor trauma that occur during normal activities, inflammatory scarring due to prior episodes of disc disease or inflammation, or as a result of previous surgery. Blikra concluded that occasionally the resulting adhesions are so resistant to disc migration that a herniated disc is forced through the dura instead, making this mechanism the primary cause of intradural lumbar disc herniations.

Unfortunately, often at the time of surgery the preoperative diagnosis of dural penetration from a disc herniation is rarely obtained. Myelography generally shows a total or subtotal block of contrast medium, making it difficult to make a diagnosis with this technique. Unenhanced CT scanning is also not useful in revealing significant abnormalities; however, contrast-enhanced (metrizamide) CT scanning may demonstrate a lobular mass and extent of herniation size. Other investigators have found that MRI was superior to myelography in visualizing all components of the herniation, including adhesions and other inflammatory tissue.

Several authors have identified other characteristics of intradural lumbar disc herniations. Smith (1981) recommended analysis of the cerebrospinal fluid (CSF) taken at the time of myelography for the presence of macrophages that contain fibrocartilage as a way to make a preoperative diagnosis of intradural disk herniation. Although rare, the presence of gas in the intradiscal space (called the vacuum phenomenon) might be indicative of intradural herniation.

Other disorders that should be considered in the differential include a neurofibroma, an ependymoma, a meningioma, a neurilemoma, an epidermoid tumor, an arachnoid cyst, and arachnoiditis.

Neurofibroma

The Schwann cell is the principal constituent of a neurofibroma and exhibits diffuse, intrafascicular growth within nerve fascicles. Several types of categories of neurofibromas exist; however, the ones commonly confused with an intradural disc herniation are those that arise directly from the nerve root itself. This variety, although intradural, is extramedullary and, as such, mimics a herniated disc. As a result, symptoms and signs of nerve root irritation including muscle weakness and perhaps muscle atrophy with decreased reflexes are often an early manifestation of its presence.

Ependymoma

Ependymal cells line the walls of the ventricles of the brain and the central portion of the spinal canal. In addition, they line the ventriculus terminalis of the conus medullaris and the filum terminale, and are present in streaks at points of acute angulation of the ventricles. Ependymomas can occur wherever ependymal cells are present. They are the most common primary tumor of the spinal cord. The most common site for a spinal cord ependymoma is in the filum terminale of the ventriculus terminalus of the conus medullaris. The reason for this predominance has yet to be explained.

Metrizamide myelography may reveal an enlarged spinal cord, contrast flow blockage in the spinal canal, and evidence of an intradural extramedullary tumor. In addition, interpediculate distance may also be increased. Metrizamide-enhanced CT scanning may also disclose enlargement of the spinal cord and, at times, a collection of metrizamide in the cystic component of the tumor. Abnormal soft tissue masses may also be apparent in the spinal canal, extending to the intervertebral foramen. The benefit of MRI is its direct visualization of the tumor and good contrast between the CSF and spinal cord.

Meningiomas

Meningiomas are extremely common primary tumors and account for a quarter of all primary spinal tumors. However, meningiomas arising in the lumbar spine represent only a small proportion of the total number of spinal meningiomas. These tumors arise from the arachnoid villi.

A characteristic MRI feature of meningiomas is their dense, homogeneous contrast enhancement. They are not usually associated with scalloping of the vertebral bodies, but flattening of the pedicles, often unilateral, may be seen.

On MRI analysis, meningiomas tend to be isointense with the spinal cord on T1- and T2-weighted images. This characteristic may be used to distinguish meningiomas from schwannomas, which tend to be brighter on T2-weighted images.

Neurilemoma

A neurilemoma is a tumor arising from Schwann cells in the nerve sheath. When these tumors occur in the spinal canal, most (67%) are intradural in location. The remaining tumors are located both intradurally and extradurally (16%) or entirely extradurally (16%).

A large neurilemoma will often affect the neighboring bone by erosion of the pedicle, enlargement of the intervertebral foramen, increase of the interpediculate distance, scalloping of the vertebral bodies, and thinning of the laminae. A positive contrast myelogram is usually diagnostic of the lesion and shows characteristic intradural and extradural defects. Without bony changes or myelographic defects, radiologic diagnosis is almost impossible. The use of intravenous contrast medium is a valuable adjunct to high-resolution CT in the evaluation of neurilemomas.

Epidermoid Tumor

Epidermoid tumors are rare, benign congenital tumors occurring within the central nervous system (CNS) less than 1% of the time. Only a small fraction of CNS epidermoid tumors occur in the spinal cord. These tumors consist of a wall of stratified squamous epithelium and contain a waxy material consisting of keratinaceous debris and cholesterol crystal.

Epidermoid tumors may either be congenital or iatrogenic. Iatrogenic induction occurs by implantation of epidermal cells into the spinal canal during diagnostic or therapeutic lumbar puncture, discography, or surgery. Congenital epidermoid tumors occur as a result of the inclusion of epithelial tissue elements during the closure of the medullary folds from the 3rd to 5th week of fetal life. The epithelial cells are included most commonly at the ends of the neuroepidermoid canal; therefore, the sacrococcygeal region is affected most frequently.

The plain radiographic findings of epidermoid tumors are those of a slowly growing intraspinal mass and consist of vertebral body scalloping and thinning of the pedicles. The myelographic findings of a lumbar intraspinal epidermoid tumor depends on the location of the tumor and may present as a complete block with intradural and/or intramedullary involvement.

On T1-weighted MRI, iatrogenic intraspinal epidermoid tumors display a signal intensity that may be similar to CSF, surrounded by a slightly increased signal intensity. On T2-weighted MRI, their signal may vary from isointense to slightly hypointense.

Arachnoid Cyst

Extradural arachnoid cysts are uncommon expanding lesions in the spinal canal and even less common in the lumbar region. These lesions typically remain in communication with the subarachnoid space via a narrow neck. They arise from a congenital defect in the dura that allows the arachnoid membrane to herniate through the adjacent dura mater. The cysts have a pedicle that connects them to the subarachnoid space, located dorsally along a root sleeve. They may cause neurologic symptoms by compressing the spinal cord or nerve roots.

The diagnosis of arachnoid cysts is usually established by myelography, which demonstrates an extradural defect with smooth displacement of the margin of the thecal sac. The correct diagnosis is contingent upon the cyst being filled by the contrast medium. Myelography in the supine position is required because of the posterior location of the cyst. The neck of the arachnoid diverticulum may be so narrow that even water-soluble contrast medium may not enter the cyst during myelography, and delayed CT may be required to demonstrate filling of the cyst.

MRI is a sensitive and specific imaging modality in identifying CSF-containing lesions. Findings on MRI include a mass posterior or posterolateral to the spinal cord with signal characteristics identical to CSF on T1- and T2-weighted images. An extradural lesion is indicated by the cysts' location within the posterior epidural fat, anterior displacement of the subarachnoid space and spinal cord, and extension into the intervertebral foramen.

Another variety of arachnoid cysts is located intradurally and can also erode bone. Intradural arachnoid cysts usually lie posterior to the spinal cord. On myelography they appear as intradural defects that may communicate with the subarachnoid space.

Arachnoiditis: Inflammatory Mass

Arachnoiditis is an irritation of the arachnoid layer of the meninges. The more common causes of arachnoiditis today are surgery, foreign materials, trauma, infection, intrathecal hemorrhage, intrathecal steroids, or anesthetic agents. The pathogenesis of arachnoiditis is a fibrous exudate with a negligible inflammatory cellular component similar to the repair process of serous membranes such as the peritoneum. This fibrinous exudate covering the nerve roots causes them to stick to themselves and to the thecal sac. The subsequent repair phase causes dense collagenous adhesions formed by proliferating fibrocytes. Inflammatory masses in the lumbar region, as may be seen with adhesive arachnoiditis, are commonly mistaken for intradural lumbar disc herniations.

MRI characteristics of arachnoiditis include large conglomerations of nerve roots residing centrally within the thecal sac with no visible peripheral dural thickening. T1-weighted images show these nerve roots as round areas of soft tissue signal, and T2-weighted images improve the definition of their shape and outline.

Occasionally the clumped nerve roots may be attached peripherally to the meninges. This appears on MRI as focal thickening of the meninges, with few or no nerve roots visible within the subarachnoid space and a centrally appearing "empty thecal sac" containing a homogeneous signal intensity consistent with CSF.

Alternative Methods of Management

Surgery is the treatment of choice in a symptomatic patient with an intradural disc herniation. Often the discal fragment is found partially outside the dural sheath, and, with gentle removal, leakage of CSF is often noted, suggesting an intradural extension. In such cases, gentle palpation of the nerve root sheath and thecal sac should be performed to exclude the presence of residual disc fragments.

Type of Management	Advantages	Disadvantages	Comments
Observation	Useful in the asymptomatic patient in which the diagnosis of an intradural disc herniation is certain	Diagnosis may be in error, resulting in the potential for spread of a malignant lesion or the occurrence of a neurologic deficit	Rarely chosen due to the fact that most patients are symptomatic as a prerequisite for obtaining the illustrative imaging study
Surgery	Useful in obtaining an accurate diagnosis and alleviating the patient's complaints of radicular pain	Potential for persistent cerebrospinal fluid (CSF) leakage, neural injury, or retained disc fragment	Often successful if properly performed with care not to avoid missing any retained disc fragments

Complications

Complications related to the surgical removal of an intradural lumbar disc herniation are several and include (1) missing a retained discal fragment, (2) neural injury during disc removal, and (3) persistent CSF leakage following dural closure. Careful preoperative assessment of all imaging modalities and a thorough inspection of the thecal sac either with ultrasonography or combined with direct palpation should minimize the reality of a retained disc fragment.

Suggested Readings

Blikra G. Intradural herniated lumbar disc. J Neurosurg 1969; 31:676–679.

Ciappetta P, Delfini R, Cantore GP. Intradural lumbar disc hernia: description of three cases. Neurosurgery 1981; 8:104–107.

Graves VB, Finney HL, Mailander J. Intradural lumbar disk herniation. AJNR 1986; 7:495–497.

Hodge CJ, Binet EF, Kieffer SA. Intradural herniation of lumbar intervertebral discs. Spine 1978; 3:346–350.

Holtas S, Nordstrom C-H, Larsson E-M, Pettersson H. MR imaging of intradural disk herniation. J Comput Assist Tomogr 1987; 11:353–356.

Koivukangas J, Tervonen O. Intraoperative ultrasound imaging in lumbar disc herniation surgery. Acta Neurochir (Wien) 1989; 98:47–54.

Smith RV. Intradural disc rupture. J Neurosurg 1981; 55:117–120.

Case 20
Spinal Meningeal or Perineural Cysts
Alexander R. Vaccaro, Kern Singh, and Janet C. Donohue

History and Physical Examination

A 57-year-old woman presented with a complaint of a long history of low back discomfort with bilateral lower extremity weakness (right > left) beginning approximately 6 years prior to her evaluation. On physical examination, the patient was noted to have marked right calf atrophy measuring 4 cm less than the left calf. Motor strength was decreased in this extremity with a grade of 4 out of 5 motor strength noted in the L4, L5, and S1 distributions. She had no sensory deficit or positive tension sign.

Radiologic Findings

A nonenhanced computed tomography (CT) scan revealed evidence of right S2 nerve root compression by an intracanal space-occupying lesion. This was read offi-

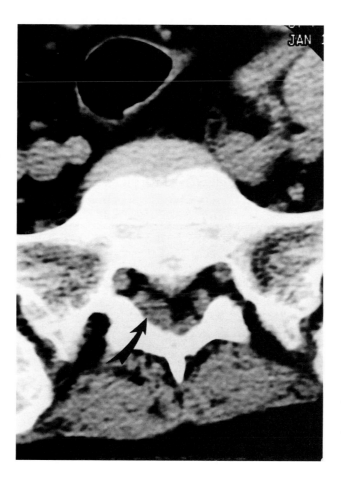

Figure 20–1. A nonenhanced computed tomography (CT) scan revealing a large intracanal space-occupying lesion of intermediate signal intensity compressing the sacral spinal roots.

cially by the neuroradiologist as a free disc fragment within the sacral spinal canal at the S1/S2 level (Fig. 20–1). In addition, multiple levels of lumbar tricompartmental stenosis localized to the L3 through L5 levels were identified.

Due to the inconsistent findings of the imaging studies (CT), indicating multiple areas of pathology down to the S1/S2 levels with the patient's symptoms predominantly localized to the L4, L5, and S1 levels, magnetic resonance imaging (MRI) was obtained to further clarify the degree of nerve root compression. The MRI findings were consistent with moderate to severe multilevel acquired spinal stenosis and neural foraminal stenosis greatest at the L3/L4 and L4/L5 levels with evidence of a L4/L5 grade 1 spondylolisthesis. At the S1/S2 level, a perineural or Tarlov's cyst was noted on the T2-weighted images consistent with the intracanal mass thought to be an extruded disc on the plain unenhanced CT scan (Fig. 20–2).

Diagnosis

A type II extradural cyst commonly referred to as a classic perineural cyst or Tarlov's cyst. The cyst was classified as type II because of its extradural location and the presence of nerve root fibers within the cyst itself.

Surgical Management

The patient subsequently underwent a posterior L3/L4, L4/L5 decompression and posterolateral fusion from L3 to L5 with marked improvement in her lower extremity pain and weakness. No exploration of the perineural cystic structure was undertaken due to the lack of clinical symptomatology.

Discussion

A spinal cyst, although infrequently the cause of neurologic symptoms, must be considered in the differential diagnosis of any patient who presents with symptoms of lower extremity pain and evidence of a space-occupying intracanal mass on a nonenhanced CT scan of the lumbar spine. The Tarlov's cyst diagnosed in this case is just one of several different cysts broadly categorized as spinal meningeal cysts.

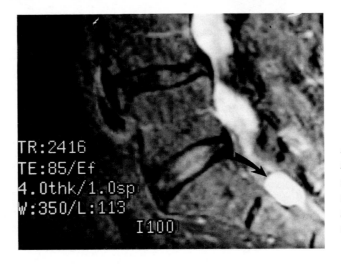

Figure 20–2. A T2-weighted sagittal magnetic resonance imaging (MRI) scan revealing a high signal intensity lesion within the sacral canal representative of a type II or Tarlov's cyst.

Much confusion has surrounded these cysts with respect to their etiology, classification, and diagnosis. Broadly, these cysts can be considered outpouchings of the meninges, arachnoid, or dura, as well as the sheath surrounding the nerve root. The classification system proposed by Nabors and colleagues in 1988 separates spinal meningeal cysts into three categories based on intraoperative and histologic examination: type I, extradural cysts, no nerve root fibers; type II, extradural cysts, including spinal root fibers; type III, intradural cysts (Fig. 20–3).

The etiology of a type I extradural cyst may be congenital, developmental, hereditary, idiopathic, or acquired. The incidence is greater in males than females. Histology demonstrates dural tissue with a variable incidence of arachnoid mater within the cyst. The location of these cysts can be anywhere along the thecal sac. Most commonly they are located in the thoracic spine (67%), followed by the lumbosacral junction (20%), with sporadic incidence in the cervical and thoracolumbar junction. Along the thecal sac these cysts are often found either midline or herniating through a neural foramen, and are dorsally located proximal to the dorsal root ganglion. These cysts have the capacity to enlarge either via a ball-valve mechanism, in which cerebrospinal fluid (CSF) enters the cyst and reflux is prevented by a one-way valve or by the active secretion of CSF from arachnoid tissue present within the cyst. Bone erosion can be present from the pulsatile CSF but is not a distinguishing factor.

Clinical presentation is variable based on the cyst location. Thoracic cysts present most commonly in the second decade of life as the cysts gradually enlarge, perhaps due to the small canal at this level. Lumbosacral cysts present in the third to fifth decades due to the larger canal at this level. Symptoms include progressive paralysis, bladder and bowel dysfunction, backache, and radiculopathy. Progressive paralysis is the most common presentation of thoracic cysts according to Naidich et al. (1983), followed by backache. Backache may be exacerbated by coughing, sneezing, or a Valsalva maneuver but may be relieved with flat bed rest, which is thought to be due to the cyst emptying in the recumbent position. Approximately 30% of patients have these positional symptoms. In many cases pain may wax and wane over several years. In some cases an acute attack of sciatica may occur and resolve with a brief period of bed rest. Bilateral symptoms are more common with the type I cyst than with the others.

Spinal Cysts

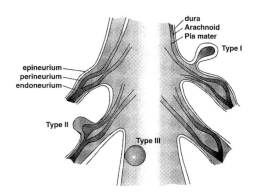

Figure 20–3. An illustration of the three types of spinal cysts as described by Nabors and colleagues (1988).

Plain radiographs do not usually assist in the diagnosis unless there is evidence of bony erosion by a space-occupying lesion. The mainstay of diagnosis is MRI and CT myelogram. On MRI, a high-intensity signal consistent with CSF is present on the T2-weighted image. CT myelogram is diagnostic for the extradural spinal cysts because they fill with contrast material. The size of the neck or pedicle connecting the cyst to the thecal sac determines the rate of filling and if it fails to fill immediately, delayed films as much as 24 hours later may demonstrate a communication. Sometimes having the patient erect and performing a Valsalva maneuver allows contrast to fill the cyst.

Management of symptomatic cysts is surgical, with observation reserved for the incidentally discovered, asymptomatic cysts. On the occasion that surgery for a disc or degenerative stenosis is needed, the cyst, if at that level, may be addressed.

Surgical management includes laminectomy for exposure, with great care taken not to puncture the cyst or dura. This may be difficult if there is a very thin shell of bone overlying the cyst. After full visualization of the cyst and pedicle, the pedicle is double-suture ligated for cyst removal. If the cyst is adherent to surrounding structures, especially the nerve roots, the cyst is drained, partially excised, and then oversewn with suture and muscle graft. Other surgical options include marsupialization and drainage into the subarachnoid space.

A poor outcome is associated with severe symptomatology and a long duration of symptoms. Remission of symptoms with surgery is possible, but the majority of patients report no change in symptoms with minimal improvement.

Type II extradural cysts are dilations of nerve root sheaths often referred to as the classic perineural cysts. Tarlov's cysts fit into this category. The etiology is considered to be either congenital or developmental. These cysts can be differentiated from type I cysts by their inclusion of nerve root fibers in the cyst wall or cyst cavity and by their location at or distal to the dorsal root ganglion. The cyst wall consists of endoneurium and perineurium derived from pia and arachnoid mater, respectively. The pedicle connecting the cyst to the subarachnoid space is obliterated by herniated nerve root fibers. This is significant because contrast dye rarely flows to these cysts, and only a pedicle defect is visualized on myelography. A connection to the subarachnoid space may be seen on the CT scan following myelography due to its sensitivity in detecting small amounts of intrathecal dye that may leach into the cyst via the nearly obliterated pedicle. These cysts are most commonly found in the sacral region, where Tarlov initially discovered them in 1938, but can occur anywhere along the spinal axis. Often these cysts are multiple and appear as a cluster. Like the extradural cysts, they also have the potential to erode bone and enlarge via a ball-valve mechanism or CSF secretion from residual arachnoid mater within the cyst walls.

Symptoms, if present, are variable depending on which nerve root is involved, but most patients have radicular symptoms, back pain, and occasional bowel and bladder symptoms. These are very similar to the symptoms for the type I cysts, but these cysts are often asymptomatic—found incidentally on myelogram or MRI. Most patients at the time of discovery are adults. MRI findings are similar to type I cysts—a high-intensity fluid-filled sac consistent with CSF on a T2 image. Myelography and CT findings are also similar to type I cysts consisting of a filling defect on myelography and a connection between the cyst and subarachnoid space visualized on CT imaging.

Treatment of type II cysts is observation unless symptomatic. Symptomatic cysts, those causing significant pain with sensory and motor deficits, require surgical management. This consists of a variety of options including complete excision, incision, and drainage supplemented by muscle or Silastic grafting to seal the subarachnoid space, and partial cyst excision followed by wall plication or marsupialization. No matter what surgical option is chosen, care must be taken during the surgical approach because of the possibility of an overlying paper-thin lamina adhering to the underlying spinal cyst. A major goal of surgery is to preserve as many nerve root fibers as possible, making complete resection of the cyst almost impossible. Intraoperative electrical stimulation to the cyst wall to elicit evoked muscle action potentials is helpful for confirmation of the diagnosis (type I or type II cyst). This may also help distinguish the type of nerve root pathology, differentiating nerve root compression from a conduction block of a degenerated nerve root.

Postoperatively patients usually manifest partial resolution of their pain with recovery of function as seen in the Nabors and colleagues (1988) series of nine type II cysts, eight of which were treated operatively. Tarlov (1970) also had good results based on his series of seven perineural cysts treated surgically either with complete excision or excision of the dome of the cyst. These patients had good relief of their symptoms, with the best results obtained from total excision. Crellin and Jones (1973) reported a series of seven extradural cysts where excision provided long-term relief of symptoms in all patients except one, whose symptoms recurred after 1 year. Reported return of neurologic function, however, was poor.

Type III cysts are intradural cysts. Their etiology is primarily congenital and is attributed to proliferation of arachnoid tissue. Other reported etiologies include proliferative arachnoid adhesions secondary to spinal trauma or meningitis. Valve mechanisms are also attributed to the potential for these cysts to expand, and they also can be associated with bone erosion. Their location can be anywhere posterior along the spinal axis, rarely occurring anteriorly. Most often they are asymptomatic like type II cysts and can occur in multiple areas as well. Symptoms are consistent with compression and are determined by their location. Imaging studies reveal an intradural defect on myelography; however, they may occasionally be missed by their blending into the surrounding tissue. MRI often shows a lesion with the same intensity as CSF compressing the cord posteriorly. Treatment of these cysts is complete excision due to the potential for recurrence with incomplete removal. If complete excision is not possible, then marsupialization is the preferred technique. Nabors et al described four type III cysts that were treated surgically with complete excision and excellent results.

In summary, the treating physician must be aware of the similarities in appearance between a free discal fragment and a fluid-filled cyst on nonenhanced CT. MRI is the imaging study of choice to diagnose a meningeal cyst as well as a herniated disc. Spinal surgeons must be careful when operating in close proximity to a meningeal cyst, due to the potential for iatrogenic injury due to the encapsulated nerve roots in the type II variety. Again, with the proper imaging studies and a knowledgeable spine surgeon, the correct diagnosis and appropriate treatment of these spinal cysts may be accomplished.

Alternative Methods of Management

Nonoperative treatment is the mainstay of management, especially for type II perineural cysts in the lumbosacral region. Often patients present with nonspecific symptoms localized to the low back with an occasional referred pain pattern (lower extremity), which is difficult to correlate conclusively as being caused by a perineural cyst. Surgery is absolutely indicated in examples of an expandable lesion located along the spinal cord level that results in a progressive neurologic deficit.

Type of Management	Advantages	Disadvantages	Comments
Excision	No recurrence	May result in sacrifice of adherent sensory fibers	Treatment of choice if able to separate from neural structures
Partial excision—oversewing edges with suture and muscle graft	Protect adhering neural structures	Potential for recurrence	Safest and easiest method of treatment with potential for recurrence
Marsupialization	Low rate of injury to adjacent neural structures	Potential for recurrence	Technically demanding

Suggested Readings

Crellin RQ, Jones ER. Sacral extradural cysts: a rare cause of low backache and sciatica. JBJS 1973; 55B:20–31.

Gortvai P. Extradural cysts of the spinal canal. J Neurol Neurosurg Psychiatry 1963; 26:223–230.

Masaryk TJ. Cystic lesions, vascular disorders, demyelinating disease and miscellaneous topics. In: Modic MT, Masaryk TJ Ross JS, eds. Magnetic Resonance Imaging of the Spine, pp. 392–399. St. Louis, MO: Mosby-Year Book, 1994.

Nabors M, Pait G, Byrd E, et al. Updated assessment and current classification of spinal meningeal cysts. J Neurosurg 1988; 68:366–377.

Naidich TP, McLone DG, Harwood-Nash DC. Arachnoid cysts, paravertebral meningoceles, and perineural cysts. In: Newton TH, Potts DG, eds. Computed Tomography of the Spine and Spinal Cord, pp. 383–396. San Anselmo, CA: Clavadel Press, 1983.

Rohrer DC, Burchiel KJ, Gruber DP. Intraspinal extradural meningeal cyst demonstrating ball-valve mechanism of formation. J Neurosurg 1993; 78:122–125.

Shinomiya K, Mutoh N, Furuya K. Giant sacral cysts with neurogenic bladder. J Spinal Disorders 1994; 5:444–448.

Tarlov IM. Spinal perineural and meningeal cysts. J Neurol Neurosurg Psychiatry 1970; 33:833–843.

Case 21
Iatrogenic Lumbar Instability
Robert J. Benz and Steven R. Garfin

History and Physical Examination

A 54-year-old man presented with a chief complaint of difficulty walking and inability to stand erect. Fourteen years ago he had undergone a lumbar laminectomy and discectomy for leg pain with resolution of his sciatica. Several years later, he developed significant back and bilateral buttock pain. Six years ago he underwent multilevel lumbar laminectomies, without significant relief of his back or leg pain. He has subsequently developed increasing back pain as well as bilateral radiating leg pain and weakness. He uses two canes to ambulate and has difficulty getting around his house. He is unable to negotiate stairs.

On physical examination he has a significant stooped posture. Motion of the lumbar spine is significantly limited, esecially in extension. With flexion he has

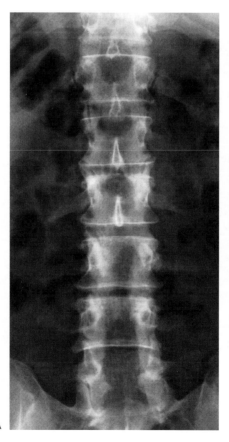

A

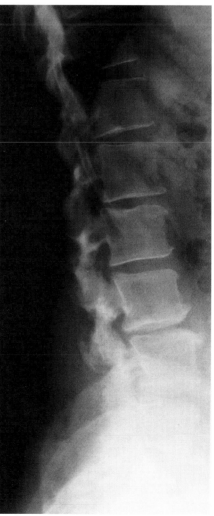

B

Figure 21–1. Anteroposterior (AP) (A) and lateral (B) radiographs taken 1 year after the patient's second decompression surgery. Note the presence of traction spurs at L2/L3 and claw osteophytes at L3/L4 with mild loss of the normal lumbar lordosis.

increased pain and a feeling of catching in the back. The previous surgical incisions are well healed. Neurologic examination of the lower extremities demonstrates diffuse weakness bilaterally with diminished deep tendon reflexes at the right knee and ankle. There are no pathologic reflexes. Straight-leg raising produces only back pain.

Radiologic Findings

Review of the radiographs taken a year after his most recent laminectomy approximately 5 years ago, reveals wide laminectomies from L3 through L5. There is disc space narrowing of the L3/L4 disc space, traction spurs at L2/L3, claw osteophytes at L3/L4, and mild loss of the normal lumbar lordosis (Fig. 21–1).

Radiographs taken at the time of presentation show marked collapse of the L2/L3 and L3/L4 disc spaces with 5 mm of anterolisthesis of L4 on L5 and 7 mm of retrolisthesis of L3 on L4. There is increased kyphosis from T12 to L5 with an apex at the L3/L4 disc (Fig. 21–2).

Magnetic resonance imaging (MRI) of the lumbosacral spine demonstrates severe spinal stenosis at L1/L2 through L4/L5 with foraminal stenosis at the lower levels (Fig. 21–3).

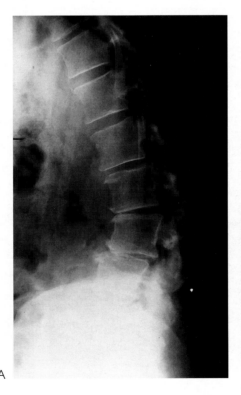

A

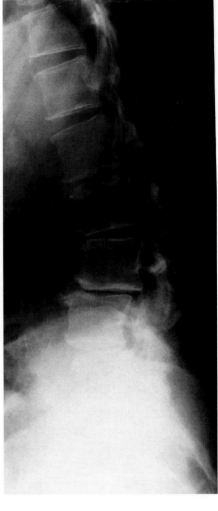

B

Figure 21–2. Flexion (A) and extension (B) lateral radiographs taken at the time of presentation. The loss of lumbar lordosis has progressed to frank kyphosis. There is retrolisthesis of L3 on L4 with anterolisthesis of L4 on L5, which is accentuated with motion.

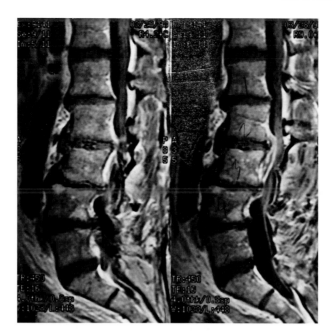

Figure 21–3. Sagittal magnetic resonance imaging (MRI) postgadolinium enhancement shows multiple levels of neural compression.

Diagnosis

Iatrogenic postlaminectomy thoracolumbar kyphosis with instability. The patient has multiple deformities. There is evidence of lumbar and thoracolumbar instability, which has resulted in progressive lumbar and thoracolumbar kyphosis. There is recurrent stenosis both centrally as well as in the foramina.

Surgical Management

The patient has kyphotic and translational deformities. To achieve correction of the sagittal deformity, along with a posterior decompression, it was felt that an anterior and posterior release and fusion procedures would best serve the patient. Although we often perform these front and back approaches on the same day, we anticipated our operating time would be long for this patient. We therefore chose to do this in a staged manner.

The patient initially underwent a posterior L1/L2 and redo L3 to L5 laminectomies and bilateral foraminotomies of L1 through L5. To prepare for the second portion of the case, osteotomies were performed posteriorly at L3/L4 and at L4/L5. The osteotomies were not fully completed so as to maintain some stability of the spine while waiting to do the anterior portion of the procedure. The pedicles were then sounded from T11 through L5 in anticipation of placing pedicle screw fixation after the anterior releases.

The patient was returned to the operating room 4 days later and placed in the lateral decubitus position. Simultaneous retroperitoneal and posterior approaches were used to access the thoracolumbar spine. Anteriorly, discectomies were performed from L1/L2 to L4/L5. Posteriorly the osteotomies were completed at the L3/L4 and L4/L5 levels. Anteriorly the disc spaces were distracted and wedge-shaped titanium cages, packed with a combination of iliac crest autograft and allograft bone, were placed in the L2/L3, L3/L4, and L4/L5 interspaces. A neutral cage was placed in the

L1/L2 interspace. This restored lumbar lordosis and the transition to neutrality at the thoracolumbar junction. Pedicle screw fixation was then used to compress the anterior devices posteriorly. Posterolateral fusion was then performed using a combination of iliac crest autograft supplemented with allograft bone (Fig. 21–4).

Postoperative Management

The patient was kept immobilized in a thoracolumbar spinal orthosis (TLSO) for 3 months. Rehabilitation included early return to light aerobic activity.

Discussion

This case is a rather extreme example of iatrogenic instability, whereas instability is often more subtle in the majority of cases. Segmental instability, as defined by the American Academy of Orthopaedic Surgeons, is an abnormal response to applied loads, characterized by motion in spinal motion segments beyond normal constraints. Controversy exists, however, over the diagnosis of segmental instability. Nachemson (1985) stated, "This clinical label has no scientific validity, the signs and symptoms are not defined, and the numerical values of the normal or abnormal motion segment mobility in any plane have not been established."

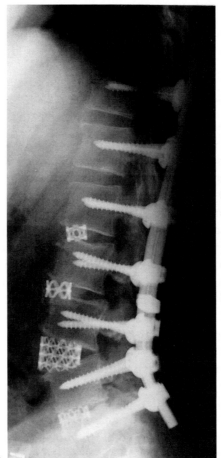

A

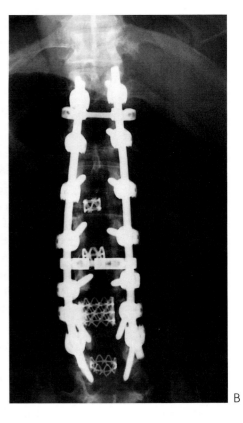

B

Figure 21–4. Postoperative AP (A) and lateral (B) radiographs demonstrating restoration of sagittal alignment.

The literature is unclear as to the true incidence of postdecompression instability, with rates ranging from 2 to 31%. Many authors believe the risk of postoperative instability is rare, and therefore arthrodesis is rarely indicated. Hanreats (1959) reported that only 2% of 6000 patients who underwent wide lumbar decompression developed spondylolisthesis severe enough to undergo spinal fusion. White and Wiltse (1976) reported only a 2% incidence of postdecompressive spondylolisthesis in 182 patients who had no evidence of preoperative spondylolisthesis. Other investigators feel postdecompression instability is common, especially if there is any evidence of preoperative instability.

Biomechanics of Instability

Studies evaluating the contribution of structures providing sagittal translation stability have found facets with intact capsules contribute 39% of the stability, an intact disc and annulus 29%, supraspinous and interspinous ligaments 19%, and the ligamentum flavum 13%. Disrupting posterior soft tissue supports may lead to anterior displacement of the internal axis of rotation. This creates increased stress and subsequent more rapid degeneration of the disc. Boden and colleagues (1994) found that a wide laminectomy with preservation of the facet joints resulted in little increased segmental motion. However, significant motion occurred when the facet capsules were removed and the joint denuded of cartilage. The importance of the facet joints in resisting sagittal translation and torsional loads has also been shown by other authors.

History and Physical Examination

Diagnosis of instability begins with a thorough history and physical examination. Typical symptoms of instability most often include low back pain, sclerotomatous pain radiating into the buttocks and upper thighs, and recurrent sciatica, which can be positional in nature. Patients often complain of an instability "catch," or a sudden onset of pain when they raise themselves from the flexed position. Pain is often relieved with lying down or sitting. On examination, patients with instability often have a dysrhythmia of lumbar spine motion. They often have a cogwheeling or rachetty motion when they go from a flexed to an erect position. In addition, a lack of reversal of the normal lumbar lordosis may be seen with bending. Neurologic examination is often normal, unless there is associated neural compression.

Radiographic Diagnosis of Instability

The radiographic diagnosis of instability is often uncertain. Many criteria have been offered. Macnab (1971) suggested that instability tends to produce characteristic traction osteophytes. The traction spur is a bony excrescence originating from the paradiscal margin 2 to 3 mm away from the endplate at the site of attachment of the outermost fibers of the annulus to bone. Friberg (1987) stated that traction spurs may be a sign of prior motion segment instability, but that no inference can be made to the current status of motion segment stability.

The absolute value of translation in the sagittal plane needed to clearly establish a diagnosis of instability is debated. Many authors define dynamic instability as 3 mm or more of translation on lateral radiographs. Spratt and colleagues (1993), however, determined intra- and interobserver errors for translational measurement and concluded that a minimum of 4 mm of displacement is needed in the lumbar region, whereas greater than 5 mm of displacement is needed at the lumbosacral junction, to define instability. Shaffer and colleagues (1990) determined that often patient positioning is not standardized during radiography and, combined with human measurement errors, translation of at least 6 mm or greater than 20 degrees of angular motion is needed to diagnose radiographic instability with certainty. Although many techniques including biplanar radiography, traction-compression radiographs, and stress-relaxation views have been used to improve the diagnostic certainty of instability, considerable controversy remains in the literature.

Controversy also exists over whether spondylolisthesis denotes an unstable condition and whether weight-bearing, lateral flexion-extension films can be relied on to diagnose instability. It has been shown that as many as 10% of women greater than 60 years of age have degenerative spondylolisthesis with a 10% slip or more, yet most of them are asymptomatic. Boden and Wiesel (1990) found 42% of asymptomatic patients had at least 3 mm of static olisthesis at one level on lumbar radiographs, whereas only 5% of the same patients demonstrated dynamic instability of 3 mm or more. This suggests the diagnosis of excessive sagittal translation be based on flexion-extension films, rather than comparing static images from different time periods.

Advanced imaging studies should generally be considered a preoperative study. Computed tomography (CT) scanning and magnetic resonance imaging (MRI) are both useful in evaluating the extent and nature of previous surgical decompressions. CT scanning can give important details of the bony anatomy, including the orientation of the remaining facet joints. MRI is also useful in determining the relative health of the intervertebral discs.

Risk Factors for Instability

Development of symptomatic instability following decompression is a relatively rare occurrence, ranging from 2 to 31% in the literature. Many factors have been implicated in predisposing a motion segment to instability. The classic teaching has been to preserve at least 50% of each facet joint to prevent instability. However, Hazlett and Kinnard (1982) reported on 33 patients who had at least one entire facet removed during decompression. Only four of these patients, all of whom had multilevel decompressions, showed radiographic evidence of instability. Only two of these four patients with radiographic instability had poor outcomes.

In addition to the absolute amount of the facet joint that remains after decompression, the orientation of the remaining facet joint also appears to be important in maintaining stability. More sagittally oriented facets predispose the motion segment to instability.

It is generally accepted that as the number of levels decompressed increases, the risk of instability increases. Although surgical violation of the disc at the time of posterior decompression has been cited as a risk factor for progression, some authors have found a decreased risk of instability following laminectomy with discectomy compared to laminectomy alone. The degenerating disc is generally thought to be a source of instability, but as the degenerative process continues and osteophytes form, the motion segment gradually stabilizes.

For those patients with some evidence of instability preoperatively, the risk of progression is relatively high, up to 70% in some series. Several factors have been associated with increased deformity. These include a near-normal disc space height at the time of decompression, the absence of large osteophytes, the removal of the disc at the time of decompression, female sex, and a younger age at the time of surgery.

Conversely, severely degenerated and collapsed disc spaces, spur formation from the vertebral body, sclerosis of the endplate, and ossification of the anterior longitudinal ligament are all generally considered to be stabilizing agents.

Indications for Fusion

One treatment for iatrogenic segmental instability is avoidance by determining which patients will become unstable and performing a concomitant fusion at the time of initial decompression.

The available literature does not give a clear indication of which patients will benefit from fusion. Although patients who develop postoperative spondylolisthesis have been shown to have an increased rate of poor clinical outcome, concomitant fusion has been shown to improve clinical outcome in some patient groups. In one of the few prospective studies available, Herkowitz and Kurz (1991) showed that in a group of patients with preexisting spondylolisthesis, decompression and concomitant fusion improved clinical outcome over decompression alone; 24 out of 25 patients treated with decompression alone showed progression of their deformity, whereas only 7 out of 25 treated with an in-situ fusion showed evidence of progression. This finding agrees with other retrospective studies of the effects of fusion in patients undergoing decompression for spinal stenosis. However, other studies have shown no clinical advantage of concomitant arthrodesis at the time of decompression.

After reviewing the literature, it seems that fusion is indicated in cases of preoperative spondylolisthesis and in cases where multilevel wide decompressions are performed with complete or subtotal facetectomies. In addition, arthrodesis should be considered for patients with significant degenerative scoliosis or lateral listhesis who are undergoing decompression.

Surgical treatment for postlaminectomy instability should be based on the patient's symptoms and the results of imaging studies. If signs of persistent stenosis are present, decompression is performed. Instability, particularly dynamic instability, is usually addressed with a posterolateral arthrodesis and segmental instrumentation. For those patients with resulting deformities, as in the case presented, restoration of spinal alignment is needed. This may involve a combination of anterior and posterior procedures to correct the associated deformity.

Alternative Methods of Management

An obvious controversy in the management of degenerative spinal conditions is in determining which patients will benefit from fusion at the time of decompression. A multitude of factors must be considered for each individual patient, including the extent of the decompression, the age of the patient and their activity level, the amount of back pain present preoperatively, the condition of the disc, and the presence of any preoperative instability. Patients can be managed with or without arthrodesis. The only clear indications for fusion include a "radical" decompression at multiple levels.

Arthrodesis can be performed with or without instrumentation. Noninstrumented fusion rates vary in the literature from 46 to 100%. Comparison studies of fusion rates with and without instrumentation have generally shown improved fusion rates with instrumentation; however, complication rates are also increased. In cases where there is progressive or dynamic instability, we use instrumentation to prevent progression of the deformity and possibly correct the deformity.

Most cases of postlaminectomy instability can be addressed from a posterior approach alone. In cases such as that presented here, where there is a significant kyphotic deformity, an anterior approach with anterior releases and correction of the deformity is needed to restore sagittal balance to the spine.

Type of Management	Advantages	Disadvantages	Comments
Decompression without fusion for spinal stenosis	Minimize complications	Risk for development or progression of deformity	Recommended approach unless there are firm indications for fusion
Decompression with fusion for spinal stenosis	May have improved clinical outcome	Increased complication rate Adjacent segment degeneration	Preferred method if there is evidence of instability preoperatively
Posterolateral fusion for iatrogenic instability	Prevents further deformity	May not be able to correct deformity Associated with higher nonunion rate than primary fusion	Typical method used for iatrogenic instability Instrumentation often used
Anterior and posterior fusion for iatrogenic instability	Allows for correction of deformity	Potentially increased complication rate with two approaches	Used when complex deformity present

Suggested Readings

Adams MA, Hutton WC. The mechanical function of the lumbar apophyseal joints. Spine 1983; 8:327–330.

Boden SD, Martin C, Rudolph R, et al. Increase of motion between lumbar vertebrae after excision of the capsule and cartilage of the facets. A cadaver study. J Bone Joint Surg 1994; 76A:1847–1853.

Boden SD, Wiesel SW. Lumbosacral segmental motion in normal individuals. Have we been measuring instability properly? [published erratum appears in Spine 1991; 16(7):855]. Spine 1990; 15:571–576.

Friberg O. Lumbar instability: a dynamic approach by traction-compression radiography. Spine 1987; 12:119–129.

Hanreats PR, Hollander ME, eds. The Degenerative Back and Its Differential Diagnosis. New York: Elsevier, 1959.

Hazlett JW, Kinnard P. Lumbar apophyseal process excision and spinal instability. Spine 1982; 7:171–176.

Herkowitz HN, Kurz LT. Degenerative lumbar spondylolisthesis with spinal stenosis. A prospective study comparing decompression with decompression and intertransverse process arthrodesis [see comments]. J Bone Joint Surg 1991; 73A:802–808.

Macnab I. The traction spur. An indicator of segmental instability. J Bone Joint Surg 1971; 53A:663–670.

Nachemson A. Lumbar spine instability. A critical update and symposium summary. Spine 1985; 10:290–291.

Shaffler WO, Spratt KF, Weinstein J, et al. 1990 Volvo Award in clinical sciences. The consistency and accuracy of roentgenograms for measuring sagittal translation in the lumbar vertebral motion segment. An experimental model. Spine 1990; 15:741–750.

Spratt KF, Weinstein JN, Lehmann TR, et al. Efficacy of flexion and extension treatments incorporating braces for low-back pain patients with retrodisplacement, spondylolisthesis, or normal sagittal translation. Spine 1993; 18:1839–1849.

White AA, Wiltse LL. Spondylolisthesis after extensive lumbar laminectomy. Presented at the annual meeting of the American Academy of Orthopaedic Surgeons, New Orleans, 1976.

Case 22

Management of Failed Back Surgery Syndrome

Christopher C. Annunziata, William C. Lauerman,
and Samuel W. Wiesel

History and Physical Examination

The patient is an active, healthy, 72-year-old woman who has an 18-month history of back and leg pain. Seven months ago she underwent a decompressive laminectomy at L4/L5 as well as right-sided foraminotomies at L3/L4 and L4/L5 for spinal stenosis. The complaint at that time was pain in the right side of her back, her right hip, and down her right leg with associated numbness. She has had improvement in her right leg pain and numbness since the surgery but, beginning about 2 weeks after the surgery, she noted recurrence and worsening of her back, right hip, and posterior thigh pain. The pain is worse with walking and standing and she is limited to about 15 minutes on her feet. The pain is moderately relieved by lying down. She has no bowel or bladder dysfunction, left leg symptoms, or any medical problems. Conservative management consisting of treatment with nonsteroidal antiinflammatory drugs, physical therapy, and two epidural injections has resulted in no significant improvement. This continues to represent a major functional disability, especially since she runs her own country store.

On physical examination her back is moderately tender and she stands off balance to the right in the frontal plane. She has good range of motion in flexion and extension of the back and has normal spinal rhythm. She is able to heel-walk and toe-

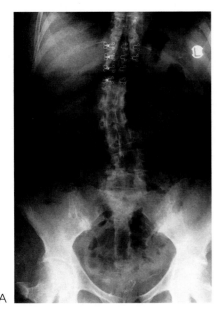 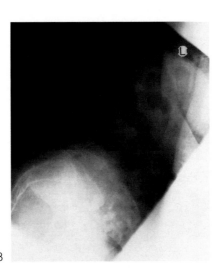 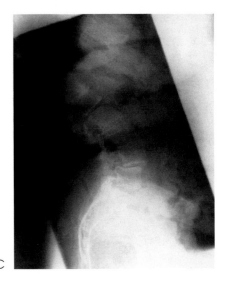

A B C

Figure 22–1. Current radiographic evaluation consisting of an anteroposterior (AP) (A) and flexion (B) and extension (C) lateral images notable for degenerative scoliosis and spondylolisthesis.

walk with assistance, and motor function is fully intact in all groups. Light-touch sensation is decreased over the medial aspect of her right leg and her right knee jerk is diminished, both of which, she notes, are unchanged since before her surgery. All other neurologic testing including that for tension signs is normal.

Radiologic Findings

Diagnostic imaging studies include her preoperative computed tomography (CT) scan as well as new standing anteroposterior (AP) and lateral lumbar spine radiographs, flexion and extension radiographs and magnetic resonance imaging (MRI) with gadolinium of her spine. The preoperative CT scan is notable for severe central and right-sided lateral recess stenosis at the L4/L5 level as well as moderate central and right-sided stenosis at L3/L4. Mild degenerative scoliosis is also noted at L3/L5, but no spondylolisthesis is seen. The postoperative radiographs (Fig. 22–1) confirm the presence of severe spondylolisthesis at L4/L5 with a worsened concave collapsing scoliosis on the right at L3/L4 and L4/L5. Her MRI is also notable for delineating a well-decompressed L4/L5 segment with no further evidence of significant stenosis, but confirms the presence of severe spondylolisthesis and degenerative scoliosis.

Diagnosis

Failed back surgery—progressive postdecompressive spondylolisthesis and degenerative scoliosis.

Surgical Management

Because conservative measures had been unsuccessful, it was recommended that the patient undergo a posterior spinal fusion from L3 to L5 with iliac crest bone graft fusion supplemented with segmental pedicle screw instrumentation (Fig. 22–2). The patient was positioned prone on a Jackson table. A straight midline incision was made utilizing the old scar. The deep fascia was incised longitudinally and subperiosteal dissection proceeded to the tips of the transverse processes of L3, L4, and L5 bilaterally. An intraoperative lateral radiograph confirmed the operative level. Once the soft tissue exposure was obtained, the previous laminectomy margins were explored. It was noted on the right side that there was a fracture of the inferior articular facet of L4, which had been significantly resected. This likely explained the subluxation of L4/L5 and the instability.

Dissection then proceeded in the subcutaneous plane to the right posterior superior iliac spine. Corticocancellous and cancellous bone graft was then harvested through a separate fascial incision. After the bone graft site was closed, attention then returned to the midline wound. The pedicle entry zones were identified bilaterally at L3, L4, and L5. The pedicles were then broached, probed, and sequentially tapped and a 7.0- $\times$ 45-mm pedicle screw was then placed into each pedicle. Intraoperative radiographs confirmed adequate placement of the screws. Decortication proceeded along each level and the bone graft was then placed over the decorticated posterior elements out to the tips of the transverse processes. A $\frac{1}{4}$-inch rod was contoured into slight lordosis and tightened into place with a modest amount of compression on the left side. In hope of improving the scoliotic deformity on the right

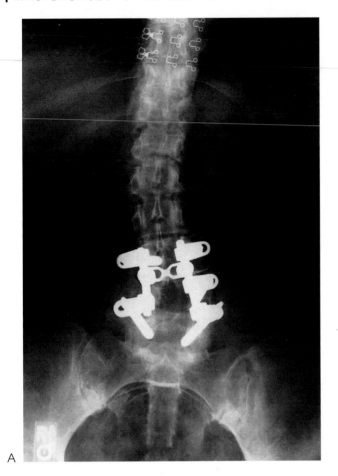 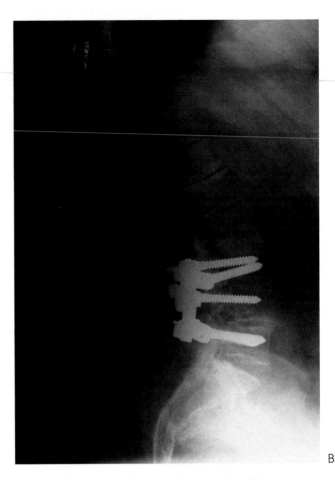

Figure 22–2. AP (A) and lateral (B) radiographs taken after an L3/L5 bilateral posterolateral fusion and segmental pedicle screw instrumentation.

side, a similar rod was contoured into lordosis but placed with slight distraction. A transverse connector was then applied in the standard fashion to lock the rods together. The wound was then copiously irrigated and closed in standard fashion over drains placed deep and superficial to the fascia.

Postoperative Management

The patient tolerated the procedure well and was noted to be neurologically intact. The drains were removed and ambulation started by the first postoperative day. She was instructed upon discharge on the third postoperative day to increase ambulation but to avoid any heavy lifting or bending. An orthosis or corset was not deemed necessary. Two weeks postoperatively she noted substantial improvement in her preoperative back and hip pain and no longer required analgesics.

Discussion

Lumbar spine surgery has become increasingly common as the population ages. Although generally successful, a significant number of patients remain disabled even after surgery. A variety of symptoms with myriad potential causes can be seen in these unfortunate individuals, but these patients all suffer from failed back surgery syndrome (FBSS).

Following failed surgery, diligent gathering of vital information is essential in determining whether current symptoms are mechanical in nature and if they can be treated effectively with surgery or nonsurgical means. Analysis of preoperative studies and operative notes is critical. A careful recapitulation of the original symptom complex and its subsequent treatment are also important in evaluating the accuracy of the previous diagnosis and the appropriateness of future surgery.

The patient's symptoms prior to the initial operation, the extent of pain relief achieved, and the length of the pain-free interval postoperatively are valuable diagnostic information. The pain-free interval can be divided into three diagnostic groups: immediately postoperative, 1 to 6 months after surgery, and greater than 6 months. If there was no relief of pain in the immediate postoperative period, assuming the correct diagnosis was made, then the symptoms are likely due to persistent neural compression at the level of the operation. When pain recurs within 1 to 6 months after surgery, it most likely arises from perineural scarring or occasionally infection. Pain reappearing more than 6 months postoperatively may have a number of causes including new disc herniation, canal stenosis, scarring, or segmental instability.

Because patients with FBSS are primarily concerned about pain rather than neurologic deficit, a detailed delineation of the pain itself must be determined. It is helpful to note whether the pain is the same or has changed since surgery. The distribution of the pain, namely leg versus back pain, and the nature of the pain, whether unremitting or intermittent with well-defined provocative and palliative factors, are helpful in determining if the patient is suffering from failure to treat the original problem effectively or if a new problem has arisen.

A thorough physical examination assessing limitation of back motion and the effect of motion on radicular symptoms may be valuable. For example, extension may worsen leg pain caused by stenosis, whereas forward flexion may exacerbate leg pain due to disc herniation. Evaluation of motor strength, sensation, deep tendon reflexes, and upper motor neuron signs is vital. Residual numbness, weakness, or reflex changes is common following successful discectomy and should not be considered significant. On the other hand, if a deficit reappears that had been previously resolved following the initial surgery, and an interval neurologic test was normal, then a recurrent herniated disc is more likely.

A tension sign is considered an essential objective preoperative finding for a disc herniation that might effectively be treated with surgery. In a previously operated patient, however, it is no longer completely specific because scarring can cause a positive test. Finally, a brief screening for inorganic findings (Waddell's signs) should be performed, including nonanatomic signs and symptoms as well as distraction findings. The presence of greater than three of these findings, even if a mechanical problem exists, suggests that surgical intervention will lead to a poor outcome.

Extraspinal medical illnesses such as abdominal aortic aneurysm, vascular diseases, diabetes, or pancreatitis must be excluded as the cause of back or leg pain. Psychosocial issues, particularly depression, are common in patients with chronic pain, and can interfere with the success of surgical or nonsurgical treatment.

Imaging studies are integral to further refining the diagnosis of FBSS. For each study there is a specific role, an appropriate indication, and a correct time during the course of evaluation. Many errors in decision making arise not from misinter-

PEARLS

- Patient selection is the most important consideration in the treatment of FBSS. The greatest potential successful outcome from lumbar spine surgery will be in those patients with significant signs and symptoms corroborated by diagnostic imaging studies, and who have failed an appropriate conservative treatment protocol.

- Vital information about the patient suffering from FBSS should include a careful review of the original symptom complex, objective findings, imaging studies, and previous operative reports to determine whether the surgery performed was indicated and, if so, appropriately performed.

- Categorizing the patient's pain into pain-free intervals is helpful in determining which of many clinical conditions may be the cause of persistent symptoms.

- Even if a true cause of the persistent pain may exist, conservative treatment should first be exhausted before proceeding with further surgery, because with each additional operation the chances of improvement decline significantly. Most patients will benefit from an adequate therapy protocol and will not need a reoperation.

pretation of the studies but rather from misuse of the imaging information. Greater than one-third of asymptomatic individuals will have abnormal findings using modern neuroradiographic imaging.

Diagnostic studies should begin with standard weight-bearing AP and lateral lumbosacral (LS) spine radiographs. These images are useful in assessing the levels of prior laminectomies and/or fusions as well as current spinal alignment. Lateral flexion and extension views can help to assess stability.

CT myelography is also useful in evaluating the size of the canal, surgical defects, and hypertrophic bone changes that may cause stenosis, particularly when deformity is present.

MRI has become increasingly useful in diagnosing stenosis, tumors, infection, and arachnoiditis. Gadolinium enhances the ability of this study to differentiate residual disc herniation from scar tissue. MRI is not reliable in the early postoperative period, however, because scar tissue may be interpreted as recurrent or residual disc material. This study is most valuable in evaluating the cause of postoperative pain occurring more than 6 months after the initial surgery. Diffuse contrast enhancement on T1-weighted images identifies scar tissue by its extensive vascularity, but the presence of an epidural mass effect without contrast enhancement is more consistent with disc material as the cause of compression. Unfortunately, abnormal findings in asymptomatic individuals are also common with this modality.

Provocative studies including discography, diagnostic facet injection, and selective nerve root infiltration have been recommended as a means of identifying a source of pain, but no study has been able to establish the predictive value of these methods in either the nonoperated or previously operated patients.

Once medical and unrelated spinal conditions are excluded, the differential diagnosis narrows to conditions that predominantly cause leg or back pain or occasionally both. Radicular pain caused by a herniated disc may propagate from a new herniation, a recurrent herniation, or possibly a residual fragment not recovered from the prior procedure. Typically patients with the latter describe no pain-free interval and continue to be bothered by the same radiculopathy in the immediate postoperative period. Objective clinical findings, including a tension sign, continue to be present. Although an MRI can be misleading in the early postoperative period, a combination of the history and clinical findings with contrast-enhanced MRI usually confirms the diagnosis. This diagnostic group is one that would likely benefit from reexploration, provided a more extensive discectomy is accomplished.

A patient who describes the recurrence of leg pain similar to that prior to the original surgery, after a period of relief lasting 6 months or longer, is likely suffering from a recurrent disc herniation.

Spinal stenosis is a frequent cause of back and leg pain in this patient population. New or residual stenosis can cause symptoms almost anywhere along the time line following surgery; unrecognized stenosis in a patient undergoing simple discectomy can result in no relief of pain following surgery, or stenosis may develop gradually, many years following a successful operation, leading to radicular symptoms.

Recurrent leg pain can also be caused by the postoperative formation of hypertrophic scar tissue either within the dural sac (arachnoiditis) or outside the sac (epidural fibrosis). Arachnoiditis and epidural fibrosis are potential causes of nerve root irritation and subsequent radicular symptomatology, which varies in severity but can occasionally mimic that which was present preoperatively. The symptoms usually appear 1 to 6 months after an initial pain-free interval. Often the pain in the leg will follow a nondermatomal distribution and be associated with neurogenic

PITFALLS

- Overinterpretation of imaging studies without appropriate clinical correlation or before completion of an adequate conservative treatment protocol may erroneously lead to further surgery for a condition that is not truly the cause of persistent pain.
- If further surgery is indicated, failure to consider performing a fusion with or without supplemental instrumentation may lead to further postoperative problems. Reoperations in the lumbar spine can result in extensive loss of supporting osseous and soft tissue structures. This can lead to a significant risk of instability or pseudarthrosis in the postoperative period.

type of symptoms such as burning and multilevel dysesthesias. The judicial use of nonoperative measures affords variable periods of symptomatic relief.

Instability may be the underlying cause of persistent back pain, particularly in those patients with excessive bone and soft tissue loss from prior surgery. The pain-free interval associated with instability is variable, but patients predominantly complain of moderate to severe back pain occurring early in the postoperative period and exacerbated by activity. Radicular symptoms may persist but the physical exam is usually unremarkable. Standard weight-bearing flexion and extension lateral radiographs remain the most useful diagnostic tools. Surgical correction via fusion in those with true instability frequently results in clinical improvement.

Pseudarthrosis is reported in 5 to 40% of fusions and may result in instability and persistent back pain. This persists as one of the most common conditions leading to FBSS, yet is one of the most difficult to treat. Standard radiography is usually diagnostic of pseudarthrosis, but its presence must correlate with symptoms because it is frequently difficult to determine if the pseudarthrosis found on radiographs is the true source of pain in a patient. Revision fusion is generally not recommended unless intervertebral motion is demonstrated on flexion and extension radiographs or progressive spondylolisthesis or scoliosis is seen on weight-bearing films.

Postoperative discitis is an uncommon yet potentially dangerous complication of lumbar spine surgery and should be considered first in a patient with increased pain early after surgery. Patients usually present with rather acute onset of severe back pain following a brief, 2- to 4-week period of relief. Severe pain at rest is characteristic and typically localized to the back and buttocks. A low-grade fever may be present.

Instrumentation has now become a common adjunct to spinal fusion. Although it improves fusion rates in certain conditions, its presence has further complicated the evaluation of patients with FBSS. Several technical considerations arise in those patients with supplemental instrumentation regarding possible screw breakage, implant loosening, incorrect placement, and infection. In patients who have pedicle screw instrumentation, a misplaced screw may cause nerve root compression. The patient commonly describes pain and paresthesias in the leg and may have a new neurologic deficit early in the postoperative period. With this presentation, positioning of the screws should be evaluated radiographically with thin-cut CT images. Close correlation must exist between the clinical and CT findings because of the high rate of asymptomatic malpositioned screws, but if a malpositioned screw is truly causing pain or a neurologic deficit, removal is indicated.

A patient with definitive signs and symptoms of nerve root compression or instability, with corroborative diagnostic studies, and who has failed conservative measures is likely to benefit from further lumbar spine surgery. Segmental instability, disc herniation, and stenosis are conditions associated with FBSS that may be resolved with further surgical intervention. Adequate decompression is required for the conditions that lead to symptomatic thecal sac or root compression.

Alternative Methods of Management

The alternatives to surgical management are limited. Arthrodesis without instrumentation or with the addition of segmental instrumentation but without pedicle screws is a viable option but is not the best option in this setting of postoperative instability and progressive degenerative scoliosis in an elderly patient.

Type of Management	Advantages	Disadvantages	Comments
Posterior spinal fusion with instrumentation	Definitive treatment; no bracing required	Surgical risk; risk of failed fusion; risk of adjacent segment degeneration	Definitive procedure for failure of nonoperative treatment
Anterior spinal fusion with instrumentation	Avoids laminectomy defect; less risk of infection	Less rigid stabilization; risk of nonunion; risk of intraabdominal or retroperitoneal complications	Effective as adjunct to posterior spinal fusion but alone is an inadequate form of stability after laminectomy
Bracing with or without exercise	Noninvasive; less costly; no risk of complications; autostabilization is possible	Relies on compliance with long-term program; frequent failure if motion segment is sufficiently unstable	Almost always the primary approach but some patients will require operative treatment

Suggested Readings

Boden SD, Davis DO, Dina TS, Patronas NJ, Wiesel SW. Abnormal magnetic resonance scans of the lumbar spine in asymptomatic subjects: a prospective investigation. J Bone Joint Surg 1990; 72A:403–408.

Boden SD, Martin C, Rudolph R, Kirkpatrick JS, Moeini SM, Hutton WC. Increase of motion between lumbar vertebrae after excision of the capsule and cartilage of the facet. A cadaver study. J Bone Joint Surg 1994; 76:1847–1853.

Finnegan WJ, Fenlin JM, Marvel JP, Nardini RJ, Rothman RH. Results of surgical intervention in the symptomatic multiply-operated back patient. J Bone Joint Surg 1979; 61A:1077–1082.

Lauerman WC, Bradford DS, Ogilvie JW, Transfeldt EE. Results of lumbar pseudarthrosis repair. J Spinal Disord 1992; 5:149–157.

Stambough JL. Causes of failed back surgery syndrome. Semin Spine Surg 1996; 8:165–176.

Vaccaro AR, Garfin SR. Pedicle-screw fixation in the lumbar spine. J Am Acad Orthop Surg 1995; 3:263–274.

Wiesel SW, Boden SD, Lauerman WC. The multiply operated low back: an algorithmic approach. In: Herkowitz HN, Garfin SR, Balderston RA, Eismont FJ, Bell GR, Wiesel SW, eds. The Spine, 4th ed., vol. 2, pp. 1741–1748. Philadelphia: WB Saunders, 1999.

Case 23
Sacroiliac Joint Dysfunction

Jeffrey B. Kleiner and Michael R. Moore

History and Physical Examination

A 47-year-old high school teacher complained of gradual onset of worsening left-sided upper buttock pain with radiation into her left anterior thigh and groin. The patient denied antecedent trauma, problems with arthritis, psychiatric disorders, a history of infection, or problems with substance abuse. She denied difficulty with prolonged sitting or bowel or bladder dysfunction. She was able to stand for about 1 hour but was unable to ambulate farther than one block because of left buttock and groin pain. She also noted pain-related sleep disturbance and several awakenings per night. She complained of an increase in her weight because of the inability to perform any vigorous exercise activity.

She had undergone a course of nonsteroidal antiinflammatory drugs (NSAIDs) without benefit, a 6-month period of physical therapy without improvement, and had been evaluated by a physical medicine specialist and two orthopaedic spinal surgeons. In addition, epidural steroid injections failed to provide any symptomatic relief. These treatments failed to alleviate her pain or provide any diagnostic information. She rated her pain as a 7 on a scale of 10.

The patient was 5'5" and weighed 145 pounds. Physical examination revealed that she had full range of motion of her lumbar spine without pain. There was pain to palpation over her left sacroiliac joint. She had normal deep tendon reflexes, negative tension signs, full range of motion of the hips, and a normal peripheral vascular examination. Supine examination revealed a markedly positive left-sided flexion, abduction, external rotation (FABER) test. Peripheral pulses were within normal limits.

Radiologic Findings

Radiographs of the lumbar spine, including anteroposterior, lateral, and oblique films, revealed mild disc space narrowing at L3/L4 and L5/S1. Magnetic resonance imaging (MRI) revealed dehydration with disc space narrowing at L2/L3 and L5/S1, a small left-sided L2/L3 foraminal herniation, and a small L5/S1 right-sided disc herniation. There was no evidence of central spinal stenosis. Computed tomography (CT) discography at L1/L2, L2/L3, L3/L5, L4/L5, and L5/S1 was negative for reproduction of her typical symptoms and revealed no evidence of bony canal stenosis or explanation for her left-sided symptoms.

Diagnosis

The patient underwent a left-sided L2 selective nerve root block to see if any component of her buttock and anterior thigh pain could be related to the foraminal herniation. This procedure produced no effective relief of her symptoms. A left-sided CT-directed sacroiliac joint injection was then administered. This alleviated all of her buttock pain and left thigh pain. The injection was repeated 2 weeks later with a

PEARL

• Preoperative review of the CT scan of the sacroiliac joint is mandatory to help determine the depth from the outer ilium to the sacroiliac joint and to help in determining the optimal screw length placed for internal fixation.

PITFALLS

• Care must be taken to avoid damage to the superior gluteal artery, as the gluteus medius musculature is stripped from the inferior aspect of the outer table of the ilium toward the sciatic notch.

• Penetration of the pelvis with screw fixation or missing the sacroiliac joint during osteotomy through the ilium can be avoided by preoperative planning and study of the CT scan.

similar effect. Review of the CT scan of the sacroiliac joint revealed degenerative changes without evidence of cyst formation, chronic osteomyelitis, or congenital anomalies.

Surgical Management

The patient underwent an additional 6 weeks of sacroiliac joint stabilization techniques and trial of a sacroiliac joint belt. Having failed to respond to nonoperative management, she elected to proceed with a posterior, sacroiliac joint arthrodesis described initially by Smith-Peterson and Rogers (1926) and modified by Moore (1994).

The patient was placed under a general anesthetic, a Foley catheter was inserted, and she was rolled into the prone position on an Andrews table. She was positioned such that image intensification could be used to visualize the sacroiliac joint obliquely, in the direct anteroposterior view, as well as inlet and outlet pelvis projections.

A curvilinear incision was made over the left sacroiliac joint just lateral to the posterosuperior iliac spine (Fig. 23–1A). Dissection through the subcutaneous tissue allowed exposure of the posterior, superior iliac spine and the cephalic extent of the sacroiliac joint. Subperiosteal dissection of the gluteus maximus over the lateral portion of the ilium and through the sling of gluteus medius attached to the sacrum was continued caudally. Care was taken to avoid damage to the superior gluteal artery as it exited from the greater sciatic notch. A Taylor retractor was used to maintain visualization of the lateral table of the ilium. The center of the cartilaginous portion of the sacroiliac joint was determined by using a preoperative CT scan and the reference of the posterosuperior iliac spine. An air burr was used to outline a rectangle over the synovial portion of the sacroiliac joint, which measured approximately 2 × 2.5 cm. Curved and straight osteotomes were used to cut through the

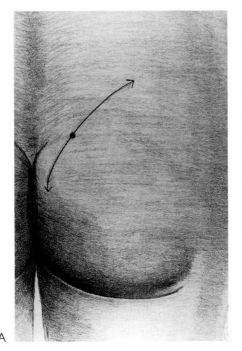
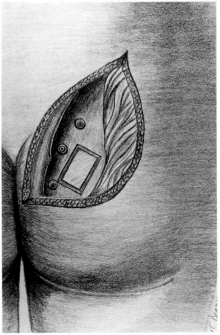

A
B

Figure 23–1. (A) A curvilinear incision is made over the left sacroiliac joint lateral to the posterior superior iliac spine. (B) The completed sacroiliac joint fusion.

ilium and into the cartilaginous portion of the sacroiliac joint. Penetration through the ilium into the sacroiliac joint was heralded by a change in the pitch of the sound of the osteotome as it cut into the harder subchondral bone and into the joint space. A 3.2-mm drill bit was then used to create drill holes into the ilium and sacrum. These were placed caudal to the osteotomized rectangle, through the center of the osteotomized rectangle, and cephalad to the osteotomized rectangle. The pathway of the drill bit was observed fluoroscopically in the anteroposterior, inlet and outlet views of the pelvis, as well as a sacroiliac joint view. The outer cortex of the ilium was tapped with a 6.5-mm AO cancellous screw tap. This was used as a corkscrew to help remove the osteotomized rectangle from the ilium. A large straight curette was used to decorticate the sacral side of the joint. The joint space was undermined circumferentially with a small angled curette. The cartilaginous surface from the iliac side of the sacroiliac joint was debrided using a rongeur and curettes.

Bone graft was harvested from the posterosuperior iliac spine using osteotomes and a Cobb gouge. The cancellous bone was impacted into the recesses developed following curetting of the joint surfaces. The bone window was then impacted and countersunk across the prepared portion of the sacroiliac joint. The appropriate-length screws were determined with a depth gauge and then 6.5-mm AO cancellous screws were added to the pretapped holes with washers. Fluoroscopic evaluation in all planes was obtained to confirm appropriate position of the implants. The wound was copiously irrigated with bacitracin and normal saline solution and a layered closure was carried out. The completed procedure is shown diagrammatically in Figure 23–1B, and Figure 23–2 shows a postoperative roentgenogram.

Postoperative Management

Patient-controlled analgesia was used for the first 18 hours postoperatively. It was discontinued, along with the Foley catheter, on postoperative day 1 and a course of physical therapy emphasizing non–weight bearing on the affected lower extremity was carried out for the ensuing 2 days in the hospital. The patient was discharged on postoperative day 3 on strict non–weight bearing on the left side, which was continued for 8 weeks. The patient was evaluated at 4 and 8 weeks after surgery and then

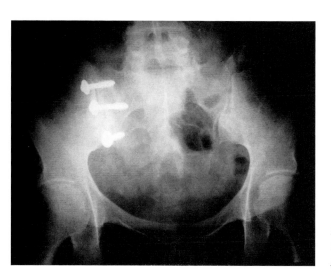

Figure 23–2. A plain radiograph of the completed sacroiliac joint fusion.

at 3 months, 6 months and 12 months, and yearly thereafter. She noted marked pain reduction and the ability to return to most of her premorbid activities.

Discussion

Sacroiliac joint dysfunction was recognized as a cause of low back pain as early as 1905. Smith-Peterson and Rogers (1926) reported an 88% clinical success rate in 26 patients with recalcitrant symptoms who were treated with arthrodesis. (As an interesting aside, Smith-Peterson performed the procedure on his wife.) The diagnosis and therapy for this disorder fell into obscurity after the discovery and description of the disc herniation by Dandy (1928) and Mixter and Barr (1934). There are sporadic references to the condition until the 1980s, when Waisbrod and colleagues (1987) reported their results of surgically treated individuals and a 70% success rate.

The key to successful treatment is the correct diagnosis. Although sacroiliac joint dysfunction may represent the cause of low back pain in up to 22% of patients, it is not commonly appreciated. This is largely due to the fact that sacroiliac joint dysfunction can resemble other maladies affecting the low back such as S1 radiculopathy. Figure 23–3 shows typical pain patterns described by patients with sacroiliac joint dysfunction.

Physical examination techniques have been found to be poorly predictive, and imaging modalities are nondiagnostic as they commonly are in the spine. Reports regarding the treatment of sacroiliac joint disease are now fairly common in both the surgical and physiatrical literature.

Once the diagnosis of sacroiliac joint dysfunction is established, treatment with NSAIDs and conditioning programs may be sufficient to reduce pain to a tolerable level. Don Tigny (1997) and Lee (1997) have described physiotherapeutic techniques with hip girdle strengthening. Mooney (1997) has demonstrated the effectiveness of a specific exercise protocol emphasizing resistive torso rotation exercises. A patient's unresponsiveness to these modalities should be reevaluated with repeat sacroiliac joint injections to confirm the diagnosis. Those with less than 90% relief of pain should be evaluated for other potential causes of low back pain, including discogenic sources, facet source arthropathy, and neoplasm. Reproducible relief of

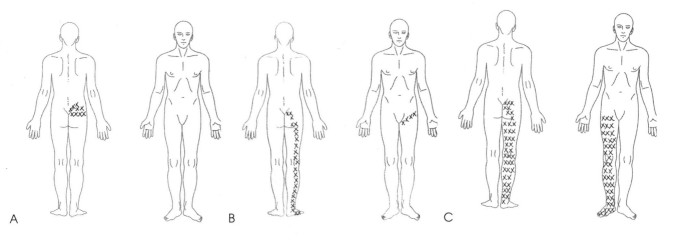

Figure 23–3. Various pain patterns often reported by patient with sacroiliac joint dysfunction. (A) Pain localized over the sacroiliac joint. (B) Pain classified as "pseudo" radicular. (C) Pain described as diffuse lower extremity discomfort and/or parasthesial often misinterpreted as "hysterical."

symptoms with injection and a negative workup for an alternative diagnosis allow a surgeon to counsel patients regarding sacroiliac joint arthrodesis. Although surgical treatment remains controversial, it is also unrealistic to assume that the sacroiliac joint is immune from pain due to arthritis or instability as opposed to every other joint in the body.

Several studies have evaluated surgically treated sacroiliac joint dysfunction. Kleiner and Weingarten (1995) and Moore (1997) have stressed the importance of a solid arthrodesis in achieving a good clinical outcome in surgically treated sacroiliac joint dysfunction. Moore reported 89% clinically successful results in a minimum follow-up of 2 years in nonsmoking patients with isolated sacroiliac joint pathology and no prior back surgery. Surgical arthrodesis should be considered a viable option for patients with severe symptoms from sacroiliac joint dysfunction.

Alternative Methods of Management

A variety of techniques in addition to those previously mentioned have been applied to sacroiliac joint dysfunction. Prolotherapy, the application of inflammatory agents into the ligamentous portion of the sacroiliac joint (upper two-thirds), has been reported as a treatment option for sacroiliac joint disease. This may be a reasonable option for a select group of patients. This process encourages the production of stiffer and more abundant ligamentous tissue. The disadvantages of this technique are that the injections are quite painful and numerous applications are necessary. No long-term results are available. Another reported technique for a sacroiliac joint stabilization involves percutaneous placement of screws across the joint without fusion. Short-term results were favorably reported in 48% of patients. Our experience with this technique and the bad outcomes associated with pseudarthrosis would not allow us to recommend this procedure.

Some orthopaedic surgeons are more comfortable with the anterior approach to the sacroiliac joint because of their experience in treatment of major trauma, such as Malgaigne fracture dislocations of the sacroiliac joint. At least one article has reported on treatment of sacroiliac joint dysfunction by elective anterior fusion. There was an

Type of Management	Advantages	Disadvantages	Comments
Antiinflammatory medication, conditioning program	Majority of patients respond favorably Minimal morbidity	Minimal	First line of treatment for degenerative spinal pathologies
Prolotherapy	Encourages the production of stiffer and more abundant ligamentous tissue	Injections are quite painful, and numerous applications are necessary	No long-term results are available
Percutaneous screw fixation	Short-term results are favorable in 48% of patients	High reported rate of dissatisfaction	Not recommended by the authors
Anterior SI fusion	Familiar surgical exposure	Complications include reflex sympathetic dystrophy (RSD), persistent causalgic pain, infection, neurologic complications	Not recommended by the authors

unacceptably high complication rate, with reflex sympathetic dystrophy (RSD), persistent causalgic pain, infection, and neurologic complications. The anterior approach for elective arthrodesis of the sacroiliac joint, therefore, cannot be recommended.

Suggested Readings

Bellamy N, Park W, Rooney PJ. What do we know about the sacroiliac joint? Semin Arthritis Rheum 1983; 12:282–313.

Bernard TN, Kirkaldy, Willis MA. Recognizing specific characteristics of non-specific low back pain. Clin Orthop Rel Res 1987; 217:266–280.

Boden SD, Davis DO, Dina TS, et al. Abnormal magnetic resonance scans of the lumbar spine in asymptomatic subjects. J Bone Joint Surg 1990; 72A:403–408.

Dandy WE. Loose cartilage from intervertebral disc simulating tumor of the spinal cord. Arch Surg 1928; 19:660–672.

DonTigny RL. Mechanics and treatment of the sacroiliac joint. J Manipulative Manual Ther 1993; 1:3–12.

DonTigny RL. Mechanics and treatment of the sacroiliac joint. In: Vleeming A, Mooney V, Doorman T, eds. Movement, Stability and Low Back Pain: The Essential Role of the Pelvis, pp. 461–476. New York: Churchill Livingstone, 1997.

Dorman T. Pelvic mechanics and prolotherapy. In: Vleeming A, Mooney V, Doorman T, eds. Movement, Stability and Low Back Pain: The Essential Role of the Pelvis, pp. 501–522. New York: Churchill Livingstone, 1997.

Dreyfuss P, Michaelson M, Pauza K, et al. The utility of the history and physical examination in diagnosing interarticular sacroiliac mediated pain as determined by intraarticular sacroiliac joint injection. Presented at the 2nd World Congress on Low Back Pain, 1995.

Fortin JD. Sacroiliac joint dysfunction. J Back Musculoskel Rehabil 1993; 3(3):31–43.

Fortin JD. Sacroiliac joint: pain referral maps upon applying a new injection/arthrography technique I and II. Spine 1994; 19(13):1475–1489.

Gaenslen, FJ. Sacroiliac joint arthrodesis. JAMA 1927; 89:2031–2135.

Goldthwaite JE, Osgood RE. A consideration of the pelvic articulations from an anatomical, pathological and clinical standpoint. Boston Med Surg J 1905; 152:593–660.

Keating FG, Avilar MD, Price M. Sacroiliac joint arthrodesis in selected patients with low back pain. In: Vleeming A, Mooney V, Doorman T, eds. Movement, Stability and Low Back Pain: The Essential Role of the Pelvis, pp. 573–586. New York: Churchill Livingstone, 1997.

Kim DH, Patel AI, Brown CW, Friermood TG. Athrodesis of the sacroiliac joint syndrome: preliminary review of results. Paper No. 76, American Academy of Orthopedic Surgeons annual meeting, scientific program, February 22, 1996.

Kleiner JB, Weingarten PL. Sacroiliac joint dysfunction as a complication of spinal fusion. Presented at the North American Spine Society 10th annual meeting, 1995.

Lee DG. Treatment of pelvic instability. In: Vleeming A, Mooney V, Doorman T, eds. Movement, Stability and Low Back Pain: The Essential Role of the Pelvis, pp. 445–459. New York: Churchill Livingstone, 1997.

Lippett AM. Percutaneous fixation of the sacroiliac joint. In: Vleeming A, Mooney V, Doorman T, eds. Movement, Stability and Low Back Pain: The Essential Role of the Pelvis, pp. 589–594. New York: Churchill Livingstone, 1997.

Mixter WJ, Barr JS. Rupture of the intervertebral disc with involvement of the spinal canal. N Engl J Med 1934; 211:210–215.

Mooney V. Understanding, examining for and treating sacroiliac joint pain. J Musculoskel Med 1993; 10(7):37–49.

Mooney V. Sacroiliac joint dysfunction. In: Vleeming A, Mooney V, Doorman T, eds. Movement, Stability and Low Back Pain: The Essential Role of the Pelvis, pp. 37–52. New York: Churchill Livingstone, 1997.

Moore MR. Diagnosis and treatment of chronic painful sacroiliac arthropathy. Orthop Trans 1994; 18(1):255.

Moore MR. Surgical treatment of chronic painful sacroiliac joint dysfunction. In: Vleeming A, Mooney V, Doorman T, eds. Movement, Stability and Low Back Pain: The Essential Role of the Pelvis, pp. 563–572. New York: Churchill Livingstone, 1997.

Moore MR. Outcomes of surgical treatment of chronic, painful sacroiliac joint dysfunction. Proceedings of the 3rd Interdisciplinary World Congress on Low Back and Pelvic Pain, Vienna, November 19–21, 1998.

Norman GF, May A. Sacroiliac conditioning simulating intervertebral disc syndrome. West J Surg Obstet Gynecol 1956; 64:461–462.

Pitkin HC, Pheasant HC. Sacrarthrogenic telagin. J Bone Joint Surg 1936; 28A:111–133.

Potter NA, Rothstein JM. Intertester reliability for selected clinical tests of the sacroiliac joint. Phys Ther 1991; 65:1671–1675.

Slipman CW, Sterenfeld MD, et al. Sacroiliac joint syndrome: the value of radionuclide imaging in the diagnosis of sacroiliac joint syndrome. Spine 1996; 21:2251–2254.

Smith-Peterson MN, Rogers WA. End result of arthrodesis of sacroiliac joint for arthritis, traumatic and non-traumatic. J Bone Joint Surg 1926; 8A:118–136.

Steindler A, Luck JV. Differential diagnosis of pain low in the back. JAMA 1938; 110:106–113.

Waisbrod H, Kainick JU, Gerbershagen HU. Sacroiliac joint arthrodesis for chronic low back pain. Arch Orthop Trauma Surg 1987; 106:238–240.

Section II

Inflammatory Disorders

Case 24
Rheumatoid Arthritis Cranial–C1/C2 Disease
Seth M. Zeidman and Thomas B. Ducker

History and Physical Examination

A 58-year-old woman with a history of early onset of rheumatoid arthritis (20 years) presented with an 8-month history of suboccipital pain that was exacerbated by any rotary head movements. Until this present acute pain she had been adequately treated with minimal doses of corticosteroids. She had only mild peripheral joint deformities. She was neurologically intact and was employed as a clerk.

Radiologic Findings

Plain radiographs demonstrated 11 mm of anterior subluxation between C1 and C2 (Fig. 24–1A). In the supine position a sagittal magnetic resonance imaging (MRI)

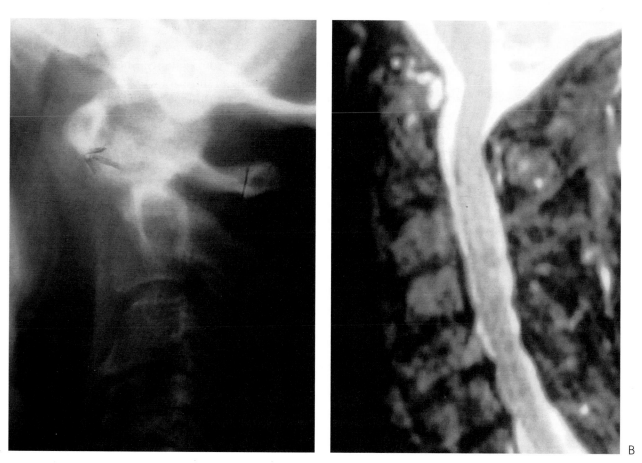

A   B

Figure 24–1. (A) Lateral plain radiograph revealing 11 mm of anterior subluxation between C1 and C2. (B) Sagittal magnetic resonance imaging (MRI) of the cervical spine revealing satisfactory alignment without cord compression and only minimal posterior indentation of the thecal sac.

revealed satisfactory alignment without cord compression and only minimal posterior indentation of the thecal sac (Fig. 24–1B) There was no evidence of significant basilar impression. Computed tomography (CT) scanning revealed no significant erosion of the C1/C2 lateral masses.

Diagnosis

C1/C2 instability (hypermobility) with persistent, severe pain interfering with the patient's normal lifestyle.

Discussion

Rheumatoid arthritis (RA) is a chronic relapsing inflammatory arthritis, affecting multiple diarthrodial joints, with variable systemic manifestations. The precise mechanism of initiation of rheumatoid arthritis remains incompletely understood, but the pathologic, inflammatory process responsible for the clinical manifestations is well delineated. Rheumatoid pannus, which is granulation tissue, forms in the inflamed joint from proliferating fibroblasts and inflammatory cells. This pannus produces collagenase and other proteolytic enzymes capable of eroding adjacent cartilage, tendons, and bone. Tendon rupture, ligamentous laxity, loss of cartilage, and bone erosion all follow. In general, joints that ultimately develop severe destruction become symptomatic within a year of disease onset.

Cervical spine involvement occurs in up to 90% of RA patients. It has been postulated that the cervical spine is the most commonly affected portion of the spinal column because of the large number of synovial joints. Rheumatoid involvement of the cervical spine generally begins early in the disease process and progresses in parallel with peripheral involvement. Within the cervical spine, RA has a particular predilection for the craniocervical junction and the atlantoaxial articulation. Prospective studies have demonstrated a mortality rate for patients with rheumatoid spondylitis that is more than twice that for matched patients without spondylitis.

At present, the only treatment that reliably increases the probability of improving overall survival is fusion. Every clinician must appreciate the potential severity of this disease and prescribe appropriate treatments. This understanding should guide all decisions regarding the necessity and role of surgical intervention.

The development and progression of neurologic disease has been described in up to 36% of patients with rheumatoid cervical spondylitis. When there are neurologic complaints, the patients often describe upper and lower extremity weakness with associated gait disturbances. Typical findings include peripheral neuropathy, symptoms of vascular insufficiency, radiculopathy, and myelopathy. These symptoms tend to progressively worsen, with regression occurring only rarely.

The overall incidence of myelopathy in RA patients is estimated to be between 10 and 40%. Myelopathy occurs in 75% of individuals with cranial settling and in 60% of patients with atlantoaxial dislocation.

Spinal cord compression at the level of the cervicomedullary junction can produce uniform weakness of all four limbs and threaten the ventilatory drive. In very advanced cases, ataxia, nystagmus, and bulbar signs all may occur. Brain stem dysfunction occurs in up to 50% of the patients with cranial settling. The cranial nerves most commonly affected include the hypoglossal, glossopharyngeal, and trigeminal nerves.

The best way to monitor the changes in the rheumatoid cervical spondylitis is radiographic evaluation because the radiologic changes of RA closely mirror the pathologic processes. The mainstay of radiologic evaluation of the cervical spine is the plain radiograph. Further information may be gained with dynamic studies including flexion and extension views.

Computed tomography allows visualization of tissues in an axial plane. CT is excellent for determining the dimensions of the spinal canal as well as the relationship of the atlas and axis. It also allows visualization and mapping of the vertebral artery, which can prove invaluable when certain surgical procedures (e.g., C1/C2 transarticular screws) are being considered. To assess the soft tissue component, dural sac, nerve roots, and spinal cord, water-soluble myelography must be performed.

Magnetic resonance imaging allows direct visualization of the cord and impinging elements, and has greatly enhanced our ability to accurately diagnose and more appropriately treat this disease.

Radiographic progression of cervical disease occurs in up to 80% of patients, but does not necessarily reflect clinical or neurologic deterioration. Nearly 50% of patients with cervical disease remain asymptomatic despite worsening radiographic appearance.

Specific Patterns of Involvement

Atlantoaxial Subluxation

Atlantoaxial subluxation is the displacement of the atlas upon the axis and is the most commonly observed lesion of the rheumatoid spine, with an incidence approaching 83% of patients with RA. Such displacement may be horizontal, vertical, or have a rotatory component, depending on the specific mechanism of destruction. The most common pattern is anterior subluxation in the horizontal or transverse plane.

A measured distance of greater than 3.5 mm between the anterior tubercle of the atlas and the odontoid is considered diagnostic of atlantoaxial subluxation, whereas a distance exceeding 12 mm denotes complete ligamentous complex failure. The flexion and extension views determine whether the subluxation is fixed or reducible. The clinically significant distance is 9 mm, with signs and symptoms of cord compression occurring only in those manifesting with more than 9 mm of subluxation.

The severity of cervical involvement parallels peripheral joint involvement and the severity of the overall systemic disease, but attempts to define a population at risk for atlantoaxial subluxation have yielded contradictory results. Atlantoaxial subluxation generally precedes the development of superior migration of the odontoid process.

Superior Migration of the Odontoid

Superior migration of the odontoid process is observed in up to one-third of RA patients. Transverse ligament laxity produces excessive dynamic loading of the lateral occipitoatlantal and atlantoaxial joints that have already been affected by the disease. Basilar invagination results from upward migration of C2 through the ring of C1 and into the foramen magnum and is due to oblique erosion of the horizontal C1/C2 facet joints. Superior migration of the odontoid is less dependent on ligamentous structural integrity than on bony support.

The radiologic changes associated with cranial settling include erosion with compression of the lateral atlantal masses; downward separation of the anterior arch of the atlas from the clivus, so that the anterior atlas arch descends onto the axis body; and displacement of the posterior arch of the atlas rostrally and ventrally, decreasing the anteroposterior spinal canal diameter.

Superior migration of the odontoid occurs relatively late in the course of the disease, typically in patients with disease duration of longer than 20 years.

Numerous craniometric techniques have been developed to diagnose superior migration of the odontoid. Chamberlain's line extends from the posterior aspect of the hard palate to the posterior border of the foramen magnum, or opisthion. The odontoid tip should not extend more than 3 mm above this line. If it extends more than 6.6 mm above this line, superior odontoid migration may be diagnosed. McGregor's line is drawn from the posterior aspect of the hard palate, but it extends to the most caudal portion of the occiput. Protrusion of the odontoid process more than 4.5 mm above this line is considered abnormal. The mean value in normal subjects, plus two standard deviations, should be used as the definitive criterion. Thus, 9 mm of extension of the odontoid above the line is diagnostic of superior odontoid migration.

Nonoperative Management

The goals of any therapeutic intervention for RA patients are reduction of symptoms, arrest of disease progression, and preservation of function. Available therapeutic strategies include observation, nonoperative management, and surgical management.

Systemic rest is effective in combating the chronic disease and the constitutional symptoms. Joint rest or limitation of joint motion is prescribed in proportion to disease severity and permits symptomatic improvement. The role of cervical collars in rheumatoid spondylitis is controversial. Although generally accepted as a means of treating cervical pain, such collars are ineffective for immobilizing an unstable cervical spine. There is even some evidence that hard cervical collars may exacerbate atlantoaxial subluxation.

Physical therapy maintains extremity muscle strength and joint mobility. However, muscle stretching and range-of-motion exercises cannot preserve functional capacity or prevent cervical deformity. Some patients benefit symptomatically from deep heat, ultrasound, and massage.

Medical management, the third component of nonoperative management, entails three classes of therapy. The first class, consisting of salicylates, nonsteroidal antiinflammatory drugs, and low-dose glucocorticoids, controls the local inflammatory process. The second class of drugs, including D-penicillamine, gold, sulfasalazine, and antimalarial agents, alters disease progression. The third class works by immunosuppression and includes methotrexate, azathioprine, and cyclophosphamide.

Surgical Management

Fundamental principles of the surgical treatment for rheumatoid spondylitis include spinal cord and brain stem decompression, realignment of mobile subluxations, and maintenance of cervical alignment with osseous fusion. Surgical intervention is generally mandated in patients with significant cord compression, significant myelopathic signs and symptoms, severe pain with obvious marked subluxations or progressive neurologic dysfunction despite maximal nonoperative therapy. It remains unclear which asymptomatic lesions pose a significant risk to the RA patient.

Despite advances in anesthetic technique and perioperative medical management, the contemporary mortality rate associated with operative stabilization ranges from approximately 5 to 15%. The probability of developing clinically evident myelopathy increases exponentially once the subluxation exceeds 8 mm. The critical element to consider and quantitate is the absolute space available for the spinal cord. Early prophylactic operative intervention with stabilization may be indicated before atlantoaxial instability progresses and appreciable neurologic deterioration occurs because once symptoms of cord compression occur, the myelopathy is often irreversible, the prognosis is poor, and the risk of sudden death is increased. Given the likelihood of progressive subluxation, operative stabilization may be indicated for surgical candidates demonstrating mobile subluxations exceeding 8 mm.

The criteria for stabilization of superior migration of the odontoid in the absence of neurologic deficit are less well defined. Evidence of upward odontoid migration with documented disease progression is an appropriate indication for operative stabilization in a neurologically intact patient. Cranial settling is generally progressive and often fatal.

Neural decompression may be obtained by direct transoral decompression of the ventral brain stem and upper cervical spinal cord, or by attempted "disimpaction" of the upwardly migrated odontoid with axial skeletal traction.

The use of traction in patients with posterior occipital-atlantal dislocations or complex rotatory subluxations can be dangerous. Any attempt at reduction with cervical traction should be performed in a monitored care setting with pulse oximetry and readily available ventilatory support. We favor application of traction by means of a halo ring, as opposed to by Gardner-Wells tongs. Traction is begun at 3 to 5 pounds and gradually increased to 15 to 20 pounds over 3 to 4 days. Periodic radiologic evaluation is essential to identify the degree of reduction and to optimize the applied vector and force of distraction. If the reduction has not occurred by the end of 5 days, the lesion is considered irreducible.

Direct transoral decompression may be performed safely and effectively as the first portion of a staged operative procedure. Concomitant vertical instability mandates an occipitocervical fusion as the stabilization procedure. Internal fixation is useful to improve the fusion outcome and to maintain proper alignment.

In individuals with gross instability or with complex forms of craniovertebral involvement, instrumentation of the craniovertebral junction is often required. There are a variety of modalities available. Anterior stabilization of the atlantoaxial complex is possible but is associated with substantial morbidity and many believe that this procedure should be augmented with a posterior fusion.

Several fusion techniques have been used for posterior stabilization of the atlantoaxial complex. Internal fixation typically involves bone graft with either midline wires (Gallie-type fusion), lateral wires (Brooks-type fusion), or posterolateral clamps (Halifax-type fusion). When wiring is required, our preference is to use a modified Brooks construct.

Transarticular C1/C2 screws immediately stabilize the atlantoaxial articulation. Transarticular screws provide direct rotational stability by immobilizing the facet joint bilaterally, in addition to translational stability due to the oblique screw angle. A CT scan detailing the C2 pedicle, facet joint, and C1 lateral mass is mandatory to delineate the vertebral artery course.

PEARL

• It is very important to get solid bony fusion posteriorly along with the transarticular screws. Fusions both anteriorly and posteriorly are sometimes required to attain a solid bony arthrodesis. Structural cortico-cancellous autografts are an integral part of the posterior arthrodesis.

When an occipitocervical fusion is required, there are a variety of instrumentation choices available. Whether one uses two parallel plates, or the newer Cervifix system (Synthes USA, Paoli, PA) or a Y plate, the choice should be based on which is most appropriate and on the surgeon's experience.

One may or may not choose to use a halo in the perioperative period but some form of bracing is certainly indicated. Overall, the patient's chances of being significantly improved are clearly in the range of 90% but these surgeries carry with them substantial associated risk.

Additional cases are presented to illustrate the full clinical spectrum of presentation. The second case is somewhat different because the patient presented with pain as well as arm and leg weakness. This patient had early myelopathic signs and symptoms with gait abnormalities. She was myelopathic with impaired hand function. Her subluxation was irreducible as shown in Figure 24–2A. It did not move on extension and when forced into extension the patient noted neurologic deterioration. MRI (Fig. 24–2B) shows an impressive pannus posterior to the dens with evidence of erosion. Significant spinal cord pathology is noted directly behind the inferior aspect of the dens. This patient did not have significant basilar impression and requires a C1 and C2 vertebra fusion with transarticular screws. Fusion will cause regression of the pannus and neurologic stabilization if not actual improvement. Placing the patient into forced extension is not recommended because the pannus

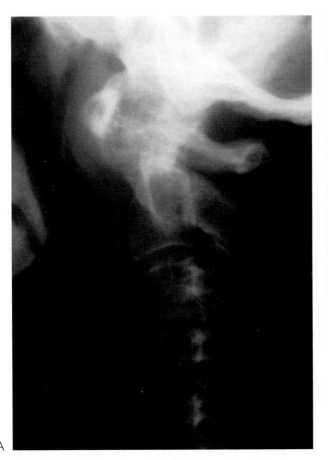 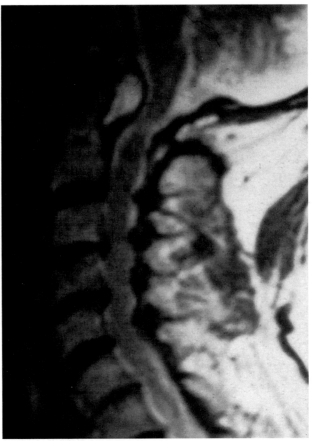

A   B

Figure 24–2. (A) Lateral plain radiograph revealing an irreducible subluxation of C1 on C2. (B) Sagittal MRI of the cervical spine revealing a large pannus posterior to the dens with evidence of odontoid erosion.

will cause spinal cord compression. This patient was fused with some residual deformity, with the ring of C1 forward on C2. If removal of the posterior portion of ring of C1 is required, the fusion should be extended to the occiput.

The third case has a fixed C1 on C2 subluxation with neurologic sequelae necessitating removal of the posterior portion of the ring of C1. A typical X-ray is shown (Fig. 24–3A). MRI reveals a fixed subluxation of C1 and C2 that is held because of pannus between the ring of C1 and the anterior aspect of the dens (Fig. 24–3B). In this case, the ring of C1 has to be removed because the subluxation cannot be reduced. This can be confirmed with flexion/extension MRI, but this must be done judiciously. In the first and second cases the flexion-extension MRI was quite helpful in demonstrating the pathology; in this third case, there was little to no movement on the flexion and extension MRI. Surgery in these patients can be significantly more risky.

The fourth case is a 64-year-old woman with a 30-year history of RA and severe deformities of the hands and feet. Cervical flexion produced transient quadriparesis, and extension made her briefly unconscious due to vertebral artery compression. MRI (Fig. 24–4) revealed superior migration of the dens through the foramen magnum with medullary stem compression. There are a variety of treatment alternatives for this patient. Many surgeons would recommend anterior odontoidectomy followed by posterior stabilization. An alternative is to put the patient through a trial

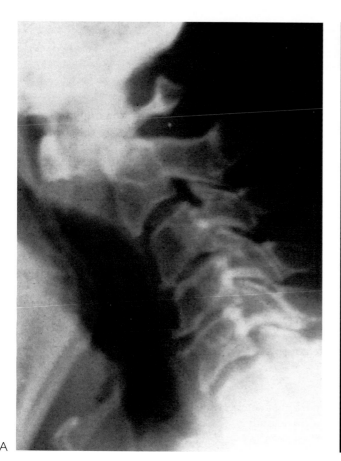
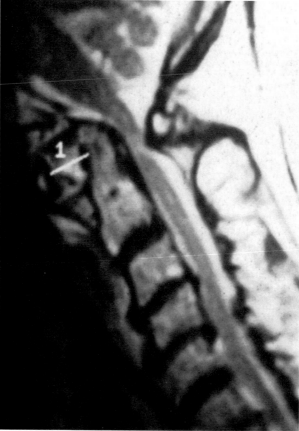

A   B

Figure 24–3. (A) Lateral plain radiograph revealing an irreducible subluxation of C1 on C2. (B) Sagittal MRI of the cervical spine reveals a fixed subluxation of C1 on C2 due to a pannus between the anterior ring of C1 and the anterior aspect of the dens.

PEARLS

- In removing the ring of C1, we use a high-speed burr initially to reduce the bone. The last bit of bone is removed with a diamond burr, and curetted away.
- The patient is held in traction using a halo ring and evoked potential monitoring is begun prior to initial positioning.
- We routinely use preoperative steroids, to potentially provide some neuroprotection.
- The posterior portion of the ring of C1 must be removed and the ligaments attached to the base of the occiput released.

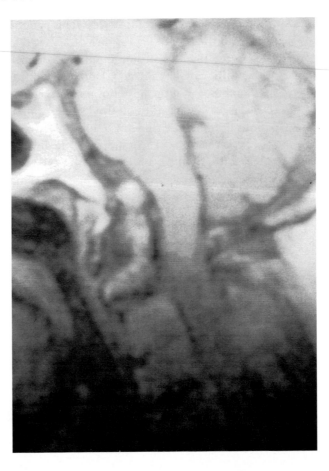

Figure 24–4. Sagittal MRI of the cervical spine revealing superior migration of the dens through the foramen magnum with medullary stem compression.

of traction to see if it is able to reduce the superiorly migrated odontoid, and then perform the posterior stabilization. This latter operative strategy was utilized in this case.

Often patients with this degree of deformity have concomitant subaxial cervical stenosis and/or subluxations. At the time of surgical stabilization the subaxial disease should also be addressed. Extending the fusion from the occiput to C5 or even lower is not uncommon.

Alternative Methods of Management

Type of Management	Advantages	Disadvantages	Comments
Observation	None	No treatment	Only useful in patients who are early in disease process or are completely asymptomatic
Nonoperative therapy	Minimal associated morbidity	Temporizing maneuver No positive result	Often very successful for an extended time period; trial of nonoperative therapy can be attempted until it fails, then proceed with surgery

Continued on next page

Continued

Type of Management	Advantages	Disadvantages	Comments
External fixation—halo	No operative risk	No real benefit to patient	Poor long-term solution
Internal posterior fixation—wiring	Decreased operative risk	Less immediate stability	Can be risky when wires are passed in sublaminar space
Internal posterior fixation—wiring with transarticular screws	Immediate stability No need for external bracing	Higher risk Increased morbidity	When instrumentation is required this is the definitive procedure
Internal posterior fixation with odontoid resection	Immediate stability Immediate decompression	Even higher risk procedure Risk of wound breakdown	Often unnecessary with rheumatoid pannus May be required with irreducible odontoid migration

Conclusion

In treating high cervical or cranial-cervical disorders in RA, it is essential that high-quality plain radiographs and MRIs be available to assess the extent of soft tissue and bony pathology. A variety of treatment modalities are available to address the myriad pathologies that exist in this patient population. However, the fundamental principles of surgical care remain consistent: thorough neural decompression with restoration of spinal alignment, rigid internal stabilization, and solid bony arthrodesis.

Suggested Readings

Casey AT, Crockard HA, Geddes JF, Stevens J. Vertical translocation: the enigma of the disappearing atlantodens interval in patients with myelopathy and rheumatoid arthritis. Part I. Clinical, radiological, and neuropathological features. J Neurosurg 1997; 87(6):856–862.

Casey AT, Crockard HA, Stevens, J. Vertical translocation. Part II. Outcomes after surgical treatment of rheumatoid cervical myelopathy. J Neurosurg 1997; 87(6):863–869.

Dunbar RP, Alexiades MM. Decision making in rheumatoid arthritis. Determining surgical priorities. Rheum Dis Clin North Am 1998; 24(1):35–54.

Fujiwara K, Fujimoto M, Owaki H, et al. Cervical lesions related to the systemic progression in rheumatoid arthritis. Spine 1998; 23(19):2052–2056.

Gurley JP, Bell GR. The surgical management of patients with rheumatoid cervical spine disease. Rheum Dis Clin North Am 1997; 23(2):317–332.

Heidecke V, Rainov NG, Burkert W. Occipito-cervical fusion with the cervical Cotrel-Dubousset rod system. Acta Neurochir (Wien) 1998; 140(9):969–976.

Kauppi M, Leppanen L, Heikkila S, Lahtinen T, Kautiainen H. Active conservative treatment of atlantoaxial subluxation in rheumatoid arthritis. Br J Rheumatol 1998; 37(4):417–420.

Keersmaekers A, Truyen L, Ramon F, Cras P, De Clerck L, Martin JJ. Cervical myelopathy due to rheumatoid arthritis. Case report and review of the literature. Acta Neurol Belg 1998; 98(3):284–288.

Mori T, Matsunaga S, Sunahara N, Sakou T. 3- to 11-year followup of occipitocervical fusion for rheumatoid arthritis. Clin Orthop 1998; 351:169–179.

Rawlins BA, Girardi FP, Boachie-Adjei O. Rheumatoid arthritis of the cervical spine. Rheum Dis Clin North Am 1998; 24(1):55–65.

Case 25
Osteomyelitis—Cervical Spine, Thoracic Spine, Lumbar Spine

M. Darryl Antonacci and Frank J. Eismont

History and Physical Examination

A 34-year-old man was referred by otolaryngology with complaints during the past 3 years of dysphagia for both liquids and solids, and a 40-pound weight loss. Six years ago the patient underwent C5/C6 anterior discectomy and fusion with plating for a cervical fracture with hemiparesis sustained during a motor vehicle accident. On examination, upper and lower extremity strength was normal on the right and decreased on the left.

Radiologic Findings

Plain radiographs demonstrated the C5/C6 anterior discectomy and fusion with plate and bone ingrowth screws. In the past, the patient had been evaluated with a computed tomography (CT) scan and magnetic resonance imaging (MRI) scan that did not show any residual neural compression. Barium swallow (Fig. 25–1) demonstrated a pharyngeal diverticulum at the level of the fixation plate on the anterior aspect of C5/C6.

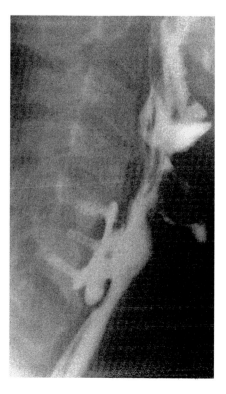

Figure 25–1. Lateral cervical spine radiograph after barium swallow.

Diagnosis

Pharyngeal diverticulum 6 years after an anterior decompression and fusion with plate fixation at C5/C6. It is likely that there is an associated vertebral osteomyelitis.

Surgical Management

The patient was taken to the operating room for repair of the pharyngeal diverticulum by the otolaryngology service in conjunction with removal of the anterior plate and screws by the spine service. After the patient underwent general endotracheal intubation, cervical esophagoscopy was performed. A broad-based posterior pharyngeal diverticulum with its introitus just above the level of the cricopharyngeus was visualized. Notably, the anterior plate and screws were visible within the lumen of the diverticulum at its posterior wall.

Preoperative antibiotics were withheld until after appropriate cultures of the wound were taken. A transverse skin incision was made through the prior operative site at the C6 level. A tremendous amount of scarring surrounding the posterior pharyngeal wall to the plate was encountered as anticipated, with a large amount of granulation tissue surrounding the anterior fixation plate. The pharynx was carefully elevated off the prevertebral fascia and the fixation plate. Entry into the lumen of the diverticulum was confirmed. The remainder of the diverticulum was sharply dissected free of the fixation plate with sufficient mobilization of adjacent mucosa to expose the entire plate.

Attention was then directed toward removal of the plate and screws prior to repair of the pharyngeal fistula. The four set screws used to lock the ingrowth screws were removed without difficulty. An additional ingrowth screw that was placed through the plate into the bone graft was noted to be loose after removal of the locking screw and was removed easily. The two superior C5 screws and two inferior C6 screws, however, were rigidly fixed, as bone had fused through the screws. Attempts at removal resulted in screw failure by shear at the junction of the screw heads and shaft. Failure of the screw heads allowed removal of the plate with approximately 6 mm of screw shafts remaining within the bone (Fig. 25–2).

After the plate was removed, a layer of purulent material could be seen overlying the vertebral cortex. The diagnosis of cervical osteomyelitis secondary to a pharyngeal fistula was confirmed. Tissue specimens for culture were taken at this time for aerobes, anaerobes, and fungus. The patient was then started on broad-spectrum intravenous antibiotics. To optimize the chance of resolving the bone infection, it was decided to remove the remaining screw shafts and to fill the bony defects using autogenous iliac crest bone graft.

A 2-mm burr was used to enlarge the area around the remaining screw shafts. A manual reamer was also used to core around the screw shafts to the screw tip. The reamer was carefully advanced until there was some toggle evident in the screw, and then a curette was used to crack the remaining attachment of the screw tip to the underlying vertebral bone. All four screws were removed in this fashion. The remaining bony defects were meticulously curetted clean of any remaining fibrous tissue or debris (Fig. 25–3).

The pharyngeal defect was repaired by the otolaryngology service prior to placement of the autogenous bone graft into the vertebral defects. A flat and smooth Blake drain was placed prior to wound closure. A Dobhoff feeding tube was placed transnasally prior to extubation.

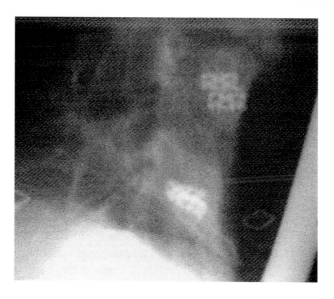

Figure 25–2. Lateral cervical spine radiograph after plate removal with evidence of shear failure of screws and residual metal.

Postoperative Management

The patient tolerated extubation well. He was kept on broad-spectrum intravenous antibiotic coverage until the culture results returned. The wound culture grew a fungus sensitive to Diflucan, and *Streptococcus viridans* sensitive to penicillin and Augmentin (amoxicillin clavulonate). The patient was fed through the Dobhoff tube and later through a gastrostomy feeding tube. The cervical drain was discontinued when the drainage was less than 10 to 15 cc in a 24-hour period. A daily

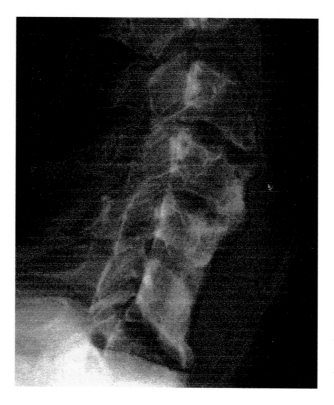

Figure 25–3. Lateral cervical spine radiograph after removal of anterior cervical plate and screws, and debridement of bone.

standing lateral radiograph was obtained after the drain was discontinued until the soft tissue swelling anterior to the cervical spine approached normal. Because the organisms were quite sensitive, and because the infection was very superficial and was debrided well at surgery, the antibiotics were discontinued after 4 weeks. At 5 weeks radiographs demonstrated no motion at C5/C6, no soft tissue swelling, and no retroesophageal air. The wound had healed well.

History and Physical Examination

The patient is a 71-year-old, previously healthy, truck driver with a 4-month history of severe back pain, a 30-pound weight loss, and fevers. Radiographs and CT scan demonstrated a T11/T12 markedly destructive process with blastic and lytic changes for which he received radiation therapy. A subsequent needle biopsy showed inflammatory changes, and cultures from the biopsy grew *Staphylococcus aureus*. Prior to referral, treatment had been begun with an intravenous cephalosporin. He was also given a thoracolumbar spinal orthosis (TLSO) for a developing kyphosis, and had placement of a gastrostomy tube to increase his nutritional intake.

On evaluation by the spine service, the patient's sedimentation rate had decreased from 140 to 60. He was afebrile. The patient had fair to good motor function in both legs. His back was not painful to palpation. Radiographs demonstrated a kyphosis of 33 degrees at T11/T12. An MRI scan was consistent with vertebral osteomyelitis at T11/T12 with minimal spinal cord impingement. Because the culture results showed sensitivity to oxacillin, it was recommended the patient be switched to maximal dose intravenous oxacillin for better disc penetration. On follow-up evaluation 4 weeks later, the patient's motor exam had worsened to poor and fair in both legs. His sedimentation rate also had increased to 120. His hematocrit was 34, his total lymphocyte count was 1400, and his albumen was 2.9. He appeared emaciated.

Radiologic Findings

Radiographs demonstrated progression of the thoracic kyphosis from 33 to 39 degrees (Fig. 25–4). The patient also had a new MRI scan that demonstrated worsening of the cord compression at T11/T12 (Fig. 25–5).

Diagnosis

Thoracic vertebral osteomyelitis. The patient developed progressive kyphosis and neurologic compromise despite treatment with antibiotics and immobilization.

Surgical Management

Because of the patient's debilitated condition, a staged anterior and posterior surgery was planned with 1 week between the procedures. The patient would also receive 2 weeks of additional intravenous hyperalimentation. The patient was taken to the operating room and was positioned, prepped, and draped in the lateral decubitus position for a left thoracic exposure under general anesthesia. The case was done with neuromonitoring and Cell Saver. He was given 30 mg/kg Solu-Medrol

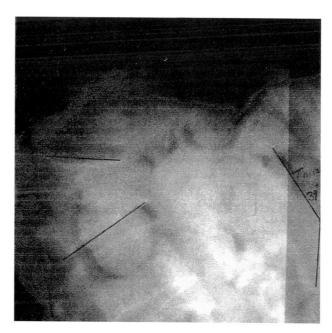

Figure 25–4. Lateral thoracic spine radiograph demonstrating 39 degrees of kyphosis with destruction at T11/T12.

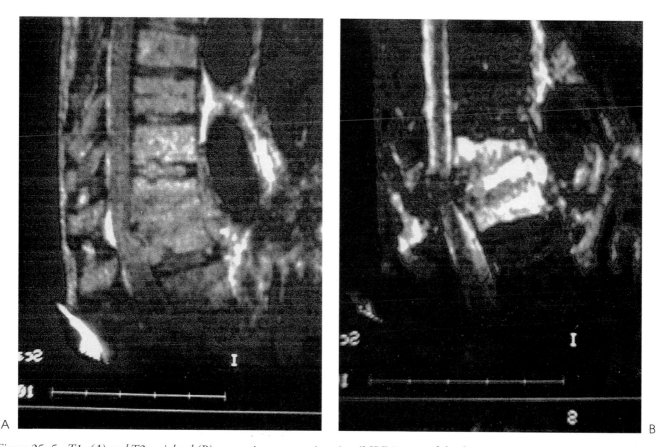

Figure 25–5. T1- (A) and T2-weighted (B) magnetic resonance imaging (MRI) images of the thoracic spine.

as a loading dose, followed by 5.4 mg/kg/hour for the duration of surgery. The use of steroids is associated with an increased risk of infection, but this was outweighed by the benefit of its use with evidence of severe compression of the spinal cord at the level of the conus medullaris. The incision was made over the 10th rib. This was taken down through the overlying fascia directly to bone. The rib was stripped subperiosteally and removed near its base. It was placed in antibiotic solution for later use as graft. A large amount of scar tissue and adherence of the lung to the posterior diaphragm and pleura were evident. The pleura was carefully dissected free of the posterior vertebral body and area of infection. Exposure necessitated partial takedown of the diaphragm posteriorly. Complete T11/T12 discectomy and subtotal corpectomies of both vertebra were undertaken. The appearance of the bone was sclerotic, but no purulence was seen. Tissue was sent to pathology and for culture. At this time gentamicin was added to antibiotic coverage of oxacillin.

The rib attachments at T11 and T12 were excised to expose the underlying pedicles. The pedicles were then removed using a Kerrison rongeur to expose the lateral dural sac. The posterior cortex of T11 and T12 was carefully removed using a combination of power burr, reverse curettes, and osteotomes. This completed the ventral decompression of the thecal sac. The area was completely debrided of any abnormal tissue, and copiously irrigated with saline with added antibiotics. Care was taken to avoid directly irrigating against the thecal sac. The rib graft was cut into approximately four equal segments and fitted as strut graft into the bony defect. The pleura was closed over the bone graft site using interrupted Vicryl suture to approximate the edges. The ribs were reapproximated using no. 2 looped chromic gut suture. Deep fascial layers were closed with 0-proline, and the skin was closed in two layers with 2-0 Vicryl and staples. Prior to closure a no. 36 chest tube was placed through a separate incision tunneled over the 11th rib. The patient was awakened, extubated, and taken to the recovery room. His motor function in his legs was unchanged and no abnormal neuromonitoring changes had been noted during the procedure.

One week after the first procedure, the patient underwent posterior instrumentation and fusion from T8 to L2. Under fluoroscopic guidance, pedicle screws were placed into L1 and L2. Each screw was tested with electromyogram (EMG) monitoring and there was no indication of any break in the pedicles. In addition, up-going laminar hooks were placed at L2 to help protect the L2 pedicle screws. The thoracic hook construct consisted of a down-going laminar hook at T8 on the right and up-going on the left; up-going at T10 on the right, and down-going on the left; and an up-going laminar hook at T9 on the right. This long construct was selected because the deformity was severe and the bone quality was suboptimal. Titanium rods were appropriately contoured and inserted. Cortical and cancellous iliac crest autograft was harvested and used for posterolateral fusion. This was done after decortication of the transverse processes, lamina, and spinous processes at each level with a burr (Figs. 25–6 and 25–7). Intraoperative neuromonitoring remained unchanged, and the wound was closed in three layers; 0-proline was used for the deep fascia, 2-0 Vicryl for the subcutaneous layer, and an interrupted 3-0 nylon vertical mattress stitch was used for the skin. A flat, smooth Blake drain was placed prior to closure.

Postoperative Management

Postoperatively after the anterior procedure, the patient was monitored in an intensive care setting. He was kept on an air mattress bed, supine and log rolled. Appro-

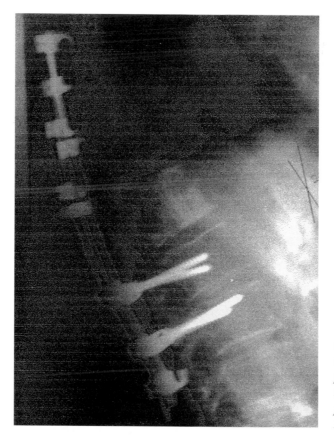

Figure 25–6. Postoperative lateral thoracic radiograph approximately 2 months after surgery demonstrating incorporation of the rib graft and 25 degrees of residual kyphosis.

priate dosing of intravenous oxacillin and gentamicin were used for antibiotic coverage. The patient's caloric intake was kept at a minimum of 3000 calories per day for a total of 4 weeks.

After the posterior procedure, the patient was transferred to a rehabilitation unit and at 6 weeks he progressed to ambulation in the parallel bars.

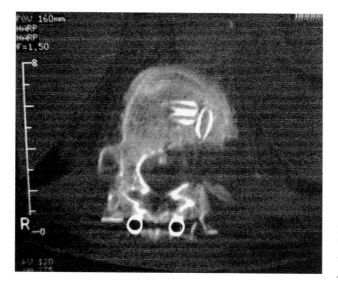

Figure 25–7. Postoperative computed tomography (CT) scan through area of decompression and bone graft.

Discussion

Presentation of vertebral osteomyelitis may be acute, subacute, or chronic, and is highly dependent on a number of factors including virulence of the organism, immune status of the host, and age. Although the majority of cases are secondary to gram-positive cocci, and in particular *S. aureus,* other frequently isolated organisms include *Escherichia coli, Pseudomonas,* and *Proteus* species. Common sources of bacteremias that can lead to hematogenous spread of infection to the spine include urinary tract infections (29%, particularly following genitourinary procedures), soft tissue infections (13%), respiratory infections (11%), and intravenous drug use (1.5%).

The objectives of current management of vertebral osteomyelitis begin with establishment of an accurate bacteriologic diagnosis, usually through either open or closed biopsy. Antibiotic therapy should be withheld until the diagnosis is made. Choice of antibiotic is based on sensitivities of the biopsy culture. Although it has been demonstrated that penetration of osteomyelitic bone parallels serum concentrations for all antibiotic classes, penetration into the disc space varies, and is highly dependent on ionic charge of the antibiotic. Vancomycin, gentamicin, tobramycin, and clindamycin penetrate the nucleous pulposus well. Cephalosporins, on the other hand, penetrate poorly. Parenteral antibiotic therapy should be continued for at least 4 to 6 weeks followed by oral antibiotics until the infection has resolved. Resolution of the disease can be monitored by the return of the erythrocyte sedimentation rate to between one-half and two-thirds of pretherapy levels.

Surgery is indicated for cases in which significant deformity or vertebral collapse occurs, or when spinal cord compression with neurologic deficit develops. Clinically significant abscesses, or cases refractory to nonoperative treatment, may also benefit from surgery.

It is very uncommon for a patient to develop an infection following an elective anterior cervical spine procedure, and if one does develop, it is necessary to assess whether there is an associated pharyngeal or esophageal fistula. A barium swallow often will demonstrate this. At the time of spine debridement, the fistula must be repaired.

Alternative Methods of Management

The mainstay of management for vertebral osteomyelitis is nonoperative. Improved pain control, minimization of deformity, and prevention of neurologic deterioration can often be achieved by immobilization in combination with maximal-dose, culture-specific, intravenous antibiotic therapy. Patients at greatest risk for progression of deformity typically have 50% vertebral body involvement at presentation. Bracing should be continued for approximately 3 to 4 months. Cervical lesions more often require surgical fixation.

Complications

Prior to the use of antibiotic therapy, the course of vertebral osteomyelitis was often fulminant, with mortalities approaching 70%. Even now, recurrent infection can occur in up to 25% of patients but is least likely in individuals treated for 4 weeks or more. In patients with impaired immune status, nonoperative treatment is less successful.

Type of Management	Advantages	Disadvantages	Comments
Nonoperative (antibiotics/bracing)	Noninvasive, improved pain control	Recurrence of infection; progression of deformity	Mainstay of treatment; requires accurate bacteriologic diagnosis
Posterior debridement (laminectomy)	Limited role for lesions below level of conus when extensive anterior debridement is not necessary	May increase instability and neurologic deterioration	Contraindicated in most cases
Anterior debridement with autogenous bone grafting	Allows direct access to the infected tissues and extensive debridement	Increased morbidity	Autogenous iliac crest and rib bone grafting reliably leads to fusion
Anterior debridement with grafting and posterior instrumentation	Effective adjunct to debridement and grafting in cases with significant deformity or instability	Long-term fate of hardware is not known; increased morbidity	May be done at same setting or as a staged procedure

Suggested Readings

Carragee EJ. Pyogenic vertebral osteomyelitis. J Bone Joint Surg 1997; 79A:874–880.

Currier BL, Banovak K, Eismont FJ. Gentamycin penetration into normal rabbit nucleus pulposus. Spine 1994; 19:2614–2618.

Currier BL, Eismont FJ. Infections of the spine. In Herkowitz HN, et al, eds. Rothman-Simeone: The Spine, 4th ed., pp. 1207–1258. Philadelphia: WB Saunders, 1999.

Eismont FJ, Bohlman HH, Soni PL, et al. Pyogenic and fungal vertebral osteomyelitis with paralysis. J Bone Joint Surg 1983; 65A:19–29.

Emery SE, Chan DPK, Woodward HR. Treatment of hematogenous pyogenic vertebral osteomyelitis with anterior debridement and primary bone grafting. Spine 1989; 14:284–291.

Frederickson B, Yuan H, Orlans R. Management and outcome of pyogenic vertebral osteomyelitis. Clin Orthop 1978; 131:160–167.

McGuire RA, Eismont FJ. The fate of autogenous bone graft in surgically treated pyogenic vertebral osteomyelitis. J Spinal Disord 1994; 7:206–215.

Riley LH, Banovac K, Martinez OV, et al. Tissue distribution of antibiotics in the intervertebral disc. Spine 1994; 19:2619–2625.

Sapico FL, Montgomerie JZ. Pyogenic vertebral osteomyelitis: report of nine cases and review of the literature. Rev Infect Dis 1979; 1:754–776.

Case 26
Postoperative Lumbar Discitis
Alan S. Hilibrand

History and Physical Examination

A 34-year-old woman presented complaining of back and bilateral lower extremity pain of 4 months duration. She had completed a 7-week trial of physical therapy and judicious use of antiinflammation drugs without any significant improvement.

The patient was in a moderate amount of distress. She had limited lumbar flexion and extension, although lateral bending was not painful. Her straight leg raise test was strongly positive at 30 degrees on the left side, and her crossed straight leg raise sign was also positive. She demonstrated weakness in left heel plantarflexion with toe-walking, as well as evertor weakness across the left ankle. Sensation was diminished across the entire posterior aspect of the calf and thigh bilaterally; perianal sensation was also diminished, although anal sphincter tone was normal. Deep tendon reflexes were diminished at both ankles but graded elsewhere at 2/4.

Radiologic Findings

Magnetic resonance imaging (MRI) of the lumbar spine was obtained 1 week prior to the patient's evaluation. As shown in Figure 26–1, there was a massive disc hernation

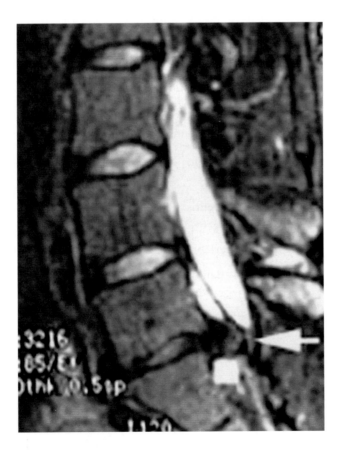

Figure 26–1. Sagittal magnetic resonance imaging (MRI) revealing a large disc herniation at the L5/S1 level.

at L5/S1, which almost completely filled the spinal canal. On the axial images through the L5/S1 disc space, the disc herniation was slightly eccentric toward the left side. Plain films were unremarkable, except for the loss of disc space height.

Diagnosis

Large lumbar disc herniation at L5/S1, with chronic cauda equina compression and bilateral S1 radiculopathies.

Surgical Management

Based on the degree of her symptoms and the apparent saddle anesthesia, as well as the concordant MRI findings of significant cauda equina compression, we strongly recommended urgent operative treatment through open microdiscectomy.

Intravenous vancomycin was administered in the preoperative holding area for antibiotic prophylaxis, due to the patient's penicillin allergy. The patient was then brought to the operating room for an open lumbar microdiscectomy at the L5/S1 level. The operation was completed without incident and the patient was discharged following a 23-hour hospital stay.

Hospital Readmission

During the next 2 weeks, the patient developed worsening of her back pain, and was forced to discontinue physical therapy. She was instructed to come to the hospital emergency room for reevaluation. Although the patient was afebrile and her white blood cell count was within normal limits, her erythrocyte sedimentation rate (ESR) and C-reactive protein (CRP) values were abnormally high at 104 and 5.9, respectively. The patient was admitted to the hospital for a presumed postoperative infection, and an MRI scan of the lumbar spine with gadolinium was obtained (Fig. 26–2). The images demonstrated a collection of fluid superficial to the deep fascia (Fig. 26–2A), as well as enhancement within the disc space and adjacent vertebral endplates (Fig. 26–2B) and in the anterior soft tissues (Fig. 26–2C). In addition, there was a question of recurrent/residual disc material anterior to the left S1 nerve root.

The MRI findings were worrisome for both a superficial wound infection as well as a deep infection with apparent discitis. Due to the signs and symptoms of a progressive infection, we recommended surgical irrigation and debridement of the entire surgical site, with reexploration of the spinal canal to remove any compressive disc material. In addition, the anterior soft tissue inflammation was biopsied under computed tomography (CT) guidance at the time of admission to the hospital prior to operative treatment.

Surgical Management, Part 2

The patient was brought to the operating room and the wound was reopened and explored. A large collection of serous fluid superficial to the deep fascia was cultured and removed, and the surrounding tissues were debrided. The deep fascia was opened and the spinal canal exposed at the L5-S1 interspace. Dense scar tissue was removed and the underlying nerve root sac dissected free. The floor of the spinal canal was cultured and explored. The previous annular defect was identified, but no

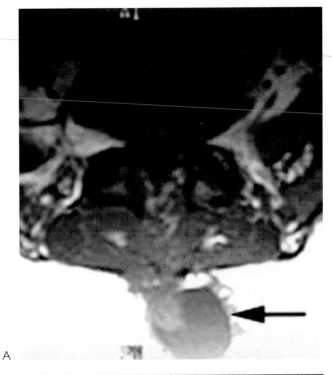

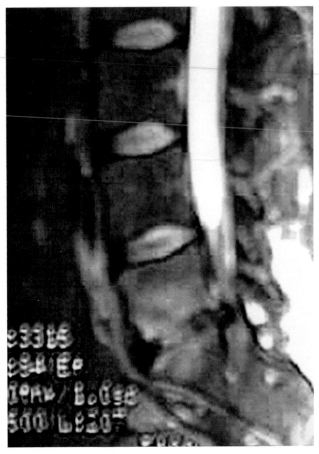

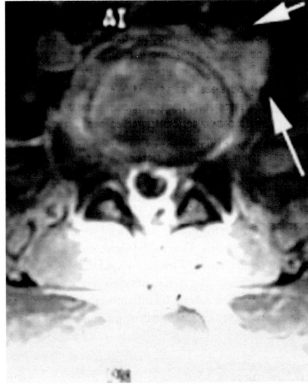

Figure 26–2. (A) Transaxial MRI of the L5/S1 interspace revealing a fluid collection superficial to the deep fascia (arrow). (B) Sagittal MRI demonstrates tissue enhancement within the disc space and vertebral endplates as well as on the anterior soft tissues on the transaxial image (C).

extruded nucleus pulposus material was present. Through the rent in the annulus the disc space was cultured and probed, although no purulent material could be expressed. The entire wound was irrigated and reapproximated in layers with monofilament suture in the deep and superficial tissues as well as interrupted nylon sutures in the skin.

Postoperative Management

The CT-guided biopsy specimens grew gram-positive cocci, as did the superficial, deep, and intradiscal culture specimens. The bacteria was identified as *Staphylococcus aureus,* and were sensitive to methicillin. The infectious disease service was consulted, and recommended 6 weeks of intravenous clindamycin treatment. The patient remained afebrile throughout her postoperative course, although her ESR and CRP values remained high (102 and 19.7, respectively) at the time of discharge. She was immobilized in a thoracolumbar spinal orthosis (TLSO) with a leg extension, but required a short course of rehabilitation due to the incapacitating back pain that made ambulation in the brace especially difficult.

The patient returned at 2-week follow-up noting improvement of her low back pain. Her wound was benign, and her nylon sutures were removed. At 4 weeks after surgery an MRI of the lumbar spine was repeated. It demonstrated increased edema within the disc space and further destructive changes at the adjacent endplates of L5 and S1 (Fig. 26–3). Plain films also suggested further disc space change, although the patient's clinical course was improving, and her ESR and CRP were approaching normal levels. By 6-week follow-up her ESR and CRP values had returned to

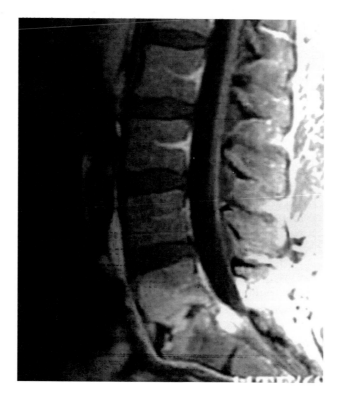

Figure 26–3. Sagittal MRI of the lumbar spine revealing increased edema within the L5/S1 disc space and further destructive changes at the adjacent endplates of L5/S1.

normal, an her back pain had almost completely resolved. She was liberated from her brace, and placed on a 6-week course of oral antibiotics.

Discussion

Disc space infection, or spondylodiscitis, results from inflammation of tissues in the disc space as well as the surrounding soft tissue and/or bone. The incidence of postoperative discitis has been reported to range from <1 to 5%. Rohde and colleagues (1998) demonstrated the important role of perioperative antibiotics in avoiding this complication. They reported a postoperative spondylodiscitis in 3.7% of 508 patients who did not receive prophylactic antibiotics, compared with no infections among another 1134 patients who had an intraoperative antibiotic sponge applied at surgery.

Our patient's clinical presentation was typical of postoperative lumbar discitis. The initial outcome was complete relief of preoperative leg and back pain, with a short uncomplicated hospital course. Iversen and colleagues (1992) retrospectively reviewed the timing of postoperative complaints in patients with spondylodiscitis, and reported an average onset of low back pain complaints during the third week following surgery. On the other hand, Lindholm and Pylkkanen (1982) suggested a more insidious onset of low back pain, averaging 5 weeks from the date of surgery. The discrepancy between these studies may reflect the difficulty in differentiating low back pain due to degenerative changes from low back pain due to inflammatory changes. As Hanley and Shapiro (1989) has shown, many patients complain of significant low back pain due to degenerative changes following lumbar discectomy, and this may delay the diagnosis of an underlying inflammatory or infectious process.

The most specific findings that confirmed the diagnosis of postoperative discitis in our patient were seen on MRI. As described by Boden and colleagues (1992), there was decreased signal in the disc space and adjacent marrow on T1-weighted images, and increased signal in these same locations on T2-weighted images. With the addition of gadolinium, T1-weighted images enhanced in the disc space and surrounding marrow. Because the images were obtained 5 weeks following the index procedure, they were felt to represent true spondylodiscitis. However, MRI performed in the immediate postoperative period must be interpreted with caution, due to the high incidence of nonspecific postoperative changes, as reported by Floris and colleagues (1997).

In the absence of an epidural abscess or postoperative fluid collection, patients with postoperative spondylodiscitis may be treated nonoperatively. However, attempts should be made to identify the offending organism through CT-guided biopsy to direct antibiotic treatment. We routinely treat postoperative spinal infections with open irrigation and debridement, as well as with 6 weeks of intravenous antibiotics followed by a variable course of an oral antibiotic, based on the patient's response to treatment.

Monitoring treatment of a disc space infection involves serial evaluation of clinical, serologic, and radiologic parameters. Clinically, patients should experience progressive improvement in their low back pain with increased mobility within the first month of treatment. The ESR and CRP usually return to near-normal levels by 1 month after initiation of antibiotic treatment, as in the present case. Plain films may be unremarkable at the time of presentation, and destructive endplate changes are often seen only after the initiation of treatment. Nielsen and colleagues (1990) reported that patients with postoperative discitis did not develop any plain radiographic abnormalities until an average of 2 months after the index procedure, with the greatest degree of destructive change evident at 4 months following lumbar discectomy. They observed a similar delay in resolution of inflammatory changes on follow-up MRI.

There were no complications following treatment of this patient's disc space infection. However, several complications are possible and require early recognition. The most serious is the development of an epidural abscess, which requires emergent surgical drainage. Another serious risk is the development of meningitis, especially in the setting of open treatment complicated by violation of the subarachnoid space due to a dural tear. Again, prompt recognition and appropriate antibiotic treatment is essential. Other adverse sequelae of postoperative discitis include the development of spinal instability at the level of the infected disc pace, pyogenic vertebral osteomyelitis of the surounding vertebral bodies, sepsis, and distant infections due to hematogenous spread of the infecting organism. In addition, anywhere from 12 to 61% of patients may have persistent back pain that prevents return to work.

Alternative Methods of Management

Alternative methods of management for a postoperative lumbar discitis include empiric antibiotics without biopsy or open irrigation and debridement, as well as extensive debridement and disc excision with interbody fusion from an anterior or posterior approach. Empiric antibiotic treatment may be effective when directed toward Staphylococcus species, which are the most common sources of postoperative spinal infections. However, failure of such treatment will subsequently require percutaneous or open biopsy to assist in redirecting antibiotic therapy, necessitate prolonged immobilization and antibiotic therapy, and increase the risk of associated complication of spondylodiscitis.

Type of Management	Advantages	Disadvantages	Comments
Empiric antibiotics and bracing	Avoids surgical risks and complications	No definitive organism No debridement	If infecting organism known or suspected If surgery contraindicated
Percutaneous biopsy and closed treatment/bracing	Obtains pathologic material Avoids surgical risks	Potential for false-negative biopsy No debridement	Most common approach Avoid in presence of wound infection
Anterior decompression and fusion	Debridement of disc space Neural decompression Obtain pathogen	No internal fixation (see comments) Anterior approach difficult (if prevertebral inflammation)	Avoid internal fixation (provides nidus for infection) May fuse without surgery (does not allow debridement of wound infection)
Posterior decompression and fusion	Rigid internal fixation Debride posterior wound Neural decompression	Dural tear possible (scar) (potential for meningitis) Difficult to debride discitis	Internal fixation if wound is clean Best for postoperative wound infection and discitis
Anterior/posterior decompression and fusion	Debridement of disc space Neural decompression Rigid internal fixation Obtain pathogen	Two surgical exposures Increased surgical risks	Recommended approach after failure of initial treatment Medically stable patient

Suggested Readings

Bircher MD, Tasker T, Crawshaw C, et al. Discitis following lumbar surgery. Spine 1988; 13:98–102.

Boden SD, Davis DO, Dina TS, et al. Postoperative discitis: distinguishing early MR imaging findings from normal postoperative disc space changes. Radiology 1992; 184:765–771.

Floris, R, Spallone A, Aref TY, et al. Early postoperative MRI findings following surgery for herniated lumbar disc. Acta Neurochir 1997; 139:169–175.

Grane P, Josephsson A, Seferlis A, et al. Septic and aseptic post-operative discitis in the lumbar spine—evaluation with MR imaging. Acta Radiol 1998; 39:108–115.

Hanley EN Jr, Shapiro DE. The development of low back pain after excision of a lumbar disc. J Bone Joint Surg 1989; 71A(5):719–721.

Heller, JG. Postoperative infection of the spine. In: Rothman RH, Simeone FA, eds. The Spine, pp. 1817–1837. Philadelphia: WB Saunders, 1992.

Iversen E, Nielsen VA, Hansen LG. Prognosis in postoperative discitis. A retrospective study of 111 cases. Acta Orhop Scand 1992; 63:305–309.

Lindholm TS, Pylkkanen P. Discitis following removal of intervertebral disc. Spine 1982; 7:618–622.

Nielsen VA, Iversen E, Ahlgren P. Postoperative discitis. Radiology of progress and healing. Acta Radiol 1990; 31:559–563.

Pilgaard S. Discitis following removal of lumbar intervertebral disc. J Bone Joint Surg 1969; 51A:713–716.

Piotrowski WP, Krombholz MA, Muhl B. Spondylodiscitis after lumbar disc surgery. Neurosurg Rev 1994; 17:189–193.

Puranen J, Makela J, Lahde S. Postoperative intervertebral discitis. Acta Orthop Scand 1984; 55:461–465.

Rohde V, Mayer B, Schaller C, et al. Spondylodiscitis after lumbar discectomy. Incidence and a proposal for prophylaxis. Spine 1998; 23:615–620.

Schulitz KP, Assheuer J. Discitis after procedures on the intervertebral disc. Spine 1994; 19:1172–1177.

Case 27

Ankylosing Spondylitis— Cervical Osteotomy

Alok D. Sharan, Alexander R. Vaccaro, and Todd J. Albert

History and Physical Examination

A 59-year-old man presented with increasing inability of maintaining a horizontal gaze. He had been diagnosed with ankylosing spondylitis 11 years previously after he was X-rayed following a motor vehicle accident. He had lost his ability to view the horizon due to a progressive cervical kyphotic deformity forcing him to walk with an assistive device.

On examination, he presented with a typical cervicothoracic kyphotic posture, with a chin on chest deformity (Fig. 27–1). He was neurologically preserved with no deficits in his motor, sensory, or reflex testing. There was no evidence of hip flexion contractures.

Radiologic Findings

A lateral plain X-ray and computed tomography (CT) with sagittal reconstruction of his cervical spine revealed complete fusion of the cervical spine from the occiput distally, consistent with ankylosing spondylitis (Fig. 27–2). There was marked

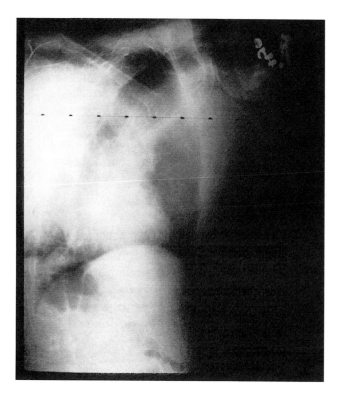

Figure 27–1. Lateral plain radiograph revealing a kyphosis at the cervicothoracic junction with a large chin-brown vertical angle (CBVA).

PEARLS

- This procedure is best performed with the patient in a sitting position wearing a halo cast.
- In assessing the degree of cervical kyphosis, it is important to examine all joints in the body that can be contributing to the flexion deformity. Sometimes adequate correction of the lumbar kyphosis or hip flexion contractures can restore overall function.
- If the patient is experiencing weakness during an awake decompression or if SSEP or MEP signals undergo significant decrement, the dura may need to be split longitudinally and transversely to decrease tension on the cord.
- Fixing patients segmentally can reduce time in the halo and significantly improve stability of the pathologic bone.
- Be aware of the need for nutritional supplementation, ulcer, and deep venous thrombosis (DVT) prophylaxis postoperatively.

PITFALLS

- Careful assessment of the cervicothoracic and craniocervical junction should be made so that osteotomies are not performed on patients with fractures in this region. These patients require reduction with a cranial halo to prevent future deformities.
- An extensive midline bony decompression must be performed above the osteotomy level to ensure that the C6 lamina does not compress the spinal cord if the vertebral body becomes displaced anteriorly. Undercutting of the C7 pedicles is a must.

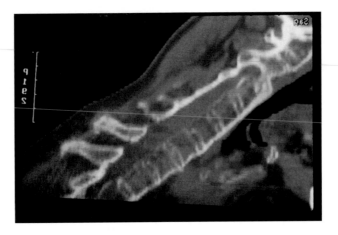

Figure 27–2. Sagittal computed tomography (CT) reconstruction revealing loss of the normal cervical lordosis with kyphosis at the cervicothoracic junction.

straightening of the cervical spine and loss of the normal lordosis. A long cassette film revealed a flattening of the normal lumbar lordosis (0 degrees) with a significant kyphotic deformity at the cervicothoracic junction.

Diagnosis

Ankylosing spondylitis with severe cervicothoracic kyphosis.

Surgical Management

After being medically cleared, the patient underwent a cervicothoracic osteotomy. Awake intubation was carried out and the patient was placed in the sitting position. The C7 lamina was removed and the C8 nerve roots were completely exposed bilaterally. Both C7 pedicles were removed to a point ventral to the C8 nerve roots. After removing the inferior portion of the lamina of C6 and the superior lamina of T1, an osteoclasis maneuver was carried out to correct the 70-degree chin-brow vertical angle (CBVA) to 10 degrees. The patient was in a halo cast (placed the day prior to surgery). After osteoclasis and correction of the deformity, the upright anterior bars of the halo were attached. The patient then underwent a C3 to T3 segmental fixation with lateral mass (C3, C4, C5) and pedicle screw fixation (T1, T2, T3) (Fig. 27–3). The patient had an uncomplicated hospital course, spending 6 weeks in the halo vest and 6 weeks in a cervicothoracic orthosis.

Discussion

Kyphosis of the cervical spine due to ankylosing spondylitis presents an uncommon but disabling problem to the patient. Initially ankylosing spondylitis causes a weakening of the posterior paraspinal muscles, which leads to an initial flexion deformity. As the disease progresses, there is a progression of facet inflammation that causes the patient to flex further to ease the pain. This flexion eventually can develop into a chin-on-chest deformity that leads to a loss of ability to see the horizon and then difficulty in swallowing, chewing, and talking. Not infrequently, the cervical kyphosis may increase acutely due to an undiagnosed spinal fracture. As the kyphosis develops, the spinal cord can become draped over the posterior elements of the vertebral bodies. However, myelopathy is rare in these patients.

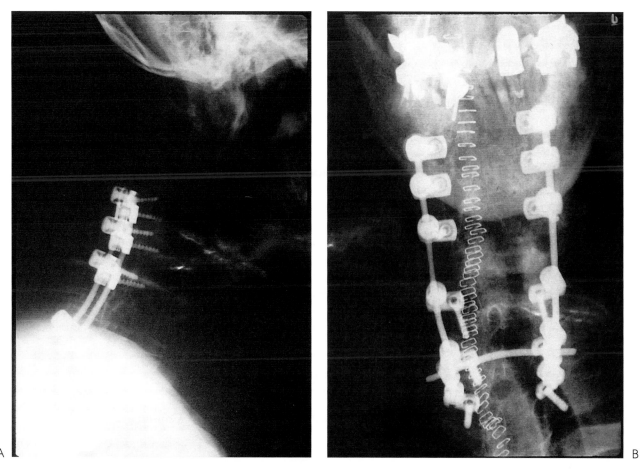

A   B

Figure 27–3. Anteroposterior (AP) (A) and lateral (B) plain radiographs following a posterior cervical osteotomy and realignment of the cervical spine.

A cervical osteotomy for patients with severe cervical kyphosis is indicated when the patient has a significant loss of function or a considerable amount of pain, and is willing to undergo surgical intervention. Careful assessment should be made to confirm that the deformity is due to ankylosing spondylitis and not due to an unrecognized fracture in the region. If a patient with long-standing ankylosing spondylitis gives a history of relatively pain-free periods with the sudden onset of pain, then it should be assumed that the patient has sustained a fracture. Cervicothoracic and craniocervical junction fractures also lead to a flexion deformity with or without pain. Therefore, it is important to use other radiologic modalities to determine if a fracture is present, that is, magnetic resonance imaging (MRI), tomography, or bone scan.

When evaluating a patient with a cervical kyphosis deformity, the surgeon must be careful to determine that the problem is not from the hips (requiring total hip arthroplasty) or lumbar spine kyphosis (requiring a preemptive lumbar osteotomy). If pathology of the hips or lumbar spine is significant, these areas should be corrected prior to a cervical osteotomy. When the surgeon feels that an osteotomy is indicated, the degree of correction required can be measured using the CBVA. Originally described by Simmons (1998), the CBVA is measured by observing from the side while the patient stands in full extension of the hips and knees. A goniometer is used to measure the angle of a line through the chin and brow with respect to a vertical line. This can also be measured from a lateral radiograph of the entire spine and head on a 36-inch cassette. A suitable angle of correction is then determined that would allow a patient to view the horizon, look at a desk, or walk outside unassisted. The angle is then transposed to a lateral X-ray of the cervical spine whereby the apex of the wedge is placed on the posterior longitudinal ligament of the C7/T1 interspace and centered over the posterior arch of C7. This method allows the surgeon to estimate the amount of bone that needs to be resected. An ideal CBVA at final correction is 10 degrees.

The technique used for operative correction of the kyphosis has not changed significantly from the original procedure described by Urist (1958). The patient is placed in a sitting position with a halo in place. We perform the operation under general anesthesia, but some surgeons still use local anesthesia. The use of local anesthesia allows the patient to assist the surgeon in determining if there is cord compression and loss of neurologic function while the neck is being extended. We have successfully performed four osteotomies under general anesthesia with somatosensory evoked potential (SSEP) monitoring, motor evoked potential (MEP) monitoring, and dermatomal evoked potential monitoring of the C8 nerves.

The exposure is carried out posteriorly over the level of C7/T1. At this level, the spinal canal is wider and the nerve roots are more mobile. In addition, this level is below the level at which the vertebral artery enters the vertebral foramen.

Alternative Methods of Management

Type of Management	Advantages	Disadvantages	Comments
Nonoperative	None	Degree of kyphosis will progress	Other therapeutic modalities may alleviate the pain, but it will not stop the progression of the structural deformity
Correction of the deformity using general anesthesia with sophisticated spinal cord and nerve monitoring and segmental internal fixation	Less discomfort for the patient	It can be difficult to assess any neurologic compromise if monitoring is not superb	Local anesthesia allows better assessment of any spinal cord compression that may occur during extension of the cervical spine
Anteroposterior cervical osteotomy	Improved ease of deformity correction	Two incision sites would be needed. Visualization anteriorly is difficult to impossible if the kyphosis is severe. Longer duration of surgery	Approaching the cervical spine posteriorly is enough to achieve an adequate osteotomy to restore adequate alignment

Complications

Cervical osteotomy for correction of kyphosis is a difficult procedure that requires significant experience and knowledge of the pitfalls. If performed on an awake patient under local anesthesia, a constant surveillance of the patient's neurologic status may be obtained to ensure that no deterioration occurs while the cervical spine is being extended. If this procedure is done under general anesthesia, superb monitoring is required. The most significant complication of this surgery is loss of neurologic function that may occur during manipulation of the cervical spine. Additional complications of nonunion, loss of fixation, recurrence of deformity, and halo-related morbidity have also been reported.

In the most recently published review of this procedure, McMaster (1997) reported neurologic complications of quadriplegia in one patient, numbness in two patients, and pain in 4 of 15 patients who underwent a cervical osteotomy. Dysphagia due to retropharyngeal swelling was experienced in three patients, which resolved on its own. Finally, subluxation of the seventh cervical vertebra on the first thoracic vertebra with subsequent pain occurred in four patients with no loss of function. Neurologic complications related to vertebral subluxation may be avoided by ensuring adequate decompression such that the lamina of C6 does not impinge on the spinal cord if the vertebral body becomes displaced.

One report described a patient who developed increasing weakness in both extremities and then difficulty in his speech during the procedure. The dura was noted to be under high tension in this individual, requiring it to be split longitudinally and deep to the arachnoid. As the decompression progressed, the patient again developed weakness requiring further splitting of the dura. To manage this complication McKenzie and Dewar (1949) recommended splitting the dura both longitudinally and transversely when compression of the cord occurs.

Other complications reported in the literature have included pulmonary embolism, perforated peptic ulcer, and cardiac dysfunction. As with any surgical procedure, the risks of the procedure need to be weighed against its benefits. These patients are generally frail and should have their airway evaluated preoperatively, and they should be watched carefully in the postoperative period for malnutrition, ulcer occurrence, and thrombophlebitis.

Suggested Readings

Lipson SJ. Ankylosing spondylitis and seronegative spondyloarthropathies. In: Clark CR, ed. The Cervical Spine, 3rd ed., pp. 721–732. Philadelphia: Lippincott-Raven, 1998.

McKenzie KG, Dewar FP. Scoliosis with paraplegia. J Bone Joint Surg 1949; 31B:162–174.

McMaster MJ. Osteotomy of the cervical spine in ankylosing spondylitis. J Bone Joint Surg 1997; 79B:197–203.

Shimizu K, Matsushita M, Fujibayashi S, Toguchida J, Ido K, Nakamura T. Correction of kyphotic deformity of the cervical spine in ankylosing spondylitis using general anesthesia and internal fixation. J Spinal Disord 1996; 9(6):540–543.

Simmons EH. Ankylosing spondylitis: surgical considerations. In: Herkowitz HN, Garfin SR, Balderston RA, Eismont FJ, Bell GR, Wiesel SW, eds. The Spine, 3rd ed., pp. 721–732. Philadelphia: Lippincott-Raven, 1998.

Urist MR. Osteotomy of the cervical spine: report of a case of ankylosing rheumatoid spondylitis. J Bone Joint Surg 1958; 40A:833–843.

Zdeblick TA. Cervical kyphosis. In: An HS, Simpson JM, eds. Surgery of the Cervical Spine, pp. 367–377. Philadelphia: Williams & Wilkins, 1994.

Zdeblick TA, Bohlman HH. Cervical kyphosis and myelopathy treatment by anterior corpectomy and stunt grafting. J Bone Joint Surg 1989; 71A:170–182.

Case 28

Postoperative Spinal Wound Infections

Steven C. Ludwig, Joseph M. Kowalski, and John G. Heller

History and Physical Examination

A 70-year-old man presented with severe abdominal pain and fever 6 months following a posterior decompression, segmental instrumentation, and fusion from L2 to L4 for junctional stenosis above a previous midline posterior fusion from L4 to S1. No specific etiology for the patient's fever was identified, but he responded to an empiric course of antibiotics. Following this episode he noticed increasing lumbar pain over the ensuing year distinct from any other he had known. The pain gradually intensified and was associated with a vague sense of illness and low-grade

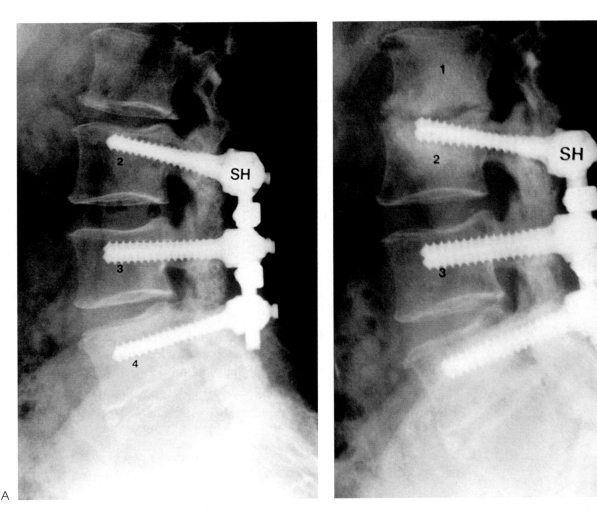

A   B

Figure 28–1. (A) Lateral radiograph made shortly after the patient's L2/L4 posterior decompression, instrumentation, and fusion procedure. Compare the L1/L2 disc space with the lateral radiograph (B) made at the time he initially presented with a wound infection. Note the loss of disc height, peridiscal erosion, and reactive bone formation. Lucencies around the screws are indicative of loose implants.

temperature. His pain intensified with activity, but was not alleviated with rest, nor with nonsteroidal pain medications. It bothered him day and night, interfering with his sleep.

On physical examination, the patient appeared to be in some distress. The neurologic examination was normal. There was no evidence of wound erythema, drainage, or swelling. Plain lumbar radiographs, when compared to previous films, revealed a marked loss of disc height at L1/L2 with erosion of the L2 endplate, as well as lucent zones around the pedicle screws (Fig. 28–1). A bone scan obtained showed increased radioisotope uptake around the L1/L2 area. Laboratory evaluation revealed a white blood cell count of 7200, erythrocyte sedimentation rate (ESR) of 70 mm/hour (normal is 0 to 20 mm/hour), and a C-reactive protein (CRP) of 1.6 mg/dL (normal is 0 to 0.8 mg/dL). A computed tomography (CT)-guided biopsy of the L1/L2 disc space grew *Staphylococcus aureus* sensitive to all antibiotics. Prompt surgical intervention was strongly recommended, but the patient and his family declined this course of action. Therefore, the patient was fitted with a thoracolumbar spinal orthosis (TLSO), placed on activity restrictions and intravenous cefazolin for 6 weeks, followed by another 6 weeks of oral antibiotics. His symptoms completely resolved and laboratory values normalized over this period. His radiographs appeared unchanged, as well.

One year later, he returned complaining of the acute onset of recurrent lumbar pain, wound erythema, swelling and drainage, fever, and diaphoresis. He remained neurologically intact without any evidence of nerve tension signs or meningeal irritation signs. Laboratory analysis at that time revealed a white blood cell count of 6900, ESR of 60 mm/hour, and CRP of 4.6 mg/dL. Recrudescence of his wound infection was evident.

Radiologic Findings

Radiographic analysis of the lumbar spine included anteroposterior and lateral views that were essentially unchanged from that shown in Figure 28–1B. Magnetic resonance imaging (MRI) revealed loss of the normal disc space signal characteristics on T1-weighted images (Fig. 28–2) consistent with the suspected infection. No significant spinal canal compromise or epidural abscess was evident, nor was there any other focus of infection evident, but a T2-weighted image was not performed. A CT myelogram done following initial debridement, which included removal of the internal fixation devices, demonstrated discitis associated with peridiscal bone erosion and sclerosis consistent with vertebral osteomyelitis (Fig. 28–3).

Diagnosis

Deep postoperative lumbar wound infection associated with L1/L2 intervertebral discitis and osteomyelitis, possibly due to hematogenous seeding from an episode of sepsis, which recurred following medical treatment.

Surgical Management

Step one included a layered reopening and debridement of the posterior surgical wound. The abnormal dermal margins were sharply excised along with any unhealthy subcutaneous tissue. Samples from this superficial layer were sent for microbiologic

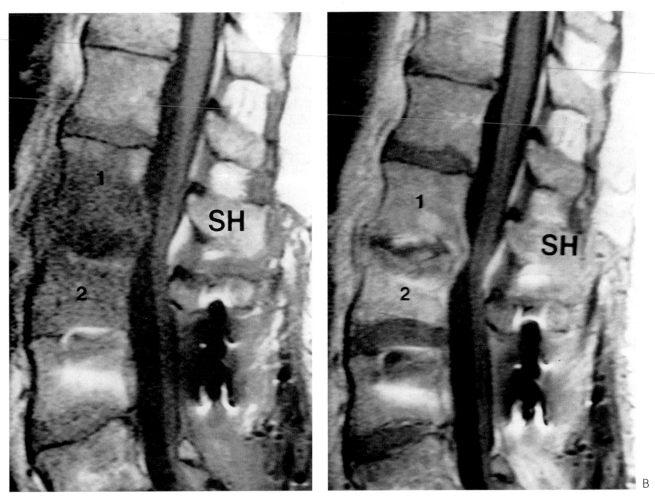

Figure 28–2. Sagittal T1-weighted magnetic resonance imaging (MRI) (A) with areas of hypointensity of the L1/L2 disc region and loss of definition of the normal subchondral landmarks. Postgadolinium image (B) with areas of hyperintensity consistent with an infectious process.

and pathologic examination. Cultures were requested for aerobic, anaerobic, acid fast, and fungal organisms. Following pulsatile lavage, the fascia was opened and the deeper layers explored and debrided. Purulence was evident both superficially and deep. The implants were noted to be loose and surrounded with inflammatory exudate. They were removed and the screw tracts curetted to remove granulation tissue. The L2/L4 fusion mass was healed despite the presence of the infection. Further debridement and lavage rendered the wound surgically clean prior to performing a layered primary closure over both superficial and deep closed-suction drains. A triple-lumen central venous line was inserted to provide for intravenous hyperalimentation as well as antibiotics.

Both superficial and deep cultures grew *Staphylococcus aureus,* which was once again sensitive to all antibiotics. In the interim, the patient was placed on intravenous cefazolin. Two days later the patient was taken back to surgery for a second-look debridement, just as one might do for an open extremity fracture. Once again, intraoperative cultures were sent for aerobic, anaerobic, fungal, and acid fast species. This time there was no evidence of purulent material. The wound was closed primarily over closed-suction drains.

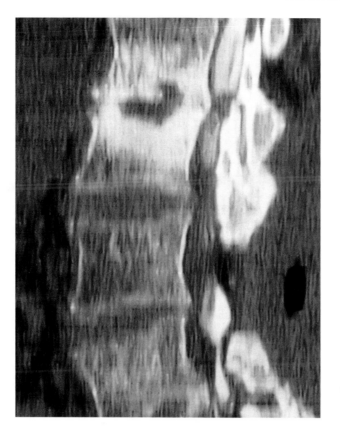

Figure 28–3. Reformatted postmyelogram computed to-mography (CT) at the L1/L2 level demonstrating disc space destruction, cavitation, and sclerotic reactive bone involving the lower half of L1 and most of L2. This information is instrumental in planning surgical debride-ment and reconstruction.

The patient was allowed out of bed in a lumbar corset. A CT myelogram was obtained to more clearly define the extent of anterior vertebral involvement (Fig. 28–3). The CT images were used to define the intended margins of debridement for the final phase of treatment. Two weeks later, following demonstration of ade-quate clinical response to the initial debridement, the patient returned to surgery for definitive treatment of the L1/L2 vertebral osteomyelitis. An L2 corpectomy and partial L1 corpectomy were performed through a 12th rib retroperitoneal ex-posure. Pieces of the bone were sent for gram stain, cultures, and biopsy. They also grew *S. aureus,* despite the previous administration of antibiotics to which they were sensitive. The upper half of the L1 vertebral body remained, but was still fairly sclerotic. The floor of the spinal canal was fully decompressed. Anterior reconstruction was accomplished with a Harms' cage packed and surrounded with a combination of morcelized rib autograft and fresh-frozen cancellous allograft (Fig. 28–4).

The remaining portion of the L1 vertebral body was judged to be too small and mechanically inadequate to apply an anterior spinal fixation device. Therefore, the decision was made to proceed with a supplemental posterior segmental instrumen-tation and fusion. After turning the patient to the prone position on a Jackson operating table, the posterior incision was reopened. A small hematoma was en-countered deep to the fascia, which was cultured. The wound was carefully debrided and irrigated with 3 L of antibiotic solution. Fluoroscopy facilitated insertion of 6.5-mm L1 pedicle screws, whereas 7.5-mm screws were inserted through the old screw tracts in L3. A posterior iliac crest bone graft was obtained through a separate incision, which was applied to the decorticated posterior elements and transverse

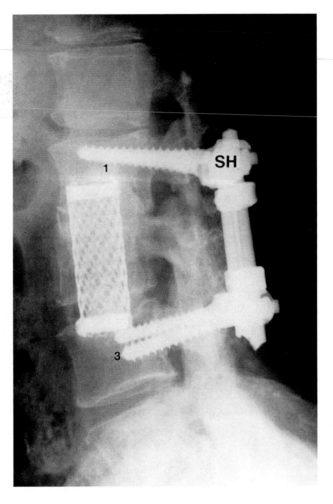

Figure 28–4. Postoperative lateral radiographs status post–L2 corpectomy, partial L1 corpectomy with anterior Harms' cage, and posterior L1/L3 segmental instrumentation.

processes from L1 to L3. Slight compression was applied across the final construct. A final primary closure proceeded over two deep drains.

Postoperative Management

Following the initial irrigation and debridement procedures, the patient was encouraged to ambulate in a lumbar corset. Intravenous hyperalimentation was maintained until he demonstrated adequate oral intake following the final procedure. After the final reconstructive procedure, the patient was allowed out of bed as comfort permitted. A TLSO was fitted, which the patient wore whenever he was out of bed during the next 3 months. Intravenous cefazolin was continued for 6 weeks after the last surgical procedure, followed by an additional 6 weeks of oral ciprofloxacin.

Discussion

Postoperative wound infection is a well-recognized and potentially devastating consequence of spinal surgery. Though steps may be taken to reduce a patient's relative risk of infection, the incidence remains finite, and varies in proportion to the magnitude of the procedure performed.

A number of classification schemes have been used for postoperative spinal wound infections. Authors have distinguished between superficial and deep infections, and early and late infections. Unfortunately, no data have emerged to support the utility of these distinctions in guiding treatment or providing a prognosis for a given patient. In the authors' opinion, the most useful concept to date has been adapted from Cierny's (1990) work with diaphyseal osteomyelitis. Thalgott and colleagues (1991) stratified hosts as class A, B, or C according to their physiology, and infections as groups 1, 2, or 3 according to their pathogens and extent of bone and soft tissue involvement. These categories correlated well with the number of procedures required to complete the treatment, the length of hospitalization, and the overall cost of treatment. Evaluating patients with these variables in mind can be helpful in planning treatment and determining the level of aggressiveness required, including the likelihood of adjunctive plastic surgical procedures to achieve a suitable healing environment.

Intraoperative measures can reduce the risk of infection. Restricting operating room traffic can decrease the number of airborne organisms and thus the inoculum. Careful attention to soft tissue handling and meticulous hemostasis can help decrease the potential for bacterial colonization by reducing the amount of necrotic material and the size of the hematoma that remains within the wound. Intermittent release of self-retaining retractors will reduce the adverse effects of local muscle ischemia. Frequent irrigation is also recommended, whether with plain saline solution or antibiotic irrigant. However, the single most effective measure is the timely administration of appropriate prophylactic antibiotics. They must be administered preoperatively to have adequate serum drug levels at the time of the incision and throughout the remainder of the procedure.

The clinical presentation of a postoperative wound infection is highly variable. Obvious infections, such as with our patient's second presentation are not the rule. The wound will appear deceptively normal while patients complain of increasing pain. They generally feel ill and often experience lethargy, anorexia, fever, chills, and/or diaphoresis.

Laboratory findings are nonspecific but suggestive of the diagnosis. The white blood count (WBC) is not often elevated unless the patient is acutely ill. The ESR and CRP are elevated in virtually all cases, and thus they provide a useful barometer for response to treatment.

Imaging techniques are helpful in many cases of postoperative wound infections. MRI with gadolinium enhancement is the modality of choice. It can readily identify most cases of postoperative discitis, vertebral osteomyelitis, as well as epidural abscesses, provided the images are not degraded by implant artifact.

Ultimately, the diagnosis rests on culture data, whether obtained by percutaneous aspiration, biopsy, or open exploration.

The goals of the surgical management of postoperative infection are (1) to eradicate the infection, (2) to close the wound, and (3) to maintain or restore the mechanical integrity of the affected motion segments. Prompt and aggressive treatment should be instituted once an infection is identified, whether superficial or deep. Surgical exploration, debridement, and irrigation proceed by layer, with each being cultured then rendered surgically clean before proceeding to the next. Open the entire incision. Well-anchored bone graft and instrumentation is left in place to promote fusion.

Primary wound closure is strongly preferred by the authors. Primary closure reduces the likelihood of superinfection, avoids contracture of the tissue margins, reduces the catabolic stress from protein loss, and simplifies nursing needs. It also tends to reduce the number of surgical procedures by one, as there is no need for a final procedure to close the wound. Reexploration and debridement is recommended at 48 hours in most patients, and potentially each 48 to 72 hours thereafter in certain circumstances. Infections that involve bone/bone grafts or implants should be treated as presumptive osteomyelitis; thus, the duration of antibiotic treatment will be a minimum of 6 weeks. The patient's clinical response and serial laboratory values will be useful in judging the effectiveness of treatment.

Alternative Methods of Management

Wound closure strategies are a matter of debate. Various authorities have published their results with open strategies or suction irrigation systems. The latter imposes significant nursing requirements without any proven benefit over closed-suction drains. They also convey some risk of superinfection. If employed, these systems should remain in place for 5 to 10 days if possible. They do not obviate the need for repeated debridement procedures. Closure over antibiotic-impregnated beads has its advocates. The clinical effectiveness has been demonstrated, but this method carries the disadvantage of requiring $N + 1$ procedures because a final operation is needed to remove the beads and reclose the wound.

Type of Management	Advantages	Disadvantages	Comments
Primary wound closure over closed suction drainage	Overall fewer complications Reduces protein losses Reduces the risk of superinfection Reduces nursing demands Potential for faster return to activities Prevents wound edge retraction, thereby facilitating wound closure	Requires meticulous and serial debridement May require plastic surgical procedures to affect primary closure	Optimal candidate: good host with a single organism cultured Allows a well-vascularized bed to cover the area providing the optimal healing environment facilitating the elimination of the bacteria
Wound closure over suction-irrigation catheter systems	Allows for a continuous antibiotic irrigation of the infected region	Should remain in place for 5 to 10 days Increased nursing demands Does not reduce the need for or number of debridements May increase the risk of nosocomial infection	A cumbersome technique that has been in use for many years Generally falling into disfavor as experience increases with closed-suction drainage and flap coverage
Wound closure over antibiotic-impregnated beads with closed-suction drainage	Improves local antibiotic concentration	Requires $N + 1$ operations to remove the antibiotic beads Does not reduce the need for or number of debridements Uncertainty about the systemic risks from erratic elution of antibiotics	This technique has been helpful in managing long bone osteomyelitis, but blood supply is less of an issue in the spine

Complications

Perhaps the worst complication to stem from such infections is failure to appreciate the diagnosis. Such an oversight can lead the physician and patient down a treatment course that is both misguided and doomed to failure (Fig. 28–5). Awareness

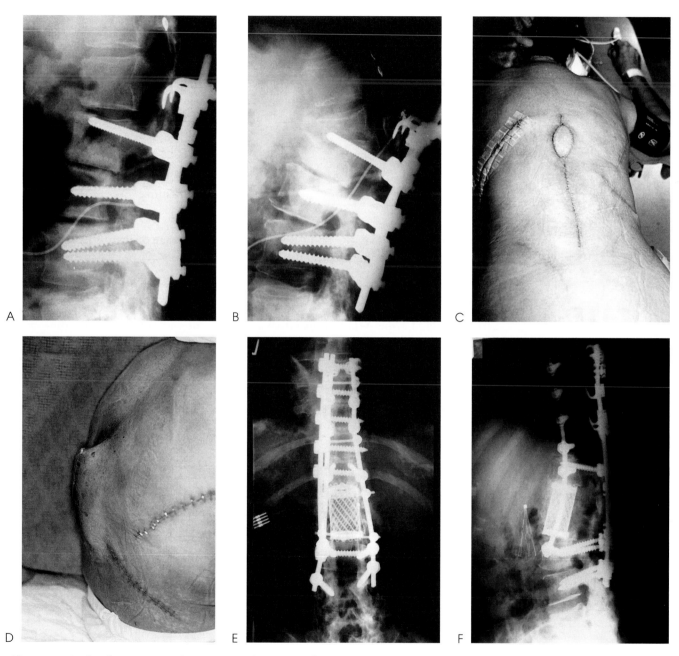

Figure 28–5. Another patient with a previous L4 to sacrum fusion ultimately required an L2/L4 instrumentation and fusion. (A) Lateral radiograph following the L2/L4 procedure. (B) Lateral radiograph taken nearly 3 months postoperatively, at which time the patient complained of escalating pain. Note the disc space destruction, collapse, and kyphosis at L1/L2, suggesting infection. The diagnosis was not appreciated, which resulted in the patient undergoing an extension of her fusion into the thoracic spine. The wound infection worsened and fixation was lost. The patient returned with her implants protruding through a latissimus dorsi flap, which had been attempted to facilitate wound healing (C and D). She was ultimately managed with four-stage procedures composed of serial debridements, anterior corpectomies, reconstruction and interbody fusions, and posterior segmental instrumentation and fusion (E and F).

of the manifestations of wound infections, careful interpretation of radiographs, other imaging technologies, and laboratory data will lead to the diagnosis. But if the possibility is never entertained, the diagnosis will await a more obvious and complex presentation.

Pseudarthrosis rates are higher among patients who have sustained a wound infection following their fusion procedure. The rationale for leaving instrumentation in place in the early stages of managing an infection within a fusion bed is not only to promote union, but also to control the pain associated with instability and to protect the neural elements.

If soft tissue coverage becomes a problem, consultation with a plastic surgeon to transfer a musculocutaneous flap will provide a well-vascularized, closed tissue bed, which facilitates healing, reduces protein loss, and increases local antibiotic concentrations.

Suggested Readings

Cierny G III. Chronic osteomyelitis. Instructional Course Lecture Series 1990; 39(62):495–508.

Glassman SD, Dimar JR, Puno RM, Johnson JR. Salvage of instrumented lumbar fusions complicated by surgical wound infection. Spine 1996; 21(18):2163–2169.

Heller JG. Postoperative infections of the spine. In: Rothman RH, Simeone FA, eds. The Spine, Vol. 2, 3d ed., pp. 1817–1837. Philadelphia: WB Saunders, 1992.

Heller JG, Levine MJ. Postoperative Infections of the Spine. Semin Spine Surg 1996; 8(2):105–114.

Ozuna RM, Delamarter RB. Pyogenic vertebral osteomyelitis and postsurgical disc space infection. Orthop Clin North Am 1996; 27:87–94.

Petty W, Spanier S, Shuster JJ, et al. The influence of skeletal implants on incidence of infection. J Bone Joint Surg 1985; 67A:1236–1244.

Stambough JL, Beringer D. Postoperative wound infections complicating adult spine surgery. J Spinal Disord 1992; 5(3):277–285.

Thalgott JS, Cotler HB, Sasso RC, et al. Postoperative infections in spinal implants—classification and analysis—a multicenter study. Spine 1991; 16(8):981–984.

Wimmer C, Gluch H, Franzreb M, Ogon M. Predisposing factors for infection in spine surgery: a survey of 850 spinal procedures. J Spinal Disord 1988; 11(2):124–129.

Section III

Metabolic Disease

Case 29
Pagetoid Disease of the Spine
Jeffrey S. Fischgrund

History and Physical Examination

A 65-year-old man presented with a 5-year history of intermittent low back pain. The patient reported pain at rest that is significantly aggravated by physical activity. The patient also noted that prolonged standing, sitting, and driving aggravated his symptoms, but the pain did not awaken him from sleep. The patient did not report any radicular leg pain but complained of episodic pain radiating to the bilateral gluteal region with rare right posterior thigh pain. There are no changes in urinary frequency or bowel habits. The patient denied any leg weakness or numbness, fevers, night sweats, or weight loss. The patient's past medical history was significant for only mild hypertension. Neither aspirin nor antiinflammatory medication relieved the pain.

Physical examination was notable for local tenderness over the lower lumbar spine. Range of motion of the spine was nearly within normal limits, with mild complaints of pain with forward flexion. There were no neurologic deficits in the lower extremities.

Radiologic Findings

Routine laboratory tests were within normal limits except serum alkaline phosphatase, which was elevated. Plain radiographs of the lumbar spine and pelvis demonstrated sclerosis and coarsened trabeculae in the pelvis, as well as the L1 vertebral body. Bone scan showed markedly increased uptake throughout L1 as well as diffusely in the pelvis.

Nonoperative Management

The patient was treated with disodium etidronate 200 mg orally twice daily. The patient noticed a gradual decline in pain after 6 months of treatment. A repeat bone scan taken 6 months after initiation of treatment showed decreased uptake in the pelvis as well as the L1 vertebral body. Plain films taken were unchanged from those 6 months prior.

Discussion

Paget's disease is a combination of excessive osteoclastic and osteoblastic activity that results in a markedly increased rate of osseous turnover. The exact cause of this disease is unknown. Proposed etiologies include inflammatory disease, a generalized disease of connective tissue, vascular disease, infectious disease, or an autoimmune disorder. More recent work has identified the possibility of a viral cause of this disease. This recent theory is based on the findings of intranuclear inclusion bodies (which may be viral) in pagetic osteoclasts.

Generally, the pathologic process of Paget's process of Paget's disease is divided into three phases. The first phase, also known as the osteolytic or hot phase, is characterized by an intense resorption of existing bone. The mixed phase follows, which is accompanied by accelerated deposition of spicules of lamellar bone in a disorganized fashion. The final phase is known as the osteoblastic or cold phase, in which bone formation is dominant and the irregular-shaped trabecular are characterized by a mosaic pattern of cement lines. These cement lines often appear haphazardly between fragments of lamellar bone. All three phases may be present within a single bone, or the disease may be in different phases throughout the body.

Laboratory evaluation of the patient with Paget's disease relies on the detection of increased remodeling of bone, which leads to a high turnover rate of the mineral and organic phases of bone. In this disease process, the increased release of mineral ions that results from increased bone resorption is closely accompanied by local re-utilization of these ions for the formation of bone. Therefore, plasma concentrations of calcium and phosphorus are usually normal. Similarly, the concentration of parathyroid hormone is also normal.

However, when bone is resorbed, not only is there release of mineral ions from the inorganic portion of bone, but there is resorption of the organic content—collagen and noncollagenous proteins—as well. During bone resorption, free hydroxylysine and hydroxyproline are released from collagen-derived peptides and are reutilized for collagen synthesis; in the process they are degraded to small carbon fragments. Specifically, hydroxylysine and hydroxyproline are excreted in the urine, with the rate of excretion roughly paralleling the rate of collagen degradation. The presence of these peptides in the urine provides a useful marker for studying the collagen turnover in patients with Paget's disease and assessing their responses to therapy.

Elevation of the serum level of alkaline phosphatase is characteristically seen in patients with Paget's disease. This level correlates well with the extent of the disease as well as with the level of the urinary hydroxyproline excretion. Markedly elevated levels do not occur in patients who had isolated involvement of a small bone such as a vertebral body, whereas those patients with involvement of larger bones have a broad range of alkaline phosphatase levels. In patients followed for several years, the levels of alkaline phosphatase tend to show a long-term upward trend with the tendency to plateau.

Patients with Paget's disease may present with either single-site involvement or multiple sites of involvement. If the patient presents with localized involvement to the vertebral column, open or computed tomography (CT)-guided biopsy may be required for definitive diagnosis. Histologic analysis of these biopsy specimens will show abnormal architecture of lamellar bone (Fig. 29–1). Normal lamellar bone results from the parallel arrangement of collagen fibers in a rectangular orientation. This type of bone is characterized by few osteocytes per unit area of matrix with a uniformity in size and shape of osteocytes. This normal arrangement of lamellar bone is generally not found in Paget's disease.

During the osteolytic phase of Paget's disease, the osteoclasts are seen to assume bizarre shapes and may contain up to 100 nuclei. Following osteoclastic resorption (Fig. 29–2), there is fibrous tissue replacement of adjacent normal fatty or hematopoietic bone marrow. At this stage of the disease there is development of vascular hypertrophy and hyperplasia and the appearance of undifferentiated mesenchymal cells adjacent to the hypertrophic osteoclasts. As bone resorption continues, there is an increase in the deposition of this fibrous stroma and the vascularity becomes more prominent. During the lytic phase, there are frequently foci of intense osteoblastic activity as well. This osteoblastic activity results in the deposition of lamellar bone, often adjacent to the areas of osteoclastic resorption.

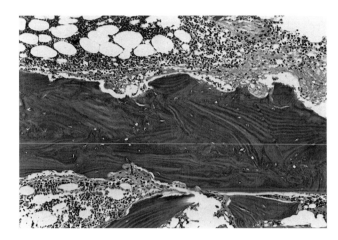

Figure 29–1. Photomicrograph demonstrates the thick, irregular plate of bone characteristic of Paget's disease. (Hematoxylin and eosin × 5)

During the mixed phase of Paget's disease, the osteoclasts become less numerous and the osteoblastic activity increases. Now, new lamellar bone formation occurs, with hypertrophic osteoblasts closely approximated to the bone (Fig. 29–3). This leads to the appearance of classic pagetic bone featuring a mosaic arrangement of the cement lines. This diagnostic feature is characterized by irregular jigsaw-shaped pieces of lamellar bone with an erratic arrangement of cement lines.

During the osteoblastic or sclerotic phase of the disease, dense irregular masses of pagetic bone are found with little cellular activity. Frequently, the marrow is nearly replaced with fibrous tissue containing irregular vessels and osteoblasts lining the bone surfaces.

Radiologic Findings

The most common vertebral presentation of Paget's disease is involvement of the lumbar spine and sacrum (Figs. 29–4 and 29–5). Thoracic and cervical disease as well as monostotic disease can also occur. Pagetoid changes of the lumbar spine are more common in the body than the posterior elements. Frequently, enlarged, coarsened trabeculae are seen with condensation of the bone usually prominent along the outer contours of the vertebral body (Fig. 29–6). When this occurs, the highlighted contour of the body resembles a picture frame. Occasionally, there can be a uniform

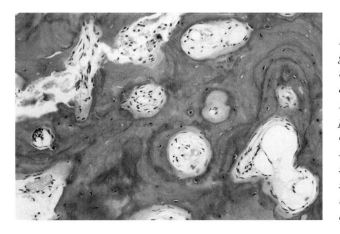

Figure 29–2. Photomicrograph demonstrates both osteoblastic and osteoclastic activity that may coexist in Paget's disease. The mosaic pattern formed by basophilic cement lines is clearly seen. Micro-cracks occur at the site of cement lines and result in weakness of Paget's bone. (Hematoxylin and eosin × 10)

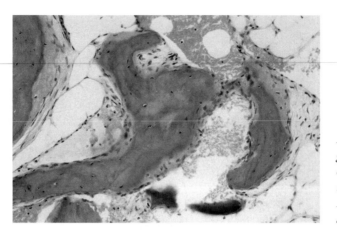

Figure 29–3. Photomicrograph demonstrates prominent osteoblastic rimming characteristics of new bone formation in Paget's disease. (Hematoxylin and eosin × 10)

increase in osseous density, producing an ivory vertebrae. The vertebral body is frequently enlarged, which assists in differentiating Paget's disease from other causes of ivory vertebrae, such as metastases and lymphoma; however, in these processes there is no enlargement of the vertebral body.

Increased bone formation in Paget's disease may lead to an increased amount of bone per unit volume. However, the bone formed is structurally unsound compared to normal bone. This structural weakness of the vertebral body can lead to alterations in shape of the involved bodies. Bi-concave deformities can occur due to compression of the softened vertebrae by the adjacent intervertebral disc. These deformities are identical to those that occur in metabolic disorders such as osteoporosis, osteomalacia, and hyperparathyroidism. Secondary degenerative alterations in the discs will frequently lead to disc space narrowing and occasional osseous bridging of vertebral bodies.

Posterior element involvement, particularly that of the pedicles, will be manifested by an increased radiodensity, which can simulate osteoblastic metastases. Additionally, alterations in the size and shape of the vertebral body can lead to an

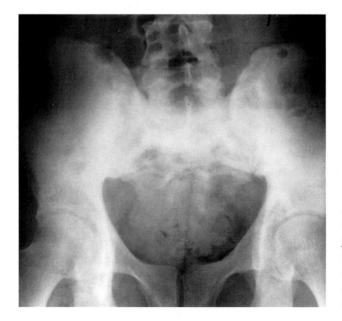

Figure 29–4. Anteroposterior (AP) radiograph of the pelvis in a patient with the diagnosis of Paget's. Note the diffuse, mottled appearance and linear areas of sclerosis with coarsened trabeculae.

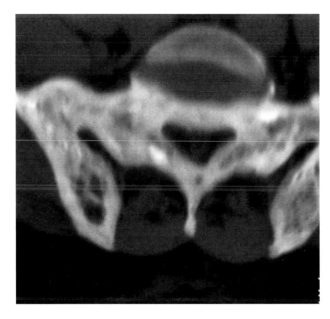

Figure 29–5. Computed tomography (CT) scan of the patient in Fig. 29–4 demonstrates thickening of the trabeculae and diffuse thickening of the cortex of the ilium and S2 vertebral segment.

increase in the interpedicular distance, which is more suggestive of Paget's disease rather than metastatic disease.

Neurologic deterioration can occur in patients with Paget's disease due to either spinal cord, cauda equina, or nerve root compression. The neural compression can be due to the disease process itself or secondary changes within the bone. Five mechanisms have been described in the pathogenesis of neurologic complications: (1) collapse of affected vertebral bodies; (2) increased vascularity of pagetic bone, which "steals" blood from the spinal cord; (3) mechanical interference with spinal cord blood supply; (4) narrowing of the spinal canal due to new bone formation or soft tissue and ligament ossification; and (5) stenosis of neural foramina resulting from involvement of the vertebral posterior elements.

Radioisotope bone scanning can also be used for evaluation of the patient with Paget's disease. Due to the increased radionucleide uptake, areas of active skeletal disease are seen to be "hot." Bone scans are generally more sensitive than radiographic evaluation, and frequently scintigraphic abnormalities can precede

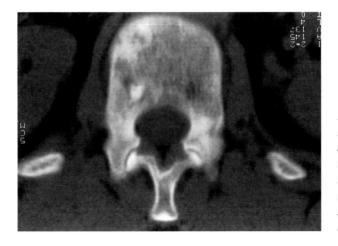

Figure 29–6. CT scan of the L1 vertebral body, which demonstrates thickening of the trabeculae and enlargement of the pedicles. Significant posterior enlargement can lead to spinal stenosis (not seen in this example).

radiographic changes. During the lytic phase of Paget's disease, increased radionucleide activity can be prominent at the advancing edge of bone lysis, which corresponds to the sites of increased vascularity and new bone formation. Serial bone scans can provide objective evidence of the effect of therapeutic regimens, which is useful when monitoring patient progress.

Generally, CT scans and magnetic resonance imaging (MRI) do not help in the radiographic diagnosis of Paget's disease. However, neurologic compromise is best shown with one of these two tests, which can help to delineate the amount of neural compression and to plan for surgical decompression.

Medical Management

Calcitonin

Calcitonin, administered intramuscularly, subcutaneously, or nasally, leads to an acute decrease in bone resorption due to its effect on the inhibition of osteoclastic activity. Generally, patients respond with a fall in urinary hydroxyproline excretion within days and a fall in serum alkaline phosphatase levels within weeks. The reported clinical benefits associated with chronic calcitonin therapy include relief of bone pain, reduction of increased cardiac output, reversal of central and peripheral neurologic deficits, stabilization of hearing deficits, healing of osteolytic lesions, reduction of skeletal blood flow, and prevention of excessive hemorrhage associated with orthopaedic surgery. The optimum dose of salmon-calcitonin is in the range of 50 to 100 Medical Research Council (MRC) units administered daily or three times weekly by subcutaneous self-injection. Side effects include nausea and facial flushing, with rare reports of significant toxicity. The preliminary results obtained with nasal spray and suppository formulations of salmon-calcitonin have produced only modest results.

There are several patterns of response to calcitonin that become apparent after long-term treatment of Paget's disease. Occasionally, there may be complete biochemical and clinical remission. More commonly, however, there is an initial decrease in the indices of bone remodeling, but normalization of bone remodeling does not take place with continued treatment. Patients who show this pattern usually maintain clinical improvement associated with biochemical evidence of decreased bone turnover. On the average, the biochemical indices in these patients are stabilized at approximately 50% of pretreatment levels.

The third pattern of response to calcitonin is characterized by an initial response comparable to that of other groups, but as treatment is continued, abnormalities recur. In this group of patients, high titers of antibodies to the species of calcitonin have been demonstrated in the circulation. Resistance to porcine, salmon, and human calcitonin, however, may also develop in the absence of detectable circulating antibodies. Since the advent of newer pharmaceutical agents, the use of parenteral salmon-calcitonin therapy has decreased.

Biphosphonates

Biphosphonates are synthetic analogues of inorganic pyrophosphate that bind to the surface of calcium phosphate minerals. This class of medications inhibits bone resorption and formation. There is a direct effect on osteoclasts and osteoclast precursors as well as indirect effects on these cells through possible interactions with osteoblasts and macrophages. The first biphosphonate used to treat Paget's disease was disodium etidronate, usually administered at a dose of 5 mg/kg of body weight, daily for 6 months. As has been found with calcitonin therapy, there are several patterns of biochemical and clinical response to disodium etidronate. Approximately half of the patients have a prolonged response after a single course of therapy. A second group of patients experienced a good response to the initial course of therapy but required treatment with disodium etidronate 3 months to 5 years after the initial therapy and then responded similarly to 20 mg/kg per day, but not as well to 5 mg/kg per day.

The desirable therapeutic effect observed histologically in patients treated with disodium etidronate is a reduction in the osteoclastic bone resorption. Ultrastructural analysis of the osteoclasts reveals evidence of cell degeneration. Bone marrow fibrosis is reduced and areas of woven bone may be replaced by lamellar bone. Side effects of disodium etidronate therapy includes increased bone pain, nausea, and diarrhea.

Since the introduction of disodium etidronate, several newer, more potent biphosphonates have been developed. These include Clodronate and Pamidronate. Alendronate is approved for all uses in Paget's disease. The most recently approved biphosphonate for treatment of Paget's disease in the United States is Tiludronate.

Alternative Methods of Management

Effective medical management can often improve the neurologic syndromes observed in Paget's disease. The rate of neurologic improvement seen with drug treatment is usually rapid and is not necessarily associated with changes in spinal canal diameter. This response is likely due to an increase in soft tissue swelling or to redistribution of blood flow. The acute onset of paraparesis or quadriparesis secondary to neural compression is an indication for urgent surgical decompression. The surgeon should be aware of the increased risk of excessive bleeding from bone during the active stage of the disease.

Type of Management	Advantages	Disadvantages	Comments
CT-guided biopsy	Useful in localized disease when the possibility of a tumerous process needs to be excluded	Minimal outside of the morbidity of the procedure	Useful procedure for diagnoses as well as histologic identification of disease staging
Calcitonin	Leads to acute decrease in bone resorption due to inhibition of osteoelastic activity	Side effects include nausea, facial flushing, and rare causes of significant toxicity	Clinical benefits include relief of some pain, reduction of increased cardiac output, reversal of central and peripheral neurologic deficits, and prevention of excessive blood loss at surgery
Biphosphonates	Inhibits bone resorption and formation Direct effect on osteoclasts and its precursors, and indirect effects on osteoblasts and microphages	Side effects include increased bone pain, nausea, and diarrhea	Histologically there is a reduction in osteoclastic bone resorption Bone marrow fibrosis is reduced and areas of woven bone may be replaced by lamellar bone

Suggested Readings

Booth RE, Simpson JM, Herkowitz HN. Arthritis of the Spine. In: Herkowitz HN, Garfin SR, Balderston RA, et al, eds. The Spine, pp. 440–441. Philadelphia: WB Saunders, 1999.

Resnick D, Niwayama G. Paget's disease. In: Resnick D, ed. Diagnosis of Bone and Joint Disorders, pp. 1923–1968. Philadelphia: WB Saunders, 1995.

Singer FR, Krane SM. Paget's disease of the bone. In: Avioli LV, Krane SM, eds. Metabolic Bone Disease, pp. 545–606. San Diego: Academic Press, 1998.

Case 30

Circumferential Surgery for Ossification of the Posterior Longitudinal Ligament in the Cervical Spine

Nancy E. Epstein

History and Physical Examination

A 58-year-old man presented with a rapidly progressive (6 months) moderate/severe spastic myeloradiculopathy (Nurick grade IV), characterized by weakness and wasting of the hands (2/5), and instability of gait. Magnetic resonance imaging (MRI) and computed tomography (CT) studies demonstrated massive continuous ossification of the posterior longitudinal ligament (OPLL) extending from the C3/C4 through the C6/C7 levels (Figs. 30–1 and 30–2). An anterior corpectomy with fusion was performed from C3 to C7 with complete removal of the OPLL, and application of an iliac crest bone graft, with placement of an Orion cervical plate. This was followed by posterior wiring and fusion from C3 to C7 using Songer cables with iliac crest autograft and halo application. Postoperatively, the patient immediately demonstrated marked neurologic improvement, and 3 months later was asymptomatic (Nurick grade 0). Radiographic studies, including 2D and 3D CT studies obtained 3 months postoperatively, confirmed complete resection of OPLL from C3 to C7, fusion of the iliac crest strut graft, and no shift in the location of the anterior plate (Figs. 30–3 through 30–7). Posteriorly, fusion of the laminae/facets was observed without failure of the Songer cables.

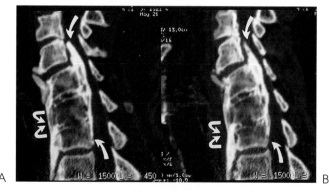

Figure 30–1. Parasagittal 2D computed tomography (CT) studies of continuous OPLL. (A) The first paramedian sagittal study demonstrates massive continuous OPLL extending from the C3/C4 level (single large arrows) all the way down to C6/C7. (B) Note the presence of ossification of the anterior longitudinal ligament (OALL) (double arrows).

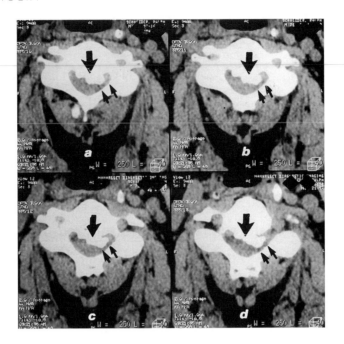

Figure 30–2. Progressive axial CT studies from mid-C4 to C4/C5 disc space level showing massive continuous OPLL. On all of these successive images obtained from the mid-C4 through the C4/C5 disc space, frank OPLL clearly occupies more than half of the spinal canal (single arrows), nearly obliterating the left C4/C5 lateral recess (double arrows).

Discussion

Circumferential surgery in this disease setting is performed using awake, nasotracheal fiberoptic intubation with awake positioning and continuous intraoperative somatosensory evoked potential (SSEP) monitoring. From 1989 to 1997, 22 patients with OPLL or spondylostenosis had multilevel anterior cervical corpectomy

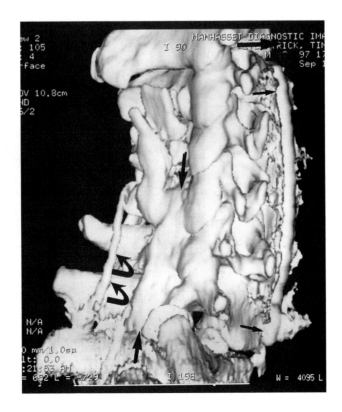

Figure 30–3. Lateral 3D CT view of cervical spine following circumferential surgery employing anterior Orion plate (3 months postoperatively). On this lateral 3D CT view, the anterior Orion plate (small single arrows) may be visualized along with the posterior wiring and fusion completed with Songer cable (double arrows). Also note the fusion mass along the posterior articular facets (large single arrows).

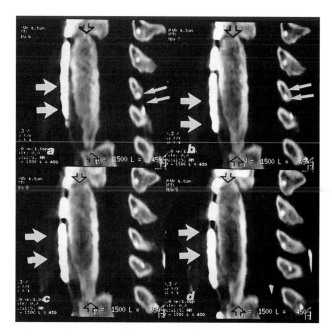

Figure 30–4. Midline and paramedian sagittal 2D CT studies demonstrating circumferential cervical C3/C7 surgery using anterior Orion plate (3 months postoperatively). These four midline and paramedian sagittal 2D CT studies readily demonstrate complete resection of OPLL, full decompression of the cervical spinal cord, adequate placement of the iliac crest strut graft (single small arrows), with cephalad/caudad fusion, the anterior Orion plate (single large arrows), with the Songer cables at the base of the spinous processes posteriorly (double small arrows).

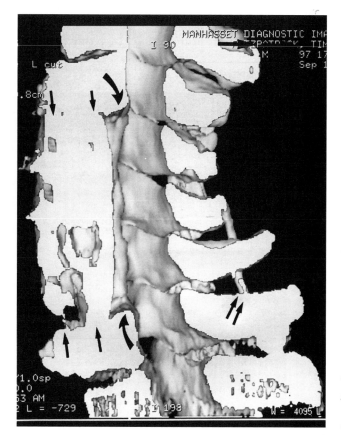

Figure 30–5. Midline sagittal 3D CT study confirming excision of OPLL following circumferential C3/C7 ACF with Orion plate placement and posterior wiring/fusion (3 months postoperatively). This midline 3D CT image reveals the full extent of OPLL resection anteriorly (small single arrows), a fused iliac crest bone graft extending from C3 to C7 (small double arrows), Orion plate placement, and posterior wiring/fusion using Songer cables (small double arrows).

PEARLS

- When performing multilevel anterior corpectomy and fusion, it is critical that the recipient cephalad and caudad endplates remain intact (i.e., they may be perforated) to avoid telescoping of the graft and fracturing of the anterior vertebral cortex with graft extrusion.
- Iliac crest autograft fuses faster than any type of fibula graft. However, the morbidity of the donor site, and graft weakening by sculpturing the graft to allow it to fit into the recipient site, may make it a weaker construct. Alternatively, straight autograft and allograft fibula may be more easily used to span longer defects, the longer time to fusion (i.e., >6 months) being compensated for by the short time for posterior fusion to occur (i.e., 3.5 months). Furthermore, both fibula grafts fuse at comparable rates, with the allograft minimizing morbidity by eliminating the donor site.

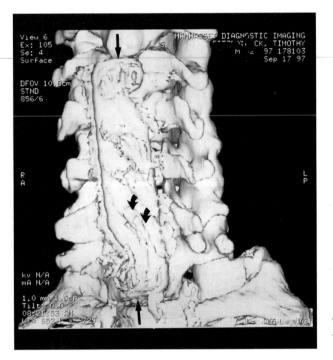

Figure 30–6. Anterior 3D CT view of incorporated Orion plate 3 months following circumferential C3/C7 surgery. This anterior 3D CT image clearly demonstrates the Orion plate in situ (small single arrows) with bony ingrowth into the oblique slots (small double arrows).

with fusion (ACF; average 2.5 levels), followed by posterior wiring and fusion (PWF; average 5 levels) or laminectomy/facet wiring and fusion with halo placement without plate instrumentation. Although 100% of these patients fused, three (14%) exhibited immediate postoperative vertebral fractures/graft extrusions requiring graft replacement, with plate application in two of the three patients. To avoid similar future vertebral fractures/graft extrusions, the next 20 patients seen

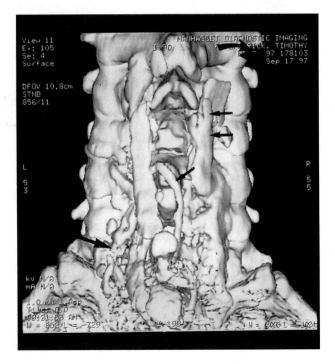

Figure 30–7. Posterior wiring using Songer cable with application of iliac crest autograft 3 months following circumferential C3/C7 surgery. This posterior 3D CT study demonstrates solid fusion 3 months following the original C3/C7 circumferential procedure. Note the Songer cable (single small arrow), iliac crest cortical strips (double small arrows), and additional cancellous bone now incorporated into the lateral fusion mass (single large arrows).

PITFALLS

- Proper patient selection is critical to the success of circumferential cervical surgery. Patients over 65 to 70 years of age, with severe cardiovascular, respiratory, or other illnesses are at increased risk from these long, stressful procedures, and may not be candidates for circumferential surgery. Additionally, patients with severe neurologic deficits, including quadriplegia, particularly of long duration, are less likely to benefit from surgery as damage is likely irreversible (e.g., necrosis, myelomalacia).
- Failure to use SSEP monitoring may result in inadvertent quadriplegia.
- The maneuvers that pose the highest risk for cord injury are distraction and tightening of the posterior wire. To address these concerns, distraction should be utilized for graft placement only after OPLL has been fully resected, and the cord decompressed. For the posterior wiring, a test tightening should be performed first for a 5-minute period, minimum, to make sure no significant SSEP changes are evolving.

between September 1997 and September 1998, in addition to having circumferential surgery as described—ACF, average 2.8 levels; PWF, average 5.4 levels—also had anterior cervical plate instrumentation. To date, none has developed vertebral fractures/graft extrusions. All 20 patients have fused without incident. Furthermore, patients having such comprehensive circumferential management of OPLL/spondylosis over the long-term should have fewer future problems requiring reoperations (reported up to 12%) for residual/recurrent disease and pseudarthrosis, and should avoid the risk of increased OPLL progression following laminectomy or laminoplasty.

MRI and CT

All patients had preoperative MRI and CT examinations, which together demonstrated the sagittal and axial extent of OPLL or spondylostenosis. MRI was superior in showing high signals within the cord indicative of myelomalacia.

Anterior Plates

Anterior cervical unicortical plates have provided up to a 100% fusion rate with limited morbidity. Indeed, in our second series in which 20 patients received plates, the plates appeared to eliminate vertebral fractures/graft extrusions, did not add to operative time or morbidity, and appeared to shorten the average time to fusion by 1 month (from 4 to 3 months).

Halo Immobilization

Although all patients from both series were originally immobilized in halo braces, three ended up being managed in cervicothoracic orthoses (hard collar/extension brace). In two patients, pins continually slipped due to the skull shape, and a third patient with severe cerebral palsy literally lunged his way out of the halo device.

Neurologic Status

Patients from both populations exhibited moderate to moderate/severe myelopathy prior to surgery (Nurick grades III to IV). Postoperatively, all improved, demonstrating either no deficit, mild radiculopathy, or mild myelopathy (Nurick grades 0 to I). No patient showed deterioration of neurologic function. There were no spinal cord injuries, and only one transient C5 root injury in a nonplated diabetic patient, which appeared 48 hours following surgery. These data compare favorably with the 2 to 10% frequency for cord and 2 to 17% frequency for root injury reported in comparable but non–SSEP-monitored studies.

Complications

There were four complications among the 22 nonplated patients. One patient incurred a fatal myocardial infarction in the setting of severe vascular disease and a rapidly evolving quadriparesis. Another patient, one who had prior multilevel anterior OPLL surgery 5 years earlier, developed a cerebrospinal fluid (CSF) fistula, requiring placement of a lumboperitoneal shunt. A third patient developed a deep venous thrombosis (DVT) requiring placement of a vena cava filter, and a fourth patient exhibited transient dysphagia for 1 month.

Among the 20 patients having surgery using plates, only one had a complication. She had a vena cava filter prophylactically placed prior to surgery because of four prior episodes of DVT, but required no further treatment when a DVT was demonstrated on Doppler studies 48 hours postoperatively.

Fusion

Using dynamic lateral radiographs and 3D CT studies, the 22 nonplated patients fused an average of 4 months (range 2 to 7 months) postoperatively, whereas 17 of the 20 plated patients fused over an average of 3 months (range 2 to 5 months). For the remaining three, operated on less than 3 months ago, fusion is awaited. The 100% fusion rate observed for circumferential surgery without and with plates has prompted us to consider limiting the use of halo devices in the future.

Operative Time

The average operative time for the first 22 circumferential procedures performed without plate instrumentation was 10 hours, requiring 3.5 units of blood (range 1 to 8). The last 20 plated procedures were completed over an average of 8 hours and have warranted 2.7 (range 0 to 6) units of blood. Of note, these procedures have been completed with limited morbidity.

Alternative Methods of Management

Type of Management	Advantages	Disadvantages	Comments
Simultaneous anterior corpectomy and fusion with posterior wiring and fusion with or without plates	Direct anterior resection of OPLL Direct posterior resection with laminectomy of stenosis or OYL Immediate maximal stability One anesthetic Plating avoids graft extrusions 100% fusion rate	Longr operative procedure: 8 hours 3 units of blood Increased risk to older patients (>70) with significant comorbidities, especially cardiovascular disease	This procedure provides the most complete and immediate management strategy for cervical OPLL, OYL, and stenosis It may be accomplished in a reasonable time frame with limited comorbidity
Anterior corpectomy and fusion with or without plates (no posterior surgery)	Direct anterior resection of OPLL Intermediate-length procedure compared with circumferential surgery	Failure to address dorsal pathology: OYL or stenosis Increased risk for graft extrusions with or without plates <100% fusion rate	This strategy results in a higher graft extrusion and lower fusion rate The longer the construct, the greater the extrusion rate It also fails to address dorsal pathology: OYL or stenosis
Laminoplasty	Shorter procedure Posterior decompression of OYL and stenosis Limited risk of instability or kyphosis Best in presence of hyperlordosis	Failure to directly resect OPLL Increased rate of ventral OPLL progression Risk of closing of the door Risk of increased radiculopathy on closed door side	Favored by some for OPLL over three or more levels; however, it results in poorer long-term outcomes Appropriate for patients with hyperlordotic curvature only

Continued on next page

Continued

Type of Management	Advantages	Disadvantages	Comments
Laminectomy with or without posterior wiring and fusion (PWF)	Shorter procedure Posterior decompression OYL and stenosis Best in presence of hyperlordosis PWF limits kyphosis	Failure to directly resect ventral OPLL Increased rate of OPLL progression	This is a shorter operation that is only appropriate for those with hyperlordosis PWF avoids kyphosis

OPLL, ossification of the posterior longitudinal ligament; OYL, ossification of the yellow ligament.

Suggested Readings

Epstein NE. The surgical management of ossification of the posterior longitudinal ligament in 51 patients. J Spinal Disord 1993; 6(5):432–454.

Epstein NE. Advanced cervical spondylosis with ossification into the posterior longitudinal ligament and resultant neurological sequelae. J Spinal Disord 1996; 9(6):477–484.

Epstein NE. Somatosensory evoked potential monitoring (SSEPs) in 173 cervical operations. Neuro-Orthopedics 1996; 20:3–21.

Epstein NE. Vertebral body fractures following extensive anterior cervical surgical procedures for ossification of the posterior longitudinal ligament. Neuro-Orthopedics 1997; 21:1–11.

Epstein NE. Circumferential surgery for the management of ossification of the posterior longitudinal ligament. J Spinal Disord 1998; 11(3):200–207.

Epstein NE. Evaluation and treatment of clinical instability associated with pseudarthrosis following anterior cervical surgery for ossification of the posterior longitudinal ligament. Surg Neurol 1998; 49(3):246–252.

Epstein NE, Danto J, Nardi D. Evaluation of intraoperative somatosensory evoked potential monitoring in 100 cervical operations. Spine 1993; 18(6):737–747.

Goto S, Kita T. Long-term follow-up of surgery for ossification of the posterior longitudinal ligament. Spine 1995; 20(20):2247–2256.

Kostuik JP, Connolly PJ, Esses SI, Suh P. Anterior cervical plate fixation with the titanium hollow screw plate system. Spine 1993; 18(10):1273–1278.

McAfee PC, Bohlman HH. One stage anterior cervical decompression and posterior stabilization with circumferential arthrodesis. A study of twenty-four patients who had a traumatic or a neoplastic lesion. J Bone Joint Surg 1989; 71A(1):78–88.

McAfee PC, Bohlman HH, Ducker TB, Zeidman SM, Goldstein JA. One-stage anterior cervical decompression and posterior stabilization. A study of one hundred patients with a minimum of two years of follow-up. J Bone Joint Surg 1995; 77A(12):1791–1800.

McNamara MJ, Devito DP, Spengler DM. Circumferential fusion for the management of acute cervical spine trauma. J Spinal Disord 1991; 4(4):4674–4671.

Saunders RL. On the pathogenesis of the radiculopathy complicating multilevel corpectomy. Neurosurgery 1995; 37(3):408–414.

Shinomiya K, Okamoto A Kamikozuru M, Furuya K, Yamamura I. An analysis of failures in primary cervical anterior spinal cord decompression and fusion. J Spinal Disord 1993; 6(4):277–288.

Yonenobu K, Hosono N, Iwasaki M, Asano MM, Ono K. Neurologic complications of surgery for cervical compression myelopathy. Spine 1991; 16(11): 1277–1282.

Case 31

Transthoracic and Transabdominal Approach to T9 to T12 Ossification of the Posterior Longitudinal Ligament with Herniated Disc/Stenosis

Nancy E. Epstein

History and Physical Examination

A 67-year-old Caucasian woman presented with an 8-month history of progressive numbness, tingling, and weakness in both lower extremities, accompanied by increasing bowel and bladder dysfunction.

On examination, she had marked difficulty ambulating even with the help of a walker and an assistant. Motor examination showed diffuse bilateral proximal and distal lower extremity weakness: iliopsoas and quadriceps (<3/5), and extensor hallicus dorsiflexor and plantar flexor function (2/5). Bilateral lower extremity hyperreflexia (4+ with clonus) and Babinski responses were present. A relative sensory level to a pin was noted from T10 downward, with the accompanying loss of vibratory and position appreciation. Cerebellar examination revealed the patient could not walk in a tandem fashion, and she exhibited poor heel to shin coordination.

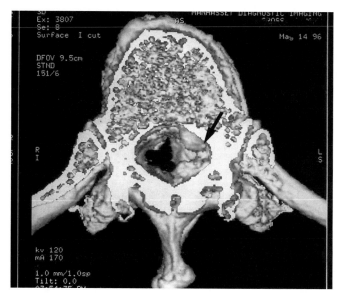

Figure 31–1. 3D transaxial noncontrast mid-T10 computed tomography (CT) of thoracic OPLL. The massive extent of OPLL occupying the entire left lateral aspect of the spinal canal is seen (arrow).

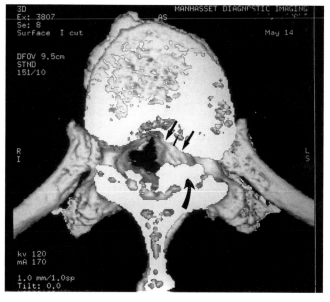

Figure 31–2. 3D midline transaxial CT of thoracic OPLL and OYL seen at the T10/T11 level. OYL (curved arrow) is clearly seen filling the left dorsolateral aspect of the spinal canal at the T10/T11 interspace. Also observe the 3D view of the left-sided OPLL filling the left-sided anterolateral aspect of the spinal canal (double arrows).

Somatosensory evoked potentials (SSEPs) showed delayed cortical latencies on stimulation of the posterior tibial nerves, and electromyography revealed lower extremity abnormalities in the L5/S1 distributions.

Radiologic Findings

The thoracic magnetic resonance imaging (MRI) study demonstrated ossification of the posterior longitudinal ligament (OPLL), ossification of the yellow ligament (OYL), high-grade spinal stenosis, and a T11/T12 disc herniation contributing to marked compression and a high signal within the distal thoracic cord and conus (myelomalacia versus edema). The complete cervical, thoracic, and lumbar myelogram computed tomography (CT) examination confirmed the presence of severe T9/T12 OPLL, OYL stenosis, and a T11/T12 disc herniation with significant accompanying L1/S1 stenosis (Figs. 31–1 through 31–4). The cervical study was unremarkable. Incidentally noted on the thoracic portion of the myelogram CT was an abnormally small and lobulated right lobe of the liver. Laboratory texts also confirmed mildly elevated liver enzymes. However, a CT scan of the abdomen and pelvis and a liver biopsy ruled out the presence of cirrhosis.

Surgical Management

In view of the patient's deteriorating neurologic status, and the predominant ventral location of the pathology, a combined transthoracic and transabdominal surgical approach to the anterior pathology alone was planned. Her fragile physical status (weight 110 pounds, small right lobe of the liver, and mild liver enzyme abnormalities) precluded the simultaneous performance of a T9/T12 laminectomy with T7/L2 fusion for the OYL, which showed only mild dorsal intrusion.

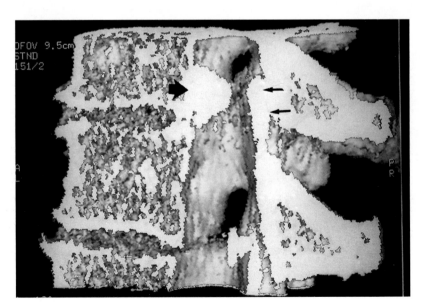

Figure 31–3. 3D midline sagittal CT showing OPLL and OYL at the T10/T11 level. The ventral ossified OPLL mass (single arrow) is seen nearly "kissing" the dorsally located OYL (double arrows). Note, neither the T11/T12 disc herniation nor hypertrophied posterior longitudinal ligament (early OPLL) is visualized on this study.

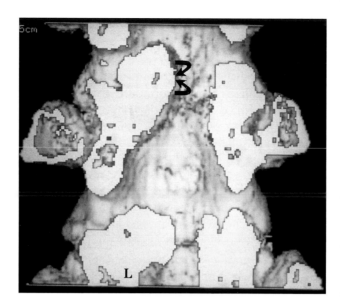

Figure 31–4. 3D coronal CT scan of thoracic OPLL at the T10/T11 level. The massive ventral and left-sided extent of OPLL at the T10/T11 levels (double arrows) are shown.

Other Specialists Involved

A thoracic surgeon first performed a left-sided transthoracic transabdominal approach, as the pathology was midline toward the left in location, and dissection around the aorta is significantly easier and associated with less morbidity than dissecting around the vena cava. The entirety of the surgery was performed under SSEP monitoring. The anesthesiologist selectively cannulated both the right and left main stem bronchi so that the left lung could be selectively collapsed, and the right lung selectively ventilated during different portions of the procedure.

Operative Approach

The incision was made between the T7 and T8 ribs, and extended inferiorly in the midline. The abdominal portion warranted an extraperitoneal exposure, which included taking down the diaphragm. Once the T9/T12 levels were fully exposed, each intercostal artery was selectively "test occluded" with a bulldog clamp to confirm that there were no significant changes in SSEPs. This avoided inadvertent ligation of the artery of Adamkiewicz, most typically found between the left-sided T9/L2 levels. As no significant SSEP changes were encountered during any of these test occlusions (or at any other time during the surgery), the T9, T10, and T11 intercostal vessels were ligated close to the aorta.

Exposure

The completed exposure afforded full visualization from above the T9/T10 disc space to below the T11/T12 disc space. The aorta was free and mobile, allowing one to place a finger between the aorta and the left more than the right side of the vertebrae. The aorta was then retracted behind wet lap pads and a wide retractor, a similar technique being used to keep the lung out of the operative field. Of note, this retraction was carefully checked and released every 20 minutes. Next, the anterior corpectomy was initiated using a high-speed cutting drill (Midas AM no. 9 bit) to remove the vertebrae and discs. Careful attention was paid to maintaining a plane of bony dissection parallel to the spinal canal, to avoid inadvertent entry into the canal. Such symmetric exposure insured that the ipsilateral dura would not pout into the wound, making dissection toward the right more difficult. This entire dissection was completed under high-power operating loupes. However, as soon as dissection approached the anterior rim of the spinal canal, all subsequent dissection was completed under the operating microscope. Additionally, the burr tip was changed to a small matchstick diamond bit (AM no. 8 diamond), completing the corpectomy with rotating small Kerrison rongeurs and curettes. Microdissectors and curettes allowed for identification and careful resection of OPLL and disc overlying the thinned dura within the narrowed spinal canal.

Grafting

Once the T9/T12 corpectomy had been completed, an iliac crest autograft and fibular allograft were applied along with a Zdeblick thoracic plate. Multiple intraoperative anteroposterior (AP) and lateral radiographs were obtained to confirm adequate graft and plate placement. Finally, the thoracic surgeon returned to close the thoracoabdominal incision. Two chest tubes were inserted.

Timing of Surgery

The entire procedure took 12 hours, required six units of transfused blood (four autologous), and 600 cc of Cell Saver blood. When examined immediately postoperatively on the operating room table, the patient's neurologic status appeared unchanged, and she was returned to the recovery room.

Intubation Period

The patient remained intubated overnight, being extubated the next postoperative day. Two days postoperatively, following removal of one of the chest tubes, a postoperative CT study was obtained to check the position of the graft. Because it showed that the femoral graft intruded somewhat into the spinal canal, an MRI study was ordered to evaluate whether this resulted in active cord compression. The MRI fortunately revealed that there was no ongoing cord compromise, and that indeed the degree of spinal cord atrophy at this level left the cord free and clear.

Follow-up MRI/CT Studies

These studies were again repeated a week later when the patient's neurologic status failed to further improve in the presence of persistent sphincteric dysfunction. MRI and CT examinations remained unchanged. However, 10 days postoperatively, when she suddenly became febrile and complained of shortness of breath, both a chest X-ray and chest CT showed a large volume of left-sided pleural fluid. On insertion of a chest tube, thin-watery fluid (500 cc) was obtained. The Gram stain revealed predominant *Streptococcus* with rare *Staphylococcus aureus*. For the former she was started on intravenous Rocephin (2 g IV q24h), and for the latter, vancomycin (750 mg IV q12h). Ten days later, the vancomycin was discontinued as the *Staphylococcus* species appeared to be a procurement contaminant. She remained on intravenous Rocephin for the next 6 weeks, followed by 6 weeks of oral Keflex (2 g/day).

Complication: Infection

Fourteen days postoperatively, a persistent fever and a left pleural effusion prompted reopening of the thoracotomy wound. Over the next 6 weeks of

PEARLS

- When dealing with thoracic myelopathy, it is critical to perform MRI and CT-based examinations (ideally a myelogram CT) to help differentiate between thoracic OPLL and more routine disc disease. Thoracic OPLL, often the continuous variant spanning multiple vertebrae and disc spaces, requires a multilevel corpectomy with instrumented strut graft fusion performed through a transthoracic or combined transthoracic-transabdominal approach.
- The use of intraoperative SSEP is critical to these procedures, and should help avoid postoperative paraplegia. Sequential test clamping of aortic segmental vessels is critical to avoid compromising the vascular supply to the cord, especially when approaching lower thoracic lesions from the left side.

hospitalization, the infection resolved, and her respiratory and neurologic status improved. She was then transferred to a rehabilitation center. Five months later X-rays and CT studies (Figs. 31–5 and 31–6) demonstrated fusion and the instrumentation well situated at the postoperative site. Ten months postoperatively, following rehabilitation, the patient was able to ambulate using a walker. Although her proximal strength is 5/5, her bilateral foot drop and loss of pin appreciation (L5/S1) continues to limit her ability to walk. Of note, hyperreflexia has largely resolved, and she remains continent.

Discussion

When reviewing this case, one has to carefully consider whether the initial operative approach was appropriately based on the requisite preoperative diagnostic studies, including both MRI and CT-based examinations. A left-sided approach was chosen due to predominant midline to left-sided pathology. A combined left-sided transthoracic-transabdominal technique was chosen due to the levels of pathology. Although this procedure carries a significant morbidity (neurologic risk, medical risk, i.e., operative time), it allows for direct visualization and resection of the multilevel OPLL and disc with assistance of an operating microscope utilized in a familiar position (ventral). The extracavitary approach does not provide comparable

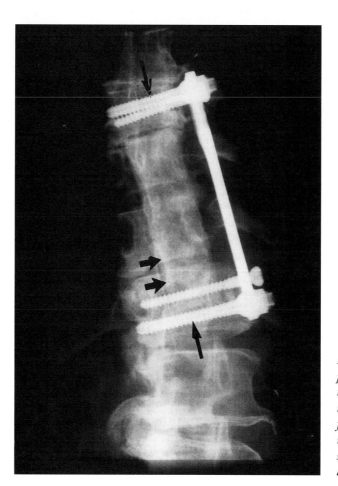

Figure 31–5. Five-month postoperative plain anteroposterior (AP) X-ray showing the intact T9/T12 fusion. The fibular allograft (double arrows) and Zdeblick plate and screws intact (single arrow) are shown.

PITFALLS

- The most common error when dealing with thoracic myelopathy is an inadequate preoperative workup. Failing to differentiate OPLL from disc disease, and inadequately demonstrating the full extent of OPLL without OYL, leads to "Band-Aid" procedures that leave the majority of the pathology behind, often making patients worse.
- Preoperatively, patients should be carefully screened for significant medical comorbidities; otherwise, postoperatively, cardiovascular or respiratory disease may lead to myocardial infarction or pulmonary decompensation.
- The use of the operating microscope when removing OPLL is critical, just as in the cervical spine; otherwise the risk of cerebrospinal fluid fistula is high with its attendant complications. Additionally, when removing the vertebral body, it is important to switch from a cutting burr to diamond burrs early in the course of dissection to limit the chance of injuring critical adjacent structures.

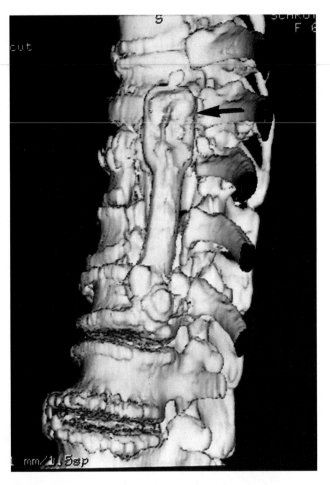

Figure 31–6. Five-month postoperative 3D left-sided anterolateral CT showing fusion. The Zdeblick plate (arrow) is shown in place with bone growing through its slots, indicating the stability of the construct.

access, and lateral thoracotomy, laminoplasty, and costotransversectomy techniques would not be appropriate.

Anterior Surgery Only

The anterior approach was a rational choice for the direct exposure and resection of T9/T12 OPLL and disc (T11/T12). Simultaneous or even sequential removal of the dorsal OYL (only mildly intruding into the spinal canal) and stenosis, via a T9/T12 laminectomy with T7/L2 Texas-Scottish Rite Hospital (TSRH) instrumented fusion, did not appear to be a reasonable option for the following reasons. First, the added dorsal surgery was not necessarily indicated, as the degree of dorsolateral compression from OYL was mild. Second, it appeared that the patient was frail and could not tolerate such extensive surgery.

Prior Case

The author previously performed a 23-hour circumferential thoracic procedure on a 450-pound, 25-year-old man with a rapidly evolving paraplegia. This procedure included a combined transthoracic, transabdominal approach for completion of a T9/T12 corpectomy for OPLL and a T10/T11 midline disc, and a T9/T12 laminectomy with T7/L2 TSRH fusion addressed the additional severe OYL and stenosis. This procedure was formidable. The patient recovered fully within one year, having also lost 150 pounds.

Indications

Because of the extent of these procedures, they should be performed therapeutically, not prophylactically. Complete identification of the extent of OPLL both locally and throughout the entire neuraxis (cervical and lumbar as well) should be made to ensure that the most symptomatic lesion is being addressed. One should not risk missing more cephalad cervical OPLL, which could render a patient quadriplegic. Because of the long duration of these operations, I recommend having a thoracic surgeon perform the approach. Stringent preoperative medical evaluation is also essential as these are long and stressful procedures, increasing the likelihood of both medical and surgical complications.

Alternative Methods of Management

Type of Management	Advantages	Disadvantages	Comments
Transthoracic-transabdominal	Direct anterior resection of OPLL	Pulmonary and/or abdominal complications including major vessel (aortic) injury	Arduous procedures to be performed in patients with limited medical comorbidity
Extracavitary	Simultaneous access to ventral OPLL and dorsal OYL with ability to complete anterior and posterior fusion	Suboptimal visualization of ventral OPLL and dorsal OYL increasing operative risk of neurologic injury	A problematic alternative to a direct anterior approach
Costotransversectomy	A familiar dorsolateral approach	Failure to adequately visualize or remove midline OPLL Increased risk of neurologic injury	Failure to adequately resect midline OPLL makes this a poor operative choice
Laminectomy	Appropriate to resect OYL	Failure to resect OPLL Dorsal decompression alone poses a high risk of postoperative paraplegia	Not an appropriate choice for the management of OPLL

OPLL, ossification of the posterior longitudinal ligament; OYL, ossification of the yellow ligament.

Suggested Readings

Enomoto H, Kuwayama N, Katsumata T, Doi T. Ossification of the ligamentum flavum. A case report and its MRI findings. Neuroradiology 1988; 30(6):571–573.

Epstein NE. Thoracic ossification of the posterior longitudinal ligament, ossification of the yellow ligament from T9–T12 with superimposed acute T10/T11 disc herniation: controversies in surgical management. J Spinal Disord 1996; 9(5):446–450.

Fujimura Y, Nishi Y, Nakamura M, Toyama Y, Suzuki N. Long-term follow up study of anterior decompression and fusion for thoracic myelopathy resulting from ossification of the posterior longitudinal ligament. Spine 1997; 22(3):305–311.

Ido K, Shimizu K, Nakayama Y, et al. Anterior decompression and fusion for ossification of the posterior longitudinal ligament in the thoracic spine. J Spinal Disord 1995; 8(4):317–323.

Mimatsu K. New laminoplasty after thoracic and lumbar laminectomy. J Spinal Disord 1997; 10(1):20–26.

Nakamura H, Crock HV, Galbally BP, Dawson J. Ossification of the posterior longitudinal ligament in the thoracic spine causing intermittent paraplegia in an Englishman: case report. Paraplegia 1992; 30(4):277–281.

Tomita K, Kawahara N, Baba H, Kikuchi Y, Nishimura H. Circumspinal decompression for thoracic myelopathy due to combined ossification of the posterior longitudinal ligament and ligamentum flavum. Spine 1990; 15(11):1114–1120.

Yonenobu K, Korkusuz F, Hosono N, Ebara S, Ono K. Lateral rhachotomy for thoracic spinal lesions. Spine 1990; 15(11):1121–1125.

Yoshino MT, Seeger JF, Carmody RF. MRI diagnosis of thoracic ossification of the posterior longitudinal ligament with concomitant disc herniation. Neuroradiology 1991; 33(5):455–457.

Case 32
Diffuse Idiopathic Skeletal Hyperostosis

Donal B. Rose and Jeffrey D. Klein

History and Physical Examination

A 63-year-old man presented with a 3-year history of worsening neck and left greater than right upper extremity pain. The pain radiated down the arm and forearm to the wrist. Intermittent numbness and tingling was noted as well. The symptoms were generally worse with activity.

The patient also reported difficulty with swallowing during the past year. He described the need to "double swallow" hard, solid food. In recent months, the patient had increasing difficulty with fine motor skills such as buttoning his shirt. He described his hands as feeling "disconnected." He also noted a recent subtle difficulty with balance and ambulation. Though he had not frankly fallen, he described a sense of unsteadiness.

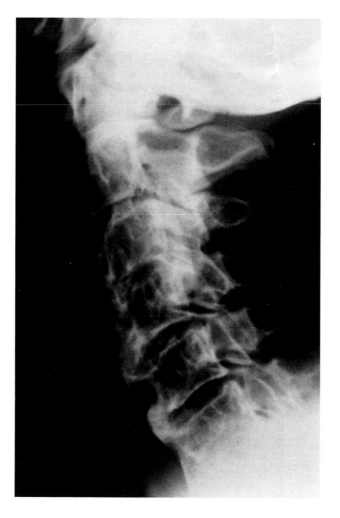

Figure 32–1. Lateral cervical spine radiograph—preoperative.

The patient denied any history of trauma. There were no symptoms with regard to bowel or bladder. Physical therapy had not offered any symptomatic relief.

Physical examination revealed a middle-aged man walking with a slow, deliberate gait. He used his hands on the wall of the corridor to help steady himself. His gate was not wide based; motor strength was normal, 5/5 throughout the upper and lower extremities. Reflexes were 3+ and symmetric at the biceps, brachioradialis, and triceps. Knee and ankle jerks were 4+ and symmetric. Hoffmann's sign was positive bilaterally. There were three beats of clonus bilaterally. Babinski's sign was equivocal.

Radiologic Findings

Anteroposterior (AP) and lateral radiographs of the cervical spine revealed marked degenerative changes at multiple levels. Large, flowing peridiscal osteophytes were noted anterolaterally (Fig. 32–1). There was relative preservation of the disc space height. Magnetic resonance imaging (MRI) of the cervical spine revealed multilevel cervical stenosis due to disc-osteophyte complexes as well as an element of ossification of the posterior longitudinal ligament (OPLL). Spinal cord and nerve root compression was noted at multiple levels (Figs. 32–2 and 32–3).

Diagnosis

Multilevel cervical spondylosis with associated myeloradiculopathy in the setting of diffuse idiopathic skeletal hyperostosis (DISH). The radiographic criteria for DISH as set forth by Resnick and Niwayama (1976) include flowing ossification along the anterolateral aspect of at least four consecutive vertebrae, preservation of the intervertebral disc height of the affected areas, relative preservation of the apophyseal joints, and absence of sacroiliac involvement. These criteria serve to help differentiate DISH from degenerative disc disease and ankylosing spondylitis. In the older patient, findings of degenerative disc disease and osteoarthritis may coexist with those of diffuse skeletal hyperostosis. Such is the case with this patient.

Surgical Management

A multilevel anterior cervical decompression was performed. Reconstruction with structural bone graft and stabilization with an anterior cervical plate followed.

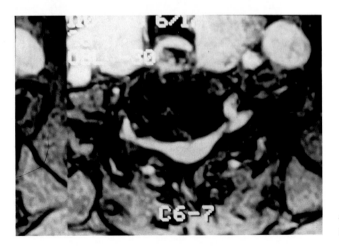

Figure 32–2. Magnetic resonance imaging (MRI)—axial.

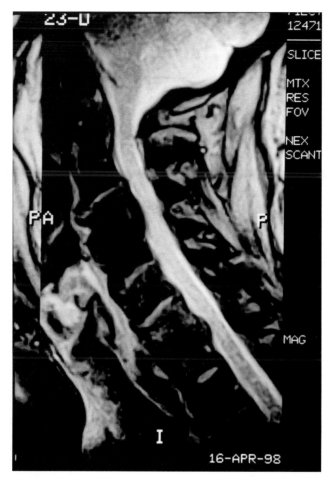

Figure 32–3. MRI—sagittal.

The patient was taken to the operating room where general endotracheal anesthesia was induced. Numerous precautions were taken at this point. In the setting of spinal cord compression and myelopathy, care must be taken not to hyperextend the neck during intubation. If necessary, an awake fiberoptic intubation should be performed with the neck neutrally aligned. Care must also be taken to maintain the mean arterial pressure throughout the induction of anesthesia and the operative case. An arterial line is preferable. This is necessary to ensure adequate perfusion of the already compromised spinal cord. Unless otherwise contraindicated, perioperative intravenous steroids are administered in cases of spinal cord compression.

A left-sided approach through a longitudinal incision was used to expose the anterior cervical spine. The left side is generally preferred as the recurrent laryngeal nerve is at less risk. Large, confluent anterior osteophytes were encountered from C3 to C7, consistent with the diagnosis of diffuse skeletal hyperostosis. These were resected, allowing visualization of the normal cortical margin of the vertebral bodies. This is necessary not only to treat dysphagia, but also to allow proper application of the anterior cervical plate along the anterior aspect of the cervical spine. This was followed by multilevel decompression and reconstruction. The construct was stabilized with an anterior cervical plate contoured into gentle lordosis to match that of the cervical spine (Fig. 32–4). The wound was then closed over a suction drainage device.

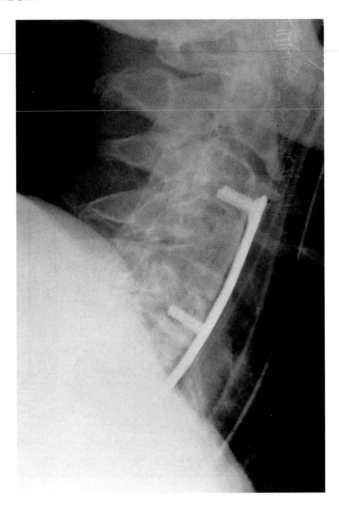

Figure 32–4. Lateral cervical spine radiograph— postoperative.

Postoperative Management

The patient was observed overnight in the surgical intensive care unit to monitor the airway. The head of the bed remained elevated at 30 degrees to assist in reducing postoperative swelling at the operative site. The Jackson-Pratt drain was removed when the drainage was less than 5 cc for an 8-hour shift. Given the long anterior construct, a Philadelphia collar was utilized for a period of 10 to 12 weeks.

The patient was mobilized rapidly. Ambulation was begun on the day of surgery. The patient was discharged on the second postoperative day.

Discussion

Diffuse idiopathic skeletal hyperostosis (DISH) was originally distinguished from ankylosing spondylitis (AS) by Forestier and Rotes-Querol (1950). They noted that whereas ossification begins in the peripheral aspect of the annulus fibrosis is AS, ossification in DISH begins at the insertion of Sharpey's fibers from the anterior longitudinal ligament to the anterior cortex of the vertebral body. In patients with DISH, ossification may progress rapidly after even minor trauma. Although metaplasia, calcification, and ossification result in a brittle disc in ankylosing spondylitis,

PEARL

• Maintain a high index of suspicion for fracture in patients with DISH after trauma. The resulting long-bone fractures are highly unstable and such patients are at high risk for immediate and delayed neurologic compromise.

PITFALLS

• There is some suggestion of a relationship between DISH and opacification of the posterior longitudinal ligament (OPLL). If present in a given patient, this may affect the preoperative plan.
• When DISH is identified in a patient with cervical trauma, one must be sure to adequately visualize the cervicothoracic junction. This is not an uncommon area for significant fractures in this patient population.

the disc height and integrity are relatively maintained in DISH. As a result of this difference, spinal fractures tend to be transdiscal in ankylosing spondylitis and transvertebral in diffuse skeletal hyperostosis. Characteristically, the middle one-third of the vertebral body is the least dense region of the hyperostosis in DISH. DISH is further distinguished from AS by a lack of sacroiliac joint involvement and a relative preservation of the apophyseal joints. There also tends to be skip areas in DISH. The relative sparing of the apophyseal joints and the skip areas tend to preserve spinal motion in these patients.

However, advanced stages of DISH are markedly hypertrophic, resulting in ankylosis and often severe stenosis. Such patients are prone, as in AS, to fracture, often with relatively minimal associated trauma. The resulting fracture is typically a transverse or long-bone fracture of the spine. Such a fracture is markedly unstable. This, together with the relatively high likelihood of significant stenosis in these patients, leads to a high rate of immediate and delayed neurologic deficit. Careful evaluation of patients with diffuse skeletal hyperostosis who sustain trauma is critical. Early treatment of such fractures is indicated, and often combined anterior and posterior procedures are needed to adequately stabilize these injuries. A low threshold for postoperative halo immobilization is warranted as well.

Those patients with significant cervical spine involvement in DISH not uncommonly present with dysphagia. This is due to very large anterior osteophytes causing partial obstruction in the posterior pharynx and proximal esophagus. Treatment of these patients requires resection of these osteophytes in addition to the decompression or fusion as clinical conditions dictate.

Lastly, numerous extraspinal manifestations of diffuse skeletal hyperostosis are commonly seen including heel spurs, epicondylitis of the elbow, generalized enthesitis, and diffuse ligament calcifications.

Alternative Methods of Management

Diffuse idiopathic skeletal hyperostosis is not an indication for surgery. Rather, the secondary manifestation of this condition often necessitates spinal surgery. In the cervical spine, significant stenosis often results in myeloradicular syndromes. When surgical decompression and stabilization are required, the anterior or posterior approach is chosen based on the same considerations as are used for cervical spondylosis. Generally, anterior procedures are more commonly employed, though the posterior approach is favored for situations involving four or more levels. In the special circumstance of DISH, the anterior approach must be utilized when dysphagia is present so as to resect the offending anterior osteophytes. When unstable long-bone fractures are encountered in DISH, often combined anterior and posterior procedures are required to obtain adequate stabilization.

Type of Management	Advantages	Disadvantages	Comments
Anterior approach	Allows resection of anterior osteophytes in dysphagia; most direct decompression, especially in the kyphotic spine	Any decompressive procedure obligates one to fusion; the older patient population is prone to postoperative dysphagia, especially with long exposures	Most common approach to treat dysphagia and neural compression
Posterior approach	May avoid the need for fusion in the lordotic spine	Cannot address anterior osteophytes; may not address the neural compression in the kyphotic spine; progressive arthrosis, recurrent foraminal stenosis, and late instability are all possible	May be preferable in expansile cases in the absence of dysphagia; limited secondary anterior procedure is always possible; may be preferred when OPLL coexists
Combined anterior and posterior approach	Advantages of both approaches; maximal stabilization	Generally excessive in elective cases unless addressing specific pathology	May be required to adequately stabilize long bone–type fracture

Complications

When diffuse skeletal hyperostosis is identified in a patient after trauma, no matter how minor, one must maintain a high index of suspicion for occult fracture. This same level of vigilance is necessary in a patient with known DISH after any trauma. Early immobilization, appropriate imaging, and stabilization are required. The unstable fracture pattern seen in DISH, together with the potential for significant pre-existing stenosis, leads to an increased likelihood of immediate and delayed neurologic deficits.

Patients with dysphagia are prone to poor nutritional status. This must be addressed preoperatively and aggressive supplementation instituted to minimize postoperative infectious complications.

When anterior osteophyte resection is undertaken for dysphagia in the absence of neural compromise, the overall degenerative pattern of the spine must be addressed in the preoperative plan. In the setting of relatively normal disc spaces and facet joints, osteophyte resection can generally be undertaken safely. In those patients with significant degenerative disc disease and facet arthrosis, even if asymptomatic, the massive osteophytes may in effect autostabilize the spine. Osteophyte resection may create a subtle instability in these patients, with associated severe neck pain. In such cases, fusion may be preferable at the time of osteophyte resection.

Lastly, patients with long anterior neck exposures, especially with significant mobilization of the esophagus, are prone to postoperative dysphagia. This is more common in the elderly and is related to disturbance of the esophageal neural plexus. This generally resolves in the days to weeks following surgery, but puts those patients at greater risk for aspiration.

Suggested Readings

Forestier J, Rotes-Querol J. Senile ankylosing hyperostosis of the spine. Ann Rheum Dis 1950; 9:321–330.

Kmucha S, Cravens R. Diffuse idiopathic skeletal hyperostosis syndrome and its role in dysphagia. Otolaryngol Head Neck Surg 1994; 110:431–436.

Mata S, Fortin P, Fitzcharles M, et al. A controlled study of diffuse idiopathic skeletal hyperostosis. Clinical features and functional status. Medicine 1997; 76:104–117.

McCafferty R, Harrison M, Tamas L, et al. Ossification of the anterior longitudinal ligament and Forestier's disease: an analysis of seven cases. J Neurosurg 1995; 83:13–17.

Resnick D, Niwayama G. Radiographic and pathologic features of spinal involvement in diffuse idiopathic skeletal hyperostosis (DISH). Radiology 1976; 119:559–568.

Case 33
Osteoporotic Fractures of the Spine
Amir Matityahu, Jeffrey D. Klein, and Frank J. Schwab

History and Physical Examination

A 67-year-old 5'4", 148-lb woman fell on her buttock while walking on a freshly waxed floor. She had immediate pain localized to her back as well as difficulty walking. She was initially seen by a chiropractor who told her that she did not need an X-ray. After 4 weeks of severe and worsening pain, she followed up with an orthopaedic surgeon. At presentation, the patient stated that her back pain increased with activity, including standing, walking, and prolonged sitting; she was currently walking with a normal gait, though with some evident discomfort. She denied night pain, as well as pain radiating to the lower extremities, numbness, and tingling. There was no bowel or bladder dysfunction.

Physical examination revealed an obvious kyphotic deformity of the thoracolumbar spine and an apparent hyperlordosis of the cervical spine to allow for a level forward gaze. The kyphotic deformity appeared to be fixed, with no correction on hyperextension. The neurologic examination was normal. Reflexes were 1+ and symmetric at the knees and ankles.

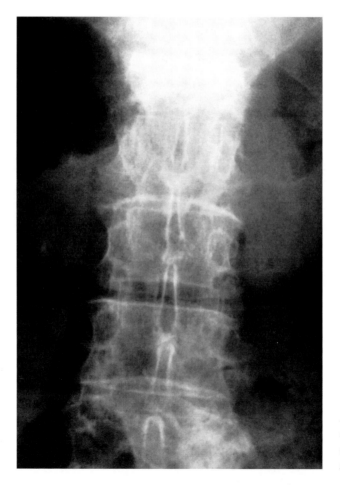

Figure 33–1. Preoperative anteroposterior (AP) radiograph of the thoracolumbar spine.

Radiologic Findings

Radiographs revealed compression fractures of T11 and L1 with bony consolidation at both of these levels and significant segmental kyphosis (Figs. 33–1 and 33–2). More specifically, at T11 there was greater than 50% anterior collapse and greater than 30 degrees of segmental kyphosis. At L1 there was no significant wedging. Computed tomography (CT) scan showed spondylosis deformans of the lower thoracic and lumbar spine with evidence of T11 and L1 collapse (Fig. 33–3). On axial images there was minimal canal compromise at the T11 and L1 levels. Extensive osteoarthritis and osteoporosis was noted at multiple levels.

Diagnosis

Osteoporotic burst fractures T11 and L1 with associated stenosis and thoracolumbar kyphosis. Severe activity-related lower back pain with marked restriction in the activities of daily living.

Surgical Management

A combined anterior and posterior decompression and stabilization was performed. A corpectomy and reconstruction at T11, the level of the more significant fracture, was followed by a posterior instrumented fusion from T7 to L3.

The patient was taken to the operating room where general endotracheal anesthesia was induced. The patient was placed in the right lateral decubitus position in

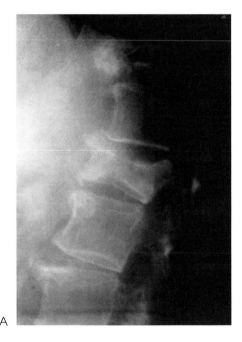

A

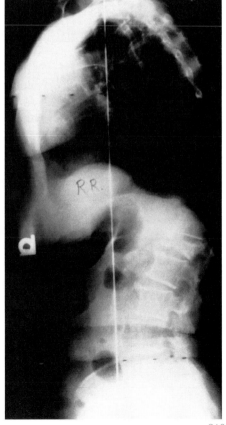

Figure 33–2. Preoperative lateral radiographs of the thoracolumbar spine.

B

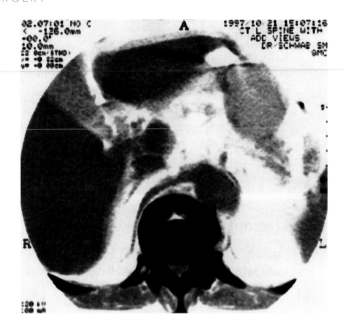

Figure 33–3. Preoperative axial computed tomography (CT) cut through the T11 vertebral body.

preparation for simultaneous anterior and posterior approaches. A T10 thoracotomy was performed to obtain exposure of the T11 vertebral body as well as the adjacent discs. A T11 corpectomy was performed, including removal of the retropulsed bone fragments. Discectomies above and below the T11 vertebrae were then performed, taking care to preserve the endplates of the adjacent vertebral bodies.

A second surgical team undertook the posterior approach simultaneously. A screw and hook construct was planned and executed from T7 to L3. Due to early consolidation at the fracture site, a chevron osteotomy was performed at the inferior aspect of the T11 posterior elements. This assisted in reduction of the kyphotic deformity. Gentle distraction was applied anteriorly and a Harms cage filled with autogenous rib bone graft placed to span T10 to T12. The posterior stabilization and fusion was then completed with hooks proximally in the thoracic region and pedicle screws distally in the lumbar region. Rods were then contoured and attached to the multiple points of fixation. Gentle compression was applied across the osteotomy site for additional correction. The wounds were then closed in standard fashion. A chest tube was placed anteriorly. Suction drainage was left deep in the posterior wound (Figs. 33–4 and 33–5).

Postoperative Management

Postoperatively, the patient was mobilized aggressively. She was logrolled every 3 hours side to side for protection of the skin. She was out of bed and sat on a chair on the first postoperative day. Progressive ambulation was begun on the second postoperative day. A custom thoracolumbosacral orthosis was fabricated and worn at all times to limit motion and provide additional support. Careful attention was paid to the perioperative nutritional status, and supplementation began preoperatively.

Discussion

The earliest symptom of osteoporosis-related spine fractures is an episode of acute back pain occurring at rest or during routine activities. In studies that reviewed

PEARLS

- One must have a low threshold for obtaining radiographs and imaging studies on older (osteoporotic) patients with back pain after trauma, no matter how seemingly trivial. The incidence of significant findings is far higher than in the general population.
- When combined anterior and posterior approaches are indicated, it is preferable, if possible, to perform them simultaneously in the lateral position with two operative teams. This decreases significantly the overall operative time. The ability to access both the anterior and posterior elements of the spine simultaneously also facilitates deformity correction and reduces the risk of neurologic injury or graft (cage) displacement that may occur with sequential procedures.
- Many of these patients are clinically malnourished at the time of presentation. Close attention must be paid to the perioperative nutritional status, and supplementation should begin as early as possible. Even those that begin with adequate nutritional status frequently become compromised in the postoperative period. Such patients are at greater risk for postoperative infections and wound-related complications.

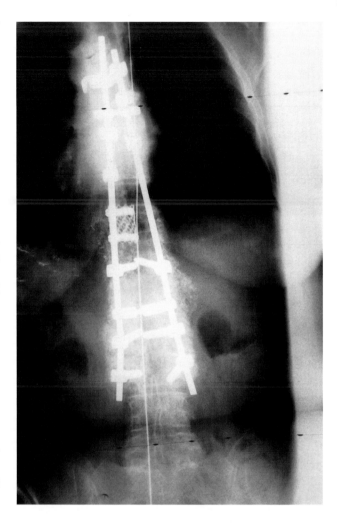

Figure 33–4. Postoperative AP radiograph of the thoracolumbar spine.

records of emergency room admissions, it was found that causative factors were falls in 30 to 50%, controlled activities (lifting, reaching overhead, opening windows, and bending over) in 10 to 20%, and 15 to 20% were found incidentally on review of X-rays. The pain usually intensifies with sitting or standing and is relieved with lying supine. Valsalva maneuvers such as coughing or straining to move the bowels increase the severity of the pain. The gait cycle is slow but usually normal. Most fractures are anterior compression fractures in the thoracic spine. They may cause a dowager's hump (thoracic kyphosis). The loss of vertebral height may be insidious and painless. It is accompanied by loss of height of the intervertebral discs. Involvement of the lumbar spine may lead to loss of the normal lordosis. Patients can have multiple fractures in a period of months followed by gradual recovery and may be able to recall each specific event and its resolution.

Involvement of the neural elements is relatively uncommon. When neurologic involvement is present, other causes such as infection, metastatic disease, primary bone tumors, Paget's disease, myeloma, and lymphoma must be ruled out.

Osteoporotic thoracolumbar burst fractures may be treated operatively or nonoperatively. An acute neurologic deficit is the most important factor that argues for surgical intervention. Loss of vertebral body height greater than 50%, kyphosis exceeding 30 degrees, and canal compromise greater than 30 to 50% are all relative

PITFALLS

• When anterior reconstruction is performed, care must be taken to preserve the intact endplates of the adjacent vertebral bodies. If the endplates are involved in the injury, or are violated during the procedure, subsidence of the construct should be expected into the soft trabecular bone. Often, such subsidence will continue until the opposite endplate is reached. In such a situation, oversizing the length of the graft at the time of surgery can minimize the amount of later subsidence.

• During posterior instrumentation in osteoporotic patients, there is a significant risk of dislodgment or failure of the instrumentation. Multiple fixation points above and below the injury level must be obtained. Even in the setting of apparently excellent fixation, strict activity limitation and bracing must be adhered to.

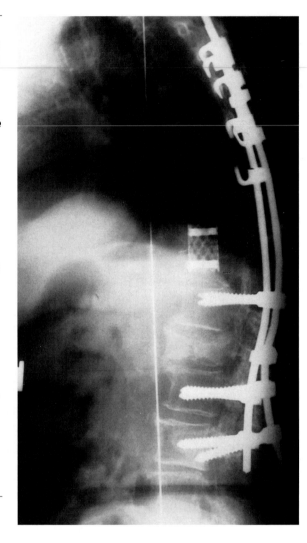

Figure 33–5. Postoperative lateral radiograph of the thoracolumbar spine.

indications for surgery. All of these are factors predispose to progressive deformity and late onset of neurologic compromise. Each case is decided individually. As this is an older patient population, comorbid medical conditions must be factored into any decision regarding possible surgical intervention.

If surgical intervention is chosen, the usual rules regarding the endpoints of spinal fixation apply. Fusion should not end on an unstable segment or at the apex of a deformity. In the specific circumstance of osteoporosis, one must make an effort to include as many points of fixation as possible to distribute the biomechanical stresses as broadly as possible and minimize the possibility of instrument failure. In addition, one may need to accept a lesser degree of deformity correction than is normally achieved. Finally, postoperative bracing is typically used as an adjunct to provide additional support and protection of the instrumentation.

Alternative Methods of Management

The treatment options for osteoporotic burst fractures include nonoperative treatment utilizing a thoracolumbosacral orthosis, anterior surgical reconstruction, posterior surgical reconstruction, and combined anterior and posterior procedures. In neurologically intact patients with relatively little deformity and tolerable pain, nonoperative treatment is entirely reasonable. In the event of deterioration, either mechanical or neurologic, surgical intervention can be undertaken secondarily. With greater deformities, especially in the presence of neurologic compromise, surgery is more likely indicated. Isolated posterior fusion with instrumentation can be undertaken. However, the risk of instrument failure, especially in the osteoporotic spine, increases with larger deformities and progressively greater anterior column insufficiency. In such cases, the addition of anterior column reconstruction becomes increasingly helpful in establishing a stable construct. In the setting of osteoporosis, isolated anterior procedures are generally not indicated. Whether cages or bone are utilized, they are prone to subsidence in the osteoporotic spine. Short-segment anterior instrumentation may not provide adequate fixation to ensure reasonable stability. A longer posterior construct with multiple points of fixation is generally more reliable in this regard.

Lastly, though decompression of the neural elements can be performed posteriorly, it is generally more complete, and preferable, if it is performed from the anterior approach. Hence, combined anterior and posterior procedures often provide the best overall result in terms of decompression and stability.

Type of Management	Advantages	Disadvantages	Comments
Nonoperative management	No risk of surgery in older medically compromised patients	No decompression of neural elements or correction of deformity	Preferred if neurologically intact and mild to moderate deformity
Posterior fusion	None of the increased morbidity associated with an anterior approach	No anterior column reconstruction; decompression is less complete	May be preferred in the neurologically intact patient with moderate deformity and significant medical comorbidities
Anterior fusion	Anterior column reconstructed	Graft subsidence, may lack stability	Not usually indicated in severe osteoporosis
Combined anterior and posterior fusion	Anterior column reconstructed	Increased amount of surgery may not be reasonable for older, sicker patients	Generally preferred in those patients with severe deformity and/or neurologic compromise

Complications

There are possible complications associated with both operative and nonoperative treatment of osteoporotic burst fractures. Those patients treated nonoperatively must be followed closely with serial X-rays to identify progressive deformity and avoid potential late neurologic compromise. Those patients treated operatively are at risk for mechanical failure as described previously. This includes the possibility of subsidence or displacement of the anterior construct. Despite all efforts, instrumentation failure is still possible due to the poor material properties of the osteoporotic spine. Lastly, there is an increased rate of postoperative infectious complications due to the generally poor nutritional status of this elderly patient population.

Suggested Readings

Biyani A, Ebraheim NA, Lu J. Thoracic spine fractures in patients older than 50 years. Clin Orthop Rel Res 1996; 328:190–193.

Hu SS. Internal fixation in the osteoporotic spine. Spine 1997; 22:43S–48S.

Jul Hayes WC, Myers ER. Biomechanical considerations of hip and spine fractures in osteoporotic bone. Instr Course Lect 1997; 46:431–438.

Koichiro O, Kozo S, Eiji A, et al. Stability of transpedicle screwing for the osteoporotic spine. Spine 1993; 18:2240–2245.

Myers ER, Wilson SE. Biomechanics of osteoporosis and vertebral fractures. Spine 1997; 22:25S–31S.

Shirado O, Kaneda K, Tadano S, et al. Influence of disc degeneration on mechanism of thoracolumbar burst fractures. Spine 1992; 17(3):286–292.

Tamayo-Orozco J, Arzac-Palumbo P, Peon-Vidales H, et al. Vertebral fractures associated with osteoporosis: patient management. Am J Med 1997; 103(2A):44S–48S.

Case 34
Spinal Deformity in the Presence of Osteogenesis Imperfecta

Fabien D. Bitan, Georges Finidori,
Marianne Pouliquen, and Gilda Forseter

History and Physical Examination

An 8-year-old nonambulatory girl presented at our osteogenesis imperfecta clinic. Her medical history was significant for several fractures of her upper and lower extremities. Previous surgeries included a Bailey rod procedure of the left tibia and femur at age $4\frac{1}{2}$, and an osteosynthesis with Luque rods and sublaminar wires from T3 to L4 without fusion at age 5 due to an early-onset thoracolumbar scoliosis.

Our initial physical examination revealed the characteristics of severe osteogenesis imperfecta (OI). The patient had a relatively large head with a prominent forehead. She had blue sclera, defective dentition, was hard of hearing, and had a strident voice. She was short of stature, which was aggravated by complex limb and trunk deformities. Her trunk was short, showing a prominent carina, an abdominal hypertrophy, and a rib hump approximately 1 inch high. The trunk was significantly shifted toward the left side. The Luque rods protruded at the upper end of the back. She had a barrel-like chest with superficial respiratory movements. Her upper limbs were severely deformed. She had bilateral 20-degrees hip flexion contractures and valgus-flexion knee deformities.

Radiologic Findings

Radiographs revealed significant pelvic obliquity. Spinal instrumentation was present extending from T3 to L4 made of Luque rods and sublaminar wires. The Cobb angle within the instrumented area was 40 degrees. The lumbopelvic angle was 25 degrees. There was no fusion mass noted. On the sagittal views the patient was dramatically kyphotic (approximately 50 degrees) due to a flat back in the instrumented area, a collapse of the spine above the rods, and severe hip flexion contractures. The vertebrae showed typical severe osteoporosis and platyspondylia.

Diagnosis

Progressive spinal and lower extremity deformities in the setting of osteogenesis imperfecta.

Nonoperative Management

Prior to considering surgery for this patient, several evaluations were performed. Her general health was determined to be good, with a normal neurologic exam and good cardiac function. Pulmonary function tests showed a restrictive syndrome with a vital capacity of 1000 cc (70% of the predictive value). An audiometric study was performed showing a stable deficit. A computed tomography (CT) scan of the head demonstrated acceptable measures of the occipital foramen. Her dentition revealed no loose teeth, and her mouth formation was deemed acceptable for intubation.

Surgical Management

The plan was to remove the spinal hardware and attempt to manage her spinal deformity nonoperatively until she reached an appropriate age for spinal fusion. Under general anesthesia, with the patient in the prone position, the spine was exposed over the entire extent of the previous procedure. The spinal instrumentation was exposed and removed. The sublaminar wire removal was done in a meticulous manner because of the risk of adherence of the wires to the dura. After all wires and rods were removed, the spine was thoroughly examined. A continuous fusion was noted, though no formal arthrodesis had been performed during the original surgery. After the procedure, radiographs showed a stable curve with the same angles and balance as preoperatively. A fiberglass cast was applied for 2 months, followed by a Boston brace with axillary supports. With extensive inpatient physical therapy, the patient began to walk using the assistance of a walker but without human assistance 3 months after surgery. Four months later she was walking independently using only a tripod cane.

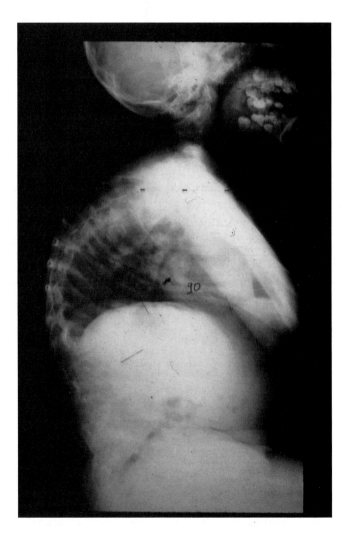

Figure 34–1. Lateral radiograph after removal of the Luque instrumentation. Marked kyphosis occurred after removal of the brace.

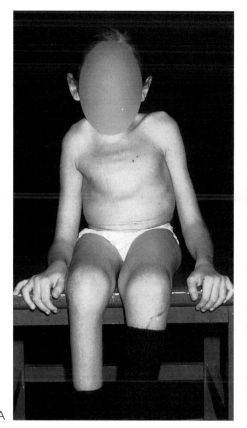 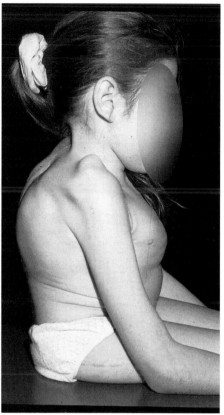

Figure 34–2. Frontal (A) and side (B) view of the patient in the prerevision surgical period.

Following brace discontinuance 3 years following surgery, the patient was noted to develop a progressive sagittal plane deformity (110 degrees of kyphosis in 5 months) (Figs. 34–1 and 34–2). Her vital capacity dropped from 1 L to 0.6 L within 6 months (demonstrating that at least a part of the restrictive syndrome in OI is a result of spine deformities). Her bone age at that time was 9 years old. The decision was made to proceed with the spinal fusion.

In preparation for the fusion, halo traction was applied to try to unfold the spine (Fig. 34–3). The weights were increased up to 50% of the patient's body weight. After 2 months, the scoliosis was still at 45 degrees but the kyphosis reduced back to 55 degrees (Fig. 34–4). At this point a posterior spinal fusion was performed. The patient was placed in a prone position on a cast bed prepared a few days prior to surgery. The spine was surgically approached in a meticulous manner because of bone fragility. Blood loss at the time of surgery was reasonable. Examination of the exposed spine revealed again a continuous fusion mass from T1 down to the sacrum. Hooks were inserted through windows dug into the graft. The instrumentation (pediatric Cotrel-Dubousset (CD) instrumentation) included hooks on the sacrum, two up-going hooks at the thoracolumbar junction, pedicle hooks on T2 on the right side, and on T1 using a connector on the left. This asymmetric construct was due to the fracture of the facet of T2 during the insertion of a hook. The spine was then carefully decorticated. This was done after insertion of the instrumentation to avoid excessive blood loss. No bone was available on the iliac crest and thus banked-bone was used. This was mixed with corticocancellous fragments harvested from the

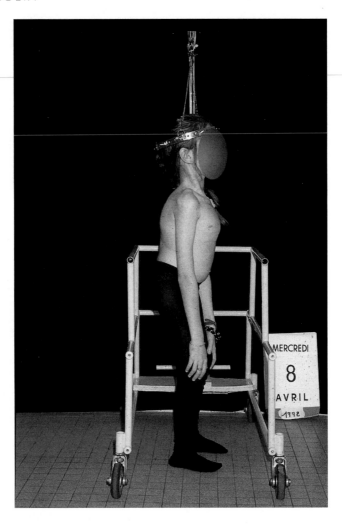

Figure 34–3. Side view of the patient under halo traction.

bone mass. The estimated blood loss of this procedure was 300 cc, and its duration was 4 hours. The halo traction was reapplied for several days postoperatively, followed by a halo cast. This cast was maintained for 3 months. After X-rays confirmed the integrity of the construct, the halo cast was removed and a brace with chin and occipital support was applied. This brace was maintained for 18 months, at which point the mandibulo-occipital support was removed. The brace itself was applied for another 6 months.

At 5-year follow-up in 1997, the patient was 17 and attending the 11th grade. She could walk independently for more than 1 hour a day. Her height was 45 inches (115 cm) standing and 24 inches (61 cm) sitting. Her vital capacity was 1 L (70%). Her spine was stable, and her curves were unchanged from the postoperative period (55 degrees scoliosis, 45 degrees kyphosis) (Figs. 34–5 and 34–6). She unfortunately developed over the years a progressive bilateral acetabular protrusio, for which there is no effective treatment.

Discussion

The incidence of scoliosis in OI varies between 39 and 80%. Osteogenesis imperfecta produces a relentlessly progressing spinal deformity causing respiratory com-

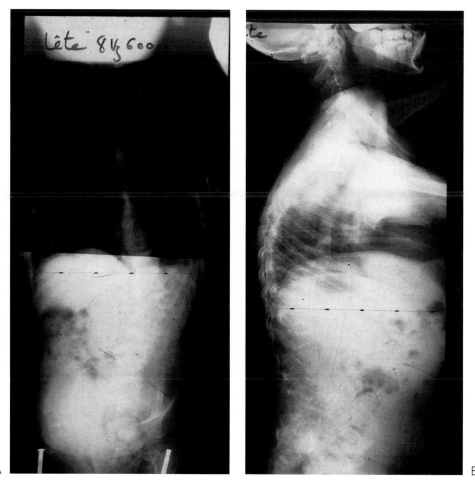

Figure 34–4. Anteroposterior (AP) (A) and lateral (B) long-cassette radiographs after halo traction. The deformity is markedly improved especially in the sagittal plane.

promise, a major cause of death in patients with OI. These spine deformities are the results of several converging factors such as platyspondylia, vertebral growth impairment, and repeated microfractures. Osteoporosis and amyotrophy are additional components of the disease, but are also dramatically accelerated by prolonged and repeated immobilization due to multiple, frequent limb fractures. Finally, pelvic and lower limb deformities, joint contractures, and constitutional hyperlaxity also contribute to this deformity. In our experience, early stabilization of the lower extremities by preventive rodding is an effective way to prevent this vicious circle.

The main respiratory consequence of OI is a restrictive pulmonary syndrome inherent to the condition, further aggravated by the trunk deformities. Paterson and colleagues (1996) have identified respiratory failure as the main cause of death in OI. Also some patients develop an additional obstructive syndrome related to various hazards such as obesity, splanchnomegaly, cigarette smoking, and asthma.

Patients must be screened for scoliosis on a regular basis with anteroposterior (AP) and lateral views of the full spine. They typically develop a kyphoscoliosis of the thoracolumbar junction. Other bony abnormalities can be encountered on the radiographs such as basilar impression, osteoporosis, platyspondylia, an elongated pars interarticularis, or an spondylolysis.

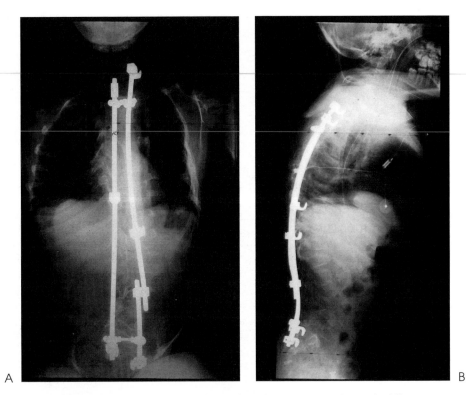

A   B

Figure 34–5. Surgical result. AP (A) and lateral (B) long-cassette radiographs following surgical stabilization.

Halo Traction

The purpose of the traction is to improve both mechanical and respiratory conditions prior to surgery. We use preoperative halo traction for a short period of time (4 to 6 weeks) prior to surgery (as suggested by Gitelis and colleagues, 1983). Magnetic resonance imaging (MRI) of the spine is performed prior to the application of halo traction to rule out a basilar impression.

Application of the halo is as follows: Eight to ten pins secure the halo and are inserted rather low on a horizontal line, just above the ears but below the prominence of the skull, avoiding the occipital area of the skull. (Pins in the occipital area often become painful in the supine position.) The pins should be tightened only by hand, cleaned every day meticulously, and checked frequently, but tightened only once. A loosened pin should be changed immediately to avoid an intracranial migration. When the child is able to sit and walk comfortably in adapted frames, the weights are rapidly increased up to 50 to 55% of body weight, reaching maximal traction in 2 to 3 weeks. The halo should not be left in place longer than 6 weeks because of the risk of pin loosening and migration. The main disadvantage of prolonged traction is increased osteoporosis.

Bracing

Most authors consider bracing dangerous and inefficient in OI patients because it can cause chest deformities with rib fractures and worsen respiratory difficulties. Additionally, most of the time bracing fails to stop progression of the curve.

Appropriate indications for bracing are cases of emerging documented progression and mild curves, with the goal of maintaining the spine until surgery. Thus, bracing should be viewed as a temporary measure.

Posterior Spinal Fusion

Patients with OI have severe growth abnormalities and the usual criteria for deciding a posterior spinal fusion are not applicable. These children tend to achieve their full growth height by age 10. At this point, surgery can be performed without any concerns regarding a crankshaft evolution.

Major criteria for surgical treatment include progression of the Cobb angle involving the coronal or sagittal planes. Often the measured Cobb angles are difficult to compare due to the degree of osteoporosis. In such cases, a lack of growth or a loss of height of the trunk may be evidence of curve progression. A worsening of respiratory function despite physical therapy should also be a warning of curve progression.

In most patients with progressive curves, spinal fusion is in theory necessary, though it has been discredited in several reports. These publications have reported

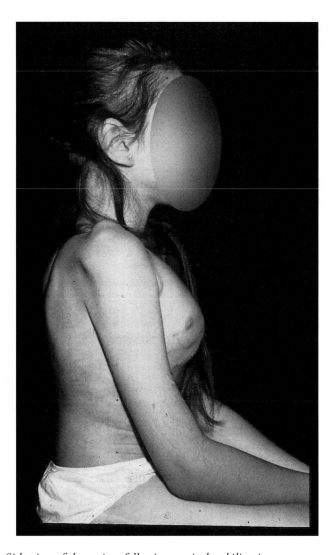

Figure 34–6. Side view of the patient following surgical stabilization.

unacceptable rates of acute and long-term complications. Yong Hing and MacEwen (1982) reported a high incidence of complications such as major intraoperative difficulties, severe bleeding, as well as a frequent loss of correction. However, techniques used in most studies were based on traditional distraction instrumentations, and the curves were often severe and kyphotic. In our experience technical difficulties of spinal surgery in OI patients have been minimized with the use of modern multisegmental instrumentation and by performing these operations on moderately deformed and well-balanced spines. Surgical treatment of kyphotic, stiff, and osteoporotic spines are fraught with many difficulties. If halo traction does not help in straightening the spine, the idea of surgery should probably be abandoned, though some authors have performed anterior releases without major complications. We do not have the experience of anterior approaches in OI.

A cast bed is prepared several days before the procedure to facilitate the positioning on the operating table. The cast is molded on the anterior aspect of the body, which is usually severely deformed, from the halo to the toes, with the patient in the supine position, hips and knees slightly bent, and with openings for the eyes and the mouth. The surgical procedure is then performed with the patient in the prone position in the cast bed, which has been dried, cut out, and padded several days in advance. The halo traction is maintained during the procedure, but no additional correction should be attempted at this stage.

The purpose of the instrumentation is essentially to maintain the correction obtained preoperatively. Any forceful maneuver is prohibited. We found in several cases that the ligamentum flavum offers a much better resistance than the laminae. It can be used as an efficient support structure for hook insertion. We have used methylmethacrylate to enhance the strength of the constructs in the past. However, since new segmental instrumentations came into use in the 1980s, methymethacrylate has been gradually abandoned.

Though the extent of the instrumentation depends on the type of deformity, sacral fusion is rarely indicated to avoid decompensation of frequent lower limb deformities. Decortication should be meticulous; most of the lamina thickness has to be harvested carefully to obtain large corticocancellous bone chips. Blood loss can become rapidly life threatening in those patients with very small blood volume. Hemostasis should be maintained throughout the case.

Conclusions

Spinal surgery in patients with osteogenesis imperfecta has been discredited because of the high incidence of short- and long-term complications. We suggest that this attitude be revised in the light of strong evidence of physical and respiratory disabilities in patients with major and progressive deformities. Appropriate steps can be taken to avoid these reported complications, such as by performing surgery on small angles, or after an appropriate preparation by halo traction to correct major curves, especially kyphosis. Segmental instrumentation needs to be applied without intraoperative correction. The patient should be immobilized until fusion is complete. Though in most cases anterior spinal fusion is not a reasonable option for respiratory reasons, in selected curves it might have an important role in cases of severe deformities.

Alternative Methods of Management

Type of Management	Advantages	Disadvantages	Comments
Bracing	Effective with mild curves and curves with emerging documented progression	May cause chest wall deformities and rib fractures, and worsen respiratory difficulties	Bracing requires strict compliance and regular medical follow-up; it may cause a psychological restriction on the child's social and educational activities
Halo traction	Useful in improving mechanical and respiratory conditions prior to surgery; applied for short period of time: 4–6 weeks prior to surgery	Prolonged traction may lead to increased osteoporosis	Allows for preoperative kyphotic correction of up to 50% and improvement in preoperative respiratory volumes
Posterior spinal fusion	Successful stabilization of progressive kyphoscoliotic curves with worsening pulmonary function	Older literature with first- and second-generation instrumentation has reported unacceptable rates of acute and long-term complications	Technical difficulties minimized with modern multisegmental instrumentation performed on moderately deformed and well-balanced spines

Suggested Readings

Barrack R, Whitecloud TS, Skinner HB. Spondylolysis after spinal instrumentation in osteogenesis imperfecta. South Med J 1984; 11:1453.

Bathgate B, Moseley CF. Scoliosis in osteogenesis imperfecta. Spine State Art Rev 1990; 4:21.

Benson DR, Donaldson DH, Millar EA. The spine in osteogenesis imperfecta. J Bone Joint Surg 1978; 60A:925.

Benson D, Newman D. The spine and surgical treatment in osteogenesis imperfecta. Clin Orthop 1981; 159:147.

Bitan FD, Finidori GF. Treatment of spinal deformities in osteogenesis imperfecta. Spine State Art Rev 1998; 12:1.

Cristofaro RL, Hock KJ, Bonett CA, Brown JC. Operative treatment of spine deformities in osteogenesis imperfecta. Clin Orthop 1979; 139:40.

Donaldson DH. Spinal deformity associated with osteogenesis imperfecta. In: Bridwell KH, DeWald RL, eds. The Textbook of Spinal Surgery, p. 491. Philadelphia: JB Lippincott, 1991.

Falvo K, Klain D, Krauss A. Pulmonary function studies in osteogenesis imperfecta. Am Rev Respir Dis 1973; 108:258.

Gitelis S, Whiffen J, DeWald RL. The treatment of severe scoliosis in osteogenesis imperfecta. Clin Orthop 1983; 175:56.

Hanscom DA, Bloom BA. The spine in osteogenesis imperfecta. Orthop Clin North Am 1988; 19:449.

Lonstein JE, Bradford DS, Winter RB, Ogilvie JW, eds. Moe's Textbook of Scoliosis and Other Spinal Deformities, 3d ed. Philadelphia: WB Saunders, 1995.

Norimatsu H, Mayuzumi T, Takahashi H. The development of spinal deformities in osteogenesis imperfecta. Clin Orthop 1982; 162:20.

Paterson CR, Ogston SA, Henry RM. Life expectancy in osteogenesis imperfecta. BMJ 1996; 312:351.

Renshaw T, Cook R, Albright J. Scoliosis in osteogenesis imperfecta. Clin Orthop 1979; 145:163.

Yong Hing K, MacEwen G. Scoliosis associated with osteogenesis imperfecta: results of treatment. J Bone Joint Surg 1982; 64B:36.

Trauma

Case 35
Spinal Cord Injury: Pharmacologic and Nonoperative Management

Terrence P. Sheehan

History and Physical Examination

A 48-year-old man stopping in his car at a red light during a wind storm sustained blunt trauma to his head and neck after a tree branch landed on the roof of his vehicle. Upon extrication from his car and physical stabilization of his head and spine by paramedics, he was found to have no sensation to touch below his shoulders and could move only his proximal left upper extremity. On admission to the emergency department of the regional spinal cord injury center, in just under 3 hours from the time of injury he was conscious and following commands, breathing independently. He re-

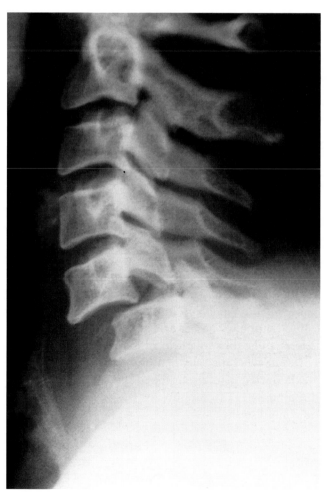

Figure 35–1. Lateral plain radiograph revealing a stage III flexion-distraction injury of the cervical spine at the C5/C5 level.

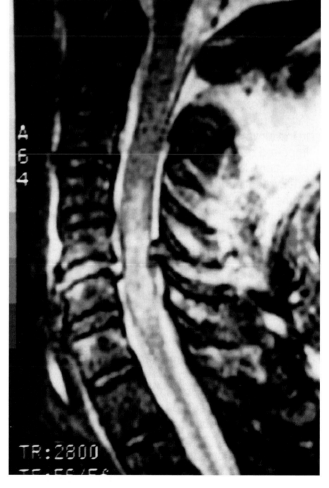

Figure 35–2. Sagittal magnetic resonance imaging (MRI) following a closer cervical reduction revealing evidence of cord edema and swelling from C4 to C7.

PEARL

- The presence of sacral motor and/or sensory function defines an "incomplete" spinal cord injury that has significantly improved functional prognosis when compared to a "complete" spinal cord injury (no sacral motor and/or sensory function).

PITFALLS

- In defining the level of neurologic injury, the C4 sensory level dips into the anterior chest and can be mistaken for the T3 sensory level. This results in confusion between classifying the patient as high quadriplegia versus high paraplegia, which has a significant functional difference.
- In quadriplegia, respiratory failure often occurs with a slow insidious onset because of progressive respiratory muscular fatigue and secretion buildup in the airways with associated impaired ability to clear these secretions. Monitoring vital capacity, continuous pulse oximetry, and early aggressive pulmonary toilet are the keys to expectant management.
- During spinal reduction and manipulation, and the application of immobilization devices, there can be a sudden subtle change in neurologic function, particularly in the sedated patient. Early neurologic baseline exam and compulsive reexamination through the stages of spinal stabilization and immobilization procedures is prudent expectant management.
- Immobilization on a spine board is common early management in those being evaluated for spine/spinal cord injury. Pressure sores often start during this period in those who

ported an inability to move his arms and legs and perceive sensation below his shoulder and upper chest. A detailed motor and sensory exam showed a 5/5 shoulder shrug bilaterally, with 1/5 right bicep, and 2/5 left bicep; there was 2/2 pinprick and light touch sensation at the C4 dermatome, and 1/2 pin and light touch appreciation at the C5 dermatome bilaterally. There was no appreciated motor strength or sensation through to the S3/S5 level. The patient had a flaccid anal sphincter and absent deep tendon reflexes in the upper and lower extremities. His vital capacity was 800-cc. He was classified as a C4 American Spine Injury Association (ASIA) A spinal cord injury.

Radiologic Findings

Plain X-ray demonstrated flexion-distraction stage III injury at the C5/C6 level (Fig. 35–1). Magnetic resonance imaging (MRI) demonstrated contusion of the spinal cord with edema from C4 to C7 with post traumatic thrombosis of the vertebral artery without distal reconstitution (Fig. 35–2). The MRI was obtained following a closed cervical reduction. The skull, brain, T-L-and S spine, chest, abdomen, and pelvis were cleared radiologically for associated injuries.

Diagnosis

Complete traumatic C4 spinal cord injury (C4 ASIA A SCI)in the setting of an advanced-stage compression flexion injury of C5 with multiple associated cervical element fractures.

Pharmacologic and Nonoperative Management

The patient was given an intravenous bolus of methylprednisolone (30 mg/kg) followed by a methlyprednisolone infusion of 5.4 mg/kg per hour for 23 hours. After mild sedation and pain control, the patient was placed in halo traction, and a Foley catheter was inserted. Following an adequate cervical reduction, the vest portion of the halo was applied and the patient was admitted to the neurology intensive care unit (ICU) for close cardiopulmonary monitoring including continuous pulse oximetry with the head of the bed kept at 30 degrees. A routine of aggressive pulmonary toilet using chest physical therapy, postural drainage, and suctioning was initiated for secretion management. Vital capacities were followed on an every 12 hour basis while in the ICU setting. A nasogastric tube was inserted, and bowel sounds were monitored closely. The nursing protocol included turning the patient every 2 hours while on a pressure relief specialty bed, and padding of pressure points of the upper and lower extremities. The distal upper and lower extremities were splinted. Deep venous thrombosis (DVT) prophylaxis was instituted. Serial neurologic exams were followed compulsively.

Discussion

Pharmacologic Intervention

In patients seen and identified within 8 hours of a spinal cord injury, high-dose methylprednisolone should be administered. An initial bolus of 30 mg/kg is given are left for extended periods on a spine board without pressure relief. The most common location is over the sacrum. Its presence is not usually recognized because the sore starts inside, next to the bone, with only nonblanchable erythema on the surface of the skin. The internal necrosis naturally extends to the skin surface over days to weeks. These sores can and do have profound impact on the early course, prolonging hospitalization and limiting rehabilitation.

intravenously for 15 minutes, followed 45 minutes later by a continuous infusion of 5.4 mg/kg per hour for 23 hours. In a prospective, randomized, double-blind, controlled study, the National Acute Spinal Cord Injury Study (NASCIS II), this regimen resulted in a statistically significant improvement in maximal motor function at 6 months postinjury. This study has since been followed by the NASCIS III trial reported in May 1997. The conclusion of this trial again supported high-dose methylprednisolone regimen but with a modification: when methylprednisolone is initiated 3 to 8 hours after injury, patients should be maintained on steroid therapy for 48 hours. With respect to the initial 24-hour recommendations, those who received the extended dosing had more severe sepsis and severe pneumonia (higher morbidity) than the patients in the 24-hour methylprednisolone group.

Traumatic injuries to the spinal cord induce breakdown of the cell membranes. This trauma ignites the enzymatic breakdown of phospholipids and release of polyunsaturated fatty acids (PUFAs) as well as platelet activating factor (PAF). The PUFAs appear to contribute to posttraumatic tissue damage, which in turn may contribute to the overall injury. Within minutes of traumatic injury, arachidonic acid is released and metabolized to these injury factors: thromboxanes, leukotrienes, and free radicals. These eicosanoids, along with PAF, are associated with the reduction of spinal cord blood flow and breakdown of the blood–brain barrier. Together, these biochemical processes that take place in the first minutes of traumatic spinal cord injury lead to irreversible tissue damage. The inflammatory and immune responses to injury begin within minutes of the trauma and continue for several days.

Several classes of pharmacologic agents help reduce the extent of secondary neuronal injury in animal models of spinal cord injury. Corticosteroids impair the process of lipid peroxidation after spinal cord injury. They promote the restoration of acid–base balance, stabilize calcium flux in/out of the cell, promote the establishment of the disrupted sodium-potassium adenosine triphosphatase (Na,K-ATPase) activity, and augment spinal cord blood flow. The major rationale for the use of steroids relates to their ability to inhibit free radical–induced lipid peroxidation. The NASCIS trials using methylprednisolone found that at doses between 30 and 50 mg/kg long-term neurologic recovery was enhanced. The 21-aminosteroids (tirilazad mesylate) have similar neuroprotective effects of inhibiting free radical–induced lipid peroxidation, but do not have the glucocorticoid and mineralocorticoid actions. These have been shown to improve spinal cord blood flow as well as motor recovery in cat models. In the NASCIS III trial, tirilazad mesylate (2.5 mg/kg bolus infusion every 6 hours for 48 hours) showed motor recovery rates equivalent to those of patients who received methylprednisolone for 24 hours.

Another class, antioxidants or free radical scavengers, act by disrupting the events that result in the process of lipid peroxidation and eventual cell membrane instability and death. Free radical production is initiated by generation of superoxide anions via purine metabolism, polymorphonuclear leukocyte activation, and prostaglandin and leukotriene synthesis. It is believed that free radical scavengers halt the highly unstable free radicals by trapping them. Other free radical scavengers such as superoxide dismutase and desferroxamine have been shown to increase the preservation of neuronal tissue and function in animal models of CNS injury.

Adjunctive Treatment

Close monitoring of the *respiratory system* should occur in all spinal cord injuries, but is most important in the cervical cord injuries. The diaphragm is supplied by the C3/C5 roots, with C4 being most important. The lung vital capacity is used to define the degree of diaphragmatic function and can be useful in conjunction with the neurologic level in predicting respiratory insufficiency. Spinal cord injury below the C5 root does not affect the function of the diaphragm, but hypoventilation will still occur because the intercostal and accessory muscles of breathing have been denervated. Thus, close monitoring through continuous pulse oximetry and serial vital capacities is paramount in identifying hypoxemia and respiratory fatigue.

Aggressive pulmonary toilet includes chest physical therapy and suctioning. This therapy entails placing the patient in multiple positions including the common lateral decubitus and Trendelenburg positions and patting the chest to loosen secretions from the dependent portions of the lungs. This is followed by deep suctioning of the larger respiratory airways to remove these loosened secretions. These secretions can become thick, especially in the dehydrated patient, and agents for thinning such as guaifenesin and improved fluid management are instituted. The secretions can be abundant and difficult to manage. The quadriplegic individual usually has an ineffective cough. The secretions should be cultured in the event of fevers, and if they consistently demonstrate pigments (i.e. green, brown, yellow), this indicates leukocyte infiltration and infection. Aerosolized bronchodilator treatments can be helpful with the bronchial irritation and bronchospasm that often occurs with these abundant poorly cleared secretions.

The impairment of the gastrointestinal system is less dramatic than the changes in other bodily functions. After a significant spinal cord injury, ileus with decreased or absent bowel sounds and no flatus or bowel movement occur because of the interruption in sympathetics and sacral parasympathetics. Ileus usually resolves in 2 to 4 days. A nasogastric tube is inserted to prevent aspiration of gastric contents and decrease gastric dilatations. As bowel sounds return, nasogastric suctioning is discontinued, swallowing function is evaluated and oral intake is increased as tolerated. In high complete cervical injuries, the early use of jejunostomy (J) feeding tube or gastric (G) feeding tube helps to meet and maintain the high caloric nutritional needs of the newly injured patient. The use of agents that promote gastric emptying and gastrointestinal motility (e.g., metoclopramide) can assist in cases of prolonged ileus. A bowel program consisting of stool softeners, bowel stimulants, and rectal suppositories is initiated at the time of feeding is successfully administered. Bowel movements are monitored very closely for return of activity (e.g., daily or every other day results).

Acute abdominal problems develop after spinal cord injury. Diagnosis of abdominal emergencies is complicated by the absence of normal symptoms and signs. Thus, close monitoring of function and investigation for causes of dysfunction (e.g., bowel obstruction, impaction, pancreatitis) are initiated early so that management can be correctly altered. Gastroduodenal ulceration, with hemorrhage or perforation, is common soon after spinal cord injury. Patients should receive prophylaxis against ulceration with (histamine) H2-blockers to diminish gastric acid secretions. Most patients experience little interruption of function when surveillance and management of the GI system is included in the management of the acute spinal cord injured patient.

Perhaps the most profound and potentially deleterious change occurring after spinal cord injury is the loss of normal genitourinary function. Because of the disruption of autonomic control over the cardiovascular system that occurs with cervical spinal cord injury. large volumes of fluid are often administered in the period following the acute injury, which subsequently leads to large urine outputs. As the control centers of bladder function are in the brain and distal half of the spinal cord, voluntary control is lost in complete injuries. The urinary bladder is usually areflexive in the acute period folllowing complete and incomplete injury. An indwelling urinary catheter (14 to 16 French) should be placed to prevent overdistention of the neurogenic bladder and to allow continuous urinary output monitoring. In males this catheter is strapped over the abdomen to prevent urethral erosion at the penoscrotal junction. This catheter can remain in place for a couple of weeks, and surveillance of the expected bacteriuria should occur as pyuria is a usual source of fever. Intermittent catheterization should be initiated after the spinal cord injured patient has been successfully remobilized. This form of drainage is recommended because of the reduced risks of bacteriuria and consequently of calculi and pyelonephritis formation.

Careful management of the *skin* in spinal cord injury is critical. Decubitus ulcers are a major cause of morbidity in the individual with spinal cord injury. A decubitus ulcer is a destruction of all tissue layers from the epithelium to the bone. It occurs almost exclusively over bony prominences. The ulcer may present as a nonblanchable redness of the skin. The greater damage is to the deeper structures, and may now show its extent until it naturally progresses to the skin surface, breaking open spontaneously. As the ulcer is a result of the compression of the vascular supply to the skin, the more sensitive tissues beneath the epithelium become ischemic and infarct.

The skin must be protected from excessive shear forces, isolated sites of increased pressure, or increased temperature. Nutrition must be adequate to maintain the soft tissue metabolic demand and promote preservation of collagen, elastin, ground material, and normal morphologic characteristics. The use of pressure relief mattresses and a turning (one-quarter turns) schedule of every 2 hours is standard in spinal cord injury management. This becomes more of a challenge in the acute, often unstable spinal cord injury patient when skin, nutrition, and noncritical anemia take a backseat to cardiovascular instability, respiratory insufficiency, and acute infection states.

Spasticity follows upper motor neuron injury. It is defined by the exaggerated deep tendon reflexes, clonus, spread of reflexes from one muscle to another or form one limb to another, spasms in response to cutaneous or visceral stimuli or without any obvious stimulus, and rigidity. The onset of spasticity and spasms is often initially recognized within days of the acute injury especially in the incompletely injured person and the older person (age 50) who was myelopathic prior to the trauma. This is addressed with a regular stretching program of limb range of motion administered by the nursing and therapy staff. If this tone becomes overriding, causing loss of normal joint range of motion and/or becomes a source of discomfort, pharmacologic intervention with antispasticity agents such as baclofen can be introduced and titrated to desired effect.

The risk of thromboembolism in the deep venous system (DVT) is a serious matter in spinal cord injury. This is likely to occur in up to 80% of the cases, with a pulmonary embolism risk of approximately 10% in those not receiving prophylaxis. The risk can be attributed to the accumulation of a number of factors of which blood stasis in the limbs from paralysis and hypercoagulability from CNS injury are at the forefront. Careful surveillance and prophylaxis constitute the most important aspects of early care. Prophylaxis with subcutaneous heparin or low molecular weight heparin *and* a mechanism to stimulate blood flow in the legs (e.g., pneumatic compression sleeves) reduce the incidence to approximately 15%. Continuous clinical monitoring through surveillance of edema is of paramount importance. The use of duplex Doppler imaging within the first days of injury and when DVT is clinically suspected is still necessary because of the group of patients that defy the current preventive measures. When a clot does occur, a full anticoagulation regimen is in order with intravenous heparin initially then oral warfarin. The low molecular weight heparins are undergoing clinical trials currently, with encouraging results. An important side effect of heparin other than bleeding is thrombocytopenia. Platelet counts need to be monitored. In those who have contraindications for full anticoagulation, such as current gastrointestinal bleeding, an intravenous venous filter is threaded into the inferior vena cava to prevent pulmonary emolism. Edema control is addressed through compressive garments (stockings). Once the patient is fully anticoagulated, remobilization can continue.

Alternative Methods of Management

Type of Management	Advantages	Disadvantages	Comments
Neurologic			
The use of a standard neurologic classification system (ASIA) defines complete vs. incomplete neurologic injuries; this should be done within 24 to 72 hours postsurgery for baseline	Defines neurologic function and identifies changes Allows early prognosis	None perceived	Standard of care
Cardiovascular			
Strict fluid monitoring (I&O's) DVT prophalaxis	Management of neurogenic shock and bradyarrhythmias	None perceived Thrombocytopenia from heparin	
Respiratory			
Continuous pulse oximetry Aggressive pulmonary toilet Follow vital capacity	Early identification of respiratory failure from infection, secretion buildup and/or fatigue	None perceived	Standard of care
Gastrointestinal			
Nasogastric tube Stress peptic ulcer prophylaxis Bowel program	Aspiration Prevent acute GI bleeding Ileus and colonic distention	Communication and swallowing are hindered Medication side effects	
Genitourinary			
Foley catheter (abdominal strap in males)	Prevents complications of genitourinary system	Urethral erosion at penoscrotal junction in males Infection	Standard of care
Skin			
Close surveillance Turn at least every 2 hours in bed	Prevent decubiti (pressure) ulcers	Disruptive to patients	Standard of care
Musculoskeletal			
Range of motion every shift Splinting of distal extremities Spasticity management	Comfort and prevents contracture formation	None perceived Sedation and subtle motor weakness	Standard of care
Pharmacologic			
High-dose steroids	Neurologic recovery	Higher morbidity	Standard of care

ASIA, American Spine Injury Association; DVT, deep venous thrombosis.

Suggested Readings

Bracken MB, Shephard MJ, Holford TR, et al. Administration of methylprednisilone for 24 or 48 hours or tirilazad for 48 hours in the treatment of acute spinal cord injury: results of the Third National Acute Spinal Cord Injury randomized controlled trial. JAMA 1997; 277:1597–1604.

Chiles BW III, Cooper PR. Acute spinal injury. N Engl J Med 1996; 334:514–520.

Ditunno JF Jr, Staas WE Jr. Traumatic spinal cord injury. Phys Med Rehabil Clin North Am 1992; 4:699.

Greene KA, Marciano FF, Sonntag VKH. Pharmacological management of spinal cord injury: current status of drugs designed to augment functional recovery of the injured human spinal cord. J Spinal Disord 1996; 9:355–366.

Case 36
Traumatic Injuries of the Occipitocervical Junction

David L. Kramer, Suken A. Shah, Gregg R. Klein,
Alexander R. Vaccaro, and Jerome M. Cotler

History and Physical Examination

A 45-year-old man was found 20 feet from his vehicle after being ejected through the windshield. The patient was apparently an unrestrained driver involved in a high-speed motor vehicle accident. The patient was appropriately immobilized at the scene with a backboard and collar and was transferred to the emergency department of a local hospital. Upon initial evaluation, the patient was noted to be confused and combative. Alcohol intoxication was suspected. He was also noted to have multiple small lacerations along his scalp and forehead as well as a contusion across the chest compatible with a steering wheel injury. Although he was able to grossly

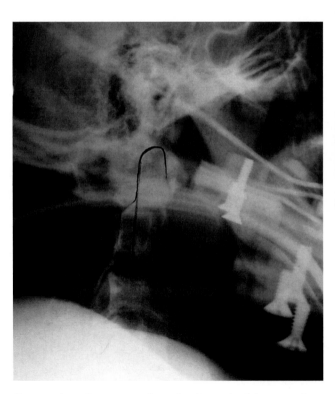

Figure 36–1. Preoperative lateral radiograph of the cervical spine demonstrating a C1/C2 dissociation.

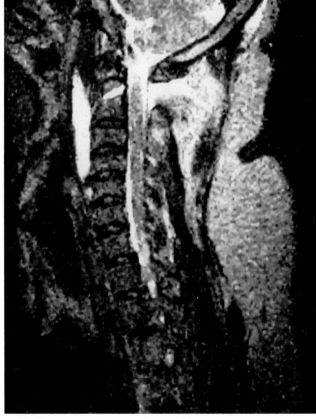

Figure 36–2. Magnetic resonance imaging (MRI) scan of the cervical spine demonstrating complete ligamentous disruption at C1/C2.

move all four of his extremities, more specific neurologic testing was difficult given his altered level of consciousness.

Radiologic Findings

Initial radiographic screening in the emergency room consisted of a lateral view of the cervical spine (Fig. 36–1). This study suggested the existence of an abnormal diastasis between C1 and C2 and possibly between the occiput and C1. The inferior endplate of C7 could not be completely visualized, and because the patient was combative, obtaining an open-mouth view of the odontoid was quite difficult. As the immobilized patient was to be brought to the computed tomography (CT) scanner for a CT scan of the head to rule out intracranial injury, it was felt that a CT scan of the cervical spine was indicated to rule out any noncontiguous spinal injuries.

The CT scan of the cervical spine with 1-mm sagittal and coronal reconstructions from the occiput to T1 revealed the C1/C2 dissociation without evidence of a subaxial vertebral fracture. Subsequent magnetic resonance imaging (MRI) of the cervical spine more accurately delineated the extent of the soft tissue injury at the occiput, C1, and C2 levels, where complete disruption of the C1/C2 articulation and posterior ligamentous complex between the occiput and C1 was noted (Fig. 36–2).

Diagnosis

Traumatic dislocation of C1 on C2 with ligamentous disruption between the occiput and C1. This injury pattern was suggestive of a distraction-extension rotational force consistent with the mechanism of injury. No other noncontiguous spinal injuries were identified. No neurologic deficit was identified on the initial limited neurologic screening.

Surgical Management

While the patient was in the emergency room, a carbon fiber halo ring was applied to the cranium through which 5 pounds of traction was initially applied to stabilize the cranium relative to the cervical spine and to allow better control of the cranium while trying to achieve a reduction of the malaligned occipitocervical junction. With a dedicated portable X-ray machine available during the reduction, a gentle closed reduction maneuver was applied with the patient awake and able to describe any change in neurologic function. The halo ring was then stabilized to the halo vest, thereby maintaining alignment of the occiput-C1, C1/C2 articulation. Once the patient was medically stable, the cervical spine radiographic survey was completed and the aforementioned MRI scan was obtained to more precisely evaluate the degree and nature of ligamentous injury.

With obvious instability noted at the occiput-C1, C1/C2 articulation in this neurologically intact patient, it was felt that stabilization of the occipital cervical junction was mandatory to protect spinal cord function. A posterior occipitocervical plate-screw construct was chosen to achieve solid fixation.

While immobilized in the halo vest, the patient was transferred supine onto a Jackson frame. An awake fiberoptic nasotracheal intubation then ensued. Baseline somatosensory evoked potentials were obtained and were subsequently monitored throughout the operation. The halo ring was then affixed to the Jackson frame. Appropriate sagittal alignment was confirmed radiographically. The patient was then rotated into the prone position.

A posterior midline approach from the occiput to C3 was then performed. The paraspinal musculature was split and subperiosteally dissected from the spinous processes and laminae out to the lateral border of the lateral masses. Care was taken to avoid dissection more than 1.5 cm laterally along the posterior laminar arch of C1 to avoid injury to the vertebral arteries as they pierce the atlanto-occipital membrane, heading toward the foramen magnum.

The appropriate-sized occipitocervical plate was selected and contoured to accommodate the angle between the occiput and C1 (Fig. 36–3). Attention was then turned to placement of 3.5-mm cancellous screws into the isthmus bilaterally of C2 to serve as the caudal anchor point of the construct. The orientation of the C2 pedicle isthmus was determined by careful palpation with a Penfield-4 elevator along the superior laminar border of C2 out laterally toward its convergence with the C2 isthmus. In this fashion, the elevator was used to palpate the medial and superior borders of the C2 pedicle or isthmus to define screw orientation during insertion. The appropriate starting point on the dorsal surface of the superior inner quadrant of the C2 lateral mass could then be determined. The surgeon must appreciate that a screw placed within the C2 isthmus or pedicle has a slight lateral-to-medial orientation when compared with screws placed into the lateral masses of the subaxial cervical vertebrae (which diverge laterally). The occipitocervical plate is designed to accommodate this difference in screw orientation between C2 and the subaxial cervical vertebrae. Once the starting point was created, a 2-mm burr was advanced in a millimeter-by-millimeter fashion coaxially down the center of the pedicle. A depth gauge was then used to determine the maximal length of the screw; the hole was then tapped. The C1/C2 facet was exposed after gently elevating the venous plexus overlying this joint with a Penfield-4 elevator. The joint was then decorticated with a burr, followed by packing with autogenous iliac crest bone graft. The appropriately sized 3.5-mm cancellous screws were then inserted through the plate and into the C2 pedicle, thereby stabilizing the construct at its most caudal level. With the cephalad portion of the plate resting flush against the occiput, three bicortical 3.5-mm cortical screws were placed between the inferior and superior nuchal lines, with screw lengths varying between 6 and 14 mm in length (Figs. 36–4 and 36–5).

Following placement of autogenous iliac crest bone graft between the occiput and C2, a tight soft tissue closure was performed. Where possible, the paraspinal musculature was reapproximated in the midline to the C2 spinous process itself. The paraspinal musculature must be reapproximated in several layers to prevent wound spreading or dehiscence.

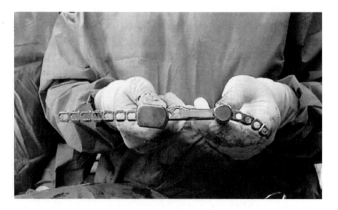

Figure 36–3. Intraoperative bending of the occipitocervical plate.

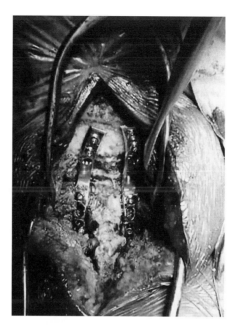

Figure 36–4. An intraoperative photograph following completion of the occipitocervical fusion.

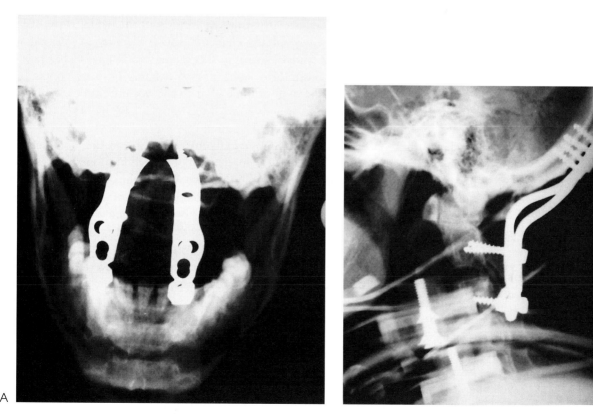

A   B

Figures 36–5. Anteroposterior (AP) (A) and lateral (B) plain radiographs demonstrating the occipitocervical fusion with a plate-screw construct.

Postoperative Management

Postoperatively, the patient remained in halo immobilization for a total of 8 weeks. He was then weaned to a sterno-occipito-mandibular immobilization (SOMI) brace for an additional month. After a total of 3 months of immobilization, progressive mobilization of the cervical spine was started. The posterior occipitocervical incision and iliac crest donor sites healed uneventfully.

Discussion

Surgical intervention for traumatic instability of the upper cervical spine has traditionally been associated with high pseudarthrosis and complication rates, prolonged halo immobilization, and fair to poor functional outcomes. Over the past decade, however, techniques for the fusion of the occiput to the subaxial spine have evolved greatly, and accordingly have decreased the morbidity and immobilization period following this procedure. Although trauma and rheumatoid arthritis are the most common causes of atlantoaxial instability, many other systemic disorders may contribute to instability patterns of the upper cervical spine. For instance, congenital, infectious, metabolic, and neoplastic processes have been known to cause instability requiring occipitocervical fusion.

Alternative Methods of Management

The type of reconstruction chosen to stabilize the occipitocervical junction is dependent on the concomitant need for a decompression of the neural elements, the presence or absence of posterior bony elements, the availability of grafting substances, and the degree of spinal instability. There are five general techniques described for performing a posterior occipitocervical fusion: (1) in situ onlay bone grafting, (2) wire or cable fixation of bone graft to the occiput and cervical spine, (3) methylmethacrylate alone or with internal fixation, (4) rod and wire or rod and screw fixation, and (5) plate and screw fixation.

The earliest and most basic technique in fusing the occiput to the upper cervical spine consisted of simple in situ onlay application of cancellous bone graft. The basic tenets of this procedure include a complete exposure of the desired posterior elements to be fused—occiput, laminae, and lateral masses of the upper cervical spine—followed by a thorough decortication before placement of the autogenous bone graft. Postoperatively, patients would typically be placed in halo immobilization for 3 to 6 months.

At present, there are two popular methods for wire fixation to the occiput. The first involves drilling holes through both cortices of the calvarium, and the second consists of burring a unicortical trough on either side of the occipital protuberance as mentioned above. The latter method penetrates only the outer cortex and thus decreases the risk of injury to the epidural veins and dura.

The technique of Wertheim and Bohlman (1987) involves the burring of a trough in the occiput starting at a point 2 cm above the foramen magnum on either side of the occipital protuberance. A towel clip is used to connect the trough for passage of 20-gauge wires, avoiding intracranial penetration. A second 20-gauge wire is looped around the atlas in the manner described by Gallie (1939). A third wire is passed through the base of the spinous process of the axis. The wires are then

PITFALLS

- If a carbon fiber halo ring is utilized, the utmost care must be taken to maintain the neutral position of the head and to prevent extremes of motion. Excessive flexion or extension of the occipitocervical junction may damage the medulla and adversely affect the respiratory center.

- The halo ring should be applied below the equator of the skull to obtain optimal bony purchase and to prevent disengagement of the pins in the skull as traction is applied. The best position for anterior halo pin placement is in the lateral quadrant of the supraorbital ridge. Posteriorly, the pins should not be directed too inferiorly as they may then extend into the mastoid process. The authors have seen two cases of deafness as the result of contact, irritation, and disruption of the electrical impulses of the auditory portion of the eighth cranial nerve.

passed through the corticocancellous struts and secured over the decorticated posterior elements of the occiput and upper cervical spine. This technique offers immediate stability, allows earlier mobilization, and is easily modified to specific deformities and various anatomic variations. Wertheim and Bohlman reported a solid arthrodesis in all 13 of their patients. Postoperatively, patients were placed in a rigid two-poster orthosis or halo for 6 to 16 weeks followed by placement in a soft cervical collar. In 1991, McAfee and colleagues reported an 84% fusion rate in 37 patients treated with this triple-wire technique.

In 1978, Luque introduced the use of a contoured steel rod attached to the upper cervical spine and occiput by wires as an alternative to wiring fixation alone. In 1966, Cregan first described the use of plate and screw fixation to the skull for obtaining an occipitocervical fusion. Roy-Camille and colleagues (1987) later developed a plate fixation device that was anatomically contoured to the occipitocervical junction. The sagittal contouring of the prebent plate was approximately 105 degrees with spacing for the cervical lateral mass screws of 16 or 19 mm.

More recently, variations on the plate-screw concept have allowed for more anatomically contoured constructs that accommodate different angular constraints when placing screws into the pedicles of C2, across the C1/C2 articular facets, or into the lateral masses of the subaxial cervical vertebrae. For instance, one such plate and screw device (Vaccaro, 1994, Medtronic Sofamor Danek, Memphis, TN) improves fixation to the occiput by medializing occipital screw placement toward the inion with bilateral plates, as well as affording ease of placement of C2 isthmus or pedicle screws through a horizontal variable screw slot design (Fig. 36–6). The subaxial portion of the plate is similar to the Axis plate design, allowing for medial, lat-

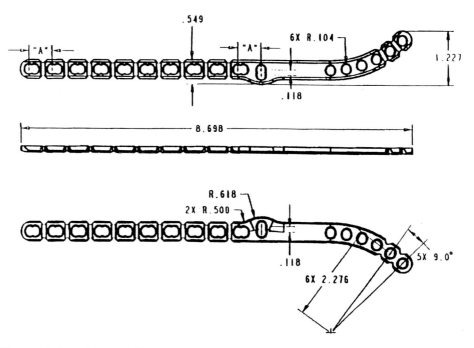

Figure 36–6. A diagram of the occipitocervical plate designed at Thomas Jefferson University by Dr. Vaccaro in 1994. Note the horizontal variable screw slot at the C2 level allowing medial screw angulation without having to obliquely align the cervical plate to achieve appropriate subaxial lateral mass screw placement. The subaxial portion of the plate is similar to the Axis plate and screw system.

eral superior, and inferior screw angular variability with the option of three screw spacing patterns (11, 13, 15 mm). The occipital portion of the plate may be shortened depending on the anatomy. This system allows for improved fixation to the occiput using newly designed 3.5-mm cortical screws with lengths as short as 6 mm. This newer generation plate-screw construct was the fixation of choice in the previously described case.

Within the past year, newer-generation constructs have been created that combine the flexibility of contoured rods with the flexibility of variable angle lateral mass screw placement. Such posterior occipitocervical rod-screw constructs are now available for use.

Type of Management	Advantages	Disadvantages	Comments
Halo immobilization	Immediate acute stabilization	Morbidity related to pin tract infections, lack of long-term stability Prolonged immobilization time	Beneficial in the acute stabilization of occipitocervical dislocations
In situ onlay bone grafting	Avoids risks of internal fixation	No inherent stability	Time-honored technique that requires prolonged postoperative immobilization
Occipitocervical fusion with wire	Immediate stabilization Technically easy	Requires intact posterior elements of the axis and atlas	Use of contoured rods in conjunction with wire allows contouring of spinal alignment
Occipitocervical fusion with plates/rods and screws	Immediate rigid fixation Allows variable angle screw placement Allows contouring of sagittal alignment	Chance of intracranial venous plexus injury with drill or screw tip Technically difficult	Late hardware loosening is a potential complication Higher fusion rate than other, more traditional techniques

Complications

Due to the proximity of the intracranial venous sinuses to the occiput, care must be taken during drill or screw penetration of the inner calvarium. Anatomically, the central venous sinus plexus lies just below the external occipital protuberance, a potential point of screw fixation. Anatomic studies have shown that the rostrocaudal level of the transverse sinus lies at the level of the superior nuchal line (SNL). Heywood and colleagues (1988) found that the thickest portion of the posterior skull is the external occipital protuberance (11 to 17 mm). The skull thickness at the level of the foramen magnum was found to be approximately 9 mm, with the thinnest portion of the skull at the level of the cerebellar fossa. Because of the proximity of the venous sinuses, some surgeons recommend unicortical screw placement below the superior nuchal line. Zipnick and colleagues (1996) confirmed the finding that the thickness of the calvarium above the SNL was significantly greater than below the SNL. Upon defining the thickness of the bone above the SNL as 45% outer table, 45% middle table, and 10% inner table, they concluded that unicortical screw purchase at or above the SNL is possible with low risk of penetration of the intracranial venous plexus. The greatest difficulty encountered in occipital screw placement above the SNL is screw head prominence. Typically, screw fixation should include a minimum of three screws on each side placed between the inferior and superior nuchal lines with screw lengths varying between 6 and 14 mm.

A thorough understanding of the anatomy of the C2 pedicle and lateral mass is imperative if one is to insert screws into these structures without damage to adjacent anatomic structures. With C2 pedicle screw or transarticular screw placement, the structure most at risk is the vertebral artery. With lateral mass screw placement, the vertebral artery and exiting nerve root are the structures most at risk.

Suggested Readings

An HS, Simpson JM. Spinal instrumentation of the cervical spine. In: An HS, Simpson JM, eds. Surgery of the Cervical Spine, pp. 379–400. United Kingdom: Dunitz, 1994.

Andreshak TG, An HS. Posterior cervical exposures. In: Albert TJ, Balderston RA, Northrup BE, eds. Surgical Approaches to the Spine, pp. 81–113. Philadelphia: WB Saunders, 1997.

Brooks AL, Jenkins EB. Atlanto-axial arthrodesis by the wedge compression method. J Bone Joint Surg 1978; 60A:279–292.

Bryan WJ, Inglis AE, Sculco TP, et al. Methylmethacrylate stabilization for enhancement of posterior cervical arthrodesis in rheumatoid arthritis. J Bone Joint Surg 1982; 64A:1045–1050.

Cregan JC. Internal fixation of the unstable rheumatoid cervical spine. Ann Rheum Dis 1966; 25:242–252.

Fehlings MG, Errico T, Cooper P, et al. Occipitocervical fusion with a five-millimeter malleable rod and segmental fixation. Neurosurgery 1993; 32:198–208.

Flint GA, Hockley AD, McMillan JJ, et al. A new method of occipitocervical fusion using internal fixation. Neurosurgery 1987; 21:947–950.

Gallie WE. Fractures and dislocations of the cervical spine. Am J Surg 1939; 46:495.

Grantham SA, Dick HM, Thompson RC, et al. Occipitocervical arthrodesis. Clin Orthop 1969; 65:118–129.

Grob D, Crisco JJ, Panjabi MM, et al. Biomechanical evaluation of four different posterior atlanto-axial fixation techniques. Spine 1992; 17:480–490.

Grob D, Dvorak J, Panjabi M, et al. Posterior occipitocervical fusion: a preliminary report of a new technique. Spine 1991; 16:S17–24.

Grob D, Dvorak J, Panjabi M, et al. The role of plate and screw fixation in occipitocervical fusion in rheumatoid arthritis. Spine 1994; 19:2545–2551.

Grob D, Jeanneret B, Aebi M, et al. Atlanto-axial fusion with transarticular screw fixation. J Bone Joint Surg 1991; 73B:972–976.

Grob D, Schmotzer H. Posterior occipitocervical fusion. Spine State Art Rev 1996; 10:275–280.

Hamblen DL. Occipito-cervical fusion. J Bone Joint Surg 1967; 49B:33–45.

Heywood AWB, Learmonth ID, Thomas M. Internal fixation for occipitocervical fusion. J Bone Joint Surg 1988; 70B:708–711.

Jeanneret B, Magerl F. Preliminary posterior fusion C1–2 and odontoid fractures: indications, technique and results of transarticular screw fixation. J Spinal Disord 1992; 5:464–475.

Kahn EA, Yglesias L. Progressive atlanto-axial dislocation. JAMA 1935; 105:348–352.

Lipscomb PR. Cervico-occipital fusion for congenital and post-traumatic anomalies of the atlas and axis. J Bone Joint Surg 1957; 39A:1289–1301.

Luque ER. Segmental correction and fixation of the spine. Proceedings of the AAOS 45th annual meeting, Dallas, TX, 1978.

MacEwen GD, King AGS. Occipito-cervical fusion. In: Cotler JM, Cotler HB, eds. Spine Fusion: Science and Techniques, pp. 253–255. New York: Springer-Verlag, 1990.

McAfee PC, Cassidy JR, Davis RF. Fusion of the occiput to the upper cervical spine. Spine 1991; 16:S490–494.

Newman P, Sweetman R. Occipito-cervical fusion. J Bone Joint Surg 1969; 51B:423–431.

O'Brien MF, Sutterlin CE III. Occipitocervical biomechanics. Spine State Art Rev 1996; 10:281–313.

Ransford AO, Crockard HA, Pozo JL, et al. Craniocervical instability treated by contoured loop fixation. J Bone Joint Surg 1986; 68B:173–177.

Roy-Camille R, Mazel C, Saillant G. Treatment of cervical spine injuries by a posterior osteosynthesis with plates and screws. In: Kehr P, Weidner A, eds. Cervical Spine, p. 163. New York: Springer-Verlag, 1987.

Sasso RC, Jeanneret B, Fischer K, et al. Occipitocervical fusion with posterior plate and screw instrumentation. Spine 1994; 19:2364–2368.

Smith MD, Anderson P, Grady S. Occipitocervical arthrodesis using contoured plate fixation. Spine 1993; 18:1984–1990.

Sutterlin CE III, Bianchi JR, Rapoff MS, et al. A biomechanical evaluation of occipitocervical fixation devices, pp. 48–49. The Cervical Spine Research Society, West Palm Beach, FL, 1996.

Wertheim SB, Bohlman HH. Occipitocervical fusion. J Bone Joint Surg 1987; 69A:833–836.

White AA, Panjabi MM. Clinical Biomechanics of the Spine. Philadelphia: JB Lippincott, 1978.

Zipnick RI, Merola AA, Gorup J. The occiput: anatomic considerations for internal fixation. Spine State Art Rev 1996; 10:269–274.

Case 37

Bilateral Cervical Facet Joint Dislocation without Neurologic Deficit

Gregg R. Klein, Suken A. Shah, and Alexander R. Vaccaro

History and Physical Examination

A 35-year-old man was involved in a high-speed motor vehicle accident while wearing a seat belt. The patient complained of severe neck pain and transient numbness and paresthesias in his upper extremities. There was no loss of consciousness or other complaints. After emergency personnel at the scene immobilized the patient's cervical spine in a collar and placed the patient on a back board, the patient was transferred to our institution for evaluation.

Physical examination revealed tenderness to palpation along the posterior aspect of the subaxial cervical spine. Neurologic examination revealed no evidence of motor weakness or sensory deficit. The patient's mental status was intact. A secondary survey revealed superficial lacerations of the lower extremities.

Radiologic Findings

A lateral plain radiograph of the cervical spine revealed the C5 vertebral body displaced anteriorly approximately 50% on C6. An anteroposterior (AP) radiograph

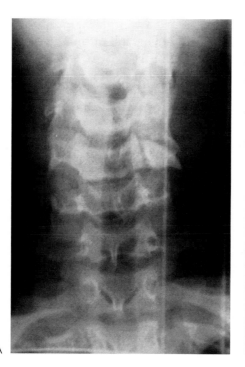
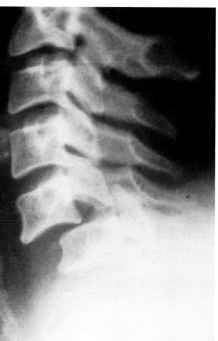

A   B

Figure 37–1. Anteroposterior (AP) (A) and lateral (B) radiographs of the cervical spine demonstrating the distraction-flexion injury and bilateral facet dislocation at the C5/C6 articulation.

revealed an increased interspinous distance at the level of the translation without any evidence of rotational malalignment (Fig. 37–1).

Computed tomography (CT) revealed bilateral dislocated facets without evidence of fracture. The inferior facets of C5 were now anterior to the superior facets of C6.

Diagnosis

This is a distractive-flexion stage 3 (DFS3) injury of the cervical spine as described by Allen and colleagues (1982).

Nonsurgical Management

It is strongly recommended that an emergent closed reduction be attempted in cases of bilateral facet injury with or without a neurologic deficit in an awake, alert, and cooperative patient.

Based on the initial plain radiographs diagnosing a distractive-flexion injury at the fifth and sixth cervical vertebrae, consistent with a bilateral facet dislocation, an attempt at an awake, closed reduction in the emergency room was undertaken.

The patient was transferred to a Stryker frame and cardiac and oxygen saturation monitoring was continued. Stainless steel Gardner-Wells tongs were placed in the cranium in a vector that would produce a slight flexion moment, and axial traction was applied to the patient's cervical spine gently and gradually, starting at 10 pounds. At each change in weight or position, a careful neurologic examination was performed and recorded, and lateral plain radiographs were obtained to evaluate the status of the reduction. At all times during the reduction, the patient was alert and cooperative with the examination. At an axial traction weight of 90 pounds, a lateral radiograph of the cervical spine demonstrated unlocking of the dislocated facet joints at C5/C6, and translation to a "perched" position. At this time, a soft towel was placed midline between the patient's scapulae, and the cervical spine was gently extended. An additional 10 pounds was added to the existing traction weight. A subsequent lateral radiograph of the cervical spine demonstrated a reduction of the flexion-distraction injury; the patient's neurologic exam remained unchanged. The weight was then gradually reduced to 15 pounds and a lateral radiograph of the cervical spine revealed maintenance of the reduction; the patient remained neurologically intact throughout the reduction procedure. The patient was placed in halo vest immobilization; a lateral radiograph of the cervical spine at this juncture confirmed adequate alignment of the cervical spine without excessive cervical extension.

The patient was then transported to the magnetic resonance imaging (MRI) suite for a cervical spine MRI to evaluate the spinal cord and presence of associated soft tissue injuries. MRI is recommended in all cases following a successful closed reduction or when awake closed reduction fails. However, closed reduction should not be delayed to obtain an MRI. The often associated time delay is not advantageous from a neurologic recovery prospective in the setting of cord compression from a maligned cervical axis. The MRI in this patient revealed no evidence of a cervical disc herniation but the presence of posterior paraspinal soft tissue and ligamentous disruption was confirmed (Fig. 37–2).

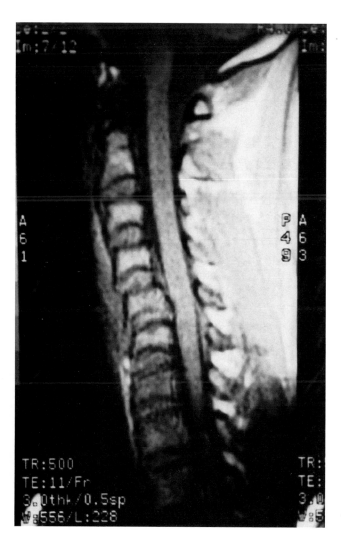

Figure 37–2. Sagittal magnetic resonance imaging (MRI) illustrating the injury to the posterior ligamentous and soft tissues.

Surgical Management

The patient subsequently underwent a posterior cervical fusion of C4 through C6 using lateral mass plates and screws with iliac crest bone graft.

The patient was brought to the operating room with his cervical spine immobilized in a halo vest. After awake intubation and induction of anesthesia, the patient was placed prone on the Stryker frame. Motor and somatosensory evoked potentials were used for intraoperative spinal cord monitoring.

A standard posterior approach was undertaken with care taken to avoid extension of exposure beyond those segments intended for fusion. Lateral mass screw placement as described by An and colleagues (1991) was used.

To place screws securely and safely in the lateral mass, the surgeon must completely determine the anatomic boundaries of the lateral mass. The superior and inferior borders are most readily identified by locating the cephalad and caudad borders of the facet joints. The medial border is defined by the depression that occurs at the junction between the lamina and lateral mass. The lateral border is simply the lateral-most edge of the lateral mass. In the technique described by An and colleagues (1991), the starting point for screw placement is located 1 mm medial to the center of the most cephalad lateral mass to be fused (see Fig. 37–4). An awl was used to create a cortical entry

PEARLS

- Gardner-Wells stainless steel tongs are preferred over carbon fiber, MRI-compatible tongs for use in an adult patient undergoing a closed reduction for bilateral facet dislocations of the cervical spine due to their high weight tolerance.
- Often in a large adult patient with a unilateral facet dislocation of the lower cervical spine without the presence of associated facet fractures, a high weight (90 to 140 pounds) may be required to unlock the dislocated facet and reduce the deformity.
- A closed reduction of a bilateral facet dislocation of the cervical spine should be attempted only by experienced personnel in an awake, cooperative patient while performing careful neurologic examinations after each weight application.

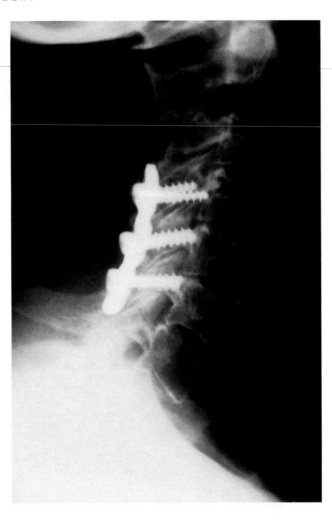

Figure 37–3. Postoperative lateral radiograph of the cervical spine demonstrating the poster cervical fusion and instrumentation with lateral mass plates and screws.

site. A 2-mm power drill was then directed approximately 15 degrees cephalad and 30 degrees laterally when using a starting point 1mm lateral to the center of the lateral mass. In this fashion, the vertebral artery, which lies anterior to the medial border of the lateral mass, and the nerve root, which exits obliquely across the anterior border of the lateral mass, will be avoided. The drill was then advanced slowly until the anterior cortex was penetrated. A depth gauge was used to confirm the depth and location of the drill hole. Bicortical purchase is preferable unless the patient has very good bone quality. Prior to placing the cervical plate, the facet joints were decorticated and packed with morcelized autogenous bone graft. Plate and screw position were then judged with a postoperative lateral X-ray (Fig. 37–3).

Discussion

A bilateral facet dislocation is an unstable injury that should be treated surgically. Studies describing nonoperative treatment of these injuries reveal poor results. Bucholz and Cheung (1989) treated 20 patients with either bilateral facet dislocations or perched facets by halo immobilization; 9 of the 20 (45%) ultimately required surgery. When surgery is contraindicated for medical reasons, halo vest immobilization is often needed for an extended period of time.

Controversy exists concerning the timing of closed reduction and the timing of obtaining an MRI. Because of the high incidence of herniated discs associated with

PITFALLS
- Neurologic deterioration during a manipulative reduction of the traumatically injured spine should alert the physician to possible etiologies of spinal cord compression such as a disc extrusion or the presence of an epidural hematoma.
- Uncontrolled manipulations without close monitoring of neurologic function are thought to be the major cause of secondary neurologic compromise.
- At our institution, given the risk of neurologic compromise in this unstable cervical spine injury with transport to the MRI scanner or operating room, we routinely perform immediate reduction and stabilization with a halo vest orthosis in the emergency room, in alert, awake, and cooperative patients.

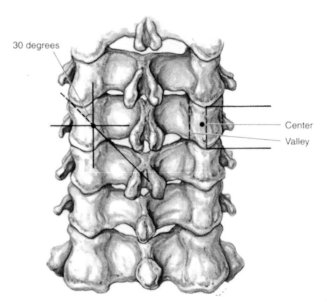

Figure 37–4. The location of the ideal point for starting lateral mass screws is 1 mm medial to the center of the lateral mass on the "hill," as described by An and colleagues (1991). The drill should be directed 30 degrees lateral and 15 degrees cephalad to avoid injuring the exiting nerve and vertebral artery. (Reprinted from Andreshak and An, 1997, with permission.)

bilateral facet dislocations, some authors recommend obtaining an MRI of the cervical spine prior to any attempt at closed reduction.

Other authors advocate emergent closed reduction prior to obtaining an MRI. This method theoretically decompresses the spinal cord as soon as possible and potentially maximizes the chance for neurologic recovery. Also, the risk of causing neurologic deterioration during transfer to the MRI scanner is eliminated. Delays in reduction, such as the time needed to obtain an MRI, may decrease the chance of recovery. Evidence shows that greater recovery in spinal cord deficits were found when patients were reduced within 8 hours of injury. Lee and colleagues (1994) reviewed 210 patients with unilateral and bilateral facet dislocations, and found that early rapid traction provided the best chance for neurologic recovery as compared to closed reduction under anesthesia. However, Ludwig and colleagues (1997) reported a case of immediate quadriparesis during awake closed reduction of a bilateral facet subluxation. The reduction maneuver was reversed and the patient regained function. Postmaneuver MRI revealed a large posterior epidural hematoma in this patient and not a herniated disc.

The method of reduction is also controversial. Some authors prefer closed reduction under general anesthesia, whereas others recommend awake-only closed reduction. Spinal cord monitoring is recommended if closed reduction under general anesthesia is performed.

At our institution we perform immediate closed reduction on all patients with bilateral facet dislocations who are awake and alert and can participate in a reliable neurologic exam. Cotler and colleagues (1992), using closed skeletal tong traction, successfully reduced 24 patients with facet dislocations or subluxations (C4–C7) without evidence of fracture using weights in the range of 10 to 140 pounds. They noted that if a closed reduction was unsuccessful or a patient developed worsening in their neurologic exam, an MRI should be performed prior to an operative reduction and stabilization procedure. If a significant herniated disc is present, an initial anterior cervical discectomy should be performed prior to cervical reduction. An MRI is recommended after all successful closed reductions, if a reduction fails or if neurologic changes occur during the reduction.

The surgical approach to stabilization of a bilateral facet dislocation that is successfully closed reduced is dependent on the presence of an associated herniated disc. A posterior spinal fusion using lateral mass plates and screws or posterior interspinous wiring is recommended in the neurologically intact patient without evidence of a herniated disc on MRI evaluation. If closed reduction is unsuccessful in the absence of a herniated disc on MRI, an open reduction and posterior spinal fusion is recommended. In the presence of a herniated disc, an anterior cervical discectomy and attempted reduction may be performed followed by either an anterior cervical plated fusion (if an anterior reduction was successful) or a posterior open reduction and spinal fusion followed by placement of an anterior bone graft. Some authors have placed a undersized Smith-Robinson bone graft anteriorly in the presence of a cervical dislocation following discectomy in anticipation of adequate settling when the subsequent posterior reduction is performed.

There is also a high incidence of unilateral vertebral artery injury associated with unilateral and bilateral facet dislocations. Using magnetic resonance angiography (MRA), Giacobetti and colleagues (1997), in their review of cervical spine trauma, found 6 vertebral artery injuries in 16 patients (38%) with facet dislocations.

Alternative Methods of Management

Until recently, posterior stabilization of the subaxial cervical spine made use of various wiring techniques. In the presence of intact posterior elements, the time-honored triple-wire technique described by Bohlman's group (McAfee and colleagues, 1985) provides fixation that resists tension while securing structural autogenous bone graft to the posterior elements.

Type of Management	Advantages	Disadvantages	Comments
Halo immobilization	Less potential for loss of alignment following a successful reduction Stabilization for patients who cannot undergo surgical intervention	Unsightly facial scars Morbidity related to skin infection and loosening	An effective means of stabilization prior to surgical intervention
Posterior cervical fusion with interspinous wiring	Technically easy Neurovascular complications rare	Biomechanically inferior to plates and screws Requires intact posterior bony elements	Time-honored, inexpensive technique requiring postoperative halo immobilization
Posterior cervical fusion with lateral mass plates and screws	Increased biomechanical strength Useful in the presence of damaged posterior elements	Risk of neurovascular injury with improper screw placement	May not need perioperative halo vest immobilization for stabilization
Posterior cervical fusion with pedicle screws	Improved purchase at ends (C2 or C7) of lateral mass plate screw constructs	Risk of vertebral artery, nerve root and spinal cord injury	Useful only at the cervicothoracic junction (C7/T1) in the absence of a vertebral artery in the C7 foramen transversarium
Anterior cervical discectomy and fusion	Direct decompression of a herniated disc	Technically difficult to perform if a successful closed reduction has not been obtained	Most efficient means of stabilization if a discectomy is required and there is adequate spinal alignment

Continued on next page

Continued

Type of Management	Advantages	Disadvantages	Comments
Anterior cervical discectomy followed by a posterior then anterior cervical fusion	Often necessary in the presence of a disc herniation in an unreduced cervical dislocation	Two incisions/approaches Operative time/morbidity	Often safer than an attempted anterior reduction, which may lead to a stretch injury to the cervical spinal cord

Suggested Readings

Abumi K, Itoh H, Taneichi H, Kaneda K. Transpedicular screw fixation for traumatic lesions of the middle and lower cervical spine: description of the techniques and preliminary report. J Spinal Disord 1994; 7:19–28.

Albert TJ, Klein GR, Joffee D, Vaccaro AR. Use of cervicothoracic junction pedicle screws for complex cervical spine pathology. Spine 1998; 23:1596–1599.

Allen BL, Ferguson RL, Lehmann R, O'Brian RP. Mechanistic classification of closed indirect fractures and dislocations of the lower cervical spine. Spine 1982; 7:1–27.

An HS, Gordin R, Renner K. Anatomic considerations for plate-screw fixation of the cervical spine. Spine 1991; 16:S548–S551.

Andreshak TG, An HS. Posterior cervical exposures. In: Albert TJ, Balderston RA, Northrup BE, eds. Surgical Approaches to the Spine, pp. 81–113. Philadelphia: WB Saunders, 1997.

Bucholz RD, Cheung KX. Halo vest versus spinal fusion for cervical injury: evidence from an outcome study. J Neurosurg 1989; 70:884–892.

Cotler JM, Herbison GJ, Nasuti JF, Ditunno JF, An H, Wolff BE. Closed reduction of traumatic cervical spine dislocation using traction weights up to 140 pounds. Spine 1993; 18:386–390.

Ebraheim NA, Hoeflinger MJ, Salpietro B, Chunk SY, Jackson WT. Anatomic considerations in posterior plating of the cervical spine. J Orthop Trauma 1991; 5:196–199.

Eismont FJ, Arena MJ, Green BA. Extrusion of an intervertebral disc associated with traumatic subluxation or dislocation of cervical facets. Case report. J Bone Joint Surg 1991; 73(A):1555–1560.

Fehlings MG, Cooper PR, Errico JJ. Posterior plates in the management of cervical instability: long term results in 44 patients. J Neurosurg 1994; 81:341–349.

Giacobetti FB, Vaccaro AR, Bos-Giacobetti MA, et al. Vertebral artery occlusion associated with cervical spine trauma: a prospective analysis. Spine 1997; 22:188–192.

Harrington JF, Likavel MJ, Smith AS. Disc herniation in cervical fracture subluxation. Neurosurgery 1991; 29:374–379.

Jeanneret B, Magerl F, Ward EW, Ward JCH. Posterior stabilization of the cervical spine with hook plates. Spine 1991; 16:56–63.

Kotani Y, Cunningham BW, Abumi K, McAfee PC. Biomechanical analysis of cervical stabilization systems. An assessment of transpedicular screw fixation in the cervical spine. Spine 1994; 19:2529–2539.

Kramer DL, Ludwig SC, Balderston RA, Vaccaro AR, Foley KF, Albert TJ. Placement of pedicle screws in the cervical spine: comparative accuracy of cervical pedicle screw placement using three techniques. Orthop Trans 1997; 21:484.

Lee AS, MacLean JC, Newton DA. Rapid traction for reduction of cervical spine dislocations. J Bone Joint Surg 1994; 76B:352–356.

Ludwig SC, Vaccaro AR, Balderston RA, Cotler JM. Immediate quadriparesis after manipulation for bilateral cervical facet subluxation. A case report. J Bone Joint Surg 1997; 79A:587–590.

McAfee PC, Bohlman HH, Wilson WL. The triple wire fixation technique for stabilization of acute cervical fracture dislocations: a biomechanical analysis. Trans Orthop 1985; 9:142.

Pratt ES, Green DA, Spengler DM. Herniated intervertebral discs associated with unstable spinal injuries. Spine 1990; 15:662–665.

Rizzolo SJ, Piazza MR, Cotler JM, Balderston RA, Schaefer D, Flanders A. Intervertebral disc injury complication of cervical spine trauma. Spine 1991; 16S:S187–189.

Roy-Camille R, Mazel C, Saillant G. Internal fixation of the unstable cervical spine by posterior osteosynthesis with plates and screws. In: Sherk HH, eds. The Cervical Spine, 2d ed., pp. 390–403. Philadelphia: JP Lippincott, 1989.

Case 38

Fixed Traumatic Atlantoaxial Rotatory Deformity

Suken A. Shah, Alexander R. Vaccaro, and Carl E. Becker II

History and Physical Examination

A 34-year-old man was involved in a bicycle accident in which he was hit by a car and thrown 10 to 15 feet off his bicycle. At the scene of the accident, the patient complained of headache, neck pain, and wrist pain, and was moving all extremities without difficulty. The patient was not seen initially at a medical center until his wife became concerned that for approximately 3 days following the accident, the patient could not turn his head, and continued to stare to the right.

Upon examination in the emergency room, the patient displayed a "cock-robin" position with his head tilted to the left and his chin rotated to the right. He complained of severe neck discomfort and spasms with any attempt at neck rotation. He

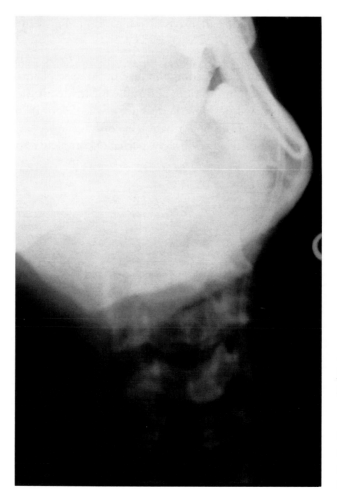

Figure 38–1. An antero-posterior (AP) plain radiograph demonstrating the "cock-robin" head posture. The patient's head is tilted to the left, but rotated to the right. There is obstruction of detail of the upper cervical spine elements.

was noted to have tenderness on palpation of his upper cervical spine and was neurologically intact.

Radiologic Findings

An anteroposterior (AP) plain radiograph (Fig. 38–1) revealed the typical cock-robin head posture with the patient's head tilted to the left, but rotated to the right. There is obstruction of detail of the upper cervical spine elements. A transaxial computed tomography (CT) scan at the level of the C1/C2 articulation (Fig. 38–2) demonstrates a fixed rotatory dislocation of the left atlantoaxial joint complex. This was further evaluated with a three-dimensional CT reconstruction (Fig. 38–3) of the upper cervical region.

The rotatory nature of this deformity is often well demonstrated on a plain AP open-mouth odontoid view. In the normal patient, looking straight ahead, the lateral masses and joint spaces should appear of equal width. Normal rotation of the atlas upon the axis results in a broader appearance of the lateral mass on the side opposite the direction of head rotation, a decrease in the distance to the odontoid, and a widened joint space. Conversely, the lateral mass on the side on which the head is rotated appears less broad, and its joint space is narrowed.

The diagnosis of a rotatory dislocation or subluxation depends on dynamic studies in which these relationships remain unchanged despite attempted rotation to the normal position. Additionally, the lateral cervical spine films should be examined for anterior atlantoaxial subluxation. This can be ruled out by measuring the predental space.

Computed tomography has proved to be extremely useful in this diagnosis. A CT scan of the patient is obtained in the axial plane in the presenting position, that is, the cock-robin position, and subsequently, with the head turned maximally to the contralateral position. Persistence of the deformity with change in head position is diagnostic of this abnormality. In contrast, however, dynamic studies of patients with benign torticollis will show partial or complete resolution of the rotational deformity.

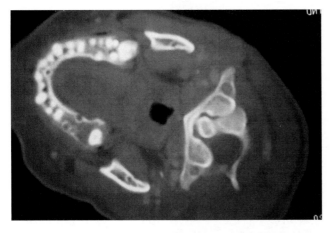

Figure 38–2. A transaxial computed tomography (CT) scan at the level of the C1/C2 articulation demonstrating a fixed rotatory dislocation of the left atlantoaxial joint complex.

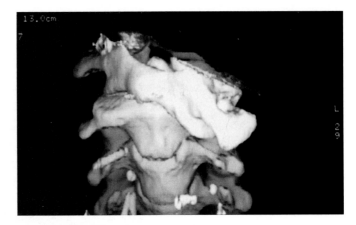

Figure 38–3. Three-dimensional CT reconstruction of the C1/C2 rotatory dislocation

Diagnosis

The diagnosis of this cervical spine deformity is a fixed atlantoaxial rotatory dislocation.

Atlantoaxial rotatory subluxation or dislocation is a relatively rare disorder that was first described by Corner in 1907. This deformity is part of a broad spectrum of injuries ranging from rotatory subluxation without translation, to rotation accompanied by subluxation implying ligamentous injury, to fixed rotatory dislocation, with or without translation. Causes may include a history of prior infection, such as otitis media, pharyngitis, viral syndromes, recent surgical procedures of the head and neck, and traumatic injury. The common thread is that all of the etiologies appear to weaken, through inflammation or force, the supporting soft tissue structures of the atlantoaxial articulation. Fixed atlantoaxial rotation deformities have also been associated with Down syndrome, Morquio syndrome, and juvenile rheumatoid arthritis, all of which are known to exhibit congenital atlantoaxial abnormalities and/or ligamentous laxity.

The patient typically will complain of neck pain and display a rotational deformity of the head and neck. The chin is rotated toward one side, and the head is tilted in the opposite direction. This is the so-called cock-robin position described by Fielding and colleagues (1978). There is frequently spasm of the sternocleidomastoid muscle on the side of the chin rotation, suggesting an attempt at reduction. Rotation of the head is restricted in both directions and causes pain. The neck discomfort may decrease over time, but the torticollis may progress. Neurologic deficits are uncommon; however, when they are present, a close, prompt investigation of the lower cervical spine should be undertaken to evaluate the presence of concomitant injuries in a patient with a traumatic mechanism.

Nonsurgical Management

Magnetic resonance imaging (MRI)-compatible tongs were placed on the patient and axial cervical traction was applied, starting at 2 lbs. Subsequently, weight was added to a total of 15 lbs over the course of a 24-hour period. At this time, there was clinical and radiographic evidence of reduction of the atlantoaxial rotatory dislocation. A cervical CT scan after reduction confirmed anatomic alignment. There was no change in the patient's normal neurologic exam during the reduction period. The patient was placed in a hard cervical collar and discharged from the hospital.

The patient returned to the emergency room 8 days after discharge with increasing neck pain. Radiographs and cervical CT scan demonstrated a recurrent atlantoaxial dislocation. A repeat reduction was performed according to the method described above, and at that point the recommendation was made for stabilization involving a C1/C2 arthrodesis.

Correction of the dislocation prior to surgery eases the technical complexity of the procedure and reduces the neurologic risk from an improper surgical reduction. Spinal surgery is technically easier in the anatomic position from the standpoints of visualization and stabilization, and allows correction of the postural deformation of the airway, allowing easier intubation for the anesthesiologist.

PEARLS

- The diagnosis of fixed atlantoaxial rotatory fixation should be confirmed with the use of a dynamic CT scan. Thin axial sections in the position of presentation, and then with the patient looking to the left, and then to the right, will clearly demonstrate the abnormality. A persistence of the deformity with a change in position of the head is diagnostic of an atlantoaxial subluxation/dislocation.
- Most rotatory deformities in the acute period can be reduced with gentle cervical traction in the alert, cooperative patient. External immobilization is then necessary to allow adequate soft tissue healing.
- Reduction of the deformity prior to surgical stabilization is desirable. Arthrodesis in the anatomic position offers predictably good results.

Surgical Management

The patient subsequently underwent a C1/C2 transarticular facet screw arthrodesis with the Magerl screw technique and a C1/C2 posterior wiring and fusion (Brooks technique) with autologous iliac crest bone graft (Fig. 38–4).

The patient was brought to the operating room in cervical traction, and after an awake, fiberoptic intubation and induction of general anesthesia, the patient was positioned prone on the operating room table using a Mayfield pin holder for cervical stabilization. Intraoperative spinal cord monitoring was performed with motor and somatosensory evoked potentials.

A posterior midline approach was used for exposure of the upper posterior elements. After denuding the posterior C1/C2 joint space of all articular cartilage, two 3.5-mm cortical screws (45 mm in length) were placed starting at the inferior C2 articular process, up through the isthmus of C2, and into the inferior articular process of the C1 lateral mass at an angulation of approximately 50 degrees to the horizontal. Care was taken not to violate the vertebral foramen transversarium laterally and the spinal canal medially with the transarticular screws. Placement of the screws was accomplished with the aid of AP and lateral fluoroscopic guidance. Following rigid stabilization of the C1/C2 joint, a posterior arthrodesis of C1/C2 was performed using a modified Brooks wiring technique and autologous iliac crest bone graft.

Postoperative Management

The patient was extubated at the conclusion of the procedure in the operating room and was immobilized in a hard cervical collar. There is often no need for halo vest immobilization due to the rigidity of the internal fixation. This allows for early mobilization and less difficult rehabilitation. The patient was discharged 3 days postoperatively with no complications.

The patient was seen for follow-up at 2, 4, 8, and 12 weeks postoperatively, and routine plain radiographs were taken. Successful C1/C2 arthrodesis was confirmed at the 12th week follow-up visit with flexion, extension lateral plain radiographs.

Discussion

Since the initial description of this rare abnormality in 1907 by Corner, there has been significant confusion regarding the cause, diagnosis, and optimal treatment of

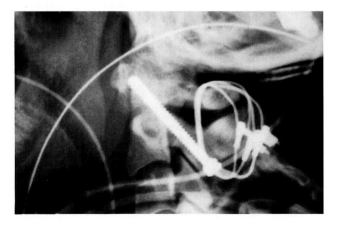

Figure 38–4. Postoperative lateral radiograph of the patient status post–closed reduction and C1/C2 arthrodesis with Magerl transarticular screw fixation and a modified Brooks wiring and autologous iliac crest bone graft.

PITFALLS

- Conditions simulating an atlantoaxial facet subluxation/dislocation include an uncooperative patient, congenital muscular torticollis, and cervical facet asymmetry. These can be ruled out with the use of dynamic CT scanning.
- A delay in diagnosis and/or treatment poses a formidable therapeutic problem. Those patients with irreducible dislocations may fail a closed reduction, and surgical interventions, such as an open reduction through the posterior, lateral, or anterior transoral approach, may be necessary.
- Although neurologic compromise is rare in these injuries, a thorough investigation of the subaxial spine should be undertaken to rule out concomitant contiguous or noncontiguous injuries in the traumatized spine patient.

rotatory abnormalities of the C1/C2 articulation. Fixed rotatory subluxation or dislocation of the atlantoaxial complex is often misdiagnosed and incorrectly managed. All patients who present with long-standing symptoms of acquired or traumatic torticollis should undergo dynamic CT imaging of the cervical spine to rule out an abnormal relation between C1 and C2, marked by a fixed rotation that fails to resolve with attempts at correction by head rotation.

Once diagnosed, most cases of acute atlantoaxial rotatory subluxation will resolve with closed treatment, such as activity restriction with collar immobilization to cervical traction followed by orthosis or halo vest immobilization. Infrequently, chronic cases, due to long-standing ligamentous, capsular, and other soft tissue changes, recur after an attempted closed reduction and often require an open reduction and stabilization procedure to restore and preserve proper alignment. In general, patients whose deformity remains unreduced for longer than 3 weeks have a higher frequency of persistent or recurrent deformity after attempted reduction.

Most reports of atlantoaxial rotatory abnormalities in the literature have involved pediatric patients, as there are several unique aspects of the pediatric cervical spine that may predispose children to this disorder. The upper cervical spine ligaments (transverse and alar), facet joint capsules, and the articulating surfaces maintain the normal alignment of the atlantoaxial joint. However, in children, the soft tissues have sufficient laxity to allow hypermobility without disruption, and the facet joints (specifically at C1/C2) are shallower and more horizontally oriented in children. Furthermore, the disproportionate size of a child's head and hypermobile cervical spine with small nuchal musculature may predispose the atlantoaxial joint to excessive forces and motion, resulting in an atlantoaxial dislocation.

During axial rotation, the size of the spinal canal is diminished because the oval vertebral foramen of C1 (spinal canal) does not conform to that of C2; however, because the spinal canal is wider at the atlas than in the subaxial cervical spine, compression of the neural elements is unlikely except in the cases of excessive rotation, congenital stenosis, or spinal dysraphism. Sometimes there is irritation of the greater occipital nerve or trigeminal branch of the facial nerve with excessive C1/C2 rotation. Occasionally, the vertebral artery may be excessively stretched with extremes in rotation, resulting in symptoms of vertebral artery insufficiency such as dizziness, nausea, and visual changes.

A description of the pathologic anatomy and classification of rotatory atlantoaxial fixation was proposed by Fielding and Hawkins in 1977. White and Panjabi (1978) submitted five patterns of abnormal displacement of the C1/C2 joint: (1) bilateral anterior or (2) posterior translatory subluxation/dislocation, (3) unilateral anterior or (4) posterior rotatory subluxation/dislocation, and (5) bilateral rotatory subluxation/dislocation.

The treatment of atlantoaxial rotatory fixation involves initial immobilization, followed by an attempted closed reduction prior to surgical stabilization. MRI can often delineate ligamentous injury (i.e., transverse ligament) with the use of a multiplanar gradient-echo technique. Rotatory dislocations, in the presence of an intact transverse ligament may be considered stable, and can be reduced and immobilized in a collar or halo vest orthosis. These injuries should be analyzed on a case-by-case basis for the need for operative stabilization. The presence of fractures, neurologic deficits, disruption of the transverse ligament, or recurrent instability necessitates internal fixation.

Alternative Methods of Management

Many authors advocate cervical immobilization alone with an orthosis (without manipulative reduction), antiinflammatory agents, and close clinical follow-up in the setting of an acute, nontraumatic atlantoaxial rotatory dislocation or subluxation. This technique may be used effectively in children with a short duration of symptoms; however, failure of the rotational deformity to resolve within 2 weeks signals the need for further intervention. The use of head halter traction with 2 to 5 lbs of weight often results in marked pain relief and a more rapid reduction of deformity. Subach and colleagues (1998) demonstrated no recurrence of subluxation in a subgroup of children that achieved reduction within 21 days of symptoms.

Following reduction, immobilization with a hard cervical orthosis for approximately 6 weeks is appropriate. Management of recurrent episodes of subluxation or dislocation may include a second trial of closed reduction (with traction) followed by prolonged cervical orthosis immobilization for up to 3 months, to avoid surgery.

Graziano and colleagues (1993) described the use of a halo-Ilizarov distraction cast for correction of various cervical deformities in the pediatric population. Three of the six patients in their series had torticollis due to atlantoaxial subluxation. This means of treatment was advocated due to its ability to achieve multidirectional correction of cervical deformities in a controlled fashion without the patient having to remain in bed. The apparatus, however, requires careful planning to apply the proper corrective forces. Complications included pin tract infection and pressure sores under the body cast.

Fixed traumatic atlantoaxial rotatory dislocations may sometimes require an open reduction to achieve reduction. An alternative approach from the standard posterior, midline dissection is the lateral retropharyngeal approach of Whitesides and McDonald (1978). This approach involves the exposure of the lateral aspect of the atlantoaxial joint through a dissection posterior to the carotid vessels, and is used in severe deformities where visualization through the anterior approach may be obscured due to the presenting deformity. This approach, however, must be performed bilaterally and screw stabilization can be difficult if an anatomic reduction is not obtained. Crockard and Rogers (1996) used an extreme lateral approach technique in two patients with fixed atlantoaxial rotatory dislocations that failed an attempted closed reduction and cervical immobilization. After the surgical exposure, the vertebral arteries were isolated and controlled, followed by a thorough debridement and reduction of the atlantoaxial joint. Intraoperative findings included abundant fibrous tissue and a segment of the transverse ligament interposed between the joint surfaces of C1/C2. Subin and colleagues (1995), in a report of 10 patients with irreducible atlantoaxial dislocations and spinal cord compression, described a transoral anterior decompression and fusion as treatment of this condition. The advantages of the transoral anterior approach include direct release of ventral compression, debridement of anterior granulation tissue (in irreducible deformities), and access to the lateral joints to allow unlocking as well as excision of articular cartilage. Postoperative treatment included skull-cervical biaxial traction in a multifunctional bed, tracheostomy care, nasal feeding, and a Minerva cast. Lee and Fairholm (1985) discussed the technique of transoral anterior decompression and posterior fusion in a small group of patients. This surgical technique allows the surgeon to address ventral pathology as well, but with the associated morbidity of speech and swallowing difficulties as well as infection. Surgical time is prolonged with this approach due to the need for a supplemental posterior stabilization procedure.

Type of Management	Advantages	Disadvantages	Comments
Collar or halo immobilization	Avoids hospitalization Less traumatic for children	Prolonged time to reduction Significant failure rate	Effective only for acute dislocations
Arthrodesis in situ	Avoids cervical traction and/or manipulative reduction	Pseudarthrosis Not anatomic	
Closed cervical reduction and external immobilization	Avoids risk of surgery Frequently successful	Significant recurrence rate Morbidity of halo vest orthosis	Effective only for acute dislocations Most frequently used method for children
Closed cervical reduction and posterior arthrodesis with internal fixation	Immediate stability Avoids recurrence Avoids halo vest if transarticular screw fixation is used	Potential surgical complications	Indicated in the setting of neural deficit, associated cervical fractures Usually required for chronic dislocations or recurrences with the above methods
Halo-Ilizarov distraction cast	Allows multidirectional correction of deformity Allows patients to ambulate during treatment	Complex apparatus Complications include pin tract infections and pressure sores	Requires experience in the Ilizarov method
Open reduction with the lateral approaches	Useful for irreducible dislocations Lower risk of infection than transoral approach	Prolonged surgical time Requires two separate incisions/approaches Risk of vertebral artery injury	Retropharyngeal lateral approach (of Whitesides) involves less risk to neural structures
Anterior decompression with the transoral approach	Useful for irreducible dislocations, myelopathic patients	Potential surgical complications Postoperative morbidity Requires two separate incisions/approaches in combination with posterior arthrodesis	

Suggested Readings

Corner ES. Rotatory dislocations of the atlas. Ann Surg 1907; 45:9–26.

Crockard HA, Rogers MA. Open reduction of traumatic atlanto-axial rotatory dislocation with use of the extreme lateral approach. J Bone Joint Surg 1996; 78A:431–436.

Curtis AD, Alexander M, Volker KHS, Burton PD. Magnetic resonance imaging of the transverse atlantal ligament for the evaluation of atlantoaxial instability. J Neurosurg 1991; 75:221–227.

El-Khoury GY, Clark CR, Gravett AW. Acute traumatic atlanto-axial rotatory dislocation in children. J Bone Joint Surg 1984; 66A:774–777.

Fielding JW, Hawkins RJ. Atlanto-axial rotatory fixation. J Bone Joint Surg 1977; 59A:37–44.

Fielding JW, Hawkins RJ, Hensinger RN, Francis WR. Atlantoaxial rotatory deformities. Orthop Clin North Am 1978; 9:955–967.

Graziano GP, Herzenberg JE, Hensinger RN. The halo-Ilizarov distraction cast for correction of cervical deformity. J Bone Joint Surg 1993; 75A:996–1003.

Kawabe N, Hirotani H, Tanka O. Pathomechanism of atlanto-axial rotatory fixation in children. J Pediatr Orthop 1989; 9:569–574.

Lee ST, Fairholm DJ. Transoral anterior decompression for treatment of unreducible atlantoaxial dislocations. Surg Neurol 1985; 23:244–248.

Lipson SJ. Posterior arthrodesis of the cervical spine. In: Bradford DS, ed. Master Techniques in Orthopaedic Surgery, The Spine, p. 265. Philadelphia: Lippincott-Raven, 1997.

Moore KR, Frank EH. Traumatic atlantoaxial rotatory subluxation and dislocation. Spine 1995; 20:1928–1930.

Niibayashi H. Atlantoaxial rotatory dislocation: a case report. Spine 1998; 23:1494–1496.

Phillips WA, Hensinger RN. The management of rotatory atlantoaxial subluxation in children. J Bone Joint Surg 1989; 71A:664–668.

Sherk HH, Nicholson JT. Rotatory atlanto-axial dislocations associated with ossiculum terminale and mongolism. J Bone Joint Surg 1969; 51A:957–964.

Subach BR, McLaughlin MR, Albright AL, Pollack IF. Current management of pediatric atlantoaxial rotatory subluxation. Spine 1998; 23:2174–2179.

Subin B, Liu J, Marshall J. Transoral anterior decompression and fusion of chronic irreducible atlantoaxial dislocation with spinal cord compression. Spine 1995; 20:1233–1240.

Van Holsbeeck EMA, MacKay NNS. Diagnosis of acute atlanto-axial rotatory fixation. J Bone Joint Surg 1989; 71B:90–91.

White AA, Panjabi MM. The clinical biomechanics of the occipitoatlanto-axial complex. Orthop Clin North Am 1978; 9:867–878.

Whitesides TE Jr, McDonald P. Lateral retropharyngeal approach to the upper cervical spine. Orthop Clin North Am 1978; 9:115.

Wilson TAS Jr, McWhorter JM. Atlantoaxial Injuries. In: Camins MB, O'Leary PF, eds. Disorders of the Cervical Spine, p. 271. Baltimore: Williams and Wilkins, 1992.

Case 39

Thoracolumbar Trauma with or without Neurologic Deficit

Glenn R. Rechtine II and Michael J. Bolesta

History and Physical Examination

A 16-year-old girl was involved in a motor vehicle collision and was transferred to Parkland Memorial Hospital 1 day postinjury. She was an unrestrained backseat passenger when the vehicle left the roadway and rolled. She suffered a mild closed head injury and a thoracolumbar injury. She remembers having paresthesias at the scene but was neurologically normal upon arrival at Parkland. She had multiple abrasions over her thorax and extremities. She was noted to have ankle tenderness and swelling with normal ankle radiographs.

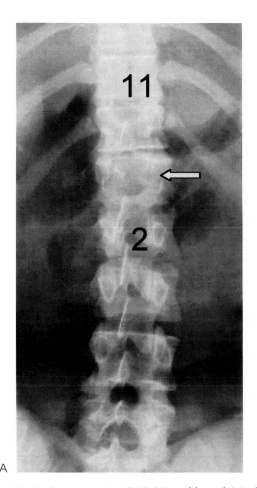 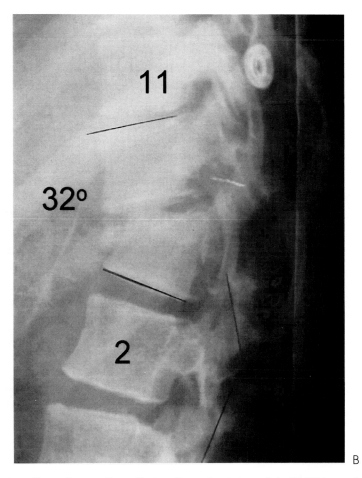

Figure 39–1. Anteroposterior (AP) (A) and lateral (B) plain radiographs revealing a flexion distraction injury of the T12/L1 vertebral bodies with communition and loss of anterior vertebral height of L1. (The arrow indicates fracture through the pedicle.) There is a 32-degree kyphotic deformity present by the Cobb method of measurement between T11 and L2 on the lateral plain radiograph.

Radiologic Findings

Supine radiographic evaluation of her thoracolumbar spine showed a T12/L1 injury (Fig. 39–1A). There was a 32-degree kyphosis over that level on the lateral plain radiograph (Fig. 39–1B). There was a combination of anterior compression, and distraction injury of the mid-body and posterior elements. This was compatible with a flexion-distraction injury, with the axis of rotation occurring through the middle of the vertebral body.

Computed tomography (CT) of the injury confirmed the flexion-distraction injury with approximately 50% canal compromise, mainly from anterior translation of T12 on L1. There was marked comminution of the body of L1, with fractures extending out into the transverse processes bilaterally (Fig. 39–2A).

Magnetic resonance imaging (MRI) was obtained to assess the extent of the ligamentous injury. There was a combined bone and ligamentous disruption. The conus appeared to be draped over the thoracolumbar kyphosis, but the canal appeared adequate (Fig. 39–2B).

Diagnosis

T12/L1 injury—flexion-distraction with anterior body compression.

Surgical Management

The patient was placed on a Roto Rest bed for initial immobilization. The closed head injury resolved. Diagnostic studies were obtained. Because of the kyphosis and

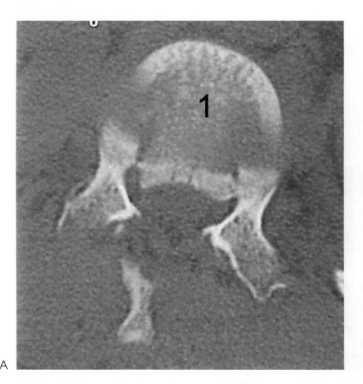
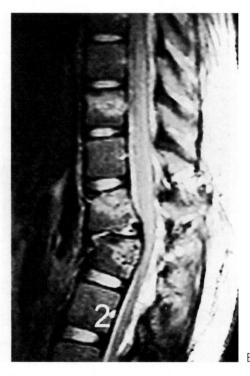

Figure 39–2. (A) Transaxial computed tomography (CT) scan revealing 50% canal occlusion with fractures extending out into the transverse processes bilaterally. (B) Sagittal magnetic resonance imaging (MRI) revealing combined bony and ligamentous disruption with the conus medullaris draped over the thoracolumbar kyphosis.

ligamentous injury, surgical reduction and stabilization was carried out on the third day postinjury (second day after transfer). Pedicle screw fixation was used for both reduction and stabilization (Fig. 39–3). The patient was mobilized on the second day after surgery in a thoracolumbar spinal orthosis (TLSO). She was discharged on the fourth day postsurgery. She was instructed to continue the TLSO for 3 months, but she was only partially compliant. Her follow-up radiographs showed no loss of correction. She returned to school in her TLSO within 4 weeks of the injury.

Discussion

The initial treatment of any trauma patient involves the airway, breathing, and circulation (ABC) to save the patient's life. Attention is given to cervical spine (c-spine) alignment. Spine immobilization is the very first action with any trauma patient. This principle is also applicable to the thoracolumbar spine. Immobilization is accomplished in the field with a back board. The board is not removed until an adequate radiographic assessment of the spine has been accomplished. Life-threatening injuries may preclude a definitive evaluation of the spine, but transfer to a kinetic bed (Roto Rest, Kinetic Concepts, Inc., San Antonio, TX) maintains immobilization.

If there is a neurologic deficit at the level of the spinal cord and the patient is seen within 8 hours of the injury, the National Acute Spinal Cord Injury Study (NASCIS III) methylprednisolone protocol should be instituted (30 mg/kg bolus then 5.4 mg/kg/hour for 24 hours if started within 3 hours of injury, and for 48

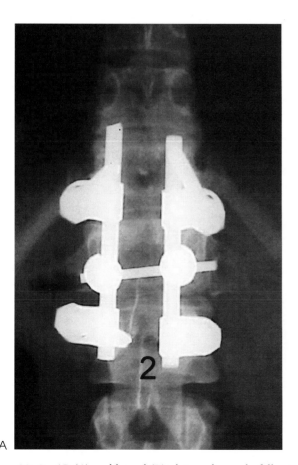
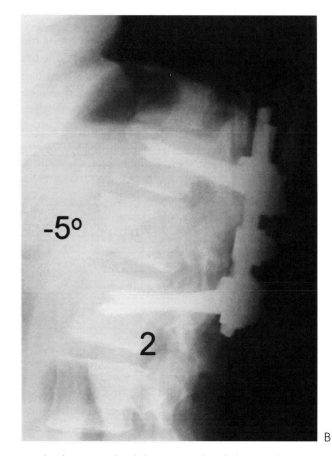

A   B

Figure 39–3. AP (A) and lateral (B) plain radiographs following surgical reduction and stabilization with pedicle screw fixation.

hours if started more than 3 and up to 8 hours postinjury). If the neurologic deficit is at root level or is the result of penetrating trauma, corticosteroids are not used. There are studies that indicate that corticosteroid use in penetrating spinal cord trauma has an adverse affect on outcome.

Long-term treatment will need to be planned. Absolute indications for emergent surgery are a progressive neurologic deficit and an associated compressive lesion. This is rare if the patient is properly immobilized. Patients on anticoagulants and those with ankylosing spondylitis are at risk for epidural hematomas, one of the most common causes of a progressive deficit. An absolute indication for surgical intervention is ligamentous instability. Complete cord injury does not require decompression.

Relative indications for surgery include spinal canal compression with associated neurologic deficit and/or unacceptable spinal alignment and deformity. Timing of surgery and definitions of unacceptable canal compromise and unacceptable deformity are extremely controversial.

Surgical Management

As with any surgery, preoperative planning is important for achieving the best surgical outcome. Having the appropriate equipment and personnel allows the surgery to proceed smoothly.

The patient is brought to the operating suite on a kinetic bed or other suitable immobilization. Anesthesia is induced, taking care to protect the cervical spine, especially if a formal clearance has not been done.

The patient is then placed prone on an appropriate frame or table. If the fracture stability will allow, having the abdomen free will make the job of ventilation easier as well as decreasing blood loss from epidural veins. An intraoperative portable radiograph is then done to assess spinal alignment.

The back is then prepared. If possible, open wounds should be draped out of the operative field to decrease the risk of wound contamination. Extra care is taken in this step, as the infection rate is much higher in trauma cases than in elective spine surgery.

As the spine is approached, soft tissues should be handled carefully. They have already been injured, so every attempt should be made to minimize surgical trauma. The retractors should be released on a regular basis to decrease paravertebral muscle ischemia.

Postoperative Management

The patient can be placed on the kinetic bed for a day or two postoperatively. This will allow for pulmonary toilet until the patient recovers enough to begin active mobilization. Good nutrition is important for wound healing, so the patient should be started on a diet or fed intravenously to prevent malnutrition.

Discussion

The treatment of thoracic and lumbar fractures has evolved over the course of the twentieth century. Initially, bed rest was the only option. With the advent of posterior instrumentation for deformity surgery, this technology was applied to trauma as well. The advance of anterior surgery has provided more options (Table 39–1).

Table 39–1
Possible Treatment Options

	Ignore	Brace	Cast	Recumbency	Surgery		
					Anterior	Posterior	Both
Spinous process fracture	X						
Transverse process fracture	X						
Single compression fracture (no ligamentous injury)	X	X	X				
Multiple compression fracture (no ligamentous injury)		X	X	X			
Burst fracture—no deficit (no ligamentous injury)		X	X	X	X	X	
Burst fracture—incomplete (deficit improving; no ligamentous injury)		X	X	X	X	X	
Burst fracture—complete deficit (no ligamentous injury)		X	X	X	X	X	
Chance (flexion-distraction) injury		X	X	X		X	
Fracture—dislocation or slice fracture				X		X	X

Anterior instrumentation has recently matured as well. Almost coming full circle, there has also been a resurgence in the use of nonoperative methods.

The critical factors with any spinal injury involve protection of the spinal cord function and restoring structural integrity of the spinal column. The treatment plan must address both. In the case of a complete cord injury, the aim is spinal stability, so that rehabilitation may proceed.

Alternative Methods of Management

There are nonoperative and operative options for the treatment of thoracolumbar injuries.

Nonoperative

Benign neglect is appropriate if assessment of the injury determines that no further treatment is necessary (e.g., isolated transverse process fractures, single-level minimal thoracic compression fracture with no kyphosis or ligamentous injury).

Bracing is used for compression fractures with no ligamentous injury. A TLSO or lumbosacral orthosis (LSO) is fit, depending on level of these stable injuries.

Reduction and casting are appropriate for fractures with deformity. Application requires a special operating table (Risser or Goldthwaite).

Recumbency is used for injuries with acute bony instability that otherwise would require surgical stabilization. A Roto Rest bed or other kinetic therapy is utilized for 4 to 6 weeks, followed by bracing until approximately 3 months postinjury.

Operative

Posterior surgery, such as decompression directly or indirectly (ligamentotaxis), is another option. Indirect reduction is effective when distraction and deformity correction is applied within 24 hours of injury. Direct decompression is technically demanding, as the compressive elements are commonly anterior.

Long rods with hook fixation are applied two levels above and two levels below the injury and provide better leverage for reduction and maintenance of reduction.

The rod-long, fuse-short option is used to fuse only the segment involved with the injury. Hardware is removed at 9 to 12 months to allow return of motion at the unfused but instrumented segments.

Short rods or plates—pedicle fixation—spares motion segments. Severe anterior column disruption is associated with failure of this type of construction.

Anterior surgery and decompression are done under direct vision.

Anterior lateral instrumentation, such as plate or rod systems, should not contact the vascular structures. Strut options include autograft (ilium, fibulae, rib), allograft (femur, tibia, humerus, fibula), or metal cage.

Combined anterior and posterior approaches are used for fracture dislocations with global instability.

Type of Management	Advantages	Disadvantages	Comments
Nonoperative			
Benign neglect	No further treatment necessary i.e., transverse process fractures	If instability is persistent and undetected—risk of deformity, neurologic deficit	
Bracing	Useful for compression fractures with no ligamentous injury	Risk of progressive deformity if ligamentous injury is present but undetected	Most frequently used method of treatment
Reduction and casting	Useful for fractures with deformity	Need for special OR table (Risser or Goldthwaite)	Especially useful in potentially uncompliant patients
Operative			
Posterior surgery	Able to decompress directly or indirectly (ligamentataxis)	Indirect decompression most effective if performed within 24 hours of injury	Direct compression is technically demanding from posterior approach
Anterior surgery	Decompression under direct vision	Not applicable in cases of fracture-dislocations	Technically more difficult than posterior approach

Complications

Thoracolumbar injuries are commonly associated with other injuries and thus encompass the multiple trauma patient. This contributes to the relatively high complication rate associated with these injuries.

Pulmonary

The most common cause of death is pulmonary emboli. Pneumonia and atelectasis are common. Adult respiratory distress syndrome (ARDS) is often associated with polytrauma.

Neurologic

Progressive neurologic deficits are rare but do occur. Proper immobilization initially is paramount to minimize the possibility of neurologic deterioration. Postoperatively, epidural hematomas and displaced bone graft fragments, from posterior, posterolateral, or transpedicular grafting, can compress the neural structures.

Vascular

For the posterior approach, vascular injuries should be extremely rare. Patients with ankylosing spondylitis are notable exceptions. In anterior surgery, the vascular structures are at greater risk during and after surgery. The instrumentation must be placed well away from the artery so that pulsation of the vessel against the implant will not erode the arterial wall. Venous contact is avoided lest thromboembolism supervene.

Infection

Postoperative wound infections occur in 7 to 15% of thoracic and lumbar fractures treated operatively. This is higher than similar surgery for degenerative spinal disease or cervical trauma.

Hardware Failure

The hardware can fail acutely or chronically. In the acute setting, the hardware can fail by loss of fixation, usually by bony failure. This results from reduction force that exceeds the strength of the patient's bone. This most commonly occurs in the patient with osteopenia.

Decubiti

Skin breakdown is much more common in the patient with a spinal cord injury. It also occurs with prolonged immobilization on a back board during transport to the hospital. Every effort should be made to remove the board as soon as medically possible.

Suggested Readings

Akbarnia B, Crandall D, Burkus K, Matthews T. Use of long rods and a short arthrodesis for burst fractures of the thoracolumbar spine. J Bone Joint Surg 1994; 76A:1629–1635.

Bracken M, Shepard M, Holford T, et al. Administration of methylprednisolone for 24 or 48 hours or tirilazad mesylate for 48 hours in the treatment of acute spinal cord injury. Results of the Third National Acute Spinal Cord Injury Randomized Controlled Trial. National Acute Spinal Cord Injury Study. JAMA 1997; 277:1597–1604.

Heary R, Vaccaro A, Mesa J, et al. Steroids and gunshot wounds to the spine. Neurosurgery 1997; 41:576–583.

Kornberg M, Rechtine G, Herndon W, Reinert C, Dupuy T. Surgical stabilization of thoracic and lumbar spine fractures: a retrospective study in a military population. J Trauma 1982; 24:140–146.

McCormack T, Karaikovic E, Gaines R. The load sharing classification of spine fractures. Spine 1994; 19:1741–1744.

Case 40
Low Lumbar Fracture with or without Neurologic Deficit
Thomas D. Kramer and Alan M. Levine

History and Physical Examination

A 46-year-old man fell 9 feet out of a deer stand, sustaining both a spine and left lower extremity injury. He did not lose consciousness but was unable to walk from the scene and was transferred to the Maryland Shock Trauma Unit. On admission, his pulse rate was 75 bpm and his blood pressure was 142/71. There was marked tenderness and edema surrounding the left ankle but intact pulses and sensation. In addition, there was diffuse lumbar spine tenderness without any palpable step-off. His motor and sensory neurologic examination in the lower extremities as well as his perirectal sensation and tone were normal.

Radiologic Findings

Radiographs of the left ankle revealed a pilon fracture with subluxation of the mortise (Fig. 40–1). Anteroposterior (AP) and lateral radiographs of the spine revealed

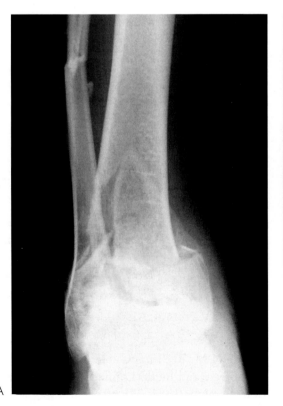
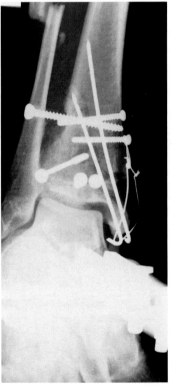

A   B

Figure 40–1. *Anteroposterior (AP) view at admission (A) of the ankle shows comminution of the distal tibial plafond. Postoperative AP view (B) shows a combination of internal fixation and an external fixateur utilized to restore the anatomic configuration of the joint.*

an L4 burst fracture, along with 10% compression fracture of L2 (Fig. 40–2A, B). Specifically, the AP radiograph showed comminution of the L4 vertebral body with no apparent interpedicular widening. The lateral radiograph revealed local kyphosis as well as retropulsed bone from the superior endplate displaced posteriorly into the neural canal. Computed tomography (CT) scan of the lumbar spine confirmed the above-mentioned findings, with evidence of 80% canal compromise at the L4 level (Fig. 40–2C).

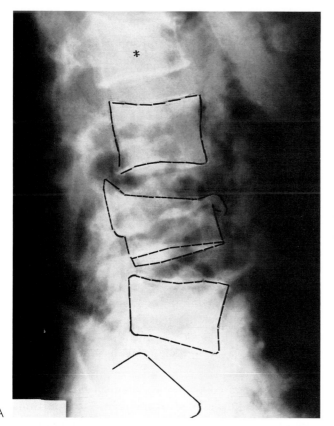

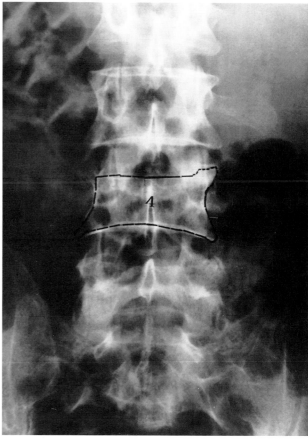

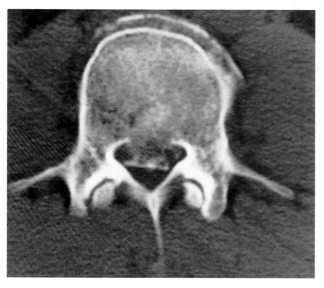

Figure 40–2. Lateral view of the spine at admission (A) shows compression of the vertical body of L4 with a kyphotic angular deformity, across the L3/L4 segmental and a reciprocal increase in lordosis across L4/L5. There is retropulsion of the posterior superior corner of L4. There is compression of the L2 body (*). The AP view (B) shows symmetrical compression of the entire L4 body. Axial computed tomography (CT) image through the L4 body (C) of the level of the pedicles shows severe retropulsion and canal compromise (80%) with intact posterior elements and pedicles.

Diagnosis

Low lumbar burst fracture without neurologic deficit.

Discussion, Part I

Low lumbar injuries are sustained by young male patients, with most in the third decade of life. The most common mechanisms are either a fall from a height or motor vehicle accident. There is a correlation between low lumbar fractures and lower extremity injury, especially those resulting from fall. The anatomic relationship of the conus and cauda equina to the lumbar spine largely determines the pattern of neurologic deficit. In the distal portion of the canal, the cauda equina occupies less than one-third of the cross-sectional area. The sacral roots lie posterior within the canal. Thus, the only indication of neurologic injury might be decreased rectal tone or sensation. Neurologic injuries related to low lumbar fractures are usually of two types. The first is a complete cauda equina syndrome. This is most commonly associated with severe burst fractures with a large fragment retropulsed within the neural canal. The second type is an isolated or combined root injury. Isolated root injury is caused by a retropulsed fragment of bone that encroaches the exiting root between it and the undersurface of the lamina. Root deficits may also be seen with lumbar burst fractures that have a sagittal split in the lamina or spinous process. These are commonly associated with dural tears.

The initial portion of the radiograph assessment of a low lumbar fracture are well-centered AP and lateral radiographs. The normal lumbar lordosis is less than 60 degrees, with segmental lordosis ranging from 11 degrees at L1/L2 to 20 degrees at L5/S1. In addition, the facet joint orientation in the lumbar spine is more sagittal, leading to progressive increases in the flexion-extension arc and decreases in the rotational arc. This fact tends to negate the flexion moment placed on the normal lordotic lumbar spine. Therefore, most low lumbar injuries are a result of axial loading rather than severe flexion mechanisms.

All burst fractures are caused by a combined mechanism of flexion and axial loading with the pattern of the injury related to the relative proportions of the forces applied. According to the Denis classification, a type A burst fracture has little kyphosis but significant axial compression of the body with comminution of both superior and inferior endplates. The body-pedicle junction is disrupted, and frequently posterior element fractures occur. This pattern occurs infrequently in the low lumbar spine. Denis type B burst fractures consist of a fracture of the superior endplate and a portion of the body, with retropulsion of the posterior superior corner of the body into the canal. The critical features on CT axial images are that the lower portions of the pedicles remain intact, are not splayed apart, and are in continuity with the body. This type includes significant anterior body compression and relative sparing of the posterior elements. This burst pattern is the most common in the low lumbar spine (L3, L4, and L5). Of particular importance is the presence of either a longitudinal laminar fracture or midsagittal split of the spinous process on CT scan. A burst fracture associated with either of the above, with the presence of any neurologic deficit and a significant degree of canal compromise, is virtually pathognomonic for a posterior dural laceration.

Nonoperative Management

There are three major groups of patients with low lumbar burst fractures: (1) those with significant deficit and/or dural laceration with varying degrees of structural disruption; (2) those with minor root deficits or who are neurologically normal with minimal structural derangement; and (3) those with minor root deficits or neurologically intact with significant canal compromise, translation, comminution, or kyphosis. Generally, those in groups 1 and 3 do better with surgical intervention and those in group 2 with nonoperative care.

There is even controversy about what constitutes nonoperative care. Certainly to immobilize L5, a thoracolumbar spinal orthosis (TLSO) (a single leg spica jacket or cast) is necessary, but the type of orthosis necessary for adequate immobilization of L4 may depend on body habitus. Some authors have advocated 3 to 6 weeks of bed rest before mobilization, whereas others mobilize the patient immediately. Generally stable low lumbar fractures can be managed in a TLSO with immediate immobilization if this does not cause severe pain.

Surgical Management

The surgical approach to most low lumbar burst fractures is from the posterior because of the difficulty in obtaining adequate fixation from an anterior approach.

The patient in this case was taken to the operating room, where he was placed under general endotracheal anesthesia. One gram of cephalosporin was administered. The patient was turned to the prone position on a Stryker frame. The back was prepped and draped in the usual sterile fashion. A longitudinal incision was made from L2 to L5 after estimating the level by reference to the iliac crest. The incision was extended sharply through the skin and subcutaneous tissue. All bleeding was controlled using electrocautery. The soft tissues were stripped off both sides of the spinous process of L4, using subperiosteal dissection. A marker was placed on L4 and lateral radiograph confirmed the position. The midline dissection was then extended proximally to the L2 spinous process and distally to the L5 spinous process. All soft tissues were also dissected out laterally on both sides until the transverse processes of L3/L5 were clearly visualized. The facet capsules were removed off L3/L4 and L4/L5 facet joints bilaterally. The L2/L3 facet capsules were identified bilaterally, and extreme caution was used not to violate these capsules. The interspinous ligaments were left intact at all levels.

Using the pars interarticularis, transverse process, and facet joints as landmarks, pedicle screws were inserted into the pedicles of L3, L4, and L5. The L3 pedicle screws were inserted slightly distal to the normal starting position to avoid damage to the L2/L3 facet joint capsules upon insertion. The screws in L4 were canted inferiorly to capture the solid uncomminuted bone in the inferior portion of the body. The positions of these screws were verified by both anteroposterior and lateral radiographs. The transverse processes of L3, L4, and L5 as well as the lateral portions of L3/L4 and L4/L5 facet joints were decorticated. A separate 1-inch vertical incision was then placed over the right posterior superior iliac crest through which corticocancellous and cancellous graft was harvested. The crest was then packed with Gelfoam soaked in thrombin. Spinal connectors were attached to the L4 pedicle screws. Two universal rods were connected to the proximal and distal pedicle screws. Slight distraction and lordosis were applied to restore the vertebral body height and sagittal alignment respectively (Fig. 40–3). A transverse connector

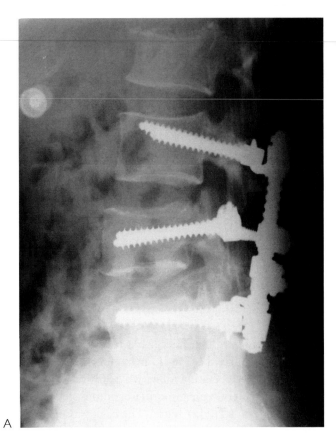
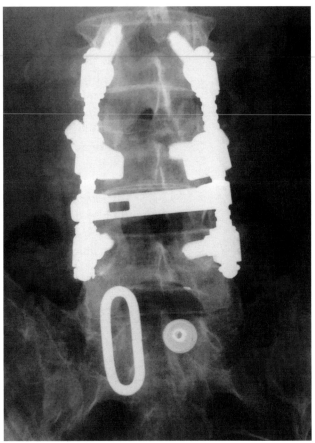

A   B

Figure 40–3. Postoperative lateral (A) and AP (B) views in an orthosis show restoration of body height and sagittal alignment. Note the screw fixation in the fractured body, which allows restoration of lordosis by an anteriorly directed force applied through that screw using a connector. Axial height is restored by the L3 and L5 screws.

was placed between the L4 and L5 screws. The iliac bone graft was placed into the lateral gutters extending from the L3 transverse processes to the L5 transverse processes. A hemovac drain was placed under the lumbodorsal fascia. The fascia was closed with interrupted 0 Vicryl sutures, reattaching it to the undisturbed interspinous ligaments. The subcutaneous tissues were closed with 2-0 Vicryl sutures, and the skin with staples.

Postoperative Management

The patient was placed in the supine position for 1 to 2 days. A postoperative TLSO was manufactured on postoperative day 2. The patient then began transfers and gait training.

The wound healed uneventfully. The patient was initially kept in the brace for 3 months. He was noncompliant with bracewear and also resumed smoking postoperatively. The brace was continued for 3 additional months, with the patient allowed to sleep without it. The fusion healed uneventfully with satisfactory alignment and clinically without pain (Fig. 40–4).

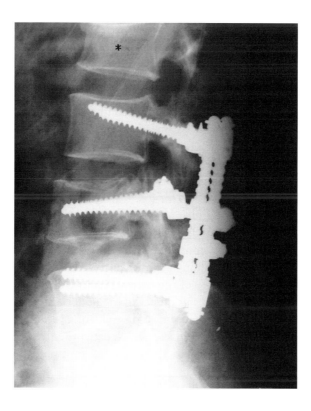

Figure 40–4. This follow-up lateral radiograph shows maintenance of alignment of the reduction at L4 as well as the L2 compression fracture level (*).

Discussion, Part II

Injuries of the lumbar spine disrupt the normal lordotic alignment of the spine, and restoration of that lordotic alignment is critical to overall vertebral mechanics. Failure to maintain or restore the normal sagittal alignment in the lower lumbar spine has led to degenerative changes and symptoms in long-term follow-up. The treatment goals are anatomic reduction of the injury; rigid fixation of the fracture; decompression of the neural elements, if applicable; maintenance of sagittal alignment; conservation of motion segments; prevention of complications.

The decision for nonoperative versus operative treatment for low lumbar spine injuries should be based on the stability of the fracture, the presence of neurologic deficit, and the sagittal/axial spinal alignment.

Stability implies that the fracture pattern created by the trauma is not likely to change position with physiologic loads. Therefore, no additional neurologic deficit or increasing deficit would be experienced.

The presence of a neurologic deficit should raise suspicion for the presence of significant instability. Nerve root involvement with localized compression may be improved by direct exploration and decompression. Patients with sagittal spinous process fractures, neurologic deficit, and dural tears with roots outside the dural sac also benefit from direct decompression and dural repair.

Maintenance of normal lumbar sagittal alignment is critical to preserve the normal weightbearing axis of the body, and therefore for optimal function and spinal mechanics.

Nonoperative Management

Nonoperative management is usually reserved for patients who are neurologically intact or who have minor degrees of root irritation and with minimal or moderate deformity (less than 25 degrees of relative kyphosis) and lesser degrees of canal compromise. This also includes compression fractures with less than 50% anterior compression. For burst fractures, the major consideration is that there is minimal disruption of the posterior elements and minimal disruption of alignment.

Improper selection of an orthosis for a desired level can lead to increased motion at the injured level by immobilizing the levels above it. In general, a TLSO should be used for immobilization for fractures above L5. For L5 fractures and below, a thigh extension must be added to successfully control fracture motion. Compliant bracewear for 3 months is mandatory for nonoperative management of these fractures. In addition, these patients must be monitored with serial radiographs for any change in fracture alignment. Although studies of patients treated nonoperatively have claimed good results, a majority of the patients had significant back pain. The proportion of patients with back pain was higher in the nonoperatively treated group than in the operatively treated group. A recent study evaluating the long-term (5- to 12-year) follow-up (mean 7.8 years) of operatively treated patients only with low lumbar burst fractures showed a 95% fusion rate and SF-36 scores comparable to a normal population sample.

Surgical Management

Surgical management of lower lumbar burst fractures is reserved for fractures with more than 25 degrees of relative kyphosis, a neurologic deficit, or a dural tear. The preferred treatment is a posterior spinal reduction and fusion using a three-level pedicle screw construct. A direct decompression via laminotomy/laminectomy along with indirect decompression via fracture reduction is added for any neurologic deficit.

Anatomic Fracture Reduction

Deforming forces of the fracture must be directly counteracted by the instrumentation system. All attempts should be made to preserve and maintain as many mobile levels as possible. The reduction and fixation should include an element of distraction and lordosis to restore the proper lumbar lordosis and sagittal alignment. This can be accomplished through a short-segment rod system or pedicle system.

Maintenance of Correction

Maintenance of correction is directly related to the rigidity of fixation and the ability to counteract both the deforming forces and normal physiologic forces of the lumbar spine. Load sharing, either with intact posterior elements or with supplemental anterior grafting, should be considered.

Decompression of Neural Elements

Debate exists as to the method of decompression for patients with neural deficit. Late spinal stenosis does not occur in patients either operated on or not operated on in whom a reasonable anatomic reduction occurs. Resorption of residual bone within the canal predictably occurs both with and without surgery. For patients with inadequate decompression with posterior instrumentation/reduction or those who present

- Mistakes are often made when evaluating sagittal alignment of the lumbar spine. The critical step is to determine the relative kyphosis at the fracture level and not the absolute kyphosis. If the absolute kyphosis is considered in the treatment rationale, an unacceptably high proportion of these patients will have significant back pain. In addition, those patients with stable low lumbar burst patterns must be followed carefully with serial radiographs to detect any progressive kyphosis.

late (more than 2 weeks after injury) and require decompression of the dural sac, an anterior corpectomy with direct decompression is the most effective approach.

Maintenance of Sagittal Alignment

Maintaining sagittal alignment is crucial to overall spinal mechanics. For low lumbar fractures, this might necessitate screw fixation into the pelvis. Instrumentation to the pelvis must preserve the normal lumbosacral angle, lumbosacral lordosis, and overall sagittal alignment of the spine, and is difficult to achieve through an anterior approach. Use of a screw in the fractured vertebral body helps load share and is preferable to only two sets of screws.

Minimizing Fixation Length

It is essential to maximize the number of mobile lumbar segments. There is a fine balance between the number of levels requiring instrumentation and stabilization and preservation of important lumbar motion segments. Hook fixation is not feasible for these fractures.

Alternative Methods of Management

An additional surgical option for low lumbar burst fractures is the anterior approach. Anterior procedures are rarely indicated except for those with inadequate decompression following a successful posterior reduction and stabilization. The only advantage of an anterior procedure is a more effective decompression of the neural elements by way of a corpectomy. Most anterior plate and rod/screw systems are not designed for fixation to the L5 or S1 segments as a result of lumbosacral plexus and iliac vessels. Thus, adequate stabilization for L4 and L5 fractures is limited anteriorly. The use of a stand alone anterior strut bone graft without instrumentation has universally provided poor correction and maintenance of spinal sagittal alignment.

Type of Management	Advantages	Disadvantages	Comments
Nonoperative/orthosis	Minimal risk	Need absolute compliance; Difficulty maintaining reduction	Useful in cases involving <25 relative kyphosis, <50% vertebral height loss, and minimal canal compromise (<30%)
Posterior instrumented reduction and fusion with/without decompression	Anatomic reduction; Rigid fixation; Ease of direct and indirect decompression with/without dural repair; Low complication rate	Loss of correction with extensive comminution of vertebral body	Indicated for unstable fractures: >25 relative kyphosis; high-grade canal compromise; neurologic deficit/dural tear
Anterior decompression and fusion	Direct decompression of neural elements	Difficulty with instrumentation due to iliac vessels; Poor correction and maintenance of sagittal alignment	Useful with fractures >2 weeks old or persistent neurologic deficit after posterior instrumented reduction and fusion

Complications

Complications are usually associated with the instrumentation of these injuries. They include pseudoarthrosis, hood dislodgment, failure of sacral fixation, and iatrogenic flatback. Complications are avoided by careful preoperative planning, meticulous surgical technique, appropriate selection of fixation, and a thorough understanding of spinal biomechanics and anatomy.

Suggested Readings

An HS, Simpson JM, Ebraheim NA, et al. Low lumbar burst fractures: comparison between conservative and surgical treatments. Orthopedics 1992; 15:367–373.

An HS, Vaccaro A, Cotler JM, et al. Low lumbar burst fractures: comparison among body cast, Harrington rod, Luque rod, and Steffee plate. Spine 1991; 16(suppl 8):S440–444.

Andreychik DA, Alander DH, Senica KM, et al. Burst fractures of the second through fifth lumbar vertebrae. Clinical and radiographic results. J Bone Joint Surg 1996; 78A:1156–1166.

Comissa FP, Eismont FJ, Green BH. Dural laceration occurring with burst fracture and associated lumbar fractures. J Bone Joint Surg 1989; 71A:44–52.

Levine AM. Low lumbar spine trauma. In: Levine AM, Eismont F, Garfin S, Zigler J, eds. Spine Trauma, pp. 452–495. Philadelphia: WB Saunders, 1998.

Mick CA, Carl A, Sachs B, et al. Burst fractures of the fifth lumbar vertebra. Spine 1993; 18:1878–1884.

Stephens GC, Devito DP, McNamara MJ. Segmental fixation of lumbar burst fractures with Cotrel-Dubousset instrumentation. J Spinal Disord 1992; 5:344–348.

Case 41
Sacral Fractures
Kirkham B. Wood and Francis Denis

History and Physical Examination

An 18-year-old man was an unrestrained passenger in a motor vehicle accident when the driver lost control at approximately 55 mph. Although the vehicle rolled several times, there was no reported loss of consciousness. On admission to the emergency room, the patient complained of pain in his buttocks, groin, right thigh, and right posterior calf. Multiple facial lacerations were present and closed primarily in the emergency room. Physical examination revealed pain with compression of the iliac wings. The ankle reflex on the right was absent, and strength of the right gastrocnemius was diminished (3/5) when compared with the left. There was no sensory deficit. The remainder of the neurologic exam of the lower extremities was within normal limits.

Radiologic Findings

Lumbosacral spine radiographs including the pelvis revealed minimally displaced fractures of the superior and inferior rami of the right hemipelvis (Fig. 41–1). A Ferguson view of the upper sacrum revealed internal disruption of the architecture of the first right sacral foramen (Fig. 41–2). Computed tomography (CT) examination of the sacrum confirmed bony compression of the right sacral ala with

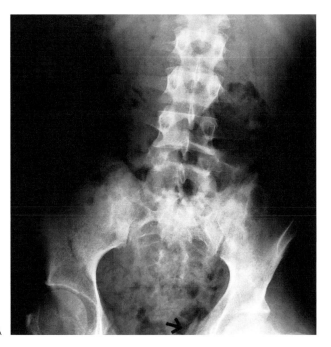
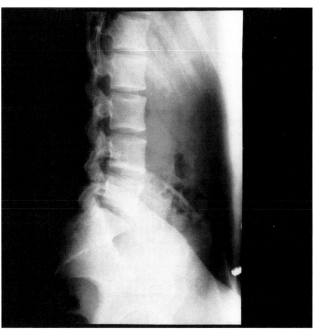

A

B

Figure 41–1. Posteroanterior (PA) (A) and lateral (B) radiographs of the lumbosacral spine and pelvis reveal fractures of the right superior and inferior pubic rami (arrow).

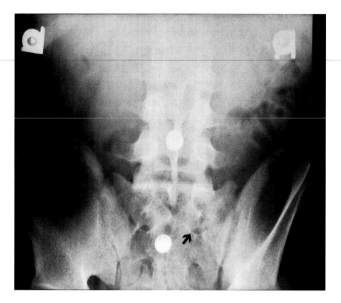

Figure 41–2. Ferguson view of the upper sacrum allows improved viewing of the upper sacrum. Some disruption of the architecture of the first sacral foramen can be seen (arrow).

extension into the S1 foramen (Fig. 41–3). Magnetic resonance imaging (MRI) examination demonstrated edematous compression of the S1 nerve root on the right side (Fig. 41–4). Cystometrography with CT follow-up also revealed extravasation of dye at the inferior pole of the bladder (Fig. 41–5).

Diagnosis

Lateral compression injury resulting in right alar and foraminal fractures involving the first sacral foramen (zones I and II) with sciatica secondary to high-energy blunt trauma and compression of the S1 nerve root. The fracture is considered to be in zone I as it originates in the lateral sacral ala, but also in zone II because it traverses the neural foramen. The patient also has right-sided rami fractures and a rupture of the neck of the bladder.

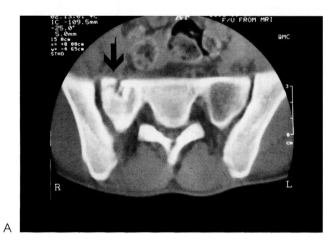

A

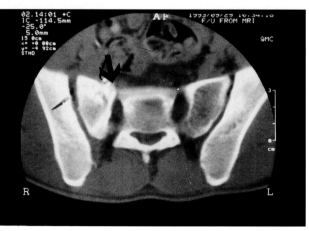

B

Figure 41–3. Two axial computed tomography (CT) images through the sacrum illustrate the fracture through the lateral ala (zone I) (A, arrow), with extension into the first sacral foramen (zone II) (B, arrow).

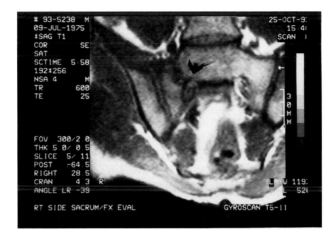

Figure 41–4. Axial magnetic resonance imaging (MRI) shows edematous compression of the S1 nerve root (arrow).

Surgical Management

The patient was medically stabilized and initially underwent surgical repair of a tear of the urethral neck of the bladder. His pelvic fractures were treated with bed rest followed by progressive touch-down ambulation. Initially, his fracture of the sacrum was managed nonoperatively with observation; however, due to persistence of weakness and pain in the right leg and local calf and hamstring tenderness with a positive straight leg raise, 6 weeks after the injury it was elected to proceed with operative decompression. (The patient's back and buttock pain had resolved.) Electromyogram (EMG) examination at 3 weeks showed decreased conduction in the right S1 nerve root.

The patient was taken to the operating theatre, where general anesthesia was administered via endotracheal intubation. The patient was placed prone on a four-poster frame, and the back and buttocks were prepped with an iodine

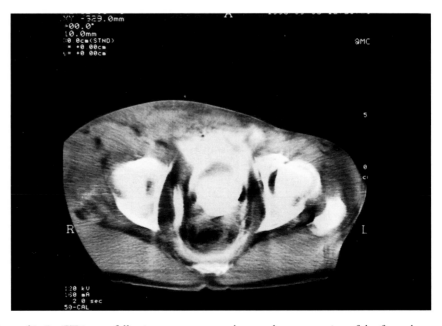

Figure 41–5. CT image following cystometrography reveals extravasation of dye from the torn bladder neck.

solution and draped in a sterile manner. An incision was made in the midline from the spinous process of L5 to the spinous process of S3. The position was radiographically verified. Subperiosteal dissection was carried out along the posterior arches of S1, S2, and S3. This revealed clear evidence of a fracture line along the right hemilaminae. The spinal canal was entered at the L5/S1 interspace by first removing the ligamentum flavum on the right side and then removing the S1 lamina using Kerrison rongeurs. At the level of the distal aspect of the medial wall of the S1 pedicle, the S1 nerve root ganglion was compressed by the bony fracture and was decompressed. Using rongeurs, the S1 nerve root was followed through to its foramen, where further bony compression was encountered. Using a combination of rongeurs and a power-driven burr to excavate bone adjacent to the foramen, bone from the compressed foramen was delivered into the created void, thus enlarging the foramen and decompressing the nerve root. The wound was closed in three layers using absorbable sutures over a Hemovac drain. Estimated blood loss was 150 cc.

Postoperative Management

The patient was allowed to ambulate without restrictions while in the hospital. The drain was removed on the second postoperative day. On the third postoperative day, he was discharged.

At 6 weeks postoperatively, the patient reported no leg pain and subjective improvement in his leg weakness. By 3 months, he was functioning in a completely normal manner with no leg pain or weakness. The only finding was a reduced ankle reflex on the right side. The patient's pelvic fracture was pain free and united, as demonstrated radiographically (Fig. 41–6).

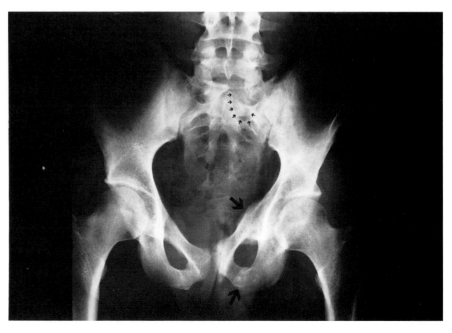

Figure 41–6. PA view of the pelvis shows the healed pelvic fractures (large arrows) as well as the laminectomy defect (small arrows) with restoration of the architecture of the S1 foramen anteriorly.

Discussion

The first step in treating patients with pelvic fractures and leg pain is recognizing that sciatica can and does occur with fractures of the sacrum, especially those involving the foraminal level and/or the central canal. Sacral fractures can result in neurologic symptoms and deficits to the lower extremities as well as to the urinary, rectal, or sexual systems.

Fractures of the sacrum can be difficult to visualize on routine radiographs, and thus the diagnosis requires a high index of suspicion. The Ferguson method often produces the best anteroposterior (AP) view of the upper sacrum and the clearest demonstration of foraminal involvement. AP or lateral tomography can be helpful as well. CT scans can provide the optimal imaging of the bony detail and is indicated whenever neurologic changes are present. MR provides exquisite information on the status of the nerve roots.

Denis and colleagues (1988) studied 236 sacral fractures in 776 pelvic injuries over a 10-year period and classified them as shown in Figure 41–7. Zone I (alar zone) involves fractures through the lateral ala and tend to be most commonly due to lateral compression. Zone II (foraminal zone) involves one or more of the sacral foramina. These commonly extend longitudinally over multiple foramina. Fractures here may also include the lateral ala, but not the central canal. Zone III (central canal) fractures involve the central nerve root canal, but usually also include zones I and II. Transverse fractures, burst fractures of the sacrum, or fracture dislocations are examples of zone III injuries.

Neurologic sequelae secondary to the sacral fractures were seen in 51 of Denis and colleagues' 236 patients (22%) and are much more common in fractures involving zone III (50 to 60%) than zones II (20 to 30%) or III (0 to 10%). Longitudinal fractures through the lateral ala or foramina are more likely to produce sciatica-type radiculopathy than bowel or bladder symptoms. Transverse fractures, which will occur more commonly in the distal two-thirds of the sacrum, are more likely to involve the distal sacral roots through the central canal and produce

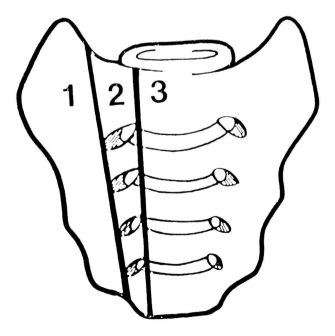

Figure 41–7. Sacral zones.

PEARLS

- Plain anteroposterior radiography of the pelvis may often miss upper sacral bony pathology due to the curved nature of the sacrum. A Ferguson view of the upper sacrum is helpful to define the anatomy, especially of the sacral foramen.
- Due to the sacrum's complex anatomy, CT scanning of the fractured sacrum may be the most helpful radiologic exam. However, it is important that the images be sectioned at 1-mm intervals as subtle foraminal pathology otherwise may be missed. Appropriate tilting of the gantry is also important, depending on the aspect of the sacrum being imaged. Sagittal and coronal reconstruction can also be very helpful.
- In cases of severe weakness of the gastrocnemius complex, it is important to assess not only the S1 nerve root but also the S2. The motor examination may be normal or nearly normal in cases of isolated S1 entrapment; however, it is much less commonly so when both roots are involved.

pathology of the bowel and bladder. Shearing of the spinal canal occurs as the trunk is displaced forward on the distal pelvis. The neurologic pattern will vary depending on the type, level of injury, and the degree of displacement.

After defining the local sacral injuries, it is important to analyze the level of concomitant pelvic ring pathology. Many isolated injuries especially to zones I and II can be treated nonoperatively with bed rest followed by progressive ambulation. However, many unstable injuries to the sacrum also involve anterior pelvic disruptions and will therefore guide the treatment planning. Diastases of the pubic symphysis may render alar fractures unstable and often require plating. Vertical shear fractures through the ala or the foramen will also typically involve disruption of the anterior pelvic ring. The L5 nerve root may become entrapped against the alar fragment or the transverse process of L5 (posttraumatic far-out syndrome). Early traction with or without follow-up open reduction and internal fixation of the pelvic fracture may relieve the radicular symptoms. Treatment of injuries involving zone III without neurologic deficit are similar to those of zones I and II, and is aimed primarily at pelvic stabilization.

When there is neurologic embarrassment of the distal sacral nerve roots, early and meticulous decompression is recommended. Attention to compression at both the central and foraminal levels is important, and both components may have to be addressed. Late decompression can be much more difficult in part due to the smallness of the central canal as well as epineural and perineural scarring. Not only is the surgery made more difficult, but the chances for functional recovery are lessened principally due to the persisting fibrous strangulation of the nerves even after decompression of the bony impingement.

Cystometrography (CMG) is quite useful in the evaluation of cauda equina damage, especially in fractures involving the proximal sacrum and those associated with neurogenic bladders. A CMG should be obtained in all patients with questionable bladder involvement and probably all patients with zone III injuries because of the very high rate of neurologic involvement.

Alternative Methods of Management

Alternatives to early decompression of a sacral fracture with radiculopathy include traction and/or bed rest followed by early ambulation, late decompression, or open reduction and internal fixation. Many injuries through zones I and/or II with isolated involvement of one or two nerve roots can be managed nonoperatively. As is the case with other acute radiculopathies (e.g., herniated lumbar disc), an initial trial of rest followed by progressive increase in activity is indicated. If after 6 to 8 weeks has passed the sciatica remains severe, or if CT scanning shows dramatic (>50%) reduction of the foramen size, surgical treatment (decompression) may be indicated. Late (>3 months) decompression remains an option if nonoperative care has not been satisfactory. However, due to the tightness of the compromised canal as well as epineural fibrosis that can follow such injuries, late decompressions can be very difficult and oftentimes less than completely successful in neural recovery. Open reduction and internal fixation is rarely indicated in the treatment of sacral fractures with or without radiculopathy, except where there has been concomitant disruption of the pelvic ring such as in vertical shear or open-book injuries. If the patient's medical condition does not allow early surgery, closed reduction of vertical shear injuries may decompress the root and keep the fracture reduced until definitive fixation can be provided.

Type of Management	Advantages	Disadvantages	Comments
Nonoperative	Minimal risk; may be appropriate for nonsurgical patients	Morbidity of bed rest; hospital cost	Many acute radiculopathies may resolve without surgery
Early decompression	Chances for neurologic recovery are greatest	May be unnecessary in some situations (e.g., minimal compression; sensory defect only)	Important to rule out other musculoskeletal pathology (spine) as source of neurologic findings
Open reduction and internal fixation	Indicated for unstable sacral fractures associated with pelvic ring disruption	Cost; surgical morbidity; risk of infection	Rarely indicated for isolated sacral pathology
Late decompression	Pathology and deficits may be more clearly defined	Epineural scarring may make dissection difficult	Neurologic recovery may be variable

PITFALL

• Acute sacral radiculopathy from fractures through zone II may resolve with a nonoperative approach. However, if too much time passes before an operative treatment is attempted, epineural scarring may make exposure and decompression of the injured nerve root difficult. Oftentimes, even with adequate bony decompression, the residual scarring may have left a permanent deformation of the exiting nerve.

Complications

Complications of a sacral fracture with radiculopathy include nerve root injury, cerebrospinal fluid leakage, bowel, bladder or sexual dysfunction, late pain, and rectal laceration in cases of gross displacement. Nerve root injuries are managed by the timely and appropriate diagnostic testing and, if treated surgically, careful manipulation of the injured structures. Cerebrospinal leakage is uncommon except in cases of severe bony disruption and can be treated as elsewhere in the spinal axis. It is important to remember that the dural sac ends at S1/S2 in most individuals. Bowel, bladder, or sexual dysfunction is most commonly seen in injuries involving the central canal (zone III), yet the neurologic pattern depends on the level of injury as well as the displacement of the fracture fragments. Fibers to and from the parasympathetic ganglia in the lower sacral roots provide motor control for the rectum and bladder wall, and sphincter inhibition at the bladder neck, as well as erection of the penis and clitoris. When present, prompt and accurate decompression of offending pathology provides the optimum environment for recovery. Late pain may result from inadequately treated pelvic pathology or neural compression. Open reduction and internal fixation can be very successful at reducing pain from bony instability, and late decompression of compromised nerves, provided extensive scarring is not present, can be helpful as well. Finally, rectal or peritoneal laceration may be seen in fractures with gross displacement and should be documented and treated urgently, to reduce the risk of sepsis.

Suggested Readings

Denis F, Davis S, Comfort T. Sacral fractures: an important problem. Clin Orthop Rel Res 1988; 227:67–81.

Fountain SS, Hamilton RD, Jameson RM. Transverse fractures of the sacrum: a report of six cases. J Bone Joint Surg 1977; 59A:486–489.

Case 42

Gunshot Wounds—Cervical Spine, Thoracic Spine, Lumbar Spine

Robert F. Heary and Christopher M. Bono

History and Physical Examination

A 33-year-old African-American man was admitted following a gunshot wound (GSW) to the left upper quadrant of the abdomen.

On physical examination, at the time of the initial spine consultation, the patient was noted to have marked weakness throughout the right lower extremity. Isolated

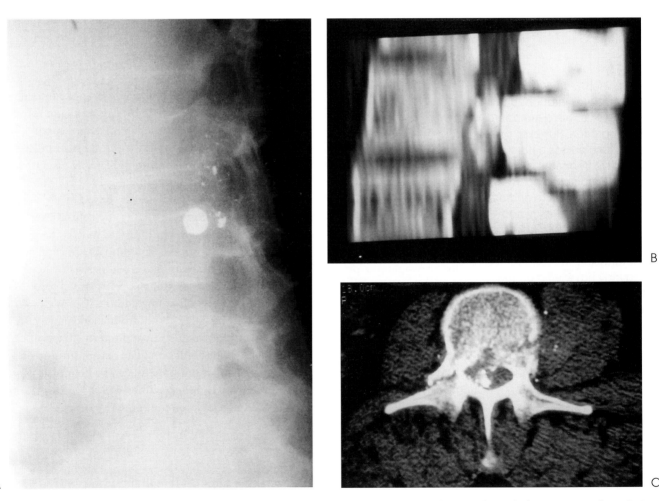

Figure 42–1. (A) Lateral lumbosacral spine radiograph of bullet lodged in soft tissues lateral to spinal canal after traversing the right L2 neural foramen. Numerous small fragments are visible above and below the principal fragment at the L2/L3 interspace. (B) Computed tomography (CT) scan (sagittal reformation) of significant bone fragment present within the spinal canal to the right of the midline. (C) CT scan (axial image) demonstrates path of bullet from posterior aspect of left L2 vertebral body to the right L2 pedicle/neural foramen region. A combination of bone fragment and bullet fragments occupies the right side of the spinal canal. All neural elements are displaced to the left side of the spinal canal.

muscle testing had the following power in the right lower extremity (LE): iliopsoas, 2/5; quadriceps, 0/5; anterior tibialis, 0/5; extensor hallucis longus, 0/5; and ankle plantar flexors, 1/5. Left LE motor exam was 5/5. The right LE was flaccid, and the left LE had normal tone. Diminished pinprick and fine-touch sensations were present throughout the right LE from the L2 dermatome distally. Left LE sensation was intact. Deep tendon reflexes were absent in the LEs bilaterally. Rectal exam demonstrated good sphincter tone; however, voluntary anal contraction was weak. The entry wound had no evidence of a cerebrospinal fluid (CSF) leak.

Radiologic Findings

Plain film radiographs demonstrated a bullet track that traversed the posterior margin of the inferiormost aspect of the L2 vertebral body (Fig. 42–1A). On the lateral view, numerous bullet fragments were demonstrated surrounding the neural foramen. A computed tomography (CT) scan demonstrated the track well and also showed displacement of the posterior margin of the L2 vertebral body into the anterior aspect of the spinal canal (Fig. 42–1B, C). The bony disruption was most noteworthy on the right side, where it extended into the neural foramen. The zygapophyseal facet joints appeared to be spared bilaterally. No evidence of intervertebral disc herniation or hematoma was identifiable within the spinal canal. A right iliopsoas muscle hematoma was well visualized.

Surgical Management

Intravenous (IV) antibiotic coverage for gram-positive, gram-negative, and anaerobic organisms was initiated empirically. An indwelling Foley catheter was placed, which yielded clear, amber urine. No steroids were administered, as the patient had a penetrating injury, and at this location the peripheral nervous system was injured. Surgical exploration and decompression of the neural elements with repair of any dural violations was recommended.

During the exposure of the lumbar spine, care was taken to avoid violating any of the facet joint capsules. Bilateral laminectomies of L1 and L2 were performed. After the ligamentum flavum was excised, two dural tears were identified. A midline vertical 1-cm dural laceration was present at the inferior portion of the L1 vertebra. A second 2-cm dural violation was present overlying the dorsal root entry zone of the right L2 nerve root. The right L2 nerve root was anatomically transected. With the aid of the operating microscope, the intradural space was inspected and copiously irrigated to remove all blood products. Numerous lumbosacral nerve roots were swollen, from the blast effect, but they remained anatomically intact.

Multiple loose bone fragments were removed, extradurally, from the right side of the spinal canal at the L2 level (Fig. 42–2). On the left side, no loose fragments were able to be removed; however, bone was able to be bluntly impacted ventrally into the L2 vertebral body. After additional irrigation to remove blood products from the intradural space, the dural tears were repaired primarily with fine, nonabsorbable, monofilament suture. Following the dural repairs, a Valsalva maneuver was performed to confirm the adequacy of the dural closures. Watertight dural closures were achieved in both locations. No attempt was made to repair the transected right L2 nerve root. A standard layered wound closure was performed. No external drains were utilized. The patient was transferred to the postanesthesia recovery room in stable condition.

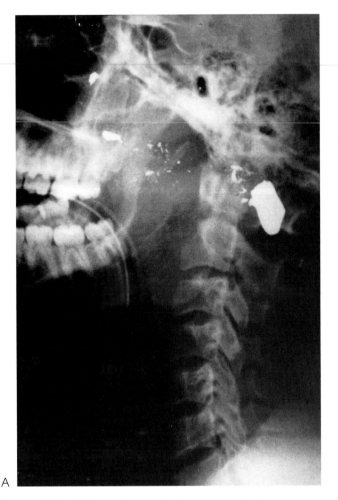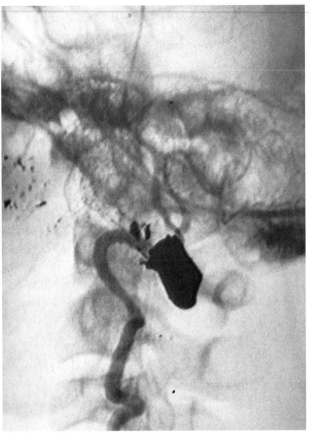

Figure 42–2. (A) Lateral cervical spine radiograph demonstrates a transoral gunshot wound with the predominant fragment lodged in the posterior arch of C1 to the right of the midline. Bullet fragments are visible in the soft tissue regions of the pharynx in this neurologically intact patient. (B) Digital subtraction angiogram, lateral cervical view, of a complete occlusion of blood flow of the right vertebral artery. Embolization of this vessel was performed angiographically to protect against late hemorrhage.

PEARLS

- Gunshot wounds to the lumbar spine are peripheral nerve injuries. As such, decompression of compressed nerve roots can lead to substantial long term neurologic improvement. Numerous studies have documented the benefits of operating on GSW victims when the lumbar spine is injured.
- In rare circumstances, if a bullet fragment or piece of bone compresses a nerve root in an ASIA class A GSW victim, then surgical decompression of the involved root may be indicated

Postoperative Management

Broad-spectrum IV antibiotic coverage was continued for the first 7 postoperative days. Steady improvement of the patient's impaired motor and sensory functions occurred during a 6-week inpatient rehabilitation. No infection occurred. By 3 months postoperatively, the patient had resumed full-time employment, and his neurologic exam was noteworthy for right hip flexor strength of 4/5 with 4+/5 power in all remaining right LE muscle groups. Bowel, bladder, and sexual function were normal. At the 1-year follow-up examination, motor and sensory function was normal throughout both lower extremities. No evidence of spinal instability was noted on lateral flexion and extension plain film radiographs.

Discussion

In the initial management of a spinal GSW victim, tetanus prophylaxis is routinely administered. Broad-spectrum intravenous antibiotics, with gram-positive, gram-to relieve pain and possibly improve nerve root function.

- In cases of CSF leak due to transdural GSWs, surgical exploration is aided by the use of the operating microscope. The benefit of improved lighting and magnification allows for better debridements and superior dural closures. Neural compression is also better appreciated and treated with the improved visualization afforded by the operating microscope.

PITFALLS

- Three-quarters of GSWs to the cervical and thoracic spines result in complete (ASIA class A) spinal cord injuries. When a complete sensorimotor neurologic deficit results from a GSW to the spinal cord above the L1 level, surgery has not been successful at improving spinal cord function.
- Regardless of the spinal level injured by a GSW, surgery is not indicated to prevent infection. In fact, in multiple large series of GSW patients, the infection rates were shown to be greater in patients who underwent surgery than in those patients who were treated conservatively.
- Steroids play no role in the management of GSW victims. Infections and GI complications are increased and no neurologic benefit can be demonstrated.

---

negative, and anaerobic coverage, are begun immediately. If a dural violation is suspected from the radiographic imaging studies, then a 7-day course of antibiotic treatment is indicated. If no dural violation has occurred, then a 2-day course of antibiotic treatment is sufficient. Glucocorticoid steroids are not indicated in the treatment of spinal GSW victims. Penetrating injuries were specifically excluded from all three National Acute Spinal Cord Injury Studies (NASCIS).

The specific treatment of the spine or neurologic injury in GSW victims is a secondary objective. A transdural lumbar GSW case was illustrated because surgical intervention plays a role in these injuries. GSWs below the L1 level cause damage to the cauda equina. These are peripheral nerve injuries that respond well to decompression of the neural elements.

There are numerous goals of surgical intervention for lumbar GSWs. The main objective is to decompress the nerve roots of any active compression resulting from intervertebral disc material, hematoma, and bone or bullet fragments. In addition to neural element decompression, debridement of devitalized tissue is performed. When a dural violation with CSF leak is detected, the dural tear should be repaired. Dural repair is performed either primarily or with a graft. Autologous tissue, such as fascia, is the preferred graft material.

The usual goals cited for operating on a spinal GSW victim are (1) improve neurologic function, (2) stabilize the spine, (3) repair dural violations, and (4) decrease the chance of infection. This reasoning is usually flawed for the following reasons: (1) complete spinal cord injuries (SCIs) usually occur following a GSW to the cervical or thoracic spines, and the neurologic function does not improve with decompressive surgery; (2) GSWs very rarely destabilize the spine—ironically, it is the surgery performed to treat these injuries that may lead to iatrogenic instability; and (3) infections are more frequent following surgery than in conservatively treated patients.

The indications for performing surgery on a spinal GSW victim are the following: (1) Treat a persistent CSF leak with a dural repair procedure to manage and/or prevent meningitis. Most CSF leaks will resolve within a week of the injury. Persistent CSF leaks will usually resolve with CSF diversion by placement of a lumbar subarachnoid drain within a week of the injury. In the small number of patients who have persistent CSF leaks despite a trial of CSF diversion, surgical treatment is indicated. (2) In cases of lumbar GSWs with cauda equina injuries, nerve root decompression has been shown to be beneficial. In the relatively rare cases of symptomatic nerve root compression following GSWs to the cervical or thoracic spines, nerve root decompression may be of benefit. (3) Stabilize the spine. GSWs very rarely cause instability significant enough to warrant a surgical procedure. (4) Treat a progressive neurologic deficit. It is not uncommon for some rostral neurologic deterioration to occur in the first week following a GSW to the spinal cord. This loss of function is usually the result of the "blast effect" from the initial injury and it is not modifiable with surgery. In the rare case of progressive rostral neurologic demise resulting from active neural compression (particularly if the compressing structure is soft, e.g., disc, hematoma), surgery may be indicated. In spite of this theoretical consideration, numerous studies have demonstrated no neurologic improvement in American Spinal Injury Association (ASIA) class A SCI GSW victims, regardless of the etiology of the compression. (5) Treat a delayed posttraumatic syrinx. Occasionally, a syrinx may develop months after a GSW to the cervical or thoracic spinal cord. If a rostral progression of the neurologic deficit is determined by serial neurologic exams in a patient with a syrinx, then a surgical procedure to decompress or shunt the syrinx is indicated.

In summary, the initial treatment of a spinal GSW victim is determined by critical care and predominantly nonspinal issues. Spine surgery is very rarely indicated in SCI patients and is frequently indicated in patients with cauda equina injuries. No large studies have proven any benefit to early surgical intervention (within 48 to 72 hours) over later surgical procedures. In SCIs at the cervical and thoracic levels, the neurologic outcome is greatly determined at the time of the initial blast injury and is infrequently modifiable with surgical procedures.

Alternative Methods of Management

Type of Management	Advantages	Disadvantages	Comments
Steroids	None proven	Increased infections; increased GI complications	GSWs were excluded from all three NASCIS trials
Antibiotics	Decrease infections (meningitis, wound)	Side effects, resistance	Clear benefit with transdural GSWs
Tetanus prophylaxis	Prevents clinical disease	None	Routinely administered
Bracing	Very rarely needed	Inhibits patient mobilization; decreases patient comfort	Not indicated unless surgery performed that destabilizes spine
Surgical decompression	No benefit in cervical and thoracic injuries; probable benefit for peripheral nerve injuries (cauda equina, cervical and thoracic nerve roots)	Morbidity of surgery not indicated with SCI at cervical and thoracic levels	Nerve root function can be improved; spinal cord function not affected
Surgical stabilization	Not necessary with cervical and thoracic injuries; only used if surgical decompression causes instability	Increased infections; no proven benefit	GSW injuries are inherently stable
Timing of surgery	After medical stabilization, nerve root decompression probably beneficial	No proof that early surgery (<48–72 hours) is necessary	Compressed peripheral nerves may be safely decompressed after critical care stabilization of the patient

GI, gastrointestinal; GSW, gun shot wound; NASCIS, National Acute Spinal Cord Injury Study; SCI, spinal cord injury.

Suggested Readings

Benzel EC, Hadden TA, Coleman JE. Civilian gunshot wounds to the spinal cord and cauda equina. Neurosurgery 1987; 20:281–285.

Bracken MB, Shepard MJ, Collins WF Jr. A randomized, controlled trial of methylprednisolone or naloxone in the treatment of acute spinal cord injury: results of the second National Acute Spinal Cord Injury Study. N Engl J Med 1990; 322:1405–1411.

Duh M-S, Shepard MJ, Wilberger JE, Bracken MB. The effectiveness of surgery on the treatment of acute spinal cord injury and its relation to pharmacological treatment. Neurosurgery 1994; 35:240–249.

Geisler FH, Dorsey FC, Coleman WP. Recovery of motor function after spinal cord injury: a randomized, placebo-controlled trial with GM-1 ganglioside. N Engl J Med 1991; 324:1829–1838.

Heary RF, Vaccaro AR, Mesa JJ, et al. Steroids and gunshot wounds to the spine. Neurosurgery 1997; 41:576–584.

Levy ML, Gans W, Wijesinghe HS, SooHoo WE, Adkins RH, Stillerman CB. Use of methylprednisolone as an adjunct in the management of patients with penetrating spinal cord injury: outcome analysis. Neurosurgery 1996; 39:1141–1149.

Prendergast MR, Saxe JM, Ledgerwood AM, Lucas CE, Lucas WF. Massive steroids do not reduce the zone of injury after penetrating spinal cord injury. J Trauma 1994; 37:576–580.

Velmanhos G, Demetriades D. Gunshot wounds of the spine: should retained bullets be removed to prevent infection? Ann R Coll Surg Engl 1994; 76:85–87.

Waters RL, Adkins RH, Yakura J, Sie I. Profiles of spinal cord injury and recovery after gunshot injury. Clin Orthop 1991; 267:14–21.

Yashon D, Jane JA, White RJ. Prognosis and management of spinal cord and cauda equina bullet injuries in sixty-five civilians. J Neurosurg 1970; 32:163–170.

Young W. Medical treatments of acute spinal cord injury. J Neurol Neurosurg Psychiatry 1992; 55:635–639.

Spinal Neoplasms

Case 43
Primary Tumor—Cervical Spine, Thoracic Spine, Lumbar Spine
Takuya Fujita, Norio Kawahara, and Katsuro Tomita

History and Physical Examination

A 16-year-old boy had a 4-month history of stiffness and severe pain in the thoracolumbar region. He was referred to our institution because of an abnormal shadow in the thoracolumbar region on plain radiographs. Physical examination at the time of admission demonstrated tenderness over the posterior elements of the 11th and 12th thoracic and first lumbar vertebrae region, without neurologic deficit.

Radiologic Findings

Plain radiographs showed an ivory 12th thoracic vertebra, and diffuse sclerotic changes in the 11th thoracic and first and second lumbar vertebrae (Fig. 43–1). Computed tomography (CT) scan showed a tumor involving the entire 12th tho-

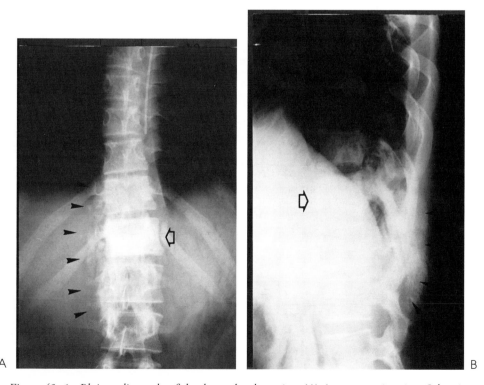

A   B

Figure 43–1. Plain radiographs of the thoracolumbar spine. (A) Anteroposterior view. Sclerotic lesion is seen in the 12th thoracic vertebra (white arrow), associated with diffuse sclerosis in the paravertebral soft tissues from the 11th thoracic to the second lumbar vertebral level (arrowheads). (B) Lateral view. Note the presence of the 12th thoracic ivory vertebra (white arrow). A large osteosclerotic mass is evident, extending into the posterior paravertebral tissues (arrowheads).

racic vertebra and segments of the 11th thoracic vertebra. There was extensive paravertebral and epidural involvement from the 11th thoracic vertebra to the first lumbar vertebra. The paraspinous muscles from the 11th thoracic vertebra to the second lumbar vertebra were invaded bilaterally (Fig. 43–2). A total body CT scan, ^{99m}Tc (technetium) scan, and gallium scan were all negative for metastases.

Diagnosis

A histologic diagnosis of osteosarcoma was established after histologic examination of an open needle biopsy specimen. A trephine 14-gauge needle was used for the biopsy. The biopsy was taken from the corpus through the right pedicle of the 12th thoracic vertebra. The biopsy track was recognized in the CT scan of the 12th thoracic vertebra (Fig. 43–2).

Surgical Management

Total en bloc spondylectomy (TES) was performed following preoperative chemotherapy using carboplatin (450 mg), pirarubicin hydrochloride (100 mg), and high-dose methotrexate (15 g) in five courses. Spinal angiography and selective embolization of the feeder segmental artery was performed 1 day prior to the operation.

En Bloc Laminectomy and Posterior Spinal Instrumentation

With the patient in a prone position, a midline posterior longitudinal incision was made. Exposure of the posterior elements was performed through healthy paraspinous muscles without exposing the biopsy track, and a wide margin of the muscle was left attached to the posterior elements. We then exposed the most lateral

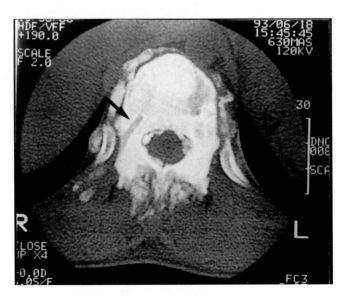

Figure 43–2. Preoperative computed tomography (CT) scan of the 12th thoracic vertebra. The entire 12th thoracic vertebra was involved. The paraspinous muscles from the 11th thoracic to the second lumbar vertebral level were invaded bilaterally. The biopsy track in the 12th thoracic vertebra is indicated by a black arrow.

aspects of the transverse processes from the 11th thoracic vertebra to the second lumbar vertebra, and the 11th and 12th ribs bilaterally. The ribs were transected from 2 to 5 cm lateral to the costotransverse joint. The parietal pleura was then separated bluntly from the lateral side of the vertebra. Next, a pediculotomy and en bloc laminectomy was performed using a T-saw (flexible multifilament threadwire saw, 0.54 mm in diameter, Fig. 43–3). The T-saw was inserted into the epidural space beneath the lamina of the 11th thoracic vertebra down to the second lumbar vertebra through the epidural catheter and was pulled through the intervertebral foramen between the 10th and 11th thoracic vertebrae and between the second and third lumbar vertebrae at each side. When both ends of this saw were pulled tightly in the lateral direction, it ran adjacent to the inner wall of the pedicles of the 11th thoracic, 12th thoracic, first lumbar, and second lumbar vertebrae. Using a reciprocating motion, thin cuts of the four pedicles were produced by the saw. After pediculotomy had been performed on both sides, the laminae of the 11th thoracic, 12th thoracic, first lumbar, and second lumbar vertebrae, with the paraspinal muscles invaded by the tumor, were removed en bloc. Posterior spinal instrumentation was then inserted. Pedicle screws of the Cotrel-Dubousset (CD) system were placed into three vertebrae above and three below the affected vertebrae. The rods, contoured to restore the normal anatomic sagittal spinal curve alignment, were attached to the pedicle screws.

En Bloc Corpectomy and Reconstruction of the Spinal Column

The pleura and insertion of the diaphragm were separated carefully from the vertebrae and ribs without damaging the pleura or the diaphragm. At the same time, the 11th and 12th intercostal and the first lumbar nerves were cut bilaterally and the 11th and 12th intercostal and the first lumbar arteries were ligated and carefully reflected. After the 11th and 12th thoracic and the first lumbar vertebrae were separated from the thoracoabdominal organs, a vertebral spatula was inserted from both sides anterior to the vertebral body to protect the large vessels and organs. The dura mater and nerve roots at the level of the affected vertebrae were separated carefully from the epidural tumor, the posterior longitudinal ligament, and the posterior wall of the vertebral bodies. Then a teethed cord protector was inserted carefully between the dura and vertebral body to protect the spinal cord during the remainder of the procedure. Next, two T-saws were introduced anterior to the vertebral body and placed at the lower endplate of the 10th thoracic vertebral body

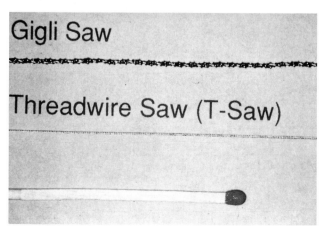

Figure 43–3. Photograph of the T-saw.

and the disc level of the first and second lumbar vertebrae. Using a reciprocating motion, these upper and lower cuts were made in an anterior to posterior direction. After the cuts were completed, the vertebral bodies of the 11th and 12th thoracic and first lumbar vertebrae were rotated carefully around the spinal cord and removed en bloc together with the tissue margin (Fig. 43–4). In the next step, the anterior spinal column was reconstructed by implanting a vertebral body allograft augmented with a fibula autograft. The implanted allograft, a portion of the thoracic spine from the fourth to the eighth thoracic vertebrae, was placed in an autoclave at 135°C for 10 minutes. After making anchoring holes in the cut vertebral surfaces of the 10th thoracic and second lumbar vertebral bodies for the fibula strut, the posterior rods were readjusted to allow compression of the bone graft. Two CD screws were inserted into the grafted bone, and a rod placed connecting the two screws. The posterior rod and anterior rod were connected using two device low-profile transverse traction (DLT) bars of the compact CD system (Fig. 43–5). Cancellous bone graft harvested from the left posterior iliac crest was placed around the strut graft and hardware.

The total operative time was 10 hours, and the estimated total blood loss was approximately 10 L. Chest tubes were not necessary.

Following the procedure, chemotherapy (carboplatin, 450 mg; pirarubicin, 100 mg; and high-dose methotrexate, 15 g) was provided for an additional five courses. A circumferential, well-molded, full-length body jacket was worn for 6 months after the operation. At 2 years postoperatively, the patient was able to walk without restriction, had no pain, and had normal neurologic function except for analgesia along the dermatomal distribution of the severed nerve roots. Radiographic examination showed a solid fusion (Fig. 43–4). Furthermore, plain radiographs, total body CT scan, ^{99m}Tc scan, and gallium scan were negative for distant metastases.

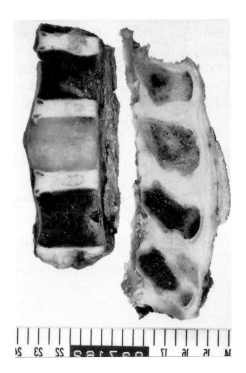

Figure 43–4. Photograph of midline sagittal section of the resected specimen.

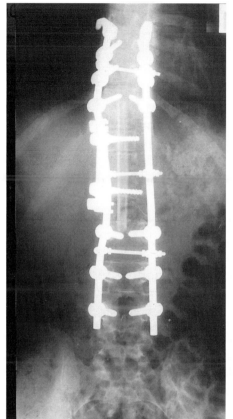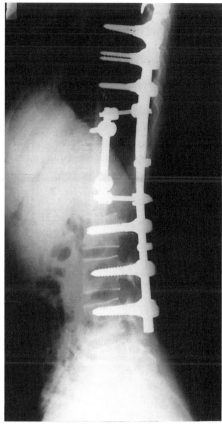

A   B

Figure 43–5. Postoperative radiographs of the thoracolumbar spine. (A) Anteroposterior view. Reconstruction of the spinal column was performed by the Cotrel-Debousset system with insertion of pedicle screws into three vertebrae above and three below the affected vertebra posteriorly, and implanting a vertebral body allograft, which was augmented with a fibula autograft between the 10th thoracic vertebra and second lumbar vertebra. (B) Lateral view. Two Cotrel-Debousset screws were inserted into the grafted bone, and a rod placed connecting the two screws. The posterior and anterior rods were connected using two device low-profile transverse traction (DLT) bars of the compact CD system.

Discussion

Spinal tumors originating in the anterior vertebral body are more likely to be malignant than lesions involving the posterior elements. Benign anterior lesions include eosinophilic granuloma, hemangioma, and aneurysmal bone cyst, and the malignant anterior lesions include lymphoma, chordoma, and all sarcomas. Lesions arising posteriorly are osteochondroma, osteoid osteoma, and osteoblastoma (Fig. 43–6).

Some tumors have a characteristic radiographic appearance. Osteoid osteoma and osteblastoma are frequently seen as sclerotic lesions in the pedicle. Aneurysmal bone cysts show progressive bone destruction and ballooning out of the cortex and periosteum to form poorly demarcated soft tissue masses. Giant cell tumors are most often expansive and lytic with cortical breakthrough and soft tissue mass associated with the lesion. Hemangiomas show striated or honeycomb texture. Eosinophilic granuloma is well known as a cause of vertebra plana. Chordomas generally appear as lytic lesions involving multiple segments with a minor amount of vague tumor

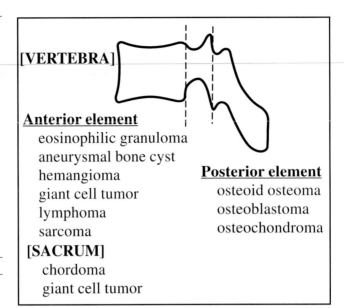

[VERTEBRA]

Anterior element
eosinophilic granuloma
aneurysmal bone cyst
hemangioma
giant cell tumor
lymphoma
sarcoma
[SACRUM]
chordoma
giant cell tumor

Posterior element
osteoid osteoma
osteoblastoma
osteochondroma

Figure 43–6. Characteristic position of vertebral tumors within the vertebra.

calcification. Chondrosarcomas are frequently calcified and lobulated. Osteosarcomas present as aggressive, osteolytic destructive lesions accompanied by variable amounts of ossification. Ewing sarcoma presents with a typical permeative pattern and is associated with soft tissue mass.

Benign spinal tumors can be classified according the staging system proposed by Enneking and colleagues (1980) as either latent (stage 1), active (stage 2), or aggressive (stage 3) lesions. Stage 1 lesions include asymptomatic lesions bordered by a true capsule. A well-defined margin around the circumference of the lesion is seen even on plain radiographs. These tumors do not require treatment (e.g., osteochondroma, hemangioma), unless pathologic fracture occurs. Stage 2 tumors grow slowly, causing mild symptoms. The tumor usually remains within the confines of the bone border of the vertebra but may expand and be bordered by a thin capsule and a layer of reactive tissue, which may be defined on plain radiograph as an expansion of the tumor's boundaries or more clearly identified on magnetic resonance imaging (MRI). These tumors are generally osteoid osteoma, eosinophilic granulomas, hemangiomas, osteochondromas, and aneurysmal bone cysts. Stage 2 lesions, in general, require en bloc excision or curettage. Stage 3 lesions include rapidly growing benign tumors, which often are associated with symptoms due to spinal cord compression or pathologic fracture. The capsule is very thin, discontinuous, or absent. The tumor invades the neighboring compartments, and a pseudocapsule is found. These lesions require en bloc excision even if only a marginal margin can be obtained. About two-thirds of osteoblastomas are stage 2, and one-third are stage 3. For stage 3 osteoblastomas, intralesional curettage is associated with a high rate of local recurrence (about 20%). Giant cell tumors have been reported to have a significant recurrence rate after curettage (50%), and a small occurrence of pulmonary metastases. Therefore, en bloc excision of affected vertebra (i.e., total en bloc spondylectomy, Fig. 43–7) is indicated, if feasible, particularly for patients with tumors expanding through the whole vertebra.

For malignant tumors, the most oncologically appropriate surgical technique is en bloc excision with wide margin. In the extremities, the technique of en bloc exci-

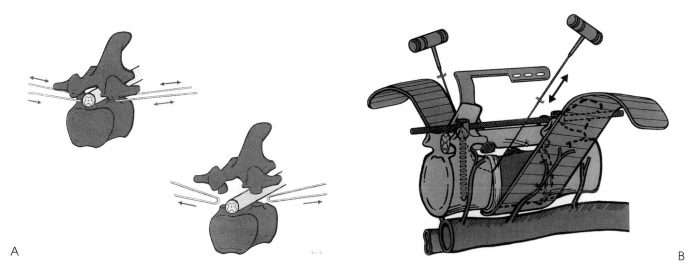

A   B

Figure 43–7. (A,B) Schematic diagrams of total en bloc spondylectomy.

sion with a wide margin was developed for primary malignant tumors, following recognition of the barrier tissues to tumor spread in bone and soft tissue sarcomas of the long bones. The operative procedure is associated with a dramatic improvement in prognosis, together with preservation of the function of the limbs. For the vertebral column, Fujita and colleagues (1997) also delineated the bony barriers in the spine that enhance and halt the spread of tumors. However, the unique anatomic structure of the vertebra makes it difficult to perform en bloc excision of the tumor with a safe margin, and thus most operations have been limited to curettage or piecemeal resection.

Alternative Methods of Management

An alternative to TES as a method of surgical management for malignant vertebral tumors is total spondylectomy in a piecemeal fashion, not en bloc. The TES procedure demands proficiency in and experience with its techniques, and thus the spine surgeon may be unable to do it. In addition, when the tumor extends to visceral organs or forms a huge mass, as seen frequently in malignant vertebral tumors, this procedure should not be applied. Therefore, piecemeal resection as an alternative to TES sometimes may be elected as the surgical management for malignant vertebral tumors. Piecemeal resection, however, results in intralesional excision from an oncologic standpoint, which would lead to poor results compared to en bloc excision, according to a large number of reports on malignant bone tumors in the extremities.

Type of Management	Advantages	Disadvantages	Comments
Piecemeal resection of tumor	Safer technically than total en bloc spondylectomy (TES)	Results in intralesional excision with contamination of remaining tissue	Used by the majority of spinal surgeons due to the technical difficulty of TES

Suggested Readings

Beltran J, Aparisi F, Bonmati LM, et al. Eosinophilic granuloma: MRI manifestations. Skeletal Radiol 1993; 22:157–161.

Boriani S, Biagini R, De Iure F, et al. En bloc resection of bone tumors of the thoracolumbar spine. Spine 1996; 21:1927–1931.

Boriani S, Capanna R, Donati D, et al. Osteoblastoma of the spine. Clin Orthop 1992; 278:37–45.

Boriani S, Chevathelley F, Weinstein JN, et al. Chordoma of the spine above the sacrum. Treatment and outcome in 21 cases. Spine 1996; 21:1569–1577.

Capanna R, Albisinni U, Picci P, Calderoni P, Campanacci M, Springfield DS. Aneurysmal bone cyst of the spine. J Bone Joint Surg 1985; 67A:527–531.

Dahlin DC, Kirshanan KU, eds. Bone Tumors, General Aspects and Data on 8542 Cases. Springfield, IL: Charles C Thomas, 1986.

Enneking WF. Spine. In: Enneking WF, ed. Musculoskeletal Tumor Surgery, p. 303. New York: Churchill Livingstone, 1983.

Enneking WF, Spanier SS, Goodmann MA. A system for the surgical staging of musculoskeletal sarcoma. Clin Orthop 1980; 153:106–120.

Fox MW, Onofrio BM. The natural history and management of symptomatic and asymptomatic vertebral hemangiomas. J Neurosurg 1993; 78:36–45.

Fujita T, Ueda Y, Kawahara N, et al. Local spread of metastatic vertebral tumors—a histologic study. Spine 1997; 22:1905–1912.

Kawahara N, Tomita K, Takahashi K, et al. Cadaveric vascular anatomy for total en bloc spondylectomy for malignant vertebral tumors. Spine 1996; 21:1401–1407.

Levine AM, Boriani S, Donati D, Campanacci M. Benign tumors of the cervical spine. Spine 1992; 17:S399–406.

Rosen G, Marcove RC, Caparros B, Nirenberg A, Kosloff C, Huvos AG. Primary osteogenic sarcoma. The rationale for preoperative chemotherapy and delayed surgery. Cancer 1979; 43:2163–2177.

Roy-Camille R, Mazel CH, Saillant G, et al. Treatment of malignant tumors of the spine with posterior instrumentation. In: Sundaresan N, Schmidek HH, Schiller AL, Rosenthal DI, eds. Tumors of the Spine. Diagnosis and Clinical Management, pp. 473–487. Philadelphia: WB Saunders, 1990.

Sanjay BKS, Sim FH, Unni KK, et al. Giant cell tumours of the spine. J Bone Joint Surg 1993; 75B:148–154.

Shives TC, Dahlin DC, Sim FH, et al. Osteosarcoma of the spine. J Bone Joint Surg 1986; 68A:660–668.

Shives TC, MacLeod MD, Uni KK, et al. Chondrosarcoma of the spine. J Bone Joint Surg 1989; 71A:1158–1165.

Stener B. Complete removal of vertebrae for extirpation of tumors. Clin Orthop 1989; 245:72–82.

Tomita K, Kawahara N. The threadwire saw: a new device for cutting bone. J Bone Joint Surg 1996; 78A:1915–1917.

Tomita K, Kawahara N, Baba H, et al. Total en bloc spondylectomy: a new surgical technique for primary malignant vertebral tumors. Spine 1997; 22:324–333.

Tsuchiya H, Yasutake H, Yokogawa A, Baba H, Ueda Y, Tomita K. Effect of chemotherapy combined with caffeine for osteosarcoma. J Cancer Res Clin Oncol 1992; 118:567–569.

Case 44
Primary Tumor of the Cervical Spine

Jed S. Vanichkachorn and Alexander R. Vaccaro

History and Physical Examination

A 58-year-old nonsmoking man, previously healthy, was evaluated for acute myelopathic symptoms. The patient reported an approximately 6-month history of unrelenting axial pain in the cervical region. The pain was described as constant and was not related to any particular physical activity. The pain was often worse at night and had recently begun to wake the patient from sleep. There was no history of radicular symptoms or referred pain. All attempts at conservative treatment, including rest, physical therapy, and nonsteroidal antiinflammatory drugs had failed to relieve the discomfort. Two days prior to the initial evaluation, the patient developed an acute increase in his discomfort level and reported new difficulties walking due to lower extremity weakness. The patient denied any bowel or bladder difficulties.

Examination of the patient revealed spasm of the paraspinal musculature in the subaxial cervical region. Range of motion of the neck was severely limited by the pa-

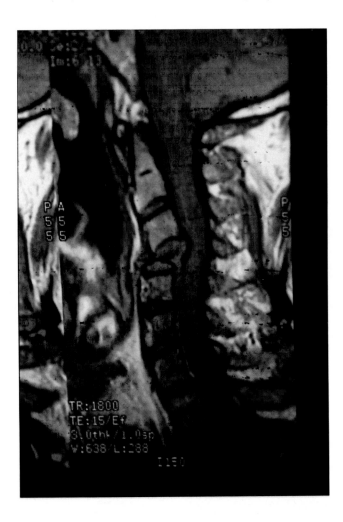

Figure 44–1. Sagittal magnetic resonance imaging (MRI) demonstrates significant anterior thecal sac compression at the C4 level.

tient's discomfort. There were no obvious skin lesions and no paraspinal masses. Palpation of the regional lymph nodes revealed no abnormal enlargement. The neurologic exam was significant for symmetrical weakness of the lower extremities. A positive Babinski sign was elicited bilaterally and three to six beats of clonus were seen in both lower extremities. The patient demonstrated a wide-based gait and could safely ambulate only with significant assistance.

Radiologic Findings

Plain anteroposterior (AP), lateral, and flexion/extension radiographs of the cervical spine were performed emergently. These radiographs demonstrated severe collapse of C4 vertebral body with a marked kyphotic deformity. Magnetic resonance imaging (MRI) of the cervical spine revealed a mass causing significant anterior thecal compression at the level of the C4 vertebral body deformity (Fig. 44–1).

Diagnosis

The patient was admitted to the hospital urgently due to acute onset of myelopathic symptoms. Flat bed rest and a rigid cervical collar were ordered for protection against further neurologic injury. Intravenous (IV) steroid therapy was begun acutely. Appropriate laboratory studies were performed and computed tomography (CT) scans of the chest, abdomen, and pelvis were performed to rule out metastatic disease. Inpatient technetium bone scan confirmed that this was indeed a solitary lesion. A CT-guided biopsy of the lesion confirmed the diagnosis of a primary non-Hodgkin's lymphoma of the C4 vertebral body. Due to the high-grade histologic nature of the lesion and the extensive bony destruction and soft tissue invasion, the tumor was staged as a IIB lesion.

Surgical Management

Lymphomas generally are extremely sensitive to chemotherapy and radiotherapy. Surgical intervention is often unnecessary in many of these cases. The patient's neurologic status, however, continued to worsen despite the immobilization and initial steroid therapy. In addition, the patient was noted to have a significant cervical deformity, which would most likely progress as the tumorous lesion was treated. As a result of those considerations an acute surgical decompression and stabilization was elected. The entire C4 vertebral body was removed through an anterior approach to the cervical spine. Reconstruction and stabilization of the spine was provided by a recently developed expanding plate/cage implant, the Telescoping Plate Spacer (Interpore Cross, Irving, CA). This device allows rigid fixation of the anterior column of the cervical spine through the plate portion of the device and provides structural support to the middle column through the expanding cage portion of the device (Fig. 44–2). Furthermore, autologuous bone graft can be placed safely and effectively within the cage portion of the implant.

The patient tolerated the surgical procedure well and was placed in a rigid cervical collar for a period of 8 weeks. All myelopathic symptoms resolved in the early postoperative period, and the patient was able to ambulate independently within 2 weeks after surgery. At approximately 6 weeks following surgery, a course of radio-

PEARLS

- Metastatic lesions are far more common than primary bone tumors of the spine. A complete workup should be done for most spinal lesions to rule out the presence of a primary lesion involving another organ system.
- Most vertebral body lesions in patients older than 21 years of age are malignant in nature and need to be worked up in an aggressive manner. Posterior element lesions are more likely to be benign in nature.
- A multidisciplinary approach for tumors of the spine needs to be taken. Successful patient outcomes during the treatment of spine bone tumors will need equal input from the surgeon, oncologist, and pathologist.
- Any patient older than 50 years of age with a spine-related complaint that persists longer than 1 month should be considered for a tumor workup. This is especially so if any of the history or physical findings are atypical.

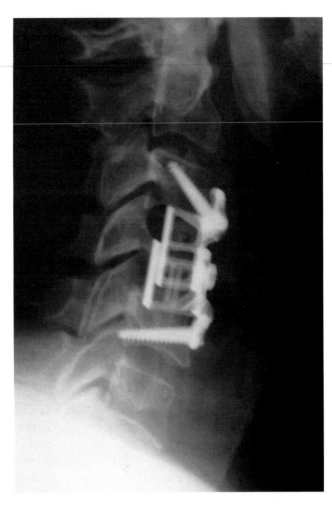

Figure 44–2. Postoperative lateral radiograph following a C4 corpectomy and reconstruction with iliac crest bone graft and a telescoping plate spacer.

therapy was begun to help eradicate any residual disease. At the most recent follow-up, the patient had no obvious tumor recurrence and is symptom free.

Discussion

Primary tumors of the spine are rare and make up less than 10% of all bone tumors. The incidence of primary spinal tumors has been estimated at between 2.5 and 8.5 tumors per 100,000 population per year. All regions of the spine can be affected, although the cervical spine is the least frequent area of involvement. This infrequency makes primary tumors of the spine difficult to distinguish from the more common benign processes in the spine. Metastatic disease of the spine, on the other hand, is a much more common process. It is estimated that metastatic disease of the spine is 40 times more common than all other forms of bone cancer combined. The higher prevalence of metastatic lesions of the spine makes primary spinal tumors a secondary consideration when managing an unknown lesion of the spine.

Common benign tumors of the spine include osteoid osteoma, osteoblastoma, and aneurysmal bone cyst. These three lesions are almost exclusively found involving the posterior elements. Common benign vertebral body lesions include hemangioma, eosinophilic granuloma, and giant cell tumors. Although considered a be-

PITFALLS

- Survival of patients with primary malignant spinal tumors is directly related to obtaining complete excision at the time of surgery. Failure to obtain adequate surgical margins often requires the use of adjuvant therapies to obtain tumor control. Adjuvant radiotherapy, when given, should be delayed to preserve graft strength and union.

- The use of nonbiologic materials such as methylmethacrylate is rarely indicated in the surgical treatment and reconstruction for primary bone tumors of the spine. Most surgical interventions for the treatment of primary bone tumors of the spine are for cure, not palliation. Nonbiologic materials have a higher long-term failure rate and a higher incidence of infection.

- The surgical approach for primary malignant bone lesions of the spine should be directed by the location of the lesion. Malignant lesions causing anterior cord compression should always be treated with an anterior approach. Posterior laminectomy and decompression for an anteriorly based lesion will fail to provide relief and will further destabilize the spine.

- Tumor staging, whether the lesion is metastatic or primary, should be carried out for all lesions before treatment is begun. Failure to adequately address the nature and extent of the tumor will produce suboptimal treatment results.

- Plain radiographs often will not show evidence of bone destruction until approximately 30 to 50% of the trabecular bone is destroyed.

nign lesion, giant cell tumors can have a poor prognosis due to the aggressive nature of the tumor's growth pattern. Common malignant primary tumors include solitary plasmacytoma, chordoma, chondrosarcoma, and lymphoma. Less commonly encountered malignant lesions include Ewing's sarcoma, osteogenic sarcoma, and fibrosarcoma.

Malignant primary tumors of the spine almost exclusively occur in the vertebral body, whereas benign tumors generally are located in the posterior elements. In a review of primary tumors of the spine by Weinstein and McLain (1987), 66% of all lesions were found to arise in the vertebral body and 34% were found to arise in the posterior elements. Of the vertebral body lesions, 76% were found to be malignant, whereas only 34% of the posterior element lesions were malignant. Approximately 80% of all malignant tumors and 42% of all benign tumors of the spine were found in the vertebral body. Malignant tumors were also more likely than benign lesions to present with a neurologic deficit.

Patients with a tumor of the spine can be divided into five categories depending on the amount of neurologic symptoms and the amount of bone destruction. Class I patients have no neurologic involvement or only mild sensory changes with minimal bone involvement. Class II patients have no neurologic symptoms but have bone involvement without any collapse or instability. Class III patients have major neurologic involvement. Class IV patients have significant bony involvement with pain and instability but minimal neurologic findings. Class V patients have significant vertebral body collapse and instability with major neurologic impairments. Class I and II patients generally respond well to irradiation and conservative treatment. Class III patients who have neurologic involvement without significant bone destruction also respond favorably to radiation therapy. Class III patients with radioresistant tumors, tumors that have already received maximum radiation, and tumors with a predicted extended survival rate may be candidates for surgical intervention. Classes IV and V with neurologic involvement due to significant mechanical instability and subsequent kyphotic deformity require surgical intervention. In general the improvement in neurologic symptoms is related to the biology of the tumor, the preoperative neurologic status of the patient, and the amount of bone destruction.

The overall prognosis for primary tumors of the spine depends largely on whether the lesion is malignant or benign. Benign lesions tend to have very little long-term morbidity; consequences of pathologic fractures, deformity, and neurologic involvement generally resolve with appropriate medical or surgical treatment. Late recurrence is not usually a complication of benign lesions. The 5-year survival rate for benign lesions has been estimated at around 86% and is not dependent on the type and extent of the surgery. The prognosis for malignant lesions, on the other hand, seems to correlate directly with the extent of tumor excision. In the study by Weinstein and McLain (1987), a 75% 5-year survival rate was seen for patients who had complete excision of their malignant lesions. This is compared to a 18.7% 5-year survival rate in patients with an incomplete excision. Often a complete resection is not a realistic possibility due to the intimate relationship of the tumor with surrounding neurovascular structures. In these situations, adjuvant radiotherapy or chemotherapy is sometimes required.

The surgical treatment of primary tumors of the spine is usually indicated for patients with tumors that (1) are resistant to and/or have failed medical therapy, (2) cause a progressive neurologic deficit or spinal instability, and (3) do not have a definitive diagnosis despite an adequate workup. Unlike the treatment of metastatic lesions of the spine, the goal of treatment for primary bone tumors of the spine is cure. Patients with primary bone tumors of the spine generally are younger and healthier than patients with a metastatic lesion. Therefore, early and complete surgical intervention is often necessary for successful outcomes. Every lesion must have a complete tumor staging prior to any definitive treatment to maximize patient outcome. Factors that must be considered include the type and location of the tumor, the presence of neurologic involvement, the mode of spinal failure, the biology/histology of the tumor, the life expectancy of the patient, and whether adjuvant therapies will be used.

Alternative Methods of Management

Type of Management	Advantages	Disadvantages	Comments
Nonoperative treatment	Avoids the potential morbidity and mortality of surgical intervention	Potential for progressive kyphotic collapse during therapy; tumor lysis syndrome	A patient with a progressive neurologic deficit is not a candidate for nonoperative treatment
Anterior surgical approach	Directly addresses the underlying pathology	Potential for surgical morbidity including neurovascular injuries and wound complications	Ideal for an anteriorly based lesion that needs subsequent anterior and middle column reconstructions
Posterior surgical approach	Less invasive surgical procedure than the anterior approach; avoids most neurovascular structures	Will destabilize the already anterior/posterior column deficient spine; fails to address anterior thecal compression	Should be reserved for benign posterior based lesions of the spine
Combined anterior and posterior surgical approach	Provides circumferential rigid fixation to the unstable spine; earlier removal of external immobilization	Increased morbidity from an additional surgical procedure; may require staged surgical procedures	More commonly needed for metastatic lesions of the spine where multiple levels of involvement exists

Suggested Readings

Bell GR. Surgical treatment of spinal tumors. Clin Orthop Rel Res 1997; 335:54–63.

Boriani S, Weinstein JN. Differential diagnosis and surgical treatment of primary benign and malignant neoplasms. In: Frymoyer JW, Ducker TB, Hadler MN, et al, eds. The Adult Spine: Principles and Practice, vol 1, pp. 951–988. New York: Raven Press, 1997.

Emery SE, Brazinski MS, Koka A, Bensusan JS, Stevenson S. The biological and biomechanical effects of irradiation on anterior spinal bone grafts in a canine model. J Bone Joint Surg 1994; 76A:540–548.

Hall DJ, Webb JK. Anterior plate fixation in Spine tumor surgery. Spine 1991; 16(suppl):S80–S83.

Harrington KD. Anterior decompression and stabilization of the spine as a treatment for vertebral collapse and spinal cord compression from metastatic malignancy. Clin Orthop Rel Res 1988; 233:177–197.

Jenis LG, Dunn EJ, An HS. Metastatic disease of the cervical spine: a review. Clin Orthop Rel Res 1999; 359:89–103.

Nicholls P, Jarecky T. The value of posterior decompression by laminectomy for malignant tumors of the spine. Clin Orthop Rel Res 1985; 201:210–213.

Ono K, Tada K. Metal prosthesis of the cervical vertebrate. J Neurosurg 1975; 42:562–566.

Rougraff BT, Kneisl JS, Simon MA. Skeletal metastases of unknown origin: a prospective study of a diagnostic strategy. J Bone Joint Surg 1993; 75A:1276–1281.

Sherk H, Nolan J, Mooar P. Treatment of tumors of the cervical spine. Clin Orthop Rel Res 1988; 233:163–167.

Siegal T, Siegel T. Current considerations in the management of neoplastic spinal cord compression. Spine 1989; 14:223–228.

Sundaresan N, Galicich JH, Lane JM, Bains MS, McCormack P. Treatment of neoplastic epidural cord compression by vertebral body resection and stabilization. J Neurosurg 1985; 63:676–684.

Weinstein JN. Differential diagnosis and surgical treatment of pathologic spine fractures. Instr Course Lect 1992; 42:301–315.

Weinstein JN, McLain RF. Primary tumors of the spine. Spine 1987; 12:843–851.

Case 45
Spinal Cord Herniation

Erol Veznedaroglu and Gregory J. Przybylski

History and Physical Examination

A 57-year-old right-handed woman described progressive right leg numbness since 1990. She subsequently developed left leg weakness manifested as difficulty ambulating and frequent tripping in 1995. Her dysfunction had slowly progressed, recently accompanied by urinary frequency and nocturia. Examination revealed no spinal tenderness, 4/5 weakness in the left lower limb, and diminished pinprick sensation below T7 on the right. She had symmetrically diminished vibratory sense in the lower limbs, although her position sense was preserved.

Radiologic Findings

Midsagittal T2-weighted magnetic resonance imaging (MRI) revealed an atrophic thoracic cord segment displaced into a posterior-superior vertebral body defect (Fig.

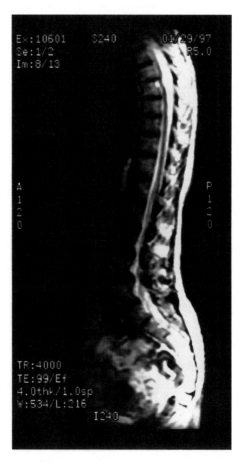

Figure 45–1. Midsagittal T2-weighted magnetic resonance imaging (MRI) demonstrates a segment of thoracic spinal cord entering a posterior-superior vertebral body defect.

45–1). Sagittal reconstruction of postmyelographic computed tomography (CT) better demonstrated an abnormality at the T7/T8 region with cerebrospinal fluid (CSF) entering the posterior superior aspect of the T8 vertebral body with displacement of the spinal cord into the defect (Fig. 45–2A). Neither study demonstrated a dorsal filling defect. However, axial postmyelographic CT revealed anterior displacement of the atrophic cord into the bony defect (Fig. 45–2B). CSF phase-contrast pulse sequences did not show an arachnoid cyst.

Diagnosis

Spinal cord herniation (SCH). This rare entity is often misdiagnosed but has several unique characteristics. The appearance of a dorsal arachnoid cyst is often thought to be the cause of spinal cord compression, prompting surgical treatment. However, the cyst is more likely a void created by the herniated cord. In the absence of trauma or prior surgery, spinal cord herniation occurs ventrally. The neurologic signs of spinal cord herniation are progressive and insidious. Patients typically develop a Brown Séquard syndrome progressing over several years with development of bowel or bladder dysfunction. Although sensory disturbances usually appear first, followed by weakness and spasticity, urinary difficulties often prompt evaluation.

Surgical Management

A transthoracic approach was chosen for exposure of the ventral herniation. Preoperative infusion of steroids and antibiotics as well as intraoperative monitoring of somatosensory and motor evoked potentials were done. After the patient was anesthetized, she was positioned (lateral decubitus) with the right side up. The posterolateral thorax was prepped with betadine, and a lumbar drain was placed prior to thoracotomy. The ribs of T8 and T9 were partially removed and an intraoperative radiograph confirmed our level. The posterior pleura was incised to expose the rib heads of T8 and T9; the segmental vessels on the T8 vertebral body were sutured

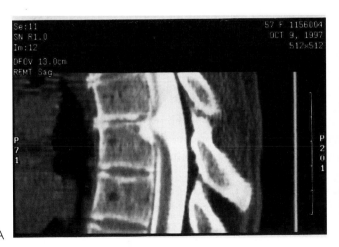

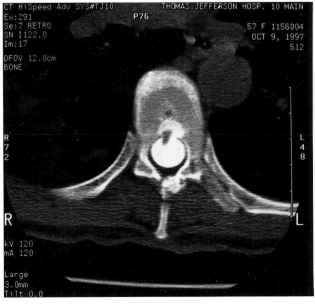

Figure 45–2. Midsagittal reconstruction (A) and axial postmyelographic computed tomography (CT) (B) demonstrate myelographic filling of the vertebral body defect. The atrophic thoracic cord segment appears displaced into the defect.

and divided. The rib attachments to the vertebral body were drilled away to uncover the underlying pedicles at T8 and T9. The T9 pedicle was then removed after identifying its edges with a curette by drilling it out, thereby allowing access to the dural sac. Dissection was continued out rostrally to identify the T8 nerve root. A posterior right-sided corpectomy of T8 was performed with a high-speed drill until an additional cortical surface was identified in the midportion of the vertebral body, which was the cavity containing the herniated spinal cord. The cortical wall of the cavity was lined with thickened arachnoid adherent to the pia.

Microdissection of the arachnoid adhesions with the intraoperative microscope allowed definition of the free dural edges around the periphery of the defect. The herniated spinal cord was then reduced with its arachnoid covering back into the thecal sac and interrupted nylon sutures were used to primarily close the dural defect. The T7 and T8 intervertebral discs were removed to expose the endplates, which were decorticated to facilitate an arthrodesis using rib graft to obliterate the bony defect. During microdissection of the spinal cord, transient reduction in the amplitudes of somatosensory and motor evoked potentials were noted, prompting continuation of high-dose methylprednisolone for 24 hours postoperatively. A chest tube was placed through a separate incision, and the patient was awakened from anesthesia and monitored in the intensive care unit overnight.

Postoperative Management

Postoperatively the patient moved her lower limbs and was extubated the following day. The lumbar drain was opened to drain approximately 225 cc of CSF daily to facilitate closure of the anterior dural defect. The patient maintained her preoperative neurologic function, and her progressive decline ceased by the time of her 12-month follow-up. Some objective improvement in left lower limb strength was observed. Postoperative MRI revealed return of the spinal cord into the spinal canal with obliteration of the cavitary bony defect (Fig. 45–3).

Discussion

Spinal cord herniation (SCH) is a rare malformation that has been described infrequently. Currently, there are approximately 30 reported cases of spinal cord herniation from various etiologies. Others may have been misdiagnosed or simply not identified. Prior to MRI, the diagnosis of SCH was difficult. Recently, we have treated two patients with spontaneous anterior thoracic SCH. Typical characteristics include a thoracic ventrolateral SCH in an adult with symptoms of a progressive Brown-Séquard syndrome, resulting in single-limb weakness with contralateral limb numbness. Imaging demonstrates anterior cord displacement without a dorsal mass and normal CSF flow behind the SCH. Stabilization or reversal of neurologic deficits can be achieved with surgical reduction of the displaced cord; neurologic decline appears progressive if untreated. The pathophysiology of this rare syndrome is uncertain but may be related to asymmetric ventrolateral spinal cord tethering within the dural defect.

Although Isu and colleagues (1991) have classified spinal cord herniation into traumatic, postoperative, and congenital groups, most reported cases are not associated with trauma or surgery. Although arachnoid cysts have also been associated with SCH, these most likely occur as a consequence rather than a cause of herniation.

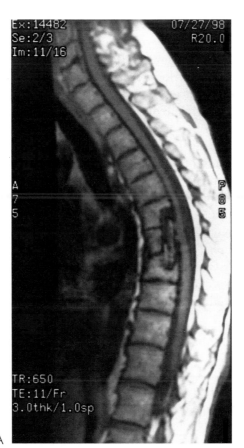

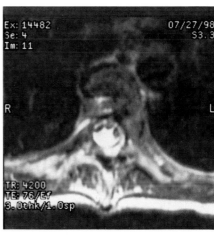

Figure 45–3. Midsaggital T1-weighted (A) and axial T2-weighted (B) MRI demonstrate the return of the thoracic cord into the thecal sac and obliteration of the vertebral body defect with an anterior autologous rib graft reconstruction.

In 1974, Wortzman and colleagues reported the first case of SCH in a 63-year-old diabetic with prior minor back trauma. The patient had progressive weakness with numbness of his left distal lower extremity and new onset of urgency and fecal incontinence. Myelography revealed a complete block at T7. A transthoracic approach was used to identify a herniated spinal cord that appeared incarcerated through a dural defect into the vertebral body of T7. The cord displacement was reduced into its normal position within the dural sac and the defect was primarily closed. Recovery occurred gradually over 2 years. Although herniation of the spinal cord through iatrogenic or traumatic dural defects has been described, idiopathic SCH is a separate identity with unique characteristics and an uncertain pathophysiology.

Alternative Methods of Management

Although progressive dysfunction without surgical treatment has been uniformly observed, the ideal surgical approach used for reduction of the SCH is uncertain.

Borges and colleagues (1995) advocate a posterolateral approach via a laminectomy; they performed one transthoracic approach among three patients treated for SCH. This familiar exposure allows treatment of a dorsal arachnoid cyst, if present. With this approach, the dentate ligaments must be divided to mobilize the spinal cord sufficiently to allow manipulation and lateral displacement of the cord to facilitate adequate visualization of the ventral defect. Placement of a dural graft patch may prevent recurrence of herniation while maintaining the cross-sectional area of the dura. Others have additionally placed a flexible rubber strip to act as a ventral sling to prevent reherniation.

Although Isu and colleagues (1991) proposed that the arachnoid cyst caused the neurologic deterioration and argued against reducing the SCH, neither patient experienced motor recovery as has been observed in other previously reported cases in which anatomic reduction was achieved. We recommend that midline ventral herniations be managed with a transthoracic approach, whereas ventrolateral dural defects are treated posterolaterally. Bony restruction of large vertebral defects may prevent recurrence. We also support the hypothesis that reduction of the displaced SCH is the primary goal of surgical treatment.

An intraoperative endoscope may aid visualization, regardless of the approach taken. Moreover, preoperative endoscopic assessment may aid in planning the surgical approach and perhaps in elucidating the pathophysiology of these unique malformations. For example, an arachnoid-like fibrous tissue present in cases of arachnoid cysts has also been observed in spinal cord herniation. Because durotomy and exploration disturb this material, successful examination and analysis of this tissue may require minimally invasive techniques like myeloscopy.

Type of Management	Advantages	Disadvantages	Comments
Transthoracic approach	Visualization of midline dural defect with less cord manipulation Allows bony reconstruction if defect is present	Difficult dural repair	Postoperative thoracic CSF effusions may be reduced with use of a lumbar drain
Posterolateral approach	Familiar anatomy Allows treatment of dorsal arachnoid cyst	Requires greater cord manipulation	Section of dentate ligaments facilitates cord mobility

Complications

Given the significant manipulation required to reduce the SCH and close the dural defect, neurologic deterioration is the most concerning postoperative complication. Inadequate exposure may preclude successful reduction and dural closure. Cerebrospinal fluid leak may cause severe headaches or preclude wound healing. Infection and bleeding are complications common to any surgical treatment, although risks of meningitis are additionally encountered after arachnoid exposure.

Suggested Readings

Borges LF, Zervas NT, Lehrich JR. Idiopathic spinal cord herniation: a treatable cause of the Brown-Sequard syndrome—case report. Neurosurgery 1995; 36:1028–1033.

Isu T, Iizuka T, Iwasaki Y, et al. Spinal cord herniation associated with an intradural spinal arachnoid cyst diagnosed by magnetic resonance imaging. Neurosurgery 1991; 29:137–139.

Miyake S, Tamaki N, Nagashima T, et al. Idiopathic spinal cord herniation. J Neurosurg 1998; 88:331–335.

Uchiyama S, Hasegawa K, Homma T, et al. Ultrafine flexible spinal endoscope (myeloscope) and discovery of an unreported subarachnoid lesion. Spine 1998; 23:2358–2362.

Wortzman G, Tasker RR, Rewcastle NB, et al. Spontaneous incarcerated herniation of the spinal cord into a vertebral body: a unique course of paraplegia. J Neurosurg 1974; 41:631–635.

Case 46
Metastatic Disease—Cervical Spine, Thoracic Spine, Lumbar Spine

Joseph M. Kowalski, Steven C. Ludwig, and John G. Heller

History and Physical Examination

A 75-year-old man presented with 6 weeks of progressive back and left flank pain associated with progressive weakness of his lower extremities. He had lost 15 pounds in the past 3 months, which was evident to inspection. Motor examination revealed bilateral grade 3/5 strength of hip flexors and quadriceps muscles, and 4/5 strength in the remaining lower extremity muscles. His deep tendon reflexes were hyperactive at the knees and ankles, with bilateral clonus at the ankles. Despite normal rectal muscle tone, his perianal sensation was reduced. His postvoid residual volume was 400 mL. A urine culture grew *Proteus mirabilis*.

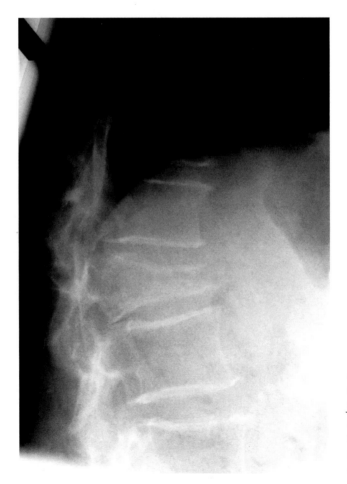

Figure 46–1. Lateral radiograph showing a pathologic fracture of L1. Note the shortening of the posterior vertebral body height, and the preservation of the adjacent disc spaces.

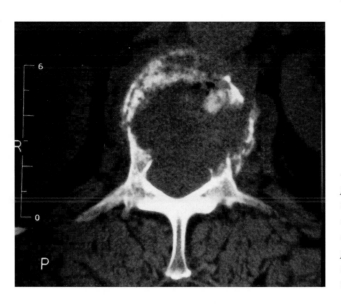

Figure 46–2. Axial computed tomography (CT) scan of L1 showing destructive lesion of vertebral body and left pedicle with increased paravertebral soft tissue thickness, and bone debris within the spinal canal.

Radiologic Findings

Plain radiographs revealed a fracture of the L1 vertebral body with loss of posterior vertebral body height, widened paraspinal soft tissue shadows, and preservation of the adjacent intervertebral disc features (Fig. 46–1). A noncontrast computed tomography (CT) scan demonstrated a lytic lesion of the L1 vertebral body and left pedicle with a mixture of bone debris and soft tissue encroaching upon the spinal canal (Figs. 46–2 and 46–3). Magnetic resonance imaging (MRI) demonstrated the extent of the paravertebral soft tissue mass and the compromise of the spinal canal with compression of the conus medullaris (Figs. 46–4 and 46–5). A staging CT scan

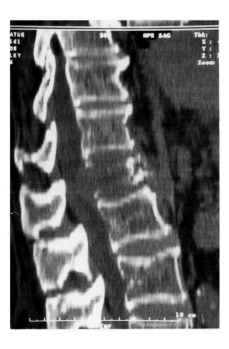

Figure 46–3. A reconstructed CT scan demonstrating local bone destruction, kyphosis, and spinal canal encroachment.

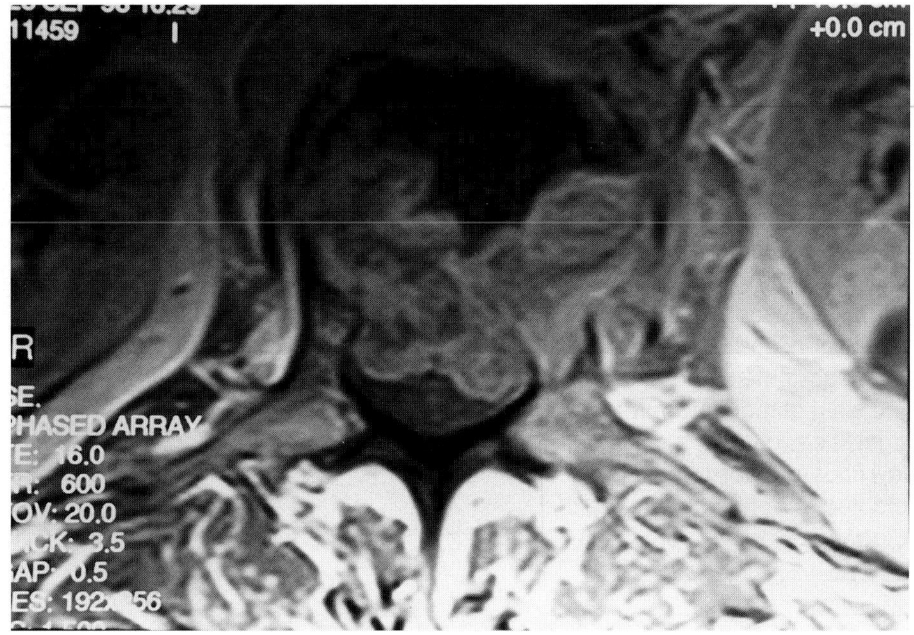

- In treating spinal metastases, one should prioritize the intended objectives of the procedure, then try to design the least complex procedure that can satisfactorily address those objectives with a favorable morbidity risk. Ideally, the patient should be rendered sufficiently stable to be rapidly mobilized, preferably brace free. Preoperative angiography and embolization can be very effective in reducing operative blood loss, thus facilitating safe resection and construction.
- It is important to recognize and address malnutrition to minimize wound healing complications, infection risk, and enhance recovery.

Figure 46–4. T1-weighted postgadolinium axial magnetic resonance imaging (MRI) of L1. Note the soft tissue lesion and extension into canal with enhancement of lesion.

PITFALLS

- Be wary of placing incisions through irradiated tissues due to the increased risk of wound dehiscence. Don't hesitate to consult a plastic surgeon to assist with a tissue flap. Prolonged wound drainage is an ominous sign.
- Try to avoid a circumstance wherein a patient leaves the operating room without sufficient spinal stability to be allowed out of bed, as this patient population is prone to complications, and a second opportunity for an anesthetic is not always assured.

of the chest, abdomen, and pelvis revealed a large lesion of the left kidney (Fig. 46–6) with no other evidence of visceral involvement. A technetium bone scan identified only the L1 area of increased activity.

Diagnosis

Pathologic fracture of L1 associated with paraparesis. The most likely cause is a metastasis from a previously undiagnosed left renal cell carcinoma, as the imaging studies are not consistent with vertebral osteomyelitis. The coexisting urinary tract infection is probably due to urinary retention from neurogenic bladder dysfunction. Malnutrition is also evident.

Surgical Management

The diagnosis of renal cell carcinoma was confirmed by a CT-guided biopsy of the renal lesion. With the primary lesion confirmed, an interdisciplinary treatment plan was devised to simultaneously address the patient's oncologic, neurologic, and skeletal needs. A Foley catheter was inserted and parenteral antibiotics were administered to address the urinary tract infection, while initiating parenteral nutritional support. Surgical intervention was indicated to (1) eradicate the primary lesion (left nephrectomy), (2) relieve spinal cord compression to arrest or reverse the progressive neurologic deficits, and (3) realign and stabilize the spine to reduce or eliminate pain and enhance the patient's quality of life.

Due to the propensity for renal cell carcinoma lesions to bleed, a preoperative arteriogram was performed for selective embolization of the L1 lesion on the day prior to surgery. A left anterior thoracoabdominal approach was performed, which simul-

PEARLS

- One can be fooled by imaging studies. Remember "to culture what you biopsy and biopsy what you culture." Be sure to specify that bacteriologic specimens be evaluated for aerobic, anaerobic, fungal, and acid-fast species, as they are all part of the differential diagnosis. A patient can develop a superinfection of a metastatic lesion.

- Routine blood studies are obtained to evaluate the patient's immunologic and nutritional status. These studies can determine the patient's physiologic status and suggest a source of the primary lesion if the metastatic lesion is the initial manifestation of the disease. Hypercalcemia is frequently encountered in metastatic disease. Prompt treatment can reduce the risk of cardiac arrhythmia and death. Renal dysfunction may result from the malignancy or from malignant calcification and may be reflected in elevated creatinine and blood urea nitrogen. An abnormal urinalysis may also be the first clue to a renal carcinoma. Most cases of multiple myeloma may be diagnosed on the basis of leukopenia, anemia, thrombocytopenia, and reversal of the albumin to globulin ratio. Serum immuno-electrophoresis may be required to guide treatment. Prostate-specific antigen (PSA) and carcinoembryonic antigen (CEA) have many shortcomings, but some physicians use them to screen and follow patients with a variety of cancers.

- If time and the patient's condition permits, oncologic staging of the lesion can be completed preoperatively. Chest radiographs and a CT of the chest,

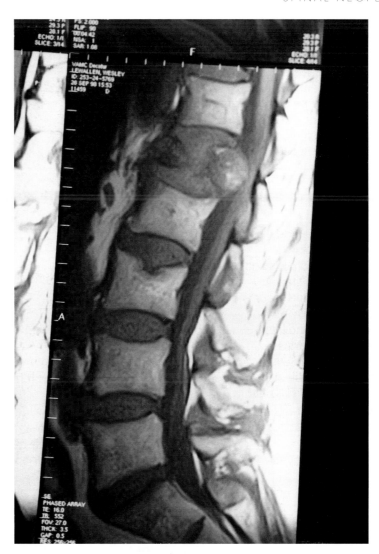

Figure 46–5. Sagittal MRI showing the degree of compression of the conus medullaris. However, MRI cannot distinguish whether the compression is due to bone or soft tissue (compare with Fig. 46–2).

taneously allowed the urologic surgeons to perform the nephrectomy and afforded appropriate access to the thoracolumbar spine. A single-stage anterior decompression, reconstruction, and instrumentation was accomplished (Figs. 46–7 and 46–8). We elected to employ a titanium mesh cylindrical cage to provide immediate anterior column support, in combination with a mixture of autogenous bone graft and morcelized fresh-frozen femoral head allograft to attempt biologic union. Supplemental anterior spinal fixation was applied for enhanced mechanical stability.

Postoperative Management

Prophylactic antibiotics are typically administered for only 24 hours postoperatively. However, they were continued in this case until sterile urine had been assured. Early mobilization was intended. In this instance the patient was out of bed

abdomen, and pelvis are performed to pursue any evidence of additional metastatic disease. If mental status changes are evident, MRI or CT of the brain should be considered, as the presence of such lesions may contraindicate aggressive treatment in certain circumstances.

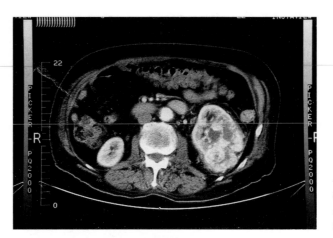

Figure 46–6. CT scan of abdomen demonstrating lesion of left kidney later proven to be renal cell carcinoma.

PITFALL

• Radiologists cannot read the surgeon's mind! Be sure to specify what levels of the spine must be included in the imaging studies. The authors recommend scanning a minimum or three levels above and three levels below any known lesions. CT scans should employ a maximum slice width of 3 mm to provide detail sufficient for intraoperative use.

once the chest tubes were removed. As fusion was intended due to the relatively favorable survival statistics associated with renal cell carcinoma with an isolated skeletal metastasis, we required that he wear a thoracolumbar spinal orthosis (TLSO) for a minimum of 3 months when he was out of bed. Local radiation therapy to the operated spinal segments and the tumor bed was delayed nearly 6 to 8 weeks to avoid untoward influence on early graft healing.

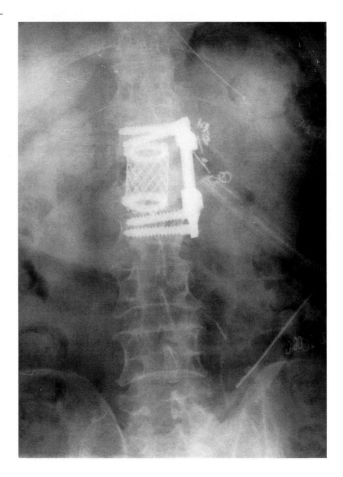

Figure 46–7. Anteroposterior radiograph showing reconstruction with anterior interbody cage and segmental fixation posteriorly with spinal hooks and pedicle screws.

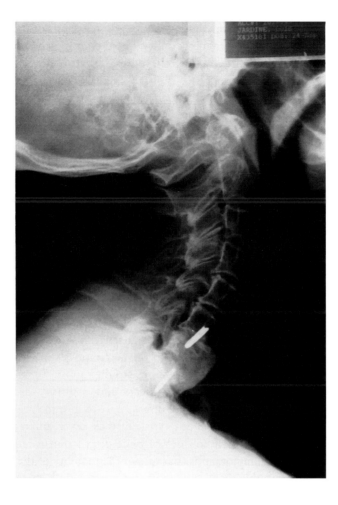

Figure 46–8. Lateral radiograph showing reconstruction of a metastasis to the cervical spine.

Discussion

Of the nearly 1 million cases of cancer diagnosed every year in this country, 50 to 70% of patients will develop skeletal metastases prior to death, with the spine being the most common site.

Within the spinal column, there are regional differences in the likelihood of metastatic involvement. Brihaye and colleagues (1988) reviewed the literature from 1959 to 1985 on the distribution of metastatic spinal tumors. Symptomatic deposits localized to the thoracic and thoracolumbar spine in 70% of cases, to the lumbar and lumbosacral spine in 22%, and to the cervical spine in 8%. Spinal cord compression most often occurs in the thoracic spine because the spinal cord is largest relative to the space available for the cord. In Gilbert and colleagues' (1978) series, 68% of patients with spinal cord compression had thoracic spinal lesions, 16% had lumbar spine lesions, and 15% had cervical spine lesions. Approximately 85% of metastatic lesions occur within the vertebral body, and the remainder are located within the posterior arch.

Clinical Presentation

Pain is by far the most common initial complaint of patients presenting with a suspected spine tumor. It may be caused by one or more of the following factors: (1)

cortical involvement (periosteal irritation) of the vertebral body, (2) pathologic fracture, (3) spinal instability, or (4) compression of the spinal cord or nerve roots. Such pain is usually not relieved by rest. It is unrelenting and may intensify at night. It tends to progress with time, in contrast to the pain associated with benign causes of vertebral fractures such as osteoporosis. In contrast, mechanical back pain is usually actively related and is relieved by rest or recumbency.

Timely diagnosis is extremely important. The neurologic status at the time of diagnosis is one of the most important prognostic factors affecting functional outcome. Patients who have significant weakness are much less likely to continue to ambulate after treatment. Of those patients who have the ability to walk at the time of diagnosis, more than 90% will retain that ability after treatment, and 30% to 60% of patients who are nonambulatory may regain the ability to ambulate. Because the compression usually occurs anteriorly in the vertebral body, the motor functions of the anterior part of the spinal cord are often compromised first. Sensory disturbances are less reliable indicators of spinal cord compression.

Plain radiographs of the spine are the initial images made due to their ready availability. However, early lesions may be difficult to detect, as 30% to 50% of trabecular bone must be destroyed before they can be seen on plain radiographs.

Technetium-99m scans are performed to survey for other bone involvement that could support a pattern of metastatic disease. Activity from tumor tissue producing bone and the host's response to the tumor can be detected, as well as reactive bone formation from fracture, infection, or arthritis. Thus, bone scans are fairly sensitive and may reveal metastatic disease 2 to 18 months prior to plain radiographic changes. The gamma camera can typically pick up a difference of 3% to 5% in bone activity, whereas 30% to 50% of bone destruction is required before changes are evident on plain radiographs. Because of the inability of the host to produce reactive bone, false-negative scans can occur, most often with myeloproliferative disorders such as myeloma, lymphoma, leukemia, reticulum cell sarcoma, and Ewing's sarcoma.

Magnetic resonance imaging facilitates characterizing the lesion on the basis of location, morphology, and signal intensity. MRI has generally displaced myelography and CT myelography as the gold standard in evaluating spinal cord compression.

Biopsy may be the final step in the workup of a spine tumor. It may confirm a metastatic lesion in a patient with a known primary tumor, evaluate a suspicious lesion, or confirm the suspected primary lesion, as in the present case. Currently, most biopsies are done percutaneously with CT or fluoroscopic guidance. The overall accuracy rate of percutaneous needle biopsy has been reported between 66% and 95% with lytic lesions and decreases to 20% to 25% with blastic lesions.

Management

The overriding goals in the treatment of spinal metastases are to provide pain control, relieve and/or prevent neural compression, and establish or maintain a quality of life that is consistent with the patient's desires. Treatment of the spinal lesion is therefore palliative. Rarely is it curative. Maintaining independence and adequate pain control can significantly impact the quality of a patient's remaining life, however long it may be.

The great majority of spinal metastases respond favorably to nonsurgical methods such as chemotherapy, radiation therapy, and hormonal manipulation. Nonsurgical therapy can be used to address the primary lesion, and possibly for local control of the spine lesion, but spinal integrity will depend on the ability of the bone to heal and remodel following radiation and or chemotherapy. Nonsurgical modalities have little or no effect on restoring spinal anatomy once fracture or deformity has occurred. The only definitive way to debulk the tumor mass, decompress neural elements, and restore and stabilize the anatomy is through surgical intervention. Thus, indications for surgical intervention in metastatic spinal disease include the need to establish a histologic diagnosis; a radioresistant or previously irradiated tumor; progressive neurologic deficit during or following nonoperative therapy; and significant spinal destruction or instability, manifested by pain, progressive deformity, and/or neurologic dysfunction.

Anterior Procedures

Because metastatic lesions primarily affect the vertebral body and compromise the spinal canal from its ventral aspect, it seems intuitive that anterior access would afford more direct decompression and reconstruction. However, widespread acceptance of anterior surgery has emerged relatively recently.

A standard ventrolateral approach along the sternocleidomastoid muscle can be used to access the majority of anterior cervical lesions. It may be combined with a median sternotomy or modified medial clavicular resection to access lesions as caudal as T4. A right thoracotomy provides ready access to the spine from T4 to L1. Thoracoabdominal or retroperitoneal exposures can be used for lesions from T12 to the sacrum. Transabdominal incisions may be most effective for lesions at the lumbosacral junction, but these are often combined with a posterior approach.

Following complete decompression of the spinal canal, it is generally possible to realign the spine by restoring normal intervertebral height. Distraction forces are applied either through an anterior internal fixation system, or specially designed instruments associated with such systems. The segmental defect must then be reconstructed, at which time the surgeon commits to either pursuing a fusion with bone graft or a palliative internal fixation with a finite life span.

Nonbiologic constructs include metallic, ceramic, or polymethylmethacrylate (PMMA) cement spacers. These constructs are intended to provide immediate mechanical integrity and compressive load bearing. PMMA cement is the least expensive and simplest technique, and it has been time tested. As bone union is not sought, there is no need to delay adjunctive radiation or chemotherapy. To prevent displacement of the spacer, a variety of techniques have been employed ranging from footings fashioned from Steinmann pins (Fig. 46–8) to more complex and expensive, but MRI compatible, titanium fixation devices.

Posterior Procedures

With adequate understanding of and experience with applicable surgical techniques, posterior procedures are not only effective but also sometimes preferable to anterior procedures for the treatment of anterior pathology.

A dorsal midline incision affords many possibilities for spinal cord decompression in metastatic disease. Laminectomy may be appropriate in limited circumstances, but it is typically restricted to multisegmental decompression of extensive disease, when combined with instrumentation techniques that realign and rigidly immobilize the spine. The same dorsal incision may be used for a circumferential decompression of the thoracic or lumbar spinal canal. This is especially true in the thoracic spine, where nerve roots may be ligated with impunity to facilitate exposure. Piecemeal removal of tumor and bone may be accomplished without manipulation of the cord. However, at least unilateral provisional instrumentation is recommended

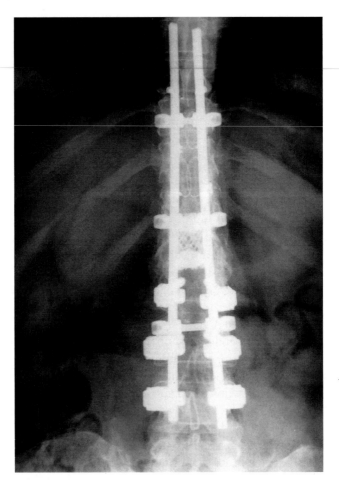

Figure 46–9. Lateral cervical radiograph 3 months after resection of a lymphoma at C7 causing severe pain with progressive radiculomyelopathy. A polymethylmethacrylate (PMMA) spacer was used for the reconstruction since immediate postoperative radiation and chemotherapy were required.

prior to the decompression to avoid inadvertent damage to the neural elements and to restore spinal alignment for the reconstruction.

In some cases all that is necessary is stabilization of the spine to prevent deformity; unfortunately, this is not often the case. Posterior segmental instrumentation techniques may employ any number of methods to grip vertebrae, such as sublaminar wires or cables, pedicle screws, and hooks attached to the pedicles, transverse processes, or beneath the laminae. The grasping elements are in turn attached to paired, cross-linked rods contoured in such a way as to affect restoration of spinal alignment (Fig. 46–9).

When bone graft is used in the reconstruction and arthrodesis is intended, radiation should be delayed 6 to 8 weeks to permit the critical early phase of graft revascularization. If delay of adjunctive medical treatment is unwise, then the authors prefer to perform a mechanical reconstruction only. The patient is advised that if all goes well with the oncologic treatment and remission is achieved, then an elective supplemental fusion may be required in 1 to 2 years.

Anterior/Posterior (360) Procedures

Circumstances that favor a combined approach in the authors' practice include lesions at the lumbosacral junction (Fig. 46–10), lesions requiring the anterior resection of two or more contiguous vertebrae, anterior resections in the face of osteopenic bone ill-suited to anterior instrumentation, and circumferential lesions that cannot be managed through a posterior exposure (e.g., the cervical spine or cervicothoracic junction).

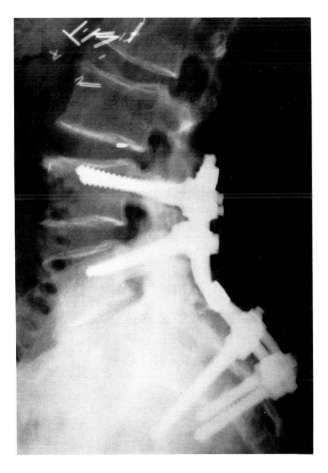

Figure 46–10. Anteroposterior radiograph showing posterior segmental fixation with sublaminar cables in thoracic spine and pedicle screws in lumbar spine. The anterior corpectomy, reconstruction, and instrumentation were accomplished through a single posterior exposure in this morbidly obese individual.

Alternative Methods of Management

Type of Management	Advantages	Disadvantages	Comments
Anterior	Directly addresses pathology in a majority of cases, i.e., tumor and compression of spinal canal Direct reconstruction of anterior and middle columns Can be used in cervical, thoracic and lumbar areas Few problems with soft tissue coverage	Not all surgeons are comfortable with these exposures/techniques Morbidity of anterior neck approach, e.g., dysphagia, and risks to cervical viscera, recurrent laryngeal nerve, thoracic duct	Versatile approaches that allow excellent view for resection of anterior and middle columns of spine May not always get adequate stability
Posterior and posterolateral	Ease and familiarity of applying instrumentation to stabilize spinal column May be performed independently of other procedures May be able to debulk and resect anterior tumor and provide anterior column support through one incision in thoracic or lumbar spine regions	Soft tissue coverage and wound healing may be difficult, especially with irradiated tissues Not able to effectively decompress or debulk cervical spine lesions Visualization and hemostasis may be difficult if attempting posterior resection of vertebral body lesions in thoracic or lumbar regions May be used to stabilize the spine independent of anterior resection and decompression	May require soft tissue coverage procedure to facilitate healing Best option for patients with significant pulmonary disease Section of dentate ligaments facilitates cord mobility

Complications

This group of patients is prone to the whole spectrum of complications. To be forewarned is to be forearmed. One should be aware of the increased relative risk of wound dehiscence, especially if the lesion has been previously irradiated. With an immunocompromised host, the relative risk of wound infection is also increased.

Intraoperatively, complications may include excessive bleeding, inadequate tumor excision, failure to achieve adequate spinal stability, and increased neurologic dysfunction. Ensuring adequate clotting capability preoperatively cannot be overemphasized. Bleeding times and platelet counts must be satisfactory before embarking on the procedure. Embolization of the lesion can be astonishingly effective at reducing blood loss. Detailed preoperative planning and adequate intraoperative visibility reduce the likelihood of inadequate tumor resection.

Suggested Readings

Asdourian PL. Metastatic disease of the spine. In: Bridwell KH, DeWald RL, eds. The Textbook of Spinal Surgery, 2d ed., pp. 2007–2050. Philadelphia: Lippincott-Raven, 1997.

Avraham E, Tadmore R, Dolly D, et al. Early MR demonstration of spinal metastasis with normal x-ray, CT and bone scans. J Comput Assist Tomogr 1987; 4:598–602.

Berg EE. The sternal-rib complex. A possible fourth column in thoracic spine fractures. Spine 1993; 18(13):1916–1919.

Boland PJ, Lane JM, Sundaresan N. Metastatic disease of the spine. Clin Orthop 1982; 169:95.

Brihaye J, Ectors P, Lemort M, Van Houtte P. The management of spinal epidural metastases. Adv Tech Stand Neurosurg 1988; 16:121–176.

DeWald RL, Bridwell KH, Prodromas C, Rodts MF. Reconstructive spinal surgery as palliation for metastatic malignancies of the spine. Spine 1985; 10:21.

Gilbert RW, Kim JH, Posner JB. Epidural spinal cord compression from metastatic tumor. Diagnosis and treatment. Ann Neurol 1978; 3(1):40.

Harrington KD. Anterior decompression and stabilization of the spine as a treatment for vertebral collapse and spinal cord compression from metastatic malignancy. Clin Orthop 1988; 233:177.

Harrington KD. The use of methylmethacrylate for vertebral-body replacement and anterior stabilization of pathologic fracture-dislocations of the spine due to metastatic malignant disease. J Bone Joint Surg 1981; 63A:36–46.

Jaffe WL. Tumors and Tumorous Conditions of the Bones and Joints. Philadelphia: Lea and Febiger, 1958.

Kaneda K, Takeda N. Reconstruction with a ceramic vertebral prosthesis and Kaneda device following subtotal or total vertebrectomy in metastatic thoracic and lumbar spine. In: Bridwell KH, DeWald RL, eds. The Textbook of Spinal Surgery, 2d ed., pp. 2071–2087. Philadelphia: Lippincott-Raven, 1997.

Kostuik JP. Anterior spinal cord decompression for lesions of the thoracic and lumbar spine, techniques, new methods of internal fixation results. Spine 1983; 8:512–531.

McAfee PC, Zdeblick TA. Tumors of the thoracic and lumbar spine: surgical treatment via the anterior approach. J Spinal Disord 1989; 2(3):145–154.

Perrin RG, McBroom RJ. Anterior versus posterior decompression for symptomatic spinal metastasis. Can J Neurol Sci 1987; 14:75–80.

Rougraff BT, Kneisl JS, Simon MA. Skeletal metastases of unknown origin. A prospective study of a diagnostic strategy. J Bone Joint Surg 1993; 75(A): 1276–1281.

Siegal T, Siegal T. Current considerations in the management of neoplastic spinal cord compression. Spine 1989; 14(2):223–228.

Siegal T, Siegal T. Surgical decompression of anterior and posterior malignant epidural tumors compressing the spinal cord: a prospective study. Neurosurgery 1985; 17(3):424.

Tatsui H, Onomura T, Morishita S, Oketa M, Inoue T. Survival rates of patients with metastatic spinal cancer after scintigraphic detection of abnormal radioactive accumulation. Spine 1996; 21:2143–2148.

Wong DA, Fornasier VL, McNab I. Spinal metastases: the obvious, the occult and the imposters. Spine 1990; 15(1):1–4.

Case 47
Spinal Intradural Intramedullary and Extramedullary Tumors

Michael K. Rosner, James M. Ecklund, and Seth M. Zeidman

History and Physical Examination

A 2-year-old girl was in her usual state of good health until 1 week prior to presentation, when she developed a fever (T_{max} = 102.5°F), neck stiffness, and inconsolable crying. Clinical and laboratory evaluation of the fever was nondiagnostic and the febrile episode subsequently resolved. Her neck stiffness, however, persisted. Comprehensive neurologic evaluation did not demonstrate any objective neurologic deficits or other findings. Diagnostic imaging included magnetic resonance imaging (MRI) scans of the brain and cervical spine, which demonstrated a well-defined radiographic abnormality within the cervical spinal cord (Fig. 47–1). Differential diagnosis included neoplasm, infection, and demyelinating conditions, though the pattern of the lesion on the images was most consistent with a neo-

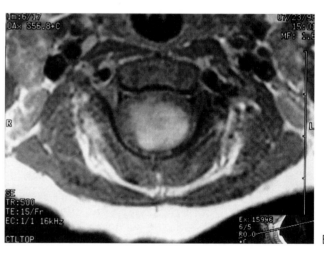

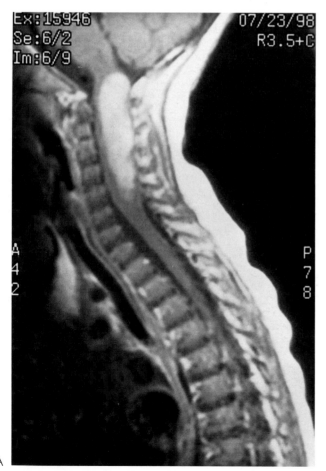

Figure 47–1. Sagittal (A) and transaxial (B) magnetic resonance imaging (MRI) of the cervical spine, revealing a focal expansile lesion of the cervical cord beginning at the level of the obex and extending inferiorly to the level of the C5/C6 disc.

plasm. The patient was subsequently transferred to the neurosurgery service for management.

Radiologic Findings

Magnetic resonance imaging of the head and screening spine demonstrated a focal expansile lesion of the cervical cord beginning at the level of the obex and extending inferiorly to the level of the C5/C6 intervertebral disc. The lesion was well circumscribed and was contained within the substance of the cord. Signal characteristics included low signal on T1, high signal on T2, and mild heterogeneous enhancement with gadolinium throughout the extent of the lesion. Maximal cord diameter and lesion diameter were 1.9 and 1.5 cm respectively. No other lesions were noted in the head or thoracolumbar spine.

Diagnosis

An intramedullary cervical spinal cord lesion was identified on MRI. The differential diagnosis was likely of glial origin (astrocytoma vs. ependymoma), as imaging characteristics and age of the patient were considered.

Surgical Management

After parentalogous blood donation, the patient was taken to the operating room and placed prone with her head on a cerebellar headrest. A midline posterior cervical incision was made with a subsequent subperiosteal dissection from the occiput to C7. An open-door laminoplasty was performed to C7 with meticulous hemostasis. The dura was opened in the midline and retracted laterally with 4-0 neurolon suture. After localization with ultrasound, a midline myelotomy was performed to identify the tumor. The mass was biopsied and sent for frozen pathology. The mass was then debulked starting from its caudal extent utilizing the ultrasonic aspirator. The patient became repeatedly bradycardic during manipulation and aspiration at the superior extent of the lesion. Margins were developed at the inferior extent and a decision was made to leave a small margin of residual tumor in an effort to avoid significant neurologic injury to the patient. A patch graft was utilized to close the dura in a watertight fashion.

The patient was extubated and followed in the intensive care unit (ICU) for several days before transfer to the regular ward. Postoperatively, the patient demonstrated no neurologic deficits. An MRI of the cervical spine obtained on postoperative day 2 (Fig. 47–2) demonstrated a small amount of residual tumor left at the superior margin.

Frozen and final pathology were consistent with low-grade astrocytoma. The patient was subsequently discharged with scheduled follow-up imaging at 3 months postoperation.

Postoperative Management

The patient was followed clinically for 3 months with no significant neurologic deficits. A routine 3-month postoperative MRI of the cervical spine demonstrated recurrence of the expansile mass from the pontomedullary junction to C6/C7 with

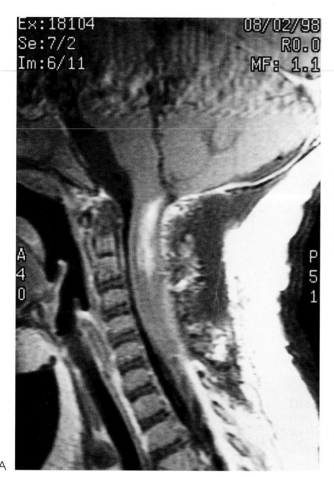

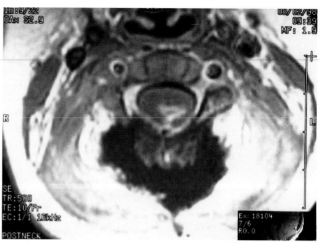

Figure 47–2. Sagittal (A) and transaxial (B) MRI of the cervical spine following surgical decompression, demonstrating a small amount of residual tumor left at the superior margin of involvement.

a large cystic component and enhancing mass (Fig. 47–3). The patient was noted to have increased episodes of crying the week prior. In light of the recurrence and questionable pathologic diagnosis from the first resection, the patient underwent re-resection of the intramedullary mass in a similar fashion utilizing ultrasound and the ultrasonic aspirator. The rostral region of the tumor was further debulked without episodes of bradycardia.

Preliminary pathology was consistent with a higher-grade glioma and a decision was made to remove grossly apparent tumor, but limit the resection at unclear margins.

Postoperatively, the patient demonstrated no motor or sensory deficits. On postoperative day 1, the patient began to leak clear fluid from her incision. A lumbar drain was placed, and the patient was started on antibiotics. The drain was removed in 5 days and no further evidence of a cerebrospinal fluid (CSF) leak was noted. A postoperative MRI demonstrated resection of approximately 85% of the total tumor volume. Final pathology was consistent with anaplastic oligoastrocytoma, grade III. In light of the higher-grade astrocytoma, the radiation and oncology services were consulted to provide additional therapy.

Discussion

Tumors involving the spinal cord or nerve roots have similarities to intracranial tumors in cellular type. They may arise from the spinal cord parenchyma, nerve roots, meningeal coverings, intraspinal vascular network, sympathetic chain, or

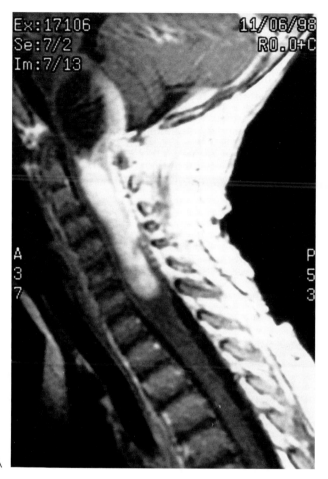

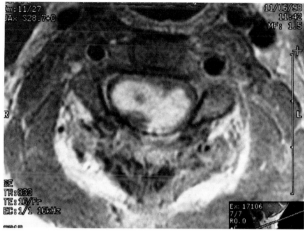

Figure 47–3. Sagittal (A) and transaxial (B) MRI of the cervical spine 3 months postoperatively, demonstrating recurrence of the expansile mass from the pontomedullary junction to C6/C7 with a large cystic component and enhancing mass.

vertebral column. Additionally, they can metastasize from elsewhere in the central nervous system or from any site within the body. The patient's signs and symptoms, the radiologic features of a spinal cord tumor, and the surgical approach to the tumor are more a function of the involved anatomic compartment than the distinct tumor histology.

Intradural tumors have been classically divided into extramedullary and intramedullary lesions. Discussion of spinal cord tumors is usually organized according to location in the spinal canal: (1) extradural, (2) intradural-extramedullary, or (3) intramedullary. Extradural (ED) tumors (55%) are the most common spine tumors. They arise outside the dura in vertebral bodies or epidural tissues. Metastatic lesions compose the majority of ED tumors (see Chapter 46). Intradural-extramedullary tumors (ID-EM) (40%) arise in leptomeninges or roots. Only 4% of metastases occur here. Intramedullary spinal cord tumors (IMSCT) (5%) arise within the substance of the spinal cord and displace or invade white matter tracts and neuron bodies. Only 2% of metastases occur in this compartment.

Intradural-Extramedullary Tumors

Included within this group are meningioma, nerve sheath tumor, and filum terminale ependymoma, which constitute approximately 85% of all ID-EM tumors. Sarcoma and lipoma account for an additional 10%. Less common entities include dermoid, epidermoid, angioma, and lymphoma.

Meningiomas

Meningiomas arise from arachnoid villi cells embedded in the dura at the nerve root sleeve, thus explaining their propensity for lateral locations. About 80% occur in the thoracic spine. Thoracic meningiomas are generally posterolateral, whereas upper cervical tumors are more commonly found in the anterolateral canal. Lower cervical and lumbar meningiomas are unusual.

The typical patient with a spinal meningioma is female (female/male ratio = 10:1), older (the majority are in the fifth to seventh decades), with a solitary (multiple tumors occur only 2% of the time) and entirely intradural (10% of lesions involve both intradural and extradural compartments) lesion.

Nerve Sheath Tumors

The classification of nerve sheath tumors is complicated by the use of the terms *neurofibroma* and *schwannoma,* and the persistence of the inaccurate terms *neuroma, neurinoma,* and *neurilemoma.* In patients with neurofibromatosis (NF-1), nerve sheath tumors are usually asymptomatic and multiple with histology consistent with neurofibromas. In the absence of neurofibromatosis, the tumors are almost always schwannomas.

Schwannomas originate from Schwann cells, but the origin of neurofibromas is uncertain. It has been postulated that neurofibromas arise from mesenchymal cells (fibroblasts). Neurofibromas produce a fusiform dilatation of the involved sensory nerve root, with no apparent plane between nerve and tumor. Occasionally they straddle the neural foramen and enlarge in the paraspinal tissues, resulting in a so-called dumbbell tumor with the narrowest portion in the foramen. Multiple neurofibromas contribute to establishing the diagnosis of NF, but the entity should be considered in any patient with even a solitary tumor.

The overwhelming majority of intraspinal nerve sheath tumors are schwannomas. They occur with approximately the same frequency as meningiomas, but in a more even distribution along the spine. They are slightly more common in men, with a peak incidence in the third to fifth decades. Like neurofibromas, schwannomas originate from sensory roots. In distinction to neurofibromas, schwannomas can often be separated from the nerve root. They are generally connected to a few fascicles without fusiform enlargement of the root.

Filum Ependymomas

Ependymomas account for only about 5% of intracranial tumors, but about 30% of intraspinal tumors. Approximately half of spinal ependymomas occur at the filum terminale, reflecting the presence of ependyma in this region. Due to their neuroectodermal origins, pathologists classify all spinal ependymomas as intramedullary, but from a clinical and surgical viewpoint the filum ependymoma is more suggestive of an extramedullary lesion. Filum ependymomas can be seen at any age, but are most common between the third and fifth decades. These patients present on average at an earlier age than those with intramedullary ependymomas.

Surgical Therapy

Because most ID-EM tumors are benign, the goal of surgery is complete removal. The treatment of intraspinal meningiomas, neurofibromas, and schwannomas is surgical excision. This may include excision of the involved portion of the dura mater (meningioma) or the involved nerve rootlets or entire root (schwannoma, neurofibroma). At the level of involvement, neurofibromas and schwannomas typically grow on the dorsal (sensory) root in preference to the ventral (motor) root, and it is generally possible to spare motor function during tumor removal. In neurofibromas, such tumors are part of a more widespread process (neurofibromatosis), in which there are similar tumors on multiple other nerve roots and nerves. Although follow-up surveillance may be needed, a majority of patients with solitary intraspinal lesions (meningioma, neurofibroma, or schwannoma) can be cured, with gross total removal of the lesion.

Intramedullary Neoplasms

Intramedullary (IM) spinal cord tumors account for 3% of all central nervous system (CNS) tumors and about 25% of spinal neoplasms. Astrocytomas and ependymomas are the most common tumors, composing 45% and 35%, respectively, of intramedullary lesions. The remaining 20% are divided among several different tumor types, including hemangioblastomas (10%), lipomas (2%), dermoids (1%), epidermoids (1%), teratomas (1%), neuroblastomas, and mixed tumors. Primary lymphoma, oligodendroglioma, cholesteatoma, and intramedullary metastases are extremely rare.

Intramedullary spinal cord tumors occur at all ages, predominantly in young or middle-aged adults and less commonly in childhood and the elderly (>60 years old). In children, astrocytomas predominate, but in adults, ependymomas and astrocytomas occur more equally. An equal distribution between males and females has been reported. Although spinal tumors are more common in the thoracic region, when the incidence is calculated as a function of actual spinal cord length, the distribution is relatively equal.

Differential Diagnosis of Intramedullary Spinal Cord Tumors

The use of MRI facilitates differentiation of intramedullary spinal cord tumors from other entities. Nevertheless, the clinical presentation of two nonneoplastic entities, multiple sclerosis (MS) and syringomyelia, can be strikingly similar to that seen with these tumors.

Management Decisions Regarding Intramedullary Spinal Cord Tumors

The presence of an intramedullary spinal cord tumor does not necessarily mandate operative removal. The decision to operate on patients with advanced neurologic deficits must be made in concert with the patient and the family, after realistic expectations have been presented. These include a desire to preserve residual sphincter function or to preserve sensation in bedridden patients who are at risk for skin breakdown. Although patients who cannot stand are unlikely to regain enough motor function to ambulate as a result of tumor resection, surgery may maintain the quality of a patient's life by preserving the ability to transfer to or to turn in bed. Patients with complete motor and sensory deficits will not improve with surgery and are not operative candidates except when the diagnosis is in doubt.

Intraoperative ultrasound is very useful for localizing tumor, identifying associated cysts, as well as delineating the extent of resection. The myelotomy should be performed at or near the posterior median septum, preferably at a point where the normal neurologic tissue appears most thinned. When an extensive myelotomy is planned, it is preferable to make a midline myelotomy even when this is not the most attenuated portion of the cord. Sometimes, being certain of the exact midline is difficult because the spinal cord anatomy may be distorted by the tumor. Therefore, because normally the midline is midway between the left and right dorsal roots, both the left and right dorsal roots should be identified before initiating the myelotomy. Extension of a myelotomy situated in the area of the dorsal root entry zone can be disastrous. The most common technical error associated with this surgery is inadequate exposure of the tumor poles.

Specific Tumor Types

Astrocytomas

Intramedullary spinal cord astrocytomas are usually located several millimeters beneath the dorsal surface of the spinal cord, and although they may be distinguished from the surrounding spinal cord, they blend imperceptibly with the spinal cord at their margins, rendering complete lesion extirpation impossible. Resection of these infiltrating lesions should be continued until the interface with the spinal cord becomes indistinguishable or until resection produces changes in the evoked potentials. An intramedullary astrocytoma ordinarily cannot be completely removed surgically. However, in some cases, especially at the cervicomedullary junction, cleavage planes can be defined and gross total resection achieved. Gross total resection can result in extended clinical (neurologic) stabilization and effective cure.

Ependymomas

Ependymomas originate from ependymal rests along the central canal. As they grow from their point of origin, they push the adjacent spinal cord aside and are distinct from the surrounding spinal cord. Ependymomas are well delineated from the surrounding parenchyma and usually can be totally excised. Cysts are frequently found at either or both ends of the tumor and aid in dissection. Ependymomas typically have a clear plane of dissection, and surgical cure is usually possible with preservation of the surrounding spinal cord. In most patients, a total resection is possible.

Hemangioblastomas

Hemangioblastomas are typically red and nodular with a clear plane of dissection, and surgical cure is usually possible with maintenance of the surrounding spinal cord. They are immediately apparent on the dorsal surface of the spinal cord, along with a collection of vessels that supply and drain the lesion. They range in size from a few millimeters in diameter to the size of a large grape and are well differentiated from the surrounding spinal cord.

No attempt should be made to enter this highly vascular tumor until its vascular supply is interrupted totally.

The arterial supply, part of which is visible on the dorsal surface of the spinal cord, should be coagulated and cut, and the tumor very slowly reduced in size with bipolar cautery. After this is done, the tumor may be dissected more easily from the adjacent spinal cord. This dissection exposes additional vascular supply, which should be interrupted sequentially, allowing total removal.

Lipomas

Lipomas of the spinal cord are seen most frequently at the level of the conus medullaris. These tumors are histologically identical to normal adipose tissue and are located on the dorsal surface of the spinal cord covered by little or no neural tissue. These lesions grow slowly, but recurrence may occur as a result of continued growth of residual tumor.

Intramedullary Metastatic Tumors

Metastases to the spinal cord are rare and represent fewer than 8% of all intramedullary spinal cord tumors. Tumors that metastasize to the spinal cord include lung and breast carcinoma. Less commonly, lymphoma, colon adenocarcinoma, head and neck carcinoma, and renal cell carcinoma may produce spinal cord metastases.

These lesions tend to be vascular and well differentiated from the adjacent spinal cord. The most effective operative strategy consists of slow bipolar coagulation of the tumor to reduce the bulk of the lesion, followed by visualization and section of the vascular supply and total removal.

Management

Prior to recent advances, the mainstay of therapy for spinal cord tumors was biopsy followed by radiation therapy. Currently, standard treatment for intradural spinal cord tumors remains microsurgical resection. Attempts at surgical resection should be performed prior to significant neurologic deterioration. Preoperative neurologic status is the best predictor of functional status postoperatively.

Neurologic outcome in the immediate postoperative period is related most closely to the patient's immediate preoperative neurologic state. Rarely, patients who have no motor function may regain a small amount of function after operation, but most likely they will not be able to walk or stand as a result of tumor resection. Similarly, patients who cannot stand are unlikely to be able to walk in the postoperative period.

Alternative Methods of Management

Type of Management	Advantages	Disadvantages	Comments
Biopsy	Simple procedure with minimal risk	Not curative, persistent neurologic deficit	Only for diagnosis
Surgical resection	Potential for complete cure	Makes deficits worse	Appropriate for most tumors
Chemotherapy	Useful for metastatic disease	No immediate relief of deficits	Limited usefulness
Radiation therapy	Metastatic disease	Does not provide decompression	Limited usefulness
Biopsy	Establish diagnosis	Not curative	Limited by biopsy field
Surgical resection	Maintain quality of life, may cure ependymoma	May increase neurologic deficit	Benefits outweigh risks
Chemotherapy	May halt progression	Limited efficacy	Limited usefulness
Radiation therapy	Smaller series describe some benefit	No established benefit for gliomas, radiation myelopathy	Efficacy difficult to evaluate

Complications of Intramedullary Spinal Cord Tumors

Exacerbation of Neurologic Deficit

Neurologic deterioration is less a function of tumor histology or the extent of surgical resection than preoperative status. Patients with severe preoperative motor deficits have the highest likelihood of sustaining a permanent neurologic deficit postoperatively. Nearly 20% of patients experience a permanent increase in their deficits.

Dorsal column injury will cause loss of proprioception and may occur as a result of the myelotomy. Lateral dissection can injure the spinothalamic tracts and produce sensory dysfunction. Diminution of somatosensory evoked potentials (SSEPs) may indicate disturbance or injury to these pathways.

Dysesthesias, hyperesthesias, and hyperpathia are terrible postoperative complications. These entities may render an otherwise functional extremity useless and prevent a patient with minimal or no motor deficit from returning to a former occupation or resuming a normal social life. Frequently, these symptoms are present preoperatively from tumor invasion of sensory pathways and persist or are exacerbated as a result of tumor removal.

Neurologic deterioration can occur several days after surgery and has been attributed to too rapid steroid taper. Subsequent increase in corticosteroid dosage does not always restore neurologic function. Potentially reversible etiologies such as postoperative hematoma and vascular insults must be considered and treated as appropriate.

Conclusions

Development of new technologies for the diagnosis and treatment of intramedullary tumors including MRI, the operating microscope, ultrasound, laser, and ultrasonic tissue aspirator have radically changed the results of surgery, perioperative management and long-term outcomes. Unsatisfactory outcomes with standard operative therapies prior to the introduction of these new technologies led many surgeons to conclude that the least harmful strategy was limited biopsy with adjuvant postoperative irradiation. These developments have allowed more accurate preoperative diagnosis and safer, more effective operative interventions.

Suggested Readings

Braverman DL, Lachmann EA, Tunkel R, Nagler W. Multiple sclerosis presenting as a spinal cord tumor. Arch Phys Med Rehabil 1997; 78(11):1274–1276.

Cusick JF, Bernardi R. Syringomyelia after removal of benign spinal extramedullary neoplasms. Spine 1995; 20(11):1289–1294.

Goh KY, Velasquez L, Epstein FJ. Pediatric intramedullary spinal cord tumors: is surgery alone enough? Pediatr Neurosurg 1997; 27(1):34–39.

Hejazi N, Hassler W. Microsurgical treatment of intramedullary spinal cord tumors. Neurol Med Chir (Tokyo) 1998; 38(5):266–271.

Horiuchi H, Yasukawa Y, Akizuki S, Takizawa T, Yamazaki I. Familial neurilemoma of the spinal cord in a mother and daughter. J Spinal Disord 1998; 11(4):359–361.

Katoh S, Ikata T, Inoue A, Takahashi M. Intradural extramedullary ependymoma. A case report. Spine 1995; 20(18):2036–2038.

Kim DS, Kim TS, Choi JU. Intradural extramedullary xanthoma of the spine: a rare lesion arising from the dura mater of the spine: case report. Neurosurgery 1996; 39(1):182–185.

Lee M, Rezai AR, Abbott R, Coelho DH, Epstein FJ. Intramedullary spinal cord lipomas. J Neurosurg 1995; 82(3):394–400.

Lee M, Rezai AR, Freed D, Epstein FJ. Intramedullary spinal cord tumors in neurofibromatosis. Neurosurgery 1996; 38(1):32–37.

Lonjon M, Goh KY, Epstein FJ. Intramedullary spinal cord ependymomas in children: treatment, results and follow-up. Pediatr Neurosurg 1998; 29(4):178–183.

Maiuri F, Iaconetta G, de Divitiis O. The role of intraoperative sonography in reducing invasiveness during surgery for spinal tumors. Minim Invasive Neurosurg 1997; 40(1):8–12.

Minami M, Hanakita J, Suwa H, Suzui H, Fujita K, Nakamura T. Cervical hemangioblastoma with a past history of subarachnoid hemorrhage. Surg Neurol 1998; 49(3):278–281.

Morota N, Deletis V, Constantini S, Kofler M, Cohen H, Epstein FJ. The role of motor evoked potentials during surgery for intramedullary spinal cord tumors. Neurosurgery 1997; 41(6):1327–1336.

Mottl H, Koutecky J. Treatment of spinal cord tumors in children. Med Pediatr Oncol 1997; 29(4):293–295.

Papadatos D, Albrecht S, Mohr G, del Carpio-O'Donovan R. Exophytic primitive neuroectodermal tumor of the spinal cord. AJNR 1998; 19(4):787–789.

Wippold FJ II, Smirniotopoulos JG, Moran CJ, Suojanen JN, Vollmer DG. MR imaging of myxopapillary ependymoma: findings and value to determine extent of tumor and its relation to intraspinal structures. AJR 1995; 165(5):1263–1267.

Xu QW, Bao WM, Mao RL, Yang GY. Aggressive surgery for intramedullary tumor of cervical spinal cord. Surg Neurol 1996; 46(4):322–328.

Adult and Pediatric Deformity

Case 48
Congenital Scoliosis
Paul E. Savas, Peter G. Gabos, and Alexander R. Vaccaro

History and Physical Examination

An 11-year-old girl was referred for evaluation of congenital scoliosis and chest wall deformities. These were noticed at birth. Previous management with a Milwaukee brace at 5 years of age failed to halt progression of the scoliosis. Presently she was premenarchal. Her family had a history of scoliosis. Back pain, neurologic symptoms, and associated cardiac and genitourinary anomalies were not present.

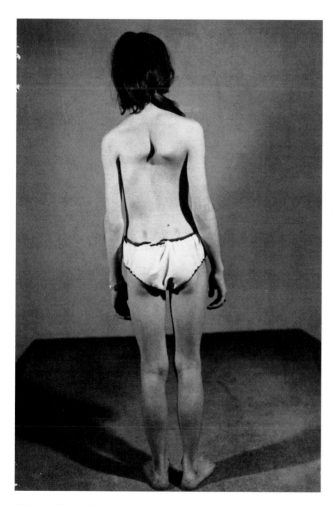

Figure 48–1. Physical examination. The patient viewed from the back to evaluate the spine deformity. There is a shift of the thorax to the left. There is shoulder tilting with right shoulder elevation. The right iliac crest appears higher secondary to the shift of the thorax.

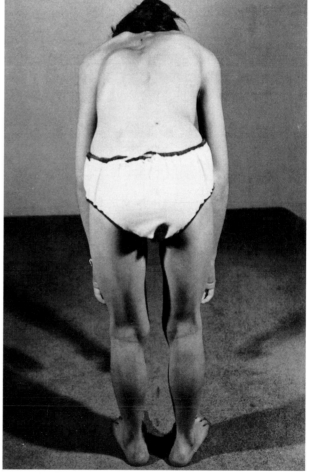

Figure 48–2. Forward-bending test. The patient stands with feet together, knees straight, and bends forward at the waist. The examiner looks down the back viewing the thoracic and lumbar areas. The right and left sides are compared. There is a left thoracolumbar hump and elevation of the left scapula.

Physical examination revealed an obvious spinal deformity, an associated marked left thoracic rib prominence, right shoulder elevation, asymmetric scapulae, and pelvic obliquity (Figs. 48–1 and 48–2). There were marked chest wall anomalies and an anterior thoracic defect over the mediastinal structures. Three supernumerary nipples were present, and there were no cutaneous lesions overlying the spine (Fig. 48–3). No neurologic deficits were demonstrated.

Radiologic Findings

A standing anteroposterior radiograph of the spine at presentation showed a 48-degree right thoracic curve due to multiple congenital spine malformations. A unilateral, unsegmented bar spanning multiple vertebrae with a contralateral, fully segmented, incarcerated hemivertebra at the apex of the thoracic curve was present. Multiple thoracic anomalies included absent and fused ribs on both sides of the curvature. A 32-degree left thoracolumbar compensatory curve had developed along with right shoulder elevation, pelvic obliquity, and a spondylolysis of the L5 vertebra (Fig. 48–4A).

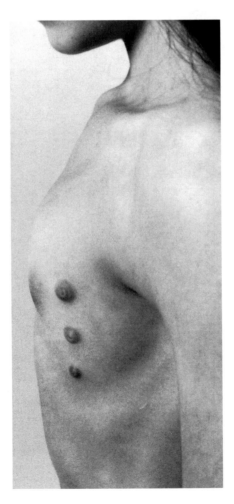

Figure 48–3. Physical examination. Left chest wall protuberance and anomalous supernumerary nipples.

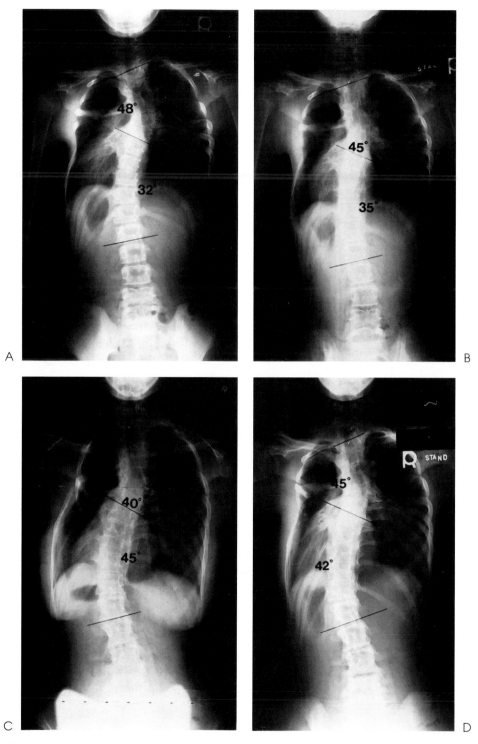

Figure 48–4. (A) Standing anteroposterior (AP) radiograph at presentation. A 48-degree right thoracic curve due to mixed anomalies. A concave, unilateral, unsegmented bar spanning multiple vertebrae with a convex, contralateral, fully segmented, incarcerated hemivertebra at the apex and a 32-degree left thoracolumbar compensatory curve have developed. There are multiple rib anomalies and spondylolysis of the L5 vertebra. (B) Radiograph at 10 months following surgery shows no progression of the curves. (C) Radiograph at 6 years following surgery shows a solid fusion and no progression of the primary curve. (D) Radiograph at 12 years following surgery; the fusion is solid and no further progression of the curves has occurred. Spinal balance is maintained.

Diagnosis

The diagnosis is *congenital scoliosis,* consisting of a unilateral, unsegmented bar with a contralateral, fully segmented, incarcerated hemivertebra, and associated marked thoracic malformations. This type of mixed spinal anomaly has the worst prognosis for progression of the spinal curvature.

Surgical Management

Surgical management was elected for curve stabilization and for prevention of curve progression prior to staged thoracoplasties for the chest wall deformities. A posterior spinal fusion without instrumentation was performed.

The technique consists of positioning the patient prone on a standard scoliosis frame. This relieves pressure on the abdomen and prevents venous congestion in the spine. Sterile preparation should include the region of the posterior iliac crests, from which autogenous bone graft is harvested.

To begin the exposure, a straight midline incision is made from at least one vertebra above and one below the vertebrae to be fused. The subcutaneous tissues are sharply divided down to the tips of the spinous processes. The tips of the spinous processes are split in the midline only in the nonanomalous spinal segments. While performing midline dissections in the region of the spinal anomalies, extreme caution must be exercised to avoid spinal injury through laminar and spinous process defects not detected on preoperative radiographs. In these regions, dissection to the midline should proceed from a lateral to a medial direction through the muscle layers until bone is encountered. Determination of the exact vertebrae to be fused may be difficult because of distorted anatomic landmarks. To confirm the correct levels prior to further exposure, an intraoperative radiograph with markers is recommended.

In the thoracic spine, subperiosteal exposure of the posterior elements should extend to the tips of the transverse processes on both sides. In the cervical and lumbar regions, exposure should be carried out laterally until the facets are well visualized. Meticulous removal of soft tissues and the facet joint capsules completes the exposure.

The concave and convex facet joints in the region to be fused are excised. The facets are decorticated. Plugs of autogenous iliac cancellous bone are impacted into the areas of the excised facet joints. The spinous processes, laminae, and transverse processes are decorticated. Large quantities of bone graft should be added to the decorticated bed to provide a thick fusion mass.

In this case, direct evaluation of the spine intraoperatively revealed large open defects at T2 and T8. The hemivertebra at T6 and the rest of the anomalous region were fused. A posterior fusion, as described, was performed on the concave and convex sides of the primary curve.

Postoperative Management

To maintain correction, a well-molded body cast with a chin-piece extension was applied 1 week after uncomplicated, postoperative recuperation and complete bed rest. Six weeks after surgery, the cast was changed to an underarm body cast and ambulation was encouraged. At 10 months following surgery, the fusion mass appeared solid radiographically, and there was no curve progression (Fig. 48–4B). After removal of the cast, an orthoplast jacket was placed. Bracing was continued to skeletal maturity to control progression of the thoracolumbar compensatory curve. At 6 years following surgery, the fusion was solid, and no progression of the primary curve occurred. The fully segmented hemivertebra was fused. Gradual progression of the secondary curve developed; this provided spinal balance (Fig. 48–4C). At 12 years following surgery, there was no progression of the curves, and spinal balance was maintained (Fig. 48–4D).

Discussion

Congenital scoliosis is a deformity of the spine caused by anomalous vertebral development; this results in a lateral curvature of the spine. Congenital vertebral anomalies may also cause isolated abnormal anterior and posterior curvatures of the spine, referred to as congenital kyphosis or congenital lordosis. A congenital scoliosis may contain an abnormal kyphotic or lordotic component, and should be termed kyphoscoliosis or lordoscoliosis. Although the anomalous vertebral defect is present at birth, clinical manifestation of the spinal defect may not be evident until later in life when progression of the curve occurs.

It is not clear what causes the vertebral defects that result in congenital scoliosis. Nongenetic factors, such as thalidomide and maternal diabetes, have been implicated. Unlike idiopathic scoliosis, where there is a strong genetic tendency, in congenital scoliosis there is a low genetic tendency.

Various associated congenital anomalies can be present in congenital scoliosis. The most common of these anomalies involves the genitourinary tract, of which approximately 6% can be life threatening. Cardiac anomalies may be present in 10 to 15% of patients. Cardiac murmurs should never be attributed to the scoliosis and must be thoroughly investigated. Rib and chest wall abnormalities are also common. Breast development, pectus excavatum, pectus carinatum, and chest expansion must be checked.

Intraspinal anomalies or spinal dysraphism can occur in 10 to 40% of patients with congenital scoliosis; this may lead to neurologic complications. Diastematomyelia is the most common intraspinal anomaly. Other intraspinal anomalies include Chiari malformations, syringomyelia, lipomas, and dermoid cysts.

Cutaneous lesions are frequently associated with intraspinal abnormalities. Inspection for hair patches overlying the spine, dimples, skin pigmentations, and hemangiomata is important.

Congenital spinal deformities may be categorized according to the region of the spine that is involved, the pattern of spinal deformity, and the specific type of vertebral malformation. Vertebral malformations may be classified as defects of segmentation, defects of formation, or a combination of defects of segmentation and formation.

A unilateral unsegmented bar, a result of unilateral failure of segmentation, can cause scoliosis. This type of defect can "malignantly" progress, resulting in severe clinical deformity (Fig. 48–5A). The rate of progression of a unilateral bar is variable; it depends on the length of the bar and the quality of convex growth. Longer bars with normal convex growth can cause a more severe rate of progression.

Anterior failure of segmentation can cause kyphosis; posterior failure of segmentation can cause lordosis (Fig. 48–5B,C). Anterolateral failure of segmentation can cause kyphoscoliosis; posterolateral failure of segmentation can cause lordoscoliosis.

Total, or circumferential, failure of segmentation results in a nonsegmented "bloc" of bone or a "bloc" vertebra (Fig. 48–5D). Lack of segmental growth can lead to a shortening of the spine without associated scoliosis.

Defects of vertebral formation result in wedge vertebrae or hemivertebrae. A hemivertebra is not an accessory vertebra. Variations of hemivertebrae are common.

Hemivertebrae may be classified as segmented, nonsegmented, incarcerated, or nonincarcerated. A fully segmented, or "free" hemivertebra, is fully separated by discs from both adjacent vertebrae (Fig. 48–6A). Curve progression may result from unbalanced growth of the wedge-oriented growth plates of the hemivertebra. A semisegmented hemivertebra is fused to one adjacent vertebra and is separated from the other adjacent vertebra by a disc (Fig. 48–6B,C). Curve progression is usually less than that of a fully segmented hemivertebra. A nonsegmented hemivertebra is not separated from adjacent vertebrae (Fig. 48–6D). There is little growth imbalance, and progression is even less common.

Hemivertebrae may be classified as incarcerated or nonincarcerated based on their position and alignment in the spine. The pedicles of an incarcerated hemivertebra maintain alignment with the pedicles of the adjacent vertebrae (Fig. 48–6E). An incarcerated hemivertebra usually does not produce abnormal spinal alignment. A nonincarcerated hemivertebra, when fully segmented and at the apex of a scoliosis, can cause distortion of the vertebral column. Pedicular alignment is not maintained, because the pedicle of the hemivertebra lies outside the line of the adjacent pedicles. The nonincarcerated hemivertebra has a more severe prognosis (Fig. 48–6F).

A hemivertebra in the lumbrosacral region may cause a significant progressive angular deformity. Because of a lack of flexible vertebrae below the defect, compensatory spinal balance cannot occur. In some cases, abnormalities in the sacrum can compensate for the L5 hemivertebra.

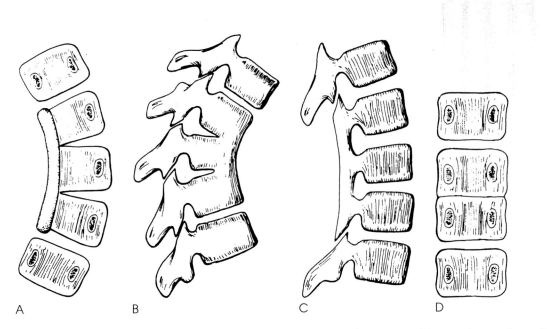

Figure 48–5. Defects of segmentation. (A) Lateral failure of segmentation, or unilateral unsegmented bar, produces scoliosis. (B) Anterior defect of segmentation results in kyphosis. (C) Posterior defect results in lordosis. (D) Total failure in segmentation; "bloc" vertebra produces shortening of the spine. (Adapted from Winter RB. Congenital Deformities of the Spine. New York: Thieme-Stratton, 1983.)

More than one hemivertebra may be present. Hemivertebrae may occur on the same side or on opposite sides of the spine, and they may be separated from or adjacent to one another (Fig. 48–7A–C). When hemivertebrae are on opposite sides of the spine, a hemimetameric shift during the somite period of fetal development may be the cause. In some cases, these hemimetameric shifts can completely rebalance the spine.

Combinations of defects from failures of formation and segmentation result in mixed spinal anomalies (Fig. 48–7D). The prognosis is difficult, because each anomaly may progress independently and/or simultaneously with the other anomaly. Progression should be monitored with careful, serial, radiographic evaluation.

Defects of formation are more progressive and consequential than defects of segmentation; they may develop anteriorly, posteriorly, and laterally. Posterior formation failures are rare and cause lordosis. Lateral failures of formation occur more frequently and produce scoliosis. Anterior defects can produce severe kyphotic deformities, which can cause paraplegia. Paraplegia occurs more commonly in upper thoracic curves and during the adolescent growth spurt.

The natural history of congenital spine deformities depends on the type of vertebral anomaly, the age of the patient at diagnosis, and the region of the spine that is involved. The most progressive anomaly with the worst prognosis is a concave, unilateral, unsegmented bar with a convex hemivertebra. Following this anomaly are a unilateral, unsegmented bar; a double-convex hemivertebra; a single, fully segmented hemivertebra; and a wedge vertebra. The rate of progression and the clinical outcome of these defects can be attributed to the extent of asymmetric growth of the affected region of the spine. With normal convex growth and abnormal concave growth, major deformity is more likely.

Curve measurement in congenital scoliosis can be difficult because of anomalous variations in vertebral anatomy. Selecting a pair of pedicles rather than the vertebral endplates may provide a more consistent definable measuring point. Although the Cobb measurement technique has become standardized, variability

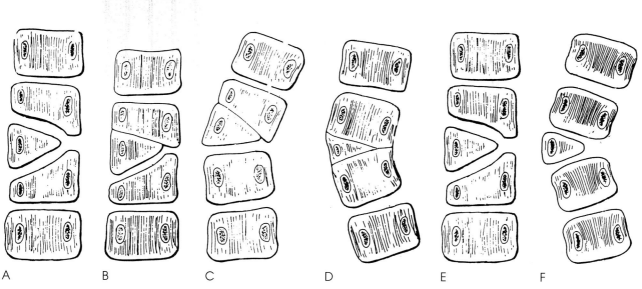

A   B   C   D   E   F

Figure 48–6. Defects of formation, hemivertebrae. (A) Fully segmented or "free" hemivertebra. (B,C) Semisegmented, fused to one adjacent vertebra. (D) Nonsegmented, not separated from adjacent vertebrae. (E) Incarcerated, pedicular alignment is maintained. (F) Nonincarcerated, the pedicle of the hemivertebra lies outside the pedicular line of the adjacent pedicles. (Adapted from Winter RB. Congenital Deformities of the Spine. New York: Thieme-Stratton, 1983.)

in measurement of angle in congenital scoliosis occurs. Intraobserver variability of ±9.6 degrees and interobserver variability of ±11.6 degrees have been noted. The most common error in curve measurement is the use of different vertebrae on different radiographs. An increase of 3 to 4 degrees, however, on each of two consecutive examinations is usually indicative of a true increase in curve progression and should be pursued. Curve progression should be monitored with careful, regular, precise follow-up. For a growing child, a return visit should be in 4 to 6 months.

Tomography and computed tomography are helpful to further define in greater detail the extent of the anomaly and the spinal canal anatomy. Magnetic resonance imaging (MRI) and or myelography are useful preoperatively to identify spinal cord dysraphism, spinal cord tethering, and diastematomyelia. A renal evaluation by MRI scans can be performed to substitute for an intravenous pyelogram or renal ultrasound.

Nonoperative treatment in congenital scoliosis has limited benefit. Few types of defects respond well to brace treatment. Congenital kyphosis and congenital lordosis do not respond to brace treatment, and if progressive, should be treated surgically. The best results with bracing are seen with mixed vertebral anomalies and with progressive secondary curves. Of these cases, the long, flexible curve (greater than eight vertebrae and greater than 50% flexibility) benefits from bracing, but the short rigid curve does not. From clinical experience, curves of less than 50 degrees with at least 50% flexibility have a definite possibility of responding to brace treatment. Curves between 50 and 75 degrees and 25 to 50% flexibility have a slight chance of responding. Curves greater than 75 degrees with less than 25% flexibility receive no benefit from bracing. In cases of mixed vertebral anomalies, where the prognosis is not well defined, bracing can be used to control progression while delaying surgery until a more optimal time.

Bracing can also be used to control progression of secondary curves. Rigid, anomalous curves may progress slowly, whereas the secondary compensatory curve may

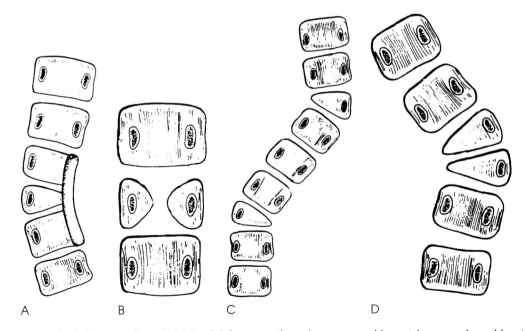

Figure 48–7. (A–C) Multiple hemivertebrae. (D) Mixed defects, a unilateral unsegmented bar with a contralateral hemivertebra. (Adapted from Winter RB. Congenital Deformities of the Spine. New York: Thieme-Stratton, 1983.)

progress more rapidly beyond the balancing point. The secondary curve may become problematic if it becomes larger than the primary curve, or if fixed rotation develops in the curve. The best method of controlling the secondary curve is to promptly control the primary curve before the secondary curve can develop into a large curve.

Surgery is the most common treatment for congenital scoliosis. Various surgical procedures can be used. The best technique for the patient should be specifically selected. Factors to consider include the age of the patient, the type of the deformity, the location of the deformity, the natural history of the defect, and the pattern of the curvature.

Fusion in patients younger than 5 years can be effective in controlling curve progression. However, surgery in infants may be technically simpler if delayed until 12 months of age when the vertebrae are larger and less cartilaginous. Posterior fusion without instrumentation is relatively safe, simple, and reliable. Disadvantages include limited correction, possible late bending, and an increased pseudarthrosis rate.

Alternative Methods of Management

Alternative methods of surgical management for congenital scoliosis include posterior fusion with instrumentation, combined anterior/posterior fusion, combined anterior/posterior convex hemiepiphysiodesis and hemiarthrodesis, and hemivertebrae excision. The standard posterior fusion technique may be supplemented with some type of metallic instrumentation. The added instrumentation can provide a slightly better correction, a lower pseudarthrosis rate, and less restrictive bracing. With the addition of instrumentation comes an increased risk of paraplegia and infection. Corrective, distraction forces by the instrumentation on the spinal cord can cause paralysis, especially in cases of cord tethering, diastematomyelia, or other types of spinal dysraphism. Gradual distraction and correction seems to be safer for the spinal cord and produces more efficient results.

An anterior procedure is not indicated in very young children with a kyphotic deformity. After posterior growth is halted by the fusion, progressive correction of the kyphosis can occur through continued anterior growth. Although a combined fusion can be performed sequentially under the same anesthesia session, there can be a higher rate of major complications than with staged procedures.

Convex growth arrest (anterior epiphysiodesis and posterior hemiarthrodesis) allows concave growth to correct the deformity as excessive convex growth is thwarted. This procedure is indicated for progressive curves, curves of less than 60 degrees, smaller curves (six segments or less), single or adjacent convex hemivertebrae, a child of age 5 or younger, and in cases where there is significant potential for bending of the fusion mass. Significant kyphosis is a contraindication. The entire curve should be fused to one vertebral segment above and below the defective area. An anterior transpedicular fusion is an alternative to a separate anterior approach. Combined with a unilateral, convex, posterior fusion, this alternative procedure appears most effective in young patients with isolated hemivertebrae and no excessive kyphosis. The convex, growth-arrest technique appears to be a reliable method for controlling progressive deformities that result from hemivertebrae.

Curves best managed by hemivertebra excision and fusion are angular curves with a hemivertebra at the apex of the curve. The most common indication is a lumbrosacral hemivertebra causing lateral spinal decompensation. The anterior procedure, excising the hemivertebra and anterior half of the pedicle back to the dura, is performed first. At a second stage, the posterior hemivertebra is removed with the posterior half of the pedicle and the transverse process. The main complication of this technique is nerve-root compression on the convexity by the proximal pedicle impinging against the nerve root in the area of resection.

Type of Management	Advantages	Disadvantages	Comments
Posterior fusion without instrumentation	Safe, simple, reliable	Minimal curve correction, potential crankshaft effect	Gold standard, brace 12–18 months postoperatively
Posterior fusion with instrumentation	Curve stabilization, added correction, lower pseudarthrosis rate	Increased risks of paraplegia, infection	Meticulous fusion technique still critical
Combined anterior/ posterior fusion	Correction of sagittal plane deformity, increase curve flexibility by anterior releases, control of crankshaft effect	Increased blood loss, may require two stages	Used with greater frequency
Convex growth arrest	Simple, low blood loss, low risk	Possible large progression at adolescent growth spurt, narrow fusion mass	Avoid when significant kyphosis is present
Hemivertebrae excision	For angular curves with hemivertebrae at apex	Convex nerve root compression, greater blood loss	May require staged procedures

Suggested Readings

Andrew T, Piggot H. Growth arrest for progressive scoliosis: combined anterior and posterior fusion of the convexity. J Bone Joint Surg 1985; 67A:193.

Hesinger R, Lang JE, MacEwen GD. Klippel-Feil syndrome: a constellation of associated anomalies. J Bone Joint Surg 1974; 56A:1246.

Leatherman KD, Dickson RA. Two-stage corrective surgery for congenital deformities of the spine. J Bone Joint Surg 1979; 61B:324–328.

McMaster MJ, Ohtsuka K. The natural history of congenital scoliosis. A study of two hundred and fifty-one patients. J Bone Joint Surg 1982; 64A(8):1128.

Winter RB. Congenital Deformities of the Spine. New York: Thieme-Stratton, 1983.

Winter RB, Moe JH, Lonstein JE. Posterior spinal arthrodesis for congenital scoliosis. J Bone Joint Surg 1984; 66A:1180–1197.

Winter RB, Moe JH, MacEwen GD, et al. The Milwaukee brace in the nonoperative treatment of congenital scoliosis. Spine 1976; 1:85–96.

Case 49
Adolescent Idiopathic Scoliosis
Peter G. Gabos

History and Physical Examination

A 14-year-old girl was referred to the orthopaedic clinic by her pediatrician for evaluation of an increasing spinal curvature. A mild spinal asymmetry had been noted at the age of 9 years. She was presently 3 years postmenarchal, and had no known family history of scoliosis. She denied back pain or neurologic symptoms. On examination, she was noted to have a thoracic spinal curvature that was convex to the right, and a lumbar spinal curvature that was convex to the left in the coronal plane. Her head was centered over the midline, but her thorax was shifted to the right and her right shoulder was slightly elevated. Her pelvis was level and her waistline was symmetric. She demonstrated a mild hypokyphosis of the thoracic region. On forward bending, a moderate right rib prominence and minimal lumbar muscular

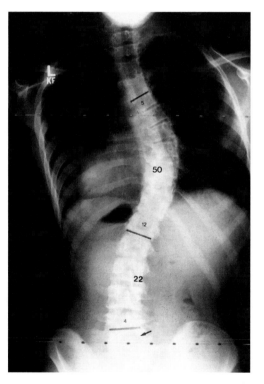

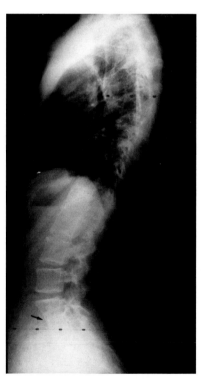

Figure 49–1. Standing anteroposterior (AP) spinal radiograph, demonstrating a 50-degree right thoracic curvature from T5 to T12, and a 22-degree left lumbar curvature from L1 to L4. The thoracic curve is more rotated than the lumbar curve. The pelvis is level, but the right shoulder is slightly elevated and the thorax is shifted to the right of the midline. A spina bifida occulta is present at L5 (arrow), and there is absence of the L4/L5 disc space.

Figure 49–2. Standing lateral spinal radiograph, demonstrating a thoracic kyphosis of 20 degrees, and a lumbar lordosis of 71 degrees. A congenital fusion of the L4 and L5 vertebrae is present (arrow).

prominence were noted. There were no cutaneous markings overlying the spine. She had no neurologic deficits.

Radiologic Findings

Standing full-length posteroanterior and lateral spinal radiographs were obtained (Figs. 49–1 and 49–2). On the posteroanterior view, the Cobb angle measured 50 degrees from T5 to T12, convex to the right, and 22 degrees from L1 to L4, convex to the left. Additional full-length spinal radiographs made with the patient bending maximally to the right and to the left in the supine position were obtained to evaluate curve flexibility. On the supine bending films, the thoracic curve corrected to 21 degrees, and the lumbar curve corrected to 4 degrees. Based on the Cobb angle of the thoracic curve and a history of progressive increase in curvature, a posterior spinal fusion from T5 to T12, using multihook segmental instrumentation and autogenous posterior iliac crest bone grafting, was recommended. Due to the presence of a congenital fusion of L4 and L5, magnetic resonance imaging (MRI) was obtained preoperatively to evaluate any spinal cord pathology.

Diagnosis

Adolescent idiopathic scoliosis, consisting of a false double major curve. Although the apices of both curves cross the midline, the curve is distinguished from a double major curve because the radiographs demonstrate that the thoracic curve is larger and less flexible, is more rotated, and its apex is more deviated from the midline than the lumbar curve. Additionally, on physical examination, the thoracic curve produced most of the deformity, the waistline was symmetric, and there was minimal lumbar muscular prominence on forward bending. The patient met the criteria for selective fusion of the thoracic component of the curve.

Surgical Management

The patient donated two units of autologous blood during the month preceding the procedure, and began oral iron supplementation. Preoperative laboratory evaluation consisted of a complete blood count (CBC), prothrombin time (PT)/partial thromboplastin time (PTT), bleeding time, serum electrolytes, and serum pregnancy test.

After induction of general anesthesia and administration of intravenous antibiotics, an additional large-bore venous line, arterial line, and indwelling urinary catheter were placed. The patient was carefully transferred to a spinal positioning frame in the prone position, taking care to pad all bony prominences and to allow the abdomen to hang free. After positioning, the monitors for recording somatosensory evoked potentials, electrocautery grounding pad, and patient warmer were placed. Predraping was performed, followed by a 10-minute surgical scrub and final sterile prepping and draping, to allow surgical access from the upper thoracic spine to the pelvis.

Attention was turned first to the posterior iliac crest. A longitudinal incision measuring approximately 7 cm in length was made to gain access to the cartilaginous apophysis, which was sharply divided along the crest. Subperiosteal dissection was used to expose the outer wall of the ilium, taking care not to injure the superior gluteal artery or superior cluneal nerves. Corticocancellous strips of bone were then obtained using an osteotome and curved gouges. Bone wax was then placed over the bleeding bony surface, and any excess wax was removed. The posterior iliac crest apophysis was then reapproximated, and the wound was closed.

The most cephalad and caudad aspects of the spinal incision were injected using an epinephrine solution (1:500,000), and a straight midline incision was made from the level of approximately T3 to L1. In making the incision, the scalpel was used to incise directly down to the thoracodorsal fascia, while digital pressure was maintained on both sides of the wound. As the incision proceeded from a cephalad to caudad direction, successive placement of self-retaining retractors was used to retract the skin margins for exposure and traction hemostasis. When the incision was completed, the lower retractors were flipped in direction. The electrocautery was then used to identify the midline raphe, while successively spreading the retractors to maintain wound tension. A curved clamp was then placed on each spinous process, and the electrocautery was used to cut through the cartilaginous caps, down to bone, and to coagulate the inferior spinous process bleeder at each level from caudad to cephalad. The cartilaginous caps were then moved to each side using the Cobb elevators, and the spinous processes were exposed subperiosteally down to the level of the lamina. A surgical sponge was packed subperiosteally on each side of the spinous processes to help complete the exposure over the lamina and to tamponade the lamina bleeders. After completing the dissection at this level, the sponges were pulled, and the retractors were repositioned to the level of the thoracodorsal fascia. A towel clamp was then placed at the base of the spinous process at approximately T12, and a temporary upgoing hook was placed into the facet joint at approximately T8 on the convex side of the curvature. The retractors were then removed from the wound, and a localizing posteroanterior radiograph was taken with the entire surgical field covered with a large sterile drape.

After checking the radiograph to verify the location of T12, the tip of the spinous process of T12 was rongeured for identification, and the towel clamp and hook were removed. The remainder of the posterior elements were then cleared from T5 to T12, out to the tips of the transverse processes. The interspinous ligament was removed at each level using a rongeur, down to the ligamentum flavum. Between T12 and L1, the interspinous ligament and facet capsules were spared, as they were not to be included in the fusion.

Attention was next turned to preparing the hook sites, beginning on the concave side. For placement of the upgoing pedicle hooks on the concave side, at T5 and T7, and on the convex side, at T6 and T8, a $\frac{1}{4}$-inch osteotome was used to remove the inferior articular process, exposing the underlying superior facet cartilage. A Harrington hook starter was then carefully inserted into the exposed facet joint. A pedicle hook was loaded onto a hook holder, and preliminary seating of the hook was performed. With the hook in place, position was verified by a firm but careful lateral translation of the hook to ensure that it was engaged on the pedicle. The hook was then impacted into place with a mallet. For placement of the down-going thoracic supralaminar hooks on the concave side, at T10 and T12, the spinous process of the vertebra cephalad to the hook site was first rongeured down to its base and removed. A small rongeur was then used to create a defect in the ligamentum flavum, and Kerrison rongeurs were used to extend the resection out laterally, removing bone from the medial portion of the inferior and superior articular processes to accommodate the hook where necessary. A thoracic laminar hook was loaded onto a hook holder, and the hook was seated. The ipsilateral lamina of the vertebra cephalad to each down-going laminar hook was thinned with a rongeur to prevent later difficulties with seating the rod due to impingement on the lamina. For placement of the lowermost up-going hook on the convex side of the curve, at T12, a "transitional" facet dictated placement of an infralaminar hook. The ligamentum flavum was carefully entered using the Harrington hook starter, and then the hook was inserted. The uppermost down-going thoracic lamina hook on the convex side of the curve was placed over the T5 transverse process. In this particular construct, the hooks at the top and bottom of the construct were all closed hooks, and the intermediate hooks were all open hooks.

A rod template was then used to match the contour of the concave side of the curve in the coronal plane, taking into account the final desired sagittal plane contour after rod rotation. The rod selected was then cut and contoured according to the template, adding a slight reverse bend at the inferior portion to accommodate transition to lordosis at the thoracolumbar junction. Next, facet joint extirpation on the concave side was performed, to include all remaining uninstrumented facet joints, using a Cobb gouge to cut into the inferior articular process and L d it out laterally, and using a Cobb curette to remove the cartilage from the exposed su rior articular process. A triangular piece of cancellous autogenous bone graft was then placed into each uninstrumented facet joint and gently impacted using a bone tamp.

The contoured rod was first inserted into the upper closed pedicle hook on the concave side, followed by insertion into the open intermediate hooks and lower closed supralaminar hook. Hook blockers and C-rings were used on the open intermediate hooks in this particular construct, to allow for seating of these hooks using segmental distraction. (Note: These steps will vary depending on the instrumentation system chosen.) Once all hooks were rechecked to ensure that they were seated, two rod holders were used to carefully and slowly rotate the rod 90 degrees, in a counterclockwise direction, toward the concave side of the curve. This allowed for simultaneous correction of the scoliosis in the coronal plane and improvement of the sagittal plane contour. The set screws were then tightened and the C-rings removed after final segmental distraction.

A second rod was then contoured for placement on the convex side. Facet joint extirpation was completed, using the technique described above. The rod was then placed into the upper claw configuration and intermediate apical pedicle hook, followed by the lower thoracic infralaminar hook. The two hooks of the upper claw were then compressed together using a hand-held compressor, and their set screws were tightened. Following this, a rod holder was placed below the intermediate apical hook, and a spreader was used to compress this hook against the upper claw configuration, and its set screw was tightened. The inferior hook was then compressed against a rod holder placed above the hook, and its set screw was tightened. Devices for transverse traction were then placed and secured, and final tightening of all screws was performed. Final decortication was then performed, followed by placement of the remainder of the autogenous graft, making sure to pack the graft directly onto bone.

The thoracodorsal fascia and subcutaneous tissue were closely reapproximated, and the skin was closed using a running subcuticular 3-0 absorbable suture. Steri-Strips and a compressive dressing were applied.

The patient was then carefully rolled onto the hospital bed while she remained intubated. Full-length anteroposterior spinal and chest radiographs were obtained to check correction and hook placement, and to evaluate for pneumothorax. The patient was brought to a conscious level by the anesthesia team, and voluntary lower extremity movement was assessed. The patient was then successfully awakened and extubated.

Postoperative Management

Intravenous antibiotics were administered every 8 hours for 48 hours. Intravenous fluids were continued until the patient was tolerating oral intake, including analgesics. The patient was allowed to sit up briefly with assistance on the first postoperative day, and to stand and transfer to a chair on the second postoperative day. Standing posteroanterior and lateral radiographs of the spine were obtained on the third postoperative day. Thereafter, under the guidance of a physical therapist, she progressed to full ambulation. She was discharged on the fifth postoperative day. Repeat standing radiographs were obtained at 4 weeks and 12 weeks after discharge, with inclusion of oblique radiographs to assess the fusion mass 6 months after the procedure. Physical activity was restricted to ambulation for the first 6 months postoperatively, with a progressive increase in allowable activities over the remainder of the year (Figs. 49–3 and 49–4).

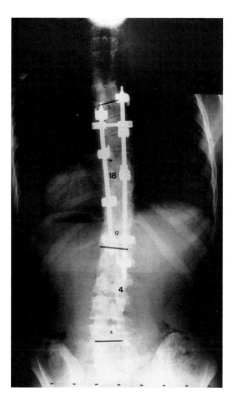

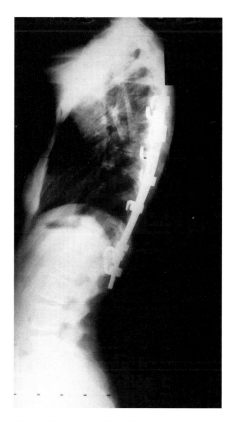

Figure 49–3. Standing AP spinal radiograph obtained 1 year after posterior spinal fusion from T5 to T12, using multihook segmental spinal instrumentation and autogenous posterior iliac crest bone grafting. The thoracic curve measures 18 degrees, and the lumbar curve has improved to 4 degrees.

Figure 49–4. Standing lateral spinal radiograph 1 year after surgery. The thoracic kyphosis measures 37 degrees, and the lumbar lordosis has been maintained at 71 degrees.

Discussion

The initial treatment of adolescent idiopathic scoliosis depends on many factors, including the size of the spinal curvature, amount of cosmetic deformity present, signs and symptoms, and the degree of skeletal maturity. A thorough history and physical examination is undertaken, paying particular attention to a positive family history of scoliosis, age at first menses, if applicable, and any symptoms of pain or neurologic involvement. Evaluation of the patient's spine in the standing position is used to evaluate the coronal and sagittal plane contours, noting the severity and location of scoliosis, kyphosis, and lordosis. As well, an assessment is made of trunkal balance and head position relative to the pelvis, shoulder and pelvic obliquity, relative limb lengths, and waist symmetry. Any cutaneous markings that might suggest an underlying congenital spinal defect or other syndrome are noted. To help assess rotation, thoracic rib or lumbar muscular prominence is evaluated with the patient in the forward-bending position. A detailed neurologic examination is performed.

Initial radiographic evaluation includes standing full-length anteroposterior and lateral spinal radiographs. On the anteroposterior radiograph, the degree of spinal curvature is determined using the Cobb method of measurement, rotation is assessed using the Pedriolle torsion meter or pedicle method, and the Risser grade is assigned. Lumbar lordosis and thoracic kyphosis are measured on the lateral radiograph. Additional studies, including an MRI in patients with neurologic signs or symptoms, unusual curve patterns, congenital anomalies, or early curve onset or rapid curve progression, and bone scans in patients with atypical back pain, are obtained when indicated.

In general, curves measuring less than 20 degrees can be observed with serial physical and radiographic examination. Curves measuring between 20 and 30 degrees that progress more than 5 degrees while under observation, or curves that measure between 30 and 40 degrees at initial presentation, can be managed with an appropriate spinal orthosis if there is skeletal growth remaining. Curves measuring more than 40 degrees, or curves in skeletally mature patients, are not appropriate for brace treatment. In general, curves that are managed surgically include curves that measure more than 50 degrees at initial presentation, and curves that progress to 50 degrees despite the use of a brace or while under a period of observation. More rarely, surgery is employed to address a smaller curvature that causes severe cosmetic deformity, or to address a painful scoliosis if the pain cannot be controlled by nonoperative means (and after thorough diagnostic investigation to find a cause of the pain other than scoliosis).

Once a patient has met the criteria for surgical treatment of the curve, careful and detailed preoperative planning is essential to determine the surgical approach to be used (anterior and/or posterior), levels to be fused, and location and type of spinal instrumentation, if applicable. Although a vast array of spinal instrumentation systems are now available for routine use, the ultimate goal of the procedure remains to safely achieve a balanced and fused spine, while allowing for the retention of as many motion segments as possible.

Determination of fusion levels will vary by curve pattern, and other factors. Preoperative standing full-length anteroposterior and lateral, and supine bending, spinal radiographs are essential. The standing radiographs allow identification of single major lumbar, thoracic, and thoracolumbar curves, combined thoracic and lumbar curves (double major curves), and double major thoracic curves. Supine bending films give an indication of curve flexibility, and help to identify false double major curves, as in the case presented above.

In the coronal plane, all pathologic curves must be included in the fusion, making sure to include all vertebrae within the measured Cobb angle. The distal level of the fusion should end within the stable zone of Harrington, and should include the most neutral (least rotated) and stable vertebra. The most stable vertebra is that which is most nearly bisected by the center sacral line on standing anteroposterior or supine bending films, and often coincides with the most neutral vertebra. As well, the distal level of the fusion is stopped at the level above disc space neutralization (the level at which the disc space height is equal on both sides, and at which the disc space opens to the right and left on supine left- and right-bending films, respectively). Inflection points (points at which the curve changes direction, as evidenced by a change in the direction of disc space opening) are recorded, making sure to include such points within the fusion. Terminating the fusion at an inflection point can lead to an increase in coronal plane deformity at the upper or lower aspects of the fusion (Fig. 49–5). In the sagittal plane, care must again be taken to identify inflection points, and to include such points within the fusion. Terminating the fusion at an inflection point in the sagittal plane can lead to a junctional kyphosis at the upper or lower aspects of the fusion.

Once the caudad and cephalad limits of the fusion have been determined, attention is given to planning of the hook location, direction, and type. In determining appropriate hook placement, consideration of the forces necessary for correction (distraction or compression) will dictate hook patterns. Distraction forces (forces directed away from the apex of the curve) typically are employed for correction of the concave side of each curve, whereas compressive forces (forces directed toward the apex of the curve) typically are employed for correc-

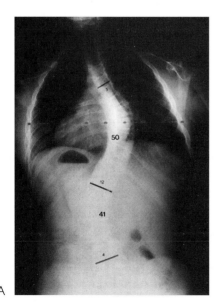
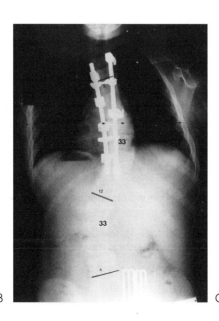
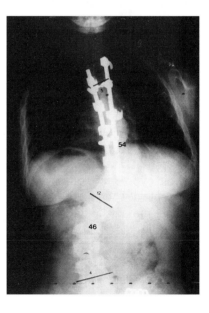

Figure 49–5. (A) *Standing AP spinal radiograph demonstrating a patient with a false double major curve consisting of a 50-degree right thoracic curvature from T5 to T12, and a 41-degree left lumbar curvature from L1 to L4. (B) Standing AP spinal radiograph obtained 1 month after selective fusion of the thoracic curvature, from T5 to T11. The fusion does not include all thoracic vertebrae within the measured Cobb angle, and ends one level cephalad to an inflection point. (C) Standing AP spinal radiograph obtained 1 year later, demonstrating a progression of both the thoracic and lumbar components of the curve below the fusion level.*

- In thoracic fusions, harvest posterior iliac crest autograft first, prior to exposing the spine. This avoids having to take the graft while the spine is widely exposed, which may help decrease overall blood loss from the spinal wound. As well, if superior gluteal artery laceration were to occur while obtaining the graft, prompt repositioning for an anterior abdominal exposure could be obtained, if necessary.
- When obtaining films of the spine intraoperatively to verify vertebral levels, use two markers at different levels (a towel clamp on the spinous process of one vertebra and an upgoing hook under the inferior articular facet of a different vertebra), to help increase accuracy of identification.
- A complete set of adequate radiographs is essential for preoperative planning.
- Pay attention to sagittal plane contour, especially when "derotation" maneuvers are to be employed.

- Avoid fusion to a level at or above inflection points in both the coronal and sagittal planes.
- Avoid hypotensive anesthesia, especially when distraction forces are anticipated.

tion of the convex side of each curve. However, sagittal plane contouring must be considered, as distraction can decrease lordosis or create kyphosis, and compression can decrease kyphosis or create lordosis. Consideration of sagittal plane contour is also critical in contouring rods, especially when "derotation" maneuvers are planned.

In the case presented here, a false double major curve was recognized, and the patient underwent selective fusion of the thoracic curve. Although the general fusion principles described above pertain to false double major curves as well, some additional considerations are necessary when planning a fusion in these cases. When selective thoracic fusion of a primary right thoracic curve with a compensatory left lumbar curve is performed, a phenomenon known as decompensation has been described. Decompensation results in a translatory shift of the thorax to the left of the patient's midline, causing a lateral prominence of the right hip and an unbalanced appearance. On the standing anteroposterior spinal radiograph, decompensation is defined as a translation of the center point of the apical vertebra of the thoracic curve on or to the left of the center sacral line.

Mason and Carango (1991) noted that when using Cotrel-Dubousset instrumentation, spontaneous correction of the compensatory lumbar curve in selective thoracic fusions occurs only in the segment between the lowest vertebral level fused and the apex of the lumbar compensatory curve. The segment below the apex of the lumbar curve remains unchanged, resulting in a straightening of the spine above the apex of the lumbar curve. The farther the apex of the lumbar curve lies to the left of the center sacral line, the farther the apex of the thoracic curve can be translated to the left, increasing the likelihood that postoperative decompensation will occur. Similarly, the farther the apex of the thoracic curve lies to the right of the center sacral line preoperatively, the less likely it is that decompensation will occur. Cotrel-Dubousset instrumentation translates the apex of the thoracic curve 1.5 cm farther to the left than Harrington instrumentation or its variants, due to the "derotation" maneuver employed. The simplest preoperative predictors of decompensation include a lumbar apical distance that is greater than 2 cm to the left of the center sacral line, a thoracic apical distance that is less than 4 cm to the right of the center sacral line, and a thoracic and lumbar Cobb angle difference of less than or equal to 12 degrees.

I have avoided the derotation maneuver when using this form of instrumentation in curves at risk for decompensation, choosing instead to contour the rod in both coronal and sagittal planes, and to correct in distraction mode only. Attempting to achieve less correction of the thoracic curve may also be helpful in preventing decompensation with these newer instrumentation systems.

Alternative Methods of Management

Posterior spinal fusion remains the gold standard for operative management of appropriately selected patients with adolescent idiopathic scoliosis. Alternatively, anterior spinal instrumentation may be utilized in appropriately selected cases. Each type of instrumentation has its advantages and disadvantages, either real or theoretical.

Type of Management	Advantages	Disadvantages	Comments
Harrington distraction rod/variants	Technically easy; less potential for "decompensation" in right thoracic false double major curves	Loss of lumbar lordosis; no correction of thoracic hypokyphosis; persistent rib prominence; postoperative immobilization required	Its simplicity may not outweigh its disadvantages
Multihook segmental instrumentation	Improvement of thoracic hypokyphosis; preservation of lumbar lordosis; improvement of rib prominence with "derotation" maneuver; no postoperative immobilization	Technically challenging; hooks can lose purchase	"Derotation" maneuver may be more of a "translatory" maneuver
Pedicle screw fixation	Increased purchase strength may allow true derotation, less risk of loss of fixation, and may allow preservation of a motion segment	Technically challenging; may increase risk of direct cord injury by screw; screw may injure visceral or vascular structures anteriorly; small or distorted pedicles may preclude use in children	Role in treatment of adolescent idiopathic scoliosis still being debated
Anterior instrumentation	Preservation of motion segments; better apical translation in lumbar curves	Requires anterior approach; requires postoperative immobilization; potential for kyphosing effect in lumbar spine; increased pseudarthrosis rates with "flexible" systems; prominent hardware can injure anterior structures	Not commonly employed for thoracic fusions

Complications

Complications from posterior spinal fusion in adolescent idiopathic scoliosis, using autogenous posterior iliac crest bone grafting and multihook segmental spinal instrumentation, can include neurologic injury, dural tear, pneumothorax, superior mesenteric artery syndrome, infection, fusing of incorrect levels, loss of lumbar lordosis, junctional kyphosis, decompensation, crankshaft phenomenon, loss or failure of fixation, and pseudarthrosis.

Detailed preoperative planning and use of intraoperative radiographs using markers to accurately identify operative level best avoids fusion of incorrect levels. Loss of lumbar lordosis is best avoided by avoiding distractive forces in the lumbar spine, and careful sagittal plane contouring of the rods. When fusing a single major lumbar curve, the convex side should be instrumented first, directing the forces toward the apex of the lumbar curve. Junctional kyphosis is best avoided by careful preoperative planning to include inflection points within the fusion, and by proper contouring of any rods that cross the thoracolumbar junction. Decompensation requires identifying patients at risk for this complication preoperatively (as described above), and by modifying technique accordingly. Crankshaft is avoided by performing concomitant anterior spinal fusion in appropriate patients. Loss of fixation can result from inadequate sagittal plane contouring of rods, and from the use of insufficient numbers of hooks, especially in the lumbar spine. The use of at least one hook on every lumbar vertebra within the fusion may discourage this complication.

Suggested Readings

Bridwell KH, McCallister JW, Betz RR, Huss G, Clancy M, Schoenecker PL. Coronal decompensation produced by Cotrel-Dubousset "derotation" maneuver for idiopathic right thoracic scoliosis. Spine 1991; 16:769–777.

King HA, Moe JH, Bradford DS, Winter RB. The selection of fusion levels in thoracic idiopathic scoliosis. J Bone Joint Surg 1983; 65A:1302–1313.

Lenke LG, Bridwell KH, Baldus C, Blanke K. Preventing decompensation in King type II curves treated with Cotrel-Dubousset instrumentation. Spine 1992; 17(8S):S274–S281.

Mason DE, Carango P. Spinal decompensation in Cotrel-Dubousset instrumentation. Spine 1991; 16(8S):S394–S403.

Case 50

Kyphosis—Round-Back Deformity, Scheuermann's Kyphosis

Gregory V. Hahn, Peter O. Newton, and Dennis R. Wenger

History and Physical Examination

A 16-year-old girl presented with a chief complaint of a round-back deformity. She was quite concerned about her posture, commenting that she was unhappy with her appearance and that it significantly affected her personal relationships. She also complained of intermittent lumbar and thoracic back pain; however, the pain was not severe enough to limit her activities. She denied radicular leg pain, numbness, paresthesias, or weakness of the lower extremities. She had no other musculoskeletal complaints, her general health was excellent, and she was approximately $3\frac{1}{2}$ years postmenarchal. There was no family history of round-back deformity or scoliosis.

Physical examination revealed an abnormal thoracolumbar posture, with a significant thoracic hyperkyphosis that did not correct with hyperextension. Clinically, the apex of the deformity appeared to be midthoracic, and there did not appear to

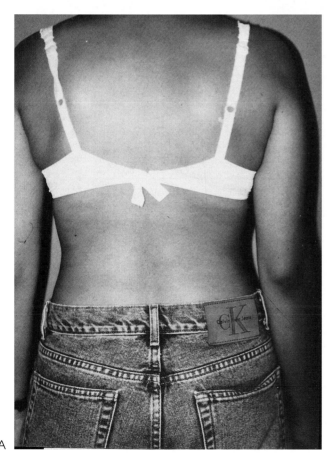 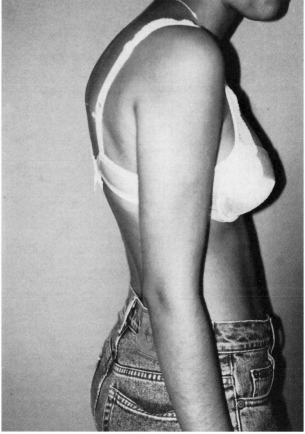

A   B

Figure 50–1. Rear (A) and side (B) view photographs revealing clinical evidence of significant thoracic round-back deformity.

be a significant scoliosis (Fig. 50–1). She walked without a limp or evidence of lower extremity weakness. She performed heel-walking and toe-walking without difficulty. Both supine and sitting straight leg raising were negative at 70 degrees bilaterally. The femoral stretch test was also negative, although her hamstring muscles were moderately tight. Motor testing revealed normal strength in all major muscle groups and deep tendon reflexes were 2+ and symmetric at the knees and ankles. Sensory examination was intact to light touch and proprioception.

Radiologic Findings

The standing posteroanterior view showed a mild scoliosis and ossification of the iliac apophysis was graded as Risser 4 (Fig. 50–2A). The standing lateral spine radiograph revealed a thoracic kyphotic curve measuring 80 degrees by the modified Cobb method, extending from T3 to T11, along with compensatory hyperlordosis of the lumbar spine (Fig. 50–2B). The spinal anatomy was normal except for anterior wedging of the thoracic vertebrae, mild disc space narrowing, and endplate irregularities. A standing hyperextension lateral radiograph illustrated reduction of the kyphosis to approximately 58 degrees, and a hyperextension lateral over a bolster revealed correction to 45 degrees.

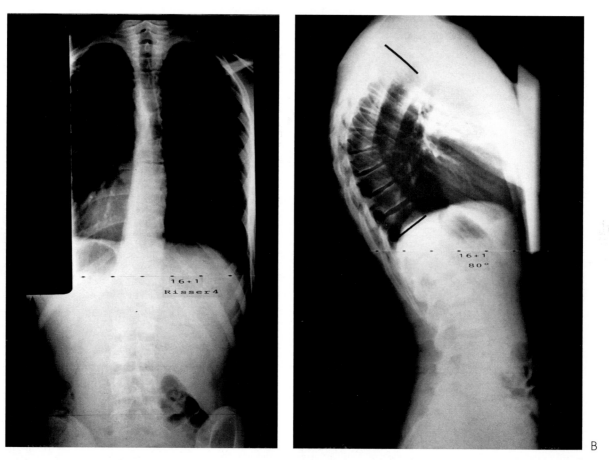

A   B

Figure 50–2. (A) A standing posteroanterior radiograph revealing mild scoliosis and ossification of the iliac apophysis graded a Risser 4. (B) A standing lateral spine radiograph revealing a thoracic kyphotic curve measuring 80 degrees by the modified cobb method, extending from T3 to T11, along with compensatory hyperlordosis of the lumbar spine.

Diagnosis

The differential diagnosis of thoracic kyphosis includes postural kyphosis, Scheuermann's kyphosis, congenital kyphosis, spondyloarthropathies, infection, and tumors. Classic Scheuermann's kyphosis is defined as hyperkyphosis (thoracic kyphosis >45 degrees) with anterior vertebral wedging of 5 degrees or more at three adjacent levels. The wedging is often associated with disc space narrowing, vertebral endplate irregularities, and Schmorl's nodes. In this patient the radiographic workup revealed most of the classic findings of Scheuermann's kyphosis. The plain radiographs showed no evidence of infection or neoplasm. She had no suggestion of a congenital deformity, and no systemic manifestations of a spondyloarthropathy. The diagnosis of Scheuermann's disease was made and she was initially treated conservatively with muscle strengthening and postural exercises. Her age and skeletal maturity precluded the use of a modified Milwaukee brace. During the course of conservative treatment, she noted a progressive increase in thoracic back pain, altering her ability to participate in vigorous physical activities. She aspired to be a fashion model and remained very unhappy with her appearance following nonoperative treatment. She and her family elected to proceed with surgical correction.

Surgical Management—Technique for Same-Day Anterior Thoracoscopic Disc Excision and Fusion Plus Posterior Instrumentation and Fusion

Preoperatively the patient underwent pulmonary function tests (within normal limits) and autodonated three units of blood. We elected to perform an anterior fusion with posterior instrumentation and fusion on the same day. Somatosensenory evoked potentials were used to monitor spinal cord function throughout the case. Following intubation with a endotrachial tube, a bronchial blocker was directed into the right main stem bronchus using flexible bronchoscopy. The patient was then turned to the lateral decubitus position (right side up) over an axillary roll. After prepping and draping the right chest, three 11.5-mm rigid thoracoscopic portals were established, centered at the apex of the deformity and in the anterior axillary line. Through these portals, a 10-mm-diameter 45-degree endoscope, a fan retractor, and working instruments were introduced. Ultrasonic shears were used to open the pleura longitudinally from T3 to T12, with the segmental vessels divided at each level allowing easier anterior retraction of the great vessels. A sponge was used to further dissect the spine anteriorly and provide additional protection of the great vessels.

The annulus of each disc was incised circumferentially with the ultrasonic scalpel, and removed with rongeurs. The cartilaginous endplates were curetted and removed, exposing bleeding bone. The discectomies were performed sequentially from proximal to distal, and each disc space was packed with cancellous allograft. The pleura was reapproximated with a running 2–0 absorbable suture using an endoscopic stitching device. The chest cavity was copiously irrigated and a chest tube was placed through the most inferior portal and tunneled subcutaneously to the middle portal, where it entered the chest and was directed to the apex of the pleural cavity. The chest tube was secured and placed to underwater suction drainage, the portals closed and sterilely dressed, the right lung reinflated, and the patient turned prone for the posterior spinal instrumentation and fusion.

The patient was repositioned on chest rolls with an additional roll placed under the sternum to encourage spine extension with all extremities appropriately positioned and padded, and the back was widely prepped and draped. A standard midline approach was used with the cartilage caps split sharply and the spine exposed subperiosteally to the tips of the transverse processes from T3 to L1. Prior to exposing the most proximal and distal aspects of the spine, intraoperative fluoroscopy confirmed the exact levels to be instrumented. Care was taken to preserve the interspinous ligament between T2 and T3, so extraperiosteal dissection was used to identify the transverse processes of T3. The decision was made to stop at L1 as this appeared to be the transitional segment; therefore, the interspinous ligament between L1 and L2 was also preserved.

The hook sites were then prepared with resection of all intervening facets. The interspinous ligaments were carefully removed at all levels. This included resecting the ligamentum flavum from the midline out to the transverse processes and partially removing the spinous processes to allow for posterior compression. The proximal construct consisted of a claw at T3 and T4 on both sides, with up-going pedicle hooks and down-going transverse process hooks, as well as up-going laminar hooks at T6 bilaterally. The distal construct consisted of up-going pedicle hooks at T8, up-going laminar hooks at T10, and pedicle screws at T12 and L1 bilaterally.

Two 6-mm rods were contoured and first placed into the proximal construct. A cantilever maneuver was used to seat the rods into the distal construct with good correction obtained. Further correction was achieved by compressing between the two proximal claw constructs and again between the laminar hooks at T10 and the proximal segment. Finally, compression was applied at the distal construct to allow for transitional lordosis.

Cross-links were then placed proximally and distally to connect the rods and provide additional stabilization. Iliac crest bone graft was harvested and carefully placed from T3 to L1. The wound was drained and closed. Estimated total blood loss was 900 cc and spinal cord monitoring was normal throughout both procedures. The patient was noted to be neurologically intact in the recovery room.

Postoperative Management

The postoperative course was uneventful with postoperative transfusion of two units of autologous blood. The chest tube was removed on postoperative day 2, and the patient was discharged on postoperative day 6. Immediate postoperative radiographs showed correction of the thoracic kyphosis to 45 degrees (Fig. 50–3). The patient wore a thoracolumbar spinal orthosis (TLSO) for 3 months and was restricted from sports activities for 1 year. On her last follow-up radiographs demonstrated a solid fusion with no loss of the initial correction. Clinically, she had a normal spinal contour and trunk alignment (Fig. 50–4) and no complaints of back pain, and she was then permitted to participate in all activities. Both she and her family were delighted with the result and felt that she had undergone a very positive physical and psychological transformation.

Discussion

Scheuermann's kyphosis or round-back deformity can be difficult to manage for even the most experienced clinician. The thoracic spine normally maintains a

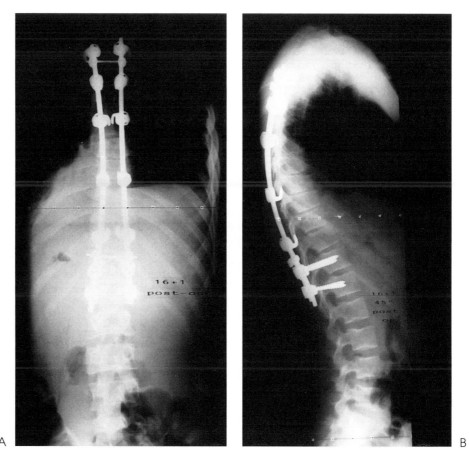

Figure 50–3. (A) A standing postoperative posteroanterior radiograph following surgical correction of the patient's kyphotic deformity with Rous, screws, and hook instrumentation. (B) A standing postoperative lateral radiograph revealing correction of the thoracic kyphosis to 45 degrees.

kyphotic curve, and the distinction between normal and abnormal can be subtle. In addition, the clinical appearance of the same magnitude curve can be substantially different, as a 60-degree thoracic hyperkyphosis may be hardly noticeable in an athletic, muscular man and yet be markedly disfiguring in a svelte, adolescent girl. The natural history of Scheuermann's disease is relatively benign in regard to back pain; however, the emotional stress from the trunk deformity is often marked and psychologically debilitating. In this case, the patient's main focus was her deformity and her subsequent increase in back pain may have also reflected her concern regarding her appearance.

When diagnosed early (Risser 0 to 3) modified Milwaukee brace treatment can provide correction of the kyphosis. As in scoliosis, brace treatment is most successful in skeletally immature patients who are Risser 3 or less. Also, as in scoliosis, compliance with brace wear is difficult for many teenagers who are experiencing the psychological stresses of adolescent maturation. Many (if not most) teenagers with Scheuermann's disease are poor candidates for brace treatment due to psychological factors. The current patient presented at age 16, $3\frac{1}{2}$ postmenarchal, Risser 4, with little skeletal growth remaining, and therefore brace treatment was not a viable option.

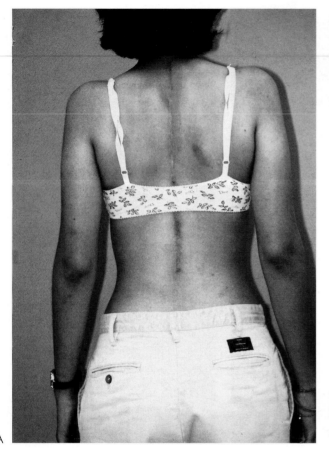
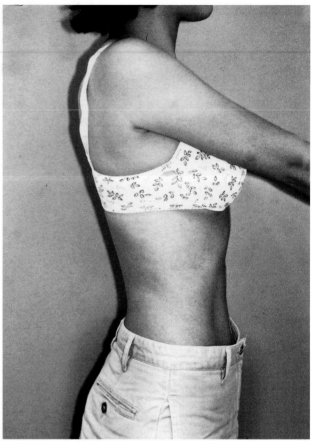

Figure 50–4. Rear (A) and side (B) view photographs revealing a clinically normal spine contour and trunk alignment.

A

B

Surgical Indications

Surgical indications for Scheuermann's kyphosis remain somewhat arbitrary for several reasons including contradictory natural history studies, failure to quantitate the lifelong burden of appearing severely round-backed, and wide variability in access to safe, excellent surgical correction. The Scoliosis Research Society advises surgical correction in patients who have progressive curves despite brace treatment, patients who have significant back pain and/or degenerative changes, and patients presenting with a curve greater than 65 degrees. These are general guidelines only, as there is no number that can be used to accurately predict progression or prognosis.

Technical Aspects

Surgical correction of Scheuermann's kyphosis is a technically demanding operation. The risk of neurologic deficit and hardware failure (instrument dislodgment) are greater than in scoliosis surgery. Attention to detail and proper preoperative planning are essential. Preoperative radiographs should include full-length standing posteroanterior and lateral spine films as well as a forced hyperextension lateral view.

Two common complications include loss of the initial postoperative correction and proximal or distal junctional kyphosis, both of which can be minimized by accurate selection of fusion levels and avoidance of surgical overcorrection.

Proximally, the fusion must extend to include all the vertebrae measured in the kyphotic deformity. The proximal extent of the curve is often difficult to ascertain as the shoulders interfere with good radiographic visualization of the proximal thoracic vertebrae; this results in the common mistake of not including the most proximal vertebra in the fusion. Ultimately, this may cause a proximal junctional kyphosis and a prominent neck thrust.

Distally the fusion must extend to include all the vertebrae measured in the kyphotic deformity as well as the first lordotic disc, representing the transitional zone. If this transitional zone is not included in the instrumentation a distal junctional kyphosis is more likely to develop. Preserving the interspinous ligaments above and below the fusion mass also aids in avoiding junctional kyphosis; therefore, it is important to confirm the levels intraoperatively to avoid inadvertently disrupting the intervertebral ligaments just proximal and distal to the planned fusion when the spine is exposed. The curve should not be corrected to more than 50% of the preoperative curve, with the postoperative kyphosis maintained at 35 degrees or greater.

Loss of the initial postoperative correction can occur. A common reason is failure to perform an anterior release and fusion. The hyperextension lateral radiograph taken over a bolster guides the surgeon as to the need for anterior release and fusion. Previously, it was felt that only severe deformity (>70°) or rigid curves that did not correct to less than 50 degrees, required anterior release. Currently, many authors recommend anterior release and fusion in almost all cases. The anterior approach, either thoracoscopically or via an open thoracotomy, allows for a more uniform correction as well as load sharing for the anterior column.

The hook pattern should consist of a double- (and occasionally triple-) claw construct proximal to the apex of the curve, and a double-claw construct distal to the apex. This allows for adequate compression at multiple levels providing good correction of the kyphotic deformity. Secure distal fixation is essential, and although hooks may be used, we recommend pedicle screw fixation especially if the bone seems osteoporotic.

We advise postoperative bracing for 3 months to protect the instrumentation and ensure the development of a complete and solid fusion. This apparent "overtreatment" is used following surgical correction of kyphosis but rarely following scoliosis instrumentation. Three months of full-time bracing is usually sufficient; however, the patient remains restricted from physical activities for 9 months to a year. The fusion mass is usually mature at 1 year, at which point the patient is released to full activity.

Alternative Methods of Management

Not all hyperkyphotic curves need to be surgically corrected. The natural history studies, although limited, have shown that no gross pulmonary compromise or severe disability occurs in curves under 100 degrees.

Brace treatment may be considered when the patient presents early in adolescence. Because the deformity may be painless, it often goes unrecognized and untreated for many years. Bracing is only effective for skeletally immature patients with a Risser sign of 3 or less. The advantage is again avoidance of surgery. The only brace shown to be truly effective is a modified Milwaukee brace that includes a neck ring (low profile).

Posterior spinal fusion and instrumentation alone can be successful. The curve in the patient presented here corrected nicely to 45 degrees and perhaps could have been done with posterior instrumentation and fusion only.

Posterior spinal fusion combined with an anterior open thoracotomy for the anterior fusion is another alternative. This approach is less technically demanding with easy availability of rib graft. The disadvantages include a second cosmetically unappealing scar and the risks of open anterior spinal surgery.

Open anterior disc release and fusion with anterior instrumentation only has also been proposed. This concept has been promoted in an era when the techniques of anterior instrumentation and fusion for thoracic scoliosis are becoming more common. Disadvantages of anterior instrumentation include the need for long instrumentation in Scheuermann's disease (probably necessitating a double thoracotomy) and the soft bone encountered in upper thoracic vertebral bodies with a high risk for screw pull-out. As a result the surgeon may err and fuse too short. A theoretical advantage is preservation of the paraspinal musculature.

Type of Management	Advantages	Disadvantages	Comments
No Treatment	No surgical risk	Persistence and possible progression of deformity	
Milwaukee Brace	No surgical risk	Poor compliance	Only useful in skeletally immature patients
Posterior Fusion and Instrumentation	No anterior surgical risks, no anterior scar	Higher rate of pseudarthrosis, greater risk of loss of correction or hardware failure	
Open Anterior Fusion and Posterior Fusion with Instrumentation	Decreased risk of loss of correction or hardware failure, easy availability of rib graft	Extensive procedure with increased surgical risk, prolonged recovery, more disfiguring scar	
Thorascopic Anterior Fusion and Posterior Fusion with Instrumentation	More cosmetic scar, quicker recovery	Technically demanding	
Anterior Fusion and Instrumentation	Preservation of spinal musculature	Technically demanding, need for double thoracotomy	Not widely used, results unproven

Suggested Readings

Bradford DS, Ahmed HB, Moe JH, et al. The surgical management of patients with Scheuermann's disease: a review of twenty-four cases managed by combined anterior and posterior spine fusion. J Bone Joint Surg 1980; 62A:705–712.

Lowe TG. Current concepts review: Scheuermann disease. J Bone Joint Surg 1990; 72A:940–945.

Lowe TG, Kasten MD. An analysis of sagittal curves and balance after Cotrel–Dubousset instrumentation for kyphosis secondary to Scheuerman's disease. Spine 1994; 19:1680–1685.

Murray PM, Weinstein SL, Spratt KF. The natural history and long-term follow-up of Scheuermann kyphosis. J Bone Joint Surg 1993; 75A:236–248.

Ponte A, Siccardi GL, Ligure P. Scheuermann's kyphosis: posterior shortening procedure by segmental closing wedge resections. J Pediatr Orthop 1995; 15:404.

Speck GR, Chopin DC. The surgical treatment of Scheuermann's kyphosis. J Bone Joint Surg 1986; 68B:189–193.

Sturm PF, Dobson JC, Armstrong GWD. The surgical management of Scheuermannn's disease. Spine 1993; 18:685–691.

Taylor TC, Wenger DR, Stephen J, et al. Surgical management of thoracic kyphosis in adolescents. J Bone Joint Surg 1979; 61A:496–503.

Case 51
Postlaminectomy Kyphosis
Todd J. Albert and Alexander R. Vaccaro

History and Physical Examination

A 70-year-old woman presented with complaints of severe neck pain, right greater than left arm pain, right arm weakness, and difficulty using her hands. One and a half years prior to presentation she had undergone a cervical laminectomy for cervical spondylotic myelopathy. After a very brief period of improvement from symptoms of right arm weakness, her neck pain began to increase, the right arm weakness returned, and her difficulty with coordination increased steadily. She also noted forward tilting of her head.

Examination showed one full grade of right wrist extensor and tricep weakness on the right compared to the left. She had hyperreflexia throughout her upper and lower extremities. She had crossed and inverted radial reflexes. She had a positive Hoffmann's reflex on the right compared to the left. She had down-going toes and normal proprioception. There was no objective sensory level discernible. The patient held her head in a flexed position and lacked 50% of cervical extension. Rotation was diminished by 20% in each direction.

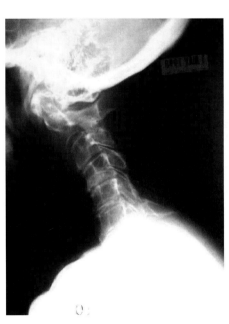

Figure 51–1. Lateral view of lateral radiograph on patient preoperatively, showing laminectomy from C3 to C7 and relative kyphotic alignment of the cervical spine.

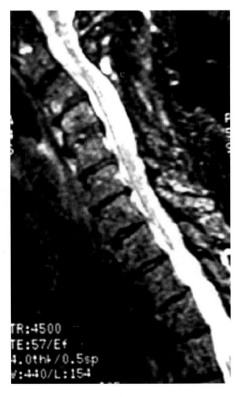

Figure 51–2. Sagittal magnetic resonance imaging (MRI) showing spondylosis at multiple levels, cervical kyphosis, and multiple disc bulging.

Radiologic Findings

X-rays in anteroposterior (AP), lateral, flexion, and extension positions of her cervical spine demonstrated no flexion-extension instability but did show a cervical kyphosis and obvious laminectomy defect from C3 to C7 (Fig. 51–1). Magnetic resonance imaging (MRI) showed neural compression due to deformity and cervical spondylosis at the disc level (Fig. 51–2).

Diagnosis

Postlaminectomy kyphosis with cervical spondylotic myelopathy and radiculopathy C6/C7 on the right.

Surgical Management

Intersegmental correction was carried out through an anterior approach. Exposure was made at the disc spaces between C3 and C7. Radical discectomies were performed, as were uncinate foraminotomies with spinal cord decompression at each level. Tricortical iliac crest autograft was placed at C3/C4, C4/C5, C5/C6, and C6/C7 in a wedged fashion, increasing cervical lordosis. Segmental fixation was obtained with a variable angled anterior plate (Fig. 51–3). Improvement in sagittal alignment was obtained.

The patient was held in a rigid surgical orthosis for 6 weeks postoperatively.

Discussion

This is a classic case of postlaminectomy kyphosis. The patient presented in a typical fashion with a short period of relief of symptoms and recurrence of symptomatology,

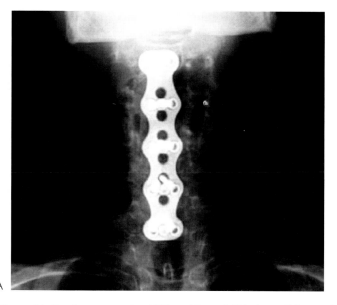
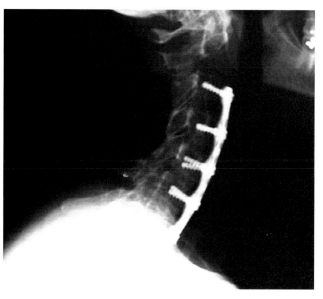

A   B

Figure 51–3. Anteroposterior (AP) and lateral (B) views of the cervical spine postoperatively, showing intersegmental correction using tricortical graft with restoration of cervical lordosis and plate fixation with variable screw anterior plating.

PEARLS

- Obtain good preoperative plain X-rays and flexion-extension cervical spine X-rays prior to a posterior decompression.
- Have a low threshold to fuse a patient following a multilevel laminectomy and foraminotomies decompression.
- Always image the spinal cord (MRI) prior to surgical correction of deformity.
- Consider the option of anterior intersegmental correction if compression of the spinal cord is due to deformity only or pathology at the disc space.

PITFALLS

- Progression of neurologic deficit.
- Lowering blood pressure without the use of very sensitive neurologic monitoring.
- Performing anterior corpectomies and strut fusion alone with inadequate internal or external fixation.

pain, and deformity. Many patients who develop a cervical deformity after a laminectomy represent a lack of attention to the sagittal plane. Preoperative x-rays are imperative prior to laminectomy to ensure that the patient has a lordotic cervical spine and no pathologic hypermobility. Any degree of facet resection in addition to a laminectomy increases the chances for cervical kyphosis. Therefore, consideration should always be given to a posterior cervical fusion with instrumentation in the face of a laminectomy or facet resection or if there is any evidence of preoperative hypermobility.

Normal alignment of the cervical spine is estimated at 14.4 degrees of lordosis from X2 to C7. This allows the weight-bearing axis in normal alignment to lie posterior to the vertebral bodies and helps maintain a normal lordotic sagittal contour. However, if cervical lordosis is lost, load transmission transfers to the anterior vertebral body, thus increasing the kyphotic deforming force. After sagittal balance is lost in the cervical spine, the cervical musculature is placed at a mechanical disadvantage, requiring constant posterior paraspinal muscle contraction to maintain an upright posture. Eventually the fatigue and pain will occur and kyphosis will progress. With progression of kyphotic deformity the spinal cord can drape over the posterior aspect of the vertebral body, thus increasing cord deformation and cord ischemia. Many patients with cervical postlaminectomy kyphosis can show severe spinal cord changes of myelomalacia or cord atrophy.

The incidence of postcervical laminectomy kyphosis is unknown. We do know the incidence is greatly increased in children, in those patients undergoing laminectomy for tumor that would require radiation, and in the face of underlying cervical kyphosis prior to the laminectomy being performed.

Clinical evaluation of these patients often requires a myriad of radiographic studies including dynamic radiographics, MRI, myelogram, postmyelogram, computed tomography (CT), and angiography6. One must first demonstrate that the deformity is not fixed by a facet ankylosis that would require a posterior osteotomy prior to anterior release. This can be done with oblique radiographs of the facets or CT scan. MRI is extremely helpful in identifying cord impingement and for cord atrophy and myelomalacia.

If there is significant cord deformation and changes within the substance of the cord, one must be extremely careful when inducing hypotension with anesthesia and in positioning the patient. CT scanning and angiography can help determine the vertebral artery anatomy. CT scanning can also help define the C7 and C2 pedicle anatomy for the placement of posterior instrumentation in the event a long fusion is necessary. Knowledge of the intertransversarial distance is useful when performing corpectomies.

In performing surgery on postlaminectomy kyphosis, deformity correction and neural decompression should occur simultaneously. Neural decompression takes precedence over the deformity correction.

The principles of kyphosis surgery apply to the neck as they do in the thoracic and lumbar regions. The anterior column is lengthened and the posterior column is shortened. Deformity correction is hinged around the posterior longitudinal ligament (PLL) or middle column. If the deformity is passively correctable, it often can be done with traction and surgical fixation following correction.

Options for both neural decompression and deformity correction include anterior discectomies and segmental correction vs. corpectomies (removal of the entire anterior bodies). Resection of the anterior bodies (corpectomies) leads to a much greater instability pattern. In the face of the posterior laminectomy, the surgeon now has created a 360-degree instability pattern. In our mind this necessitates anterior fusion fixation and posterior instrumentation as well. Depending on the degree of kyphosis correction or anterior column lengthening, despite anterior and posterior fixation, halo vest external mobilization may still be required for protection of the graft and instrumentation. If compression occurs due to posterior vertebral or soft tissue prominence, for example, ossification of the PLL (OPLL), vertebral body removal is often necessary. If the compression of the spinal cord is related to the deformity and pathology remains at the disc space, anterior multilevel discectomy can be used, as in this case, to both correct the deformity and obtain neural decompression.

Alternative Methods of Management

The alternative methods of management are anterior corpectomy, fibular strut grafting, and posterior fusion instead of the anterior procedure alone. This entails more surgery with a greater creation of instability than was performed on the patient presented here. Posterior surgery alone in this patient is not an option. The deformity was not fully correctable and the neurologic compressive pathology was anterior. The natural history, once myelopathic symptoms occur, is poor for spontaneous improvement. With onset of myelopathy, we are hesitant to recommend observation, as we fear the patient's symptoms may progress.

Type of Management	Advantages	Disadvantages	Comments
Nonoperative	None	Myelopathy and deformity will progress	Not an option unless the patient refuses surgery
Anterior segmental correction with interbody grafts	Only an anterior approach is needed Good correction with more inherent stability	Many graft junctions to heal	Treatment of choice in this case Treatment of choice if cord compression is due to deformity or pathology is limited to the disc space
Anterior corpectomy and strut with plate fixation	Only an anterior approach is needed Often good correction of deformity can be achieved	360-degree instability is created with the laminectomy posteriorly High risk of graft and/or plate failure	Rarely use this option anymore
Anterior corpectomies, fibular strut with junctional plating, and posterior segmental instrumentation with autograft fusion posteriorly	Strongest fixation for this problem Can alleviate compression posterior to the body Gain good correction of deformity and maximize fixation	Longer surgery Higher risk for dural tear posteriorly with open lamina More neck pain with posterior operation	This is our construct of choice for anyone who has deformity requiring anterior corpectomies over more than one level in postlaminectomy kyphosis

Complications

These surgeries are fraught with complications. These include neurologic injury, loss of fixation, postoperative neck pain, swallowing dysfunction, voice problems, and dural tear.

To prevent a neurologic injury, we always carefully survey the MRI for evidence of spinal cord for edema, myelomalacia, or other signs of cord wasting. In these patients great care must be taken to use high-quality intraoperative neurologic monitoring and keep the blood pressure at an adequate level (above a mean arterial pressure of 70 mm Hg). We have found that adequate neurologic monitoring can help significantly with positioning of the patient and with blood pressure control for perfusion of the cord.

Fixation failure is prevented with attention to good bone grafting technique, maximum anterior and posterior fixation (usually a buttress plate anteriorly), and segmental instrumentation with lateral mass and/or pedicle screws posteriorly (using maximum external fixation as needed). Even with an anterior and posterior fusion we often put postlaminectomy kyphosis patients into a halo orthosis.

If a revision anterior approach is needed, the patient's vocal cords are surveyed prior to surgery. If both are functional, we use a contralateral anterior exposure for ease and safety. If one vocal cord is nonfunctional due to prior anterior exposure, we expose through the same side to avoid the potential for a bilateral recurrent laryngeal nerve palsy.

Attention to detail and knowledge of the potential downfalls in this disease process help to avoid these complications.

Suggested Readings

Albert TJ, Vaccaro AR. Post-laminectomy kyphosis. Spine 1998; 23(4):2738–2745.

Mikaw Y, Shikata J, Tamamuro T. Spinal deformity and instability after multi-level cervical laminectomy. Spine 1987; 12:6–11.

Munechika Y. Influence of laminectomy on the stability of the spine: an experimental study with special reference to the extent of laminectomy and the resection of the intervertebral joint. J Jpn Orthop Assoc 1973; 47:111–125.

Nolan JP, Sherk HH. Biomechanical evaluation of the extensor musculature of the cervical spine. Spine 1988; 13:9–11.

Nowinski GP, Visarious H, Nolte LP, Herkowitz HN. A biomechanical comparison of cervical laminoplasty and cervical laminectomy with progressive facetectomy. Spine 1993; 18:1995–2004.

Pal GP, Sherk HH. The vertical stability of the cervical spine. Spine 1988; 13: 447–449.

Raynor RB, Moskovich T, Zidel P, Pugh J. Alterations in primary and coupled neck motions after facetectomy. Neurosurgery 1987; 21:681–687.

Saito T, Yamamuro T, Shikata J, Oka M, Tsutsumi S. Analysis and prevention of spinal column deformity following cervical laminectomy. I. Pathogenetic analysis of postlaminectomy deformities. Spine 1991; 16:494–502.

Sim FH, Suien HJ, Bickel WH, Janes JM. Swan-neck deformity following extensive cervical laminectomy: a review of twenty-one cases. J Bone Joint Surg 1974; 56A:564–580.

Yasouka S, Peterson HA, Laws ER, MacCarty CS. Pathogenesis and prophylaxis of postlaminectomy deformity of the spine after multiple level laminectomy: difference between children and adults. Neurosurgery 1995; 9:145–152.

Yasouka S, Peterson HA, MacCarty CS. Incidence of spinal deformity after multilevel laminectomy in children and adults. J Neurosurg 1982; 57:441–445.

Zdeblick TA, Abitbol JJ, Kunz DN, McCabe RP, Garfin S. Cervical stability after sequential capsule resection. Spine 1993; 18:2005–2008.

Zdeblick TA, Bohlman HH. Myelopathy, cervical kyphosis and treatment by anterior carpectomy and strut grafting. J Bone Joint Surg 1989; 71A:170–182.

Zdeblick TA, Zou D, Warden KE, McCabe R, Kunz D, Vanderby R. Cervical stability after foraminotomy: a biomechanical in vitro analysis. J Bone Joint Surg 1992; 74A:22–27.

Case 52
Fixed Pelvic Obliquity

Jean-Pierre C. Farcy, Brian D. Hoffman, and Frank J. Schwab

History and Physical Examination

A 6-year-old girl in excellent health and no significant medical history was involved in a head-on automobile collision. The patient was a backseat passenger and was wearing her seat belt at the time of the accident. There was no head trauma or loss of consciousness. The patient was immediately found to have complete flaccid paraplegia with a T10 sensory level. Initial radiologic evaluation revealed an L2 bony Chance-type fracture. A computed tomography (CT) myelogram additionally revealed cord disruption at T10 and a syrinx extending from T8 to T10.

Three months after her injury the patient underwent a T12/L2 posterior fusion with CD (Cotrel-Dubousset) instrumentation. Over the following year the patient

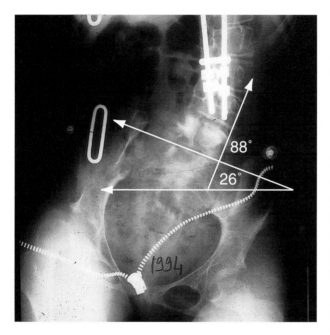

Figure 52–1. Preoperative anteroposterior radiograph of the lumbar spine demonstrating 26 degrees of pelvic obliquity. The iliolumbar angle (ILA) is 88 degrees, and the pelvis follows the lumbar curvature [type 2 fixed pelvic obliquity (FPO)].

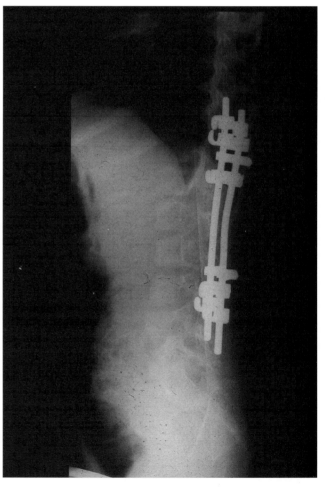

Figure 52–2. Preoperative lateral radiograph demonstrating complete loss of lumbar lordosis at the fusion mass, from T11 to L4.

developed a progressive kyphotic deformity caudal to the fused levels. She underwent an extension of her fusion from T10 to L4 and did well postoperatively, achieving wheelchair independence.

Over the next 4 years an increasing pelvic obliquity was noted with an associated thoracolumbar scoliosis refractory to bracing. Her other deformities included bilateral flexion contractures of the knees and hips with subluxation of the left hip. At that time, the patient presented to the senior author (J.-P.C.F.) for further treatment.

Radiologic Findings

Radiographs of the spine and pelvis indicated the pelvic obliquity angle (POA) was 26 degrees, the iliolumbar angle (ILA) was nearly normal, and lateral translation (LT) was minimal (Fig. 52–1). Her fusion mass was intact, although there was no lordosis from T11 to L4 (Fig. 52–2). There was also a 30-degree dextroscoliosis of the thoracic spine and a 45-degree levoscoliosis of the lumbar spine continuous with the pelvic obliquity.

Diagnosis

Posttraumatic paralytic scoliosis with fixed pelvic obliquity.

Surgical Management

Nine years after her injury and almost 8 years after her extended fusion, the patient was returned to the operating room. The goal of surgery was to correct the pelvic obliquity and offer her a balanced spine in transverse, coronal, and sagittal planes. A two-stage procedure was planned. In the first stage, a left flank incision with a retroperitoneal approach was used to access the lower lumbar spine. After ligation of the segmental vessels from L2 to L5, the aorta, left iliac vessels, and left ureter were mobilized to expose the L5/S1 disc. After complete L5/S1 discectomy, this level was found to be quite mobile. An L4/L5 discectomy was then similarly performed, with excellent resulting mobility of this segment. An L3/L4 discectomy was also performed, but this level remained rigid due to the existing posterior fusion mass. Morcelized cancellous bone from the left iliac crest was packed into the prepared disc spaces. Additional bone graft was also harvested and set aside for the subsequent posterior procedure.

At the time of bone harvest the left hip flexion contracture was released. The sartorius was detached from the anterior superior iliac spine and the rectus femoris was detached from the anterior inferior iliac spine. To complete the procedure, an iliopsoas release was also performed.

The patient was then repositioned prone on a Wilson frame. The spine was approached via an incision from T3 to the sacrum. First, the sacrum was exposed subperiosteally to the ala, and mobility was confirmed. Using Cobb elevators and electrocautery, dissection was extended superiorly to expose the existing instrumentation. The rods were cut and the hardware was removed in a caudal-to-cranial fashion. Additional freeing of the L5/S1 level was then achieved by osteotomy and subsequent rongeur excision of the inferior facets of L5. Obliquity reduction could then be tested with a spreader placed between the laminae of L5 and S1. However,

- Use two foundations (thoracolumbar and lumbosacral) and four-rod technique for ideal correction.
- Anterior release is essential for proper correction in three planes, even if the curve appears supple.
- It is essential to consider the pelvis and sacrum together as a functional end-vertebra. The "pelvic vertebra" (PV) must be moved as an entity, together with L5 and, if possible, L4.

PITFALLS

- Attempt at complete correction with two long rods is not possible. The PV must be independently secured and its obliquity considered separately from spinal deformities above it. For this reason, Luque-Galveston technique will not offer sufficient control of the pelvis to achieve and maintain adequate correction.
- If the sacral screw does not penetrate the endplate of S1, the foundation of the construct will not have strength for obliquity correction and maintenance of reduction. Also, when placing the K-wire for the sacral screws, be sure not to angle too medially. This error will place the screw tip too posteriorly, possibly penetrating the spinal canal.

after a similar facetectomy was performed at L4, mobilization was still insufficient to achieve overall balance of the spine.

Attention was then directed to the placement of the iliosacral screws. On the right side, exposure was extended to the posterior superior iliac spine (PSIS) and to the area immediately inferiolateral to the S1 facet, approaching the sacroiliac joint. The Kirschner wire (K-wire) was then oriented such that it followed a 45-degree medial angulation, slightly level to the L5/S1 disc in the axial plane. The entry point for the K-wire was located along this plane at its intersection with the small bony ridge approximately 1 cm below the PSIS. The K-wire was then slowly advanced such that it passed through a right Beurrier connector placed between the ilium and sacrum. As with any cannulated screw technique, placement of the guide wire is a critically important step, and accurate placement of the wire was confirmed with anteroposterior and lateral radiographs. Penetration of the S1 endplate was also confirmed, having advanced the K-wire approximately 45 mm within the body of the sacrum. Care was also taken, however, not to cross the midline. The path of the iliosacral screw was then hand-tapped and the screw was hand-driven through the PSIS, the Beurrier connector, and the sacrum. A second set of radiographs confirmed proper orientation and penetration of the iliosacral screw, and the K-wire was withdrawn. This procedure was then repeated on the left side.

Short (10-cm) CD rods were passed through the Beurrier connectors, dominoes for later connection to the thoracolumbar rods, and to firmly engaged closed hooks below the L4 laminae. With distraction primarily on the left side, a good L4/L5/S1 foundation was established by creating a solid symmetric construct from L4 to the pelvis.

The thoracic spine was then exposed subperiosteally, and a fusion mass osteotomy at the apex of the thoracic scoliosis (T12/L1) was performed. Left-side instrumentation was then placed, consisting of a laminopedicular claw at T3/T4, a closed supralaminar hook at T3, a closed pedicle hook at T4, and an open laminar hook at T8. The right-side construct was similar, using a down-going laminar hook at T4, an up-going laminar hook at T5, and an up-going pedicle hook at T9. Then, 36-cm precontoured CD rods were placed bilaterally, through the connecting dominoes at their distal ends. Due to good mobility of the lumbosacral junction, pelvic obliquity improvement was noted as the long rods were seated. The convex sides of the thoracic and lumbar curves were compressed, the concave sides were distracted. With axial rotation of the precontoured rods, improvement was seen in the coronal plane and sagittal plane curves, and the rods were secured to the thoracolumbar instrumentation.

Final correction of the pelvic obliquity was accomplished by applying compression on the left (high) side between the lumbopelvic construct and the thoracolumbar construct and distraction on the right (low) side. Devices for transverse traction (DTTs) were then placed at T5 and L4. Finally, the bone craft was matchsticked and laid across the decorticated laminae and spinous processes along the instrumented spine.

Postoperative Management

The patient was placed on bed rest, and intravenous antibiotics were continued for 3 days. On the second postoperative day the patient was mobilized from bed to chair. Radiographs at that time showed a POA of 4 degrees and an ILA of 89 degrees (Fig. 52–3). Residual thoracic and lumbar scolioses were 31 degrees and 36 degrees, but the curves appeared to be balanced (Fig. 52–4). No brace wear was prescribed, and the patient was transferred in good condition to the rehabilitation service on the fifth postoperative day.

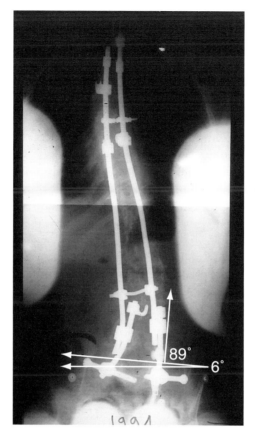

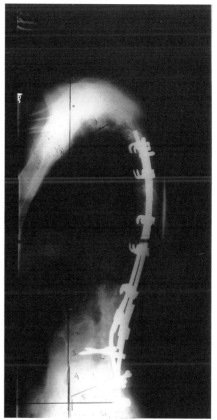

Figure 52–3. Postoperative anteroposterior radiograph demonstrating correction of FPO. The pelvic oblique angle (POA) is 6 degrees and the ILA is 89 degrees.

Figure 52–4. Postoperative lateral radiograph shows restoration of a normal sagittal contour.

One year postoperatively, radiographs showed incomplete lumbosacral fusion. However, clinically there was no gross motion and the instrumentation did not loosen. Her activity was limited to better allow fusion, and an electromagnetic bone growth stimulator was applied. One year later her fusion had improved significantly. As of the last examination, her spine is balanced, pelvis and shoulders remain level, and she continues to be very active.

Discussion

The primary objective in treating a paraplegic patient with fixed pelvic obliquity (FPO) is in achieving an overall balanced spine. Although it is tempting to address the obvious pelvic deformity, correction will likely fail if global spine alignment is not achieved. FPO is not a coronal plane tilting of the pelvis under the spinal column, but rather the result of axial rotation, which occurs in scoliosis and accelerates in growing patients with posterior fusions. Often there is also sagittal imbalance and lateral translation of the thoracic spine with respect to the sacral midline. These are important considerations in planning surgery because, as Dubousset has noted, pelvic obliquity correction cannot be achieved by instrumentation forces acting solely in the coronal plane.

Wheelchair-dependent patients with FPO have particular clinical considerations. Correction of pelvic obliquity minimizes the risk of eventual chronic pressure ulcers. It is essential to level the shoulders as well as the pelvis. This allows the patient to achieve her highest level of functional independence, allowing adequate upper extremity power for mobility and support.

In the presented patient a premenarchal tethering fusion resulted in progression of the crankshaft phenomenon. Recent studies suggest that if a posterior fusion is carried out when the patient is Risser grade 0 with absolutely no secondary sex characteristics, crankshaft progression is inevitable, although the degree of progression varies. Continuing anterior spinal growth occurs even in the presence of a rigid posterior fusion mass, which prevents progressive deformity in the sagittal plane alone. As vertebral height is added by the body endplates, the increased anterior length of the spinal column obligates it to rotate around the axis of the fusion mass. In canines transpedicular instrumentation and fusion without an anterior procedure has experimentally overcome the asymmetrical forces of vertebral body growth, but this has yet to be demonstrated clinically.

After thorough clinical and radiologic evaluation of the spine and PV in all three planes, we classify the FPO pattern into one of three types. In type 1 FPO, the concavity reverses at the thoracolumbar junction (Fig. 52–5). Type 2 FPO, exhibited in this patient, is characterized by a lumbar spine and pelvis that follow the same scoliotic curve (Fig. 52–6). Type 3 FPO follows a similar curve pattern to that in type 2; however, there is rotation and tilt of L5 with respect to the sacrum (Fig. 52–7). The relevant radiographic parameters, in addition to scoliotic curves, are the POA, the ILA, which is formed by the lateral edge of the L5 body and the transverse pelvic axis, and the degree of LT from the highest visualized thoracic vertebra to the sacral midline. In general, types 1 and 2 FPO have a normal or nearly normal ILA.

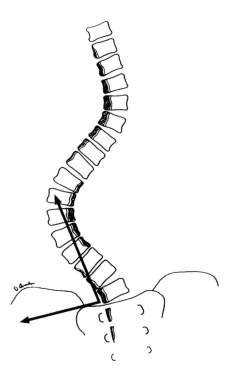

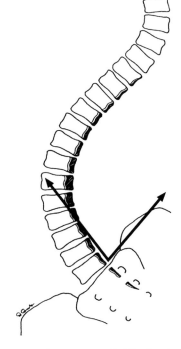

Figure 52–5. Type 1 FPO. The distal lumbar spine and pelvis create a compensatory curve opposite the lumbar scoliosis. ILA (indicated by arrows) approaches normal.

Figure 52–6. Type 2 FPO. The lumbar spine and pelvis are continuous with the thoracolumbar scoliosis. ILA (indicated by arrows) approaches normal.

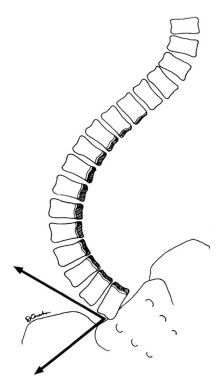

Figure 52–7. Type 3 FPO. L5 is subluxed on S1. There may be a combination of rotation, tilting, and translation. ILA (indicated by arrows) is abnormal. (Modified from Farcy J-PC, Weidenbaum M, Roye D. Fixed pelvic obliquity. In: Farcy J-PC, ed. Spine: Start of the Art Reviews, pp. 576–577. Philadelphia: Hanley & Belfus, 1994.)

When fixing a long construct to the pelvic vertebra, we agree with Camp that iliosacral fixation provides a better anchor than sacral fixation alone. Screw purchase is secure and the lever arm is long, offering greater derotational and anti-tilt moments. Iliosacral screws as described above are used by the senior author on patients who are paraplegic. In ambulatory patients, often adults, the iliac screw nail is preferred not only because it provides fixation as stable as the Galveston rod technique but because it could be removed after 18 months if the windshield-wiper phenomenon develops. Generally, we prefer CD instrumentation because it affords superior rotational correction as well as stable correction in the coronal and sagittal planes. CD-Galveston instrumentation is sufficient for more supple forms of neuromuscular scoliosis, such as Duchenne's muscular dystrophy, but in spastic cases the Galveston rods alone have insufficient distal stability and tend to move within the ilium over time. The Galveston rod extends from the ilium to the thoracolumbar spine in a single unit; only in cases of supple paralysis can the spine and pelvis be molded to the rods in the correct position. In contrast, iliosacral screws with their short connecting rods provide a second distal construct that can be precisely manipulated in relation to the thoracolumbar spine, overpowering spastic muscle moments.

In this case two constructs were made independent from each other; one thoracolumbar and one lumbosacral. The L4 sublaminar hooks were placed to create a strong hardware bridge anchored to the PV distally and to L4 proximally. Note that in patients with an abnormal and rigid ILA (type 3 FPO), this construct cannot be made without first correcting the alignment of the lumbosacral junction. When the long CD rods were introduced into the connectors on the short lumbosacral rods, much of the pelvic obliquity corrected. With compression on the low side and distraction on the high side, correction of the remaining obliquity was achieved.

Alternative Methods of Management

Generally, spastic FPO requires spinal instrumentation and fusion to the pelvis for adequate long-term results. If a patient has no L5/S1 derangement, no hip contractures, a completely correctable lumbar curve, and a corrected or balanced thoracic curve, then fusion to the PV may not be necessary. In paraplegic patients, however, this represents a small subgroup.

There are numerous systems available for the treatment of FPO. Most of the major systems are outlined in the table below, although not all of these are able to hold reduction in spastic cases. Some of these instruments, such as the Chopin block and the Jackson Liberty technique, are good in addressing FPO but work less well in conjunction with a long thoracolumbar fusion. Other systems are currently available, such as the Texas Scottish Rite Hospital (TSRH) system and Isola instrumentation, which have also been used in the treatment of FPO.

Type of Management	Advantages	Disadvantages	Comments
CD with iliosacral screws	Wide base on the pelvis provides strong fixation Excellent independent control of obliquity reduction Excellent rotational rigidity	Difficult to apply if S1 screw is not properly engaged May have less flexion pullout strength than Galveston technique	Extremely useful in spastic paralytic children and adults
Chopin block/plate	Three screws on each side Good strength Excellent rotational rigidity	Difficult to apply	Long learning curve Excellent for adult scoliosis or short lumbosacral fusion Not recommended for pelvic obliquity with long fusions
Luque-Galveston	Simpler procedure	Suboptimal rotational control Iliac rod insertions may sweep in spastic paralysis (windshield-wiper phenomenon)	Requires a supple deformity Reserved for paralytic children without too much spasticity
Harrington iliosacral bar	Easier to apply	Possible dural injury Very poor sacral purchase	Not often used
Cotrel sacro-alar screw	Less dissection	Poor sacral bone quality	Only recommended for neutralization when no major force is applied
Liberty technique (Roger Jackson)	Screw engages the S1 endplate Rod inside the sacrum to the level of the sciatic notch	Difficult to apply	Recommended by the senior author for short fixation only

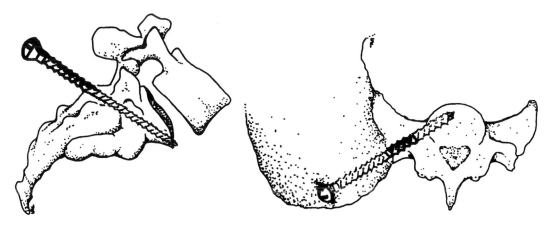

Figure 52–8. Proper placement of iliosacral screws. Note that the screw engages the S1 endplate. (Modified from Farcy J-PC, Margulies JY. Iliosacral screw fixation. In: Margulies JY, et al, eds. Lumbosacral and Spinopelvic Fixation, p. 605. Philadelphia: Lippincott-Raven, 1996.)

Complications

Complications of instrumentation for FPO are largely the same as for all spine instrumentation surgery. These include wound infection, early hardware failure, late hardware failure, and progression of deformity. Inherent in the anterior approach for intervertebral release is the risk of injury to the bowel or great vessels.

Placement of the iliosacral screws must be precise (Fig. 52–8). Overpenetration risks injury to structures that lie along the ventral surface of the sacrum. These include the rectosigmoid junction, approximately at S3, the sacral artery anastomoses, the internal iliac veins, and the S1 nerve trunk. The sacral foramina, formed by lateral fusion of the transverse processes, have a larger diameter ventrally than dorsally. As a result, the extent of the foramina cannot be fully visualized. The sacral nerve roots, spinal ganglion, and sacral arteries that course along the medial aspect of the sacral pedicle may easily be injured as hardware is inserted.

Adequate preoperative nutritional status and perioperative antibiotics are paramount in preventing infection. Also, postoperative nutrition must be monitored to optimize healing, reduce the risk of infection, and maximize the patient's tolerance for physical therapy.

Suggested Readings

Camp JF, Caudle R, Ashmun RD, Roach J. Immediate complications of Cotrel-Dubousset instrumentation to the sacro-pelvis. Spine 1990; 15(9):932–941.

Dubousset J. Pelvic obliquity correction. In Margulies JY, et al, eds. Lumbosacral and Spinopelvic Fixation, pp. 39–49. Philadelphia: Lippincott-Raven, 1996.

Dubousset J, Herring JA, Shufflebarger H. The crankshaft phenomenon. J Pediatr Orthop 1989; 9(5):541–550.

Farcy J-PC, Margulies JY. Iliosacral screw fixation. In: Margulies JY, et al, eds. Lumbosacral and Spinopelvic Fixation, pp. 601–609. Philadelphia: Lippincott-Raven, 1996.

Farcy J-PC, Weidenbaum M, Roye D. Fixed pelvic obliquity. In Farcy J-PC, ed. Spine: State of the Art Reviews, pp. 573–588. Philadelphia: Hanley & Belfus, 1994.

Kioschos HC, Asher MA, Lark RG, Harner EJ. Overpowering the crankshaft mechanism: the effect of posterior spinal fusion with and without stiff transpedicular fixation on anterior spinal column growth in immature canines. Spine 1996; 21(10):1168–1173.

Shufflebarger HL, Clark CE. Prevention of the crankshaft phenomenon. Spine 1991; 16(suppl 8):S409–411.

Stagnara P, ed. Spinal Deformity. London: Butterworths, 1988.

Case 53

Klippel-Feil Syndrome

Peter O. Newton

History and Physical Examination

A 6-year-old boy presented with the complaint of a head tilt and neck pain. The head tilt had been noted early in life, and the neck discomfort had been increasing over the prior year. The boy was born deaf and had a congenital cardiac defect that was surgically repaired in the first year of life. A cardiac pacemaker was required to maintain his heart rhythm. He had a moderate learning disability and a behavioral problem.

His physical examination was significant for a 15-degree lateral head tilt to the right. His neck flexion and extension motion was full, and his axial rotation was limited to 45 degrees in each direction. His hair line was low, although his neck was neither webbed nor particularly short. His neurologic exam was normal.

Radiologic Findings

Initial radiographs included an anteroposterior (AP), odontoid, as well as flexion and extension lateral views (Fig. 53–1) of the cervical spine. They demonstrated a congenital bony malformation as the cause of the head tilt. In addition, instability between the occiput and C1 was noted. The cranium subluxated posteriorly 12 mm with the head extended. The clivus line fell well posterior to the dens in extension and became more normally aligned with the head in flexion.

A magnetic resonance imaging (MRI) study obtained with the neck in both flexion and extension was desired, but because of the child's cardiac pacemaker, this could not be obtained. Instead a computed tomography (CT) scan was obtained with the head positioned in neutral, flexion, and extension. Due to the boy's behavioral difficulties, general anesthesia was required. He tolerated the imaging in the neutral and flexed positions but suffered apnea when his neck was extended. Spontaneous breathing resumed when the neck was flexed. Three-dimensional (3D) reconstruction of the images was performed (Fig. 53–2). These demonstrated a hemivertebra between C3 and C4 on the left with wedged vertebrae caudal to this. In addition, the left half of C1 was fused to the right half of C2, whereas the right half of C1 was fused to the occiput.

A renal ultrasound examination to identify any associated renal abnormalities demonstrated normal anatomy.

Diagnosis

The diagnosis of Klippel-Feil syndrome with occipitocervical instability was made. Although no neurologic signs could be found on examination, the patient's neck pain and episode of apnea during anesthesia with the neck in extension (the position of maximum subluxation) suggested intermittent spinal cord compression. The congenital malformations at the occiput-C1 level resulted in an altered joint configuration at this level that was mechanically incompetent. The patient's head tilt was

MASTERCASES: SPINE SURGERY

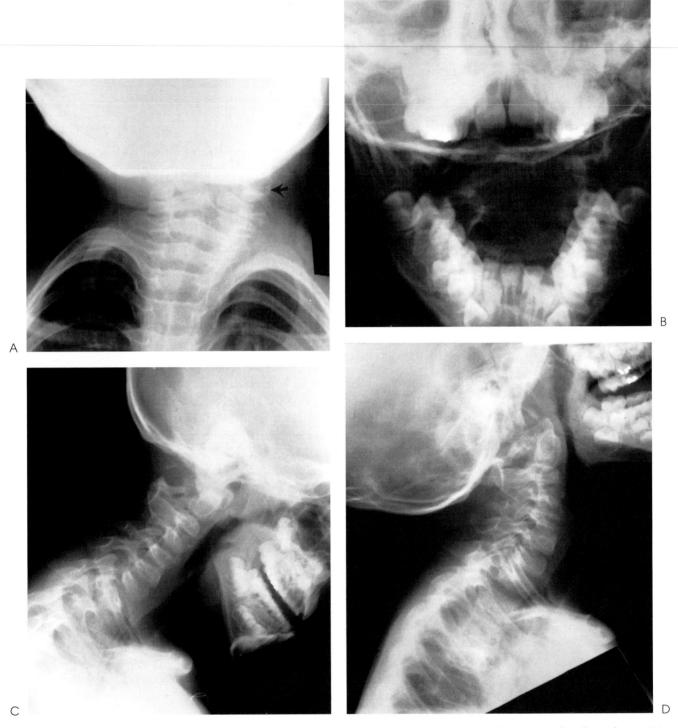

Figure 53–1. Anteroposterior (AP) radiograph (A) suggests a midcervical hemivertebra on the left side (arrow). The odontoid view (B) suggests asymmetry of the lateral masses of C1. The flexion-extension views (C,D) demonstrate posterior subluxation of the occiput in extension with the clivus line projecting posterior to the dens. In addition, when the neck is flexed, separation between C1 and C2 does not develop, suggesting congenital fusion at this level. There was no instability noted caudad to this fused level.

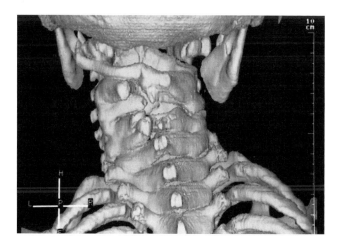

Figure 53–2. Three-dimensional computed tomography (CT) scan clarifies the congenital anomalies present. The abnormalities of formation and segmentation at the occipitocervical junction and midcervical spine can be appreciated.

related primarily to the left-sided hemivertebra and wedged segments between C3 and C5.

Surgical Management

Due to the severe occipitocervical instability, pain, and apnea, a decision was made to proceed with surgical stabilization by performing a posterior cervical arthodesis from the occiput to C5. Proximally, the arthodesis was performed to stabilize the occiput-C1 level, whereas distally the arthodesis was designed to limit further deformity due to growth of the hemivertebra. Under general anesthesia, the patient had a halo ring fixed to the skull with two pins in each quadrant tightened to 4 inch-pounds of torque. Somatosensory evoked potential monitoring was established and the patient was turned prone onto a Mayfield headrest attaching directly to the halo ring. The head was positioned and the occiput-C1 relationship visualized with an image intensifier. The clivus line was restored to a normal anatomic relationship by proper head positioning.

A midline posterior approach was made exposing the base of the skull and upper cervical vertebrae. Careful dissection splitting the midline raphe was performed to avoid bleeding from the paraspinous musculature. The spinous processes were identified and the lamina stripped in the subperiosteal plane. The 3D CT scan aided in the exposure by allowing the abnormal structure of the posterior elements to be anticipated. The lateral extent of the exposure was limited to avoid injury to the vertebral arteries. This is particularly important at the C1 level. A periosteal flap from the occiput was reflected and drill holes were placed in the outer table of the skull. Wire was passed through adjoining holes and used to secure autogenous corticocancellous iliac crest bone to the decorticated skull. Additional sublaminar and spinous process wires were utilized to fix the graft to the remaining cervical segments. A large amount of cancellous bone was placed at the occiput-C1 level. The arthodesis spanned all of the abnormal segments.

Following wound closure, a body cast was applied from the waist to over the shoulders. Uprights were fixed to the cast and connected to the halo ring. The alignment of the spine and the position of the bone graft are seen in Figure 53–3. There were no changes in the sensory evoked potentials and the wake-up test was normal.

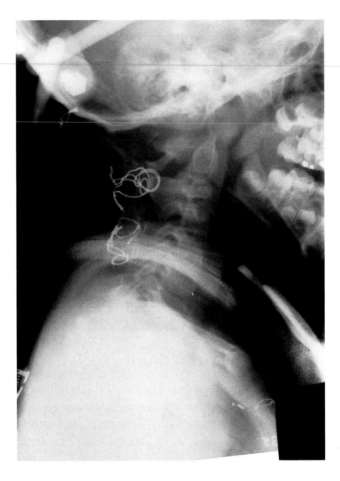

Figure 53–3. Postoperative lateral radiograph demonstrates the occipitocervical alignment as well as the position of the iliac crest bone graft.

Postoperative Management

Postoperatively, the patient was gradually mobilized in his halo-cast device. The halo pins were retightened to 4 inch-pounds the day after application. He was discharged from the hospital with sedating medications to control his behavior. He was seen at regular intervals to ensure halo stability. His pins eventually loosened 3 months postoperatively. The device was removed, and he was placed into a cervical orthosis for an additional 2 months. Interval radiographs suggested graft resorbtion at the upper level and flexion-extension views 9 months postoperatively confirmed a pseudarthrosis and persistent instability at the occiput-C1 level (Fig. 53–4).

The patient was returned to the operating room and a second attempt at fusion was undertaken. Positioning the head with image intensifier control confirmed the marked instability that remained at the occiput-C1 level. The skull abruptly subluxated posteriorly with neck extension. The exposure of the spine was performed, and a large mobile nonunion was noted between the occiput and C1. The fibrous tissue was excised, and a large bicortical iliac crest graft was shaped to fit within the bony defect. The fusion mass attached to the skull, which resulted from the first procedure, was large and allowed secure wiring with stainless steel cable to provide compression of the bone graft within the nonunion site (Fig. 53–5). A halo-cast was maintained for 4 months after the second procedure and was successful in attaining a solid arthrodesis. The lateral radiographs in Figure 53–6 demonstrate the

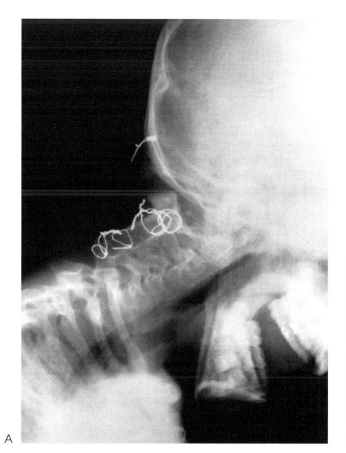 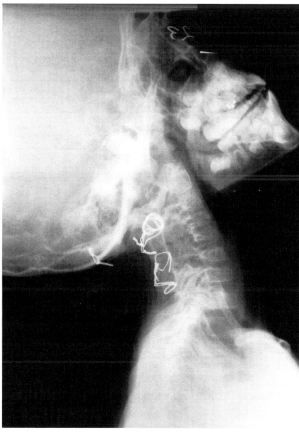

A   B

Figure 53–4. Flexion-extension lateral radiographs (A,B) 9 months postoperatively demonstrate a pseudarthrosis between the occiput and C1 with excessive motion remaining at this level.

appearance 8 months after the second procedure. The fusion mass is robust, and there is no abnormal motion with flexion or extension. His neck pain had resolved.

Discussion

The Klippel-Feil syndrome entails one or more congenitally fused motion segments in the cervical spine. The reported incidence varies between 0.2 and 0.8/1000. The original description in 1912 by Klippel and Feil was of a patient with six unsegmented cervical vertebrae. They reported the clinical features of a short neck, low hair line, and decreased cervical motion, which have become the classic findings of this syndrome. It has since become clear that often these features are absent in less severely involved cases. Pizzutillo and colleagues (1994) reported a 67% incidence of decreased cervical motion, 41% incidence of short neck, and 34% incidence of a low hair line in 111 patients diagnosed with Klippel-Feil syndrome.

Important associated anomalies of the musculoskeletal and other organ systems have been identified in these patients. Scoliosis is one of the most common, occurring in 60 to 78% of patients. The incidences of other frequent associations include renal malformations (30 to 35%), Sprengel's deformity (26 to 30%), hearing impairment (27 to 30%), and congenital heart defects (10 to 14%). Hensinger and

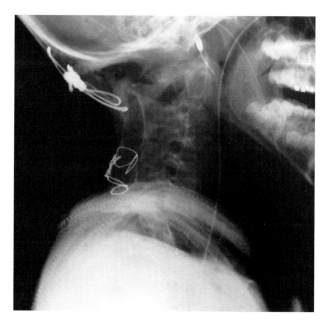

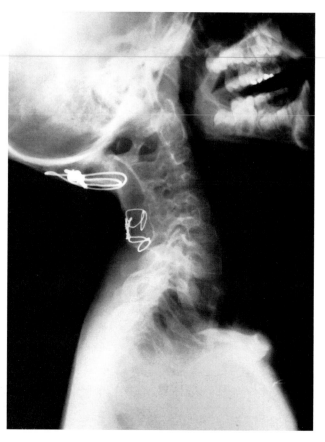

Figure 53–5. Lateral radiograph demonstrates the fixation and graft position immediately after repair of the nonunion site.

Figure 53–6. Eight months following the second procedure the fusion mass has matured. There is no abnormal motion with flexion or extension.

PEARLS
- Evaluate the remainder of the spine for potential associated congenital anomalies, and monitor for the development of scoliosis.
- Obtain a screening renal ultrasound on all patients with congenital vertebral anomalies.
- Use the 3D CT scan to better define the abnormal vertebral elements.
- An MRI with the neck positioned in flexion and extension may be useful in identifying instability and spinal cord compression.

colleagues (1974) emphasized the importance of renal screening to identify anomalies that may require treatment to preserve renal function.

The natural history of patients with Klippel-Feil syndrome is largely dependent on the location and number of fused motion segments. The major concern for these patients early in life relates to cervical instability with potential neurologic compromise. The subsequent development of painful degenerative changes in the open motion segments becomes a concern in later years. It has been postulated that congenital fusion between the occiput and C1 predisposes to increased motion and neurologic risk at the C1/C2 level. Similarly, fusion between C2 and C3 has been associated with increased motion at either the occiput-C1 or C1/C2 levels. Other features that may adversely affect stability include hypoplastic vertebral elements or failures of formation; this is particularly the case at the C1/C2 level with underdevelopment of the dens or ring of C1.

Neurologic sequelae have been reported in many patients with Klippel-Feil syndrome and associated cervical instability. These have ranged from transient paresthesias to fatal spinal cord injury. It is the risk of permanent neurologic injury that is the indication for surgical treatment or for recommending activity limitation in these patients. It is difficult, unfortunately, to predict in which patients this risk is substantial enough to warrant such intervention. Torg and Ramsey-Emrhein (1997)

* Do not overlook instability at the occiput-C1 level. It is easy to focus attention on the C1/C2 level, ignoring the occipitocervical junction. The clivus line is a useful landmark that normally intersects the dens in positions of flexion and extension. When instability at this level is suspected, a flexion-extension MRI of CT scan can be helpful. At times, the extent of neck motion is limited in these scanners and may be better visualized fluoroscopically during active motion.

have made recommendations regarding absolute contraindication for participation in contact sports. In patients with Klippel-Feil syndrome, these include occipitocervical anomalies, long cervical fusions, fused vertebrae proximal to C3, instability on flexion-extension, and disc degeneration. Patients with instability and neurologic signs are thought by most to be best treated by surgical stabilization. Those with instability but no neurologic signs are much more controversial. Certainly, they should be restricted from contact sports; however, when to recommend cervical fusion remains less well defined.

The indication for cervical fusion in this case further illustrates the lack of adequate surgical guidelines in the neurologically intact patient with cervical instability. Although the patient presented here had marked instability with occipitocervical malformations, prior to his CT scan no clear neurologic abnormalities to confirm spinal cord compression were identified. During his CT scan, neck extension resulted in cessation of spontaneous breathing. This finding in association with neck pain and increased motion was the indication for arthrodesis in this case.

Alternative Methods of Management

The alternatives to posterior cervical fusion in this case include observation and activity modification. The risk of observation has been discussed above. With marked upper cervical instability, the risk of catastrophic neurologic injury after minor trauma exists. Modifying activity to limit the risk of neck hyperextension is an option. This is an appropriate measure for those patients with less severe instability and those without other indications for surgical treatment. It is impossible, however, to completely eliminate the risk of spinal cord injury.

Alternative surgical methods of stabilization include the use of internal fixation. Segmental wiring or use of lateral mass/occipital screws fixed to rods or plates may provide secure internal fixation. These methods may be used to supplement the halo or as an alternative to the halo cast.

Type of Management	Advantages	Disadvantages	Comments
Observation	Simple	Risk of neurologic injury if the neck is unstable	Indicated for patients with single-level fusions below C4 and no evidence of instability
Activity restriction	Limits risk of neurologic injury	Risk of accidental injury not completely eliminated	Appropriate for most patients with Klippel-Feil syndrome
Cervical fusion without instrumentation	Decreased the risk of neurologic injury due to minor trauma	Further decreases neck motion; increases motion/stress on the unfused levels; intraoperative risk of spinal cord injury	Indicated for patients with neurologic signs and instability
Cervical fusion with instrumentation	Decreased the risk of neurologic injury due to minor trauma; avoid halo pin complications	As above for fusion without instrumentation; technically more demanding	Indicated for patients with neurologic signs and instability

Suggested Readings

Elster AD. Quadriplegia after minor trauma in the Klippel-Feil syndrome. A case report and review of the literature. J Bone Joint Surg 1984; 66A:1473–1474.

Hall JE, Simmons ED, Danylchuk K, et al. Instability of the cervical spine and neurological involvement in Klippel-Feil syndrome. A case report. J Bone Joint Surg 1990; 72A:460–462.

Hensinger RN, Lang JE, MacEwen GD. Klippel-Feil syndrome. A constellation of associated anomalies. J Bone Joint Surg 1974; 56A:1246–1253.

Nagib MG, Maxwell RE, Chou SN. Identification and management of high-risk patients with Klippel-Feil syndrome. J Neurosurg 1984; 61:523–530.

Pizzutillo PD, Woods M, Nicholson L, et al. Risk factors in Klippel-Feil syndrome. Spine 1994; 19:2110–2116.

Sherk HH, Dawoud S. Congenital os odontoideum with Klippel-Feil anomaly and fatal atlanto-axial instability. Report of a case. Spine 1981; 6:42–45.

Torg JS, Ramsey-Emrhein JA. Management guidelines for participation in collision activities with congenital, developmental, or postinjury lesions involving the cervical spine. Clin J Sports Med 1997; 7:273–291.

Case 54
Chiari Malformations
William Mitchell and Gregory J. Przybylski

History and Physical Examination

Case 1

An 8-year-old girl was diagnosed with scoliosis at age 3. She began brace treatment at age five when her curvature progressed to 25 degrees. Her curve has not progressed with active brace treatment. She denied symptoms of pain, weakness, paresthesias, bowel or bladder difficulties, abnormal balance, swallowing difficulties, diplopia, or headaches. Physical examination revealed a prominent right thoracic rib hump. Her spinal range of motion was normal. She did not have spinal tenderness or cutaneous lesions. Her neurologic examination was unremarkable.

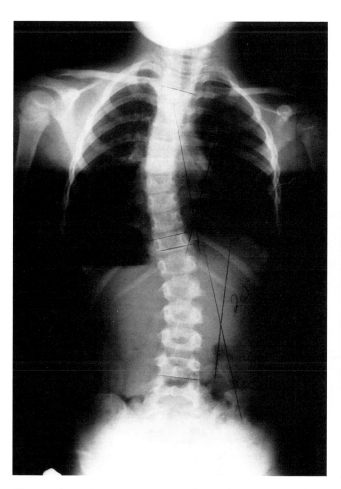

Figure 54–1. An anteroposterior radiograph in a patient with type I Chiari malformation who has an associated thoracolumbar scoliosis.

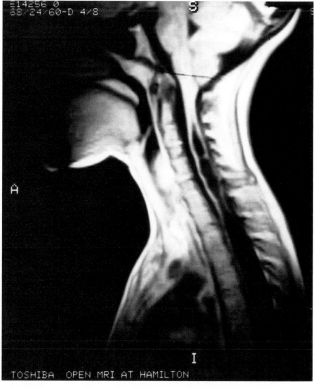

Figure 54–2. Midsagittal T1-weighted magnetic resonance imaging (MRI) reveals a type I Chiari malformation with caudal displacement of the cerebellar tonsils below the plane of the foramen magnum (line). A moderate cervicothoracic syrinx is also observed.

Case 2

A 3-year-old boy with a high lumbar myelomeningocele repair at birth and hydrocephalus treated with a ventriculoperitoneal shunt 2 days later developed progressive breathing difficulties and bradycardia. Imaging revealed a type II Chiari malformation that was treated with a suboccipital decompression at 8 months of age. His breathing subsequently improved. However, he began having transient right arm weakness, dysphagia, bradycardia, and apnea 1 year later. Symptoms progressed despite shunt revision, subtemporal decompression, untethering of his spinal cord, and syringosubarachnoid shunting. Examination revealed a lethargic and bradycardic infant with brief periods of apnea. His shunt valve pumped and refilled slowly, whereas his subtemporal decompression was sunken. He had a diminished gag reflex. Paraplegia and absent sensation were present since birth.

Case 3

A 39-year-old woman described 3 years of intractable headaches without vertigo or swallowing difficulties. She had no papilledema and a normal neurologic examination with the exception of a bilaterally decreased gag reflex and impaired tandem gait.

Radiologic Findings

An anteroposterior (AP) radiograph of the spine in case 1 (Fig. 54–1) revealed a right-sided thoracic scoliosis. Midsagittal magnetic resonance imaging (MRI) revealed a type I Chiari malformation (Fig. 54–2) with caudal displacement of the cerebellar vermis below the foramen magnum. An associated large cervicothoracic syrinx was also seen. In contrast, MRI in case 2 (Fig. 54–3) revealed a type II Chiari malformation with caudal displacement of the cerebellar vermis and medulla associated with a large cervicothoracic syrinx. Finally, MRI in case 3 (Fig. 54–4) revealed a type I Chiari malformation with a smaller associated syrinx.

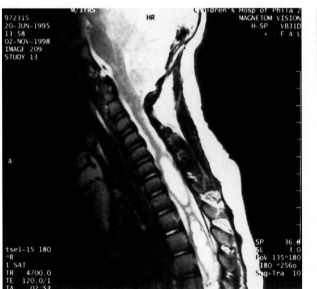
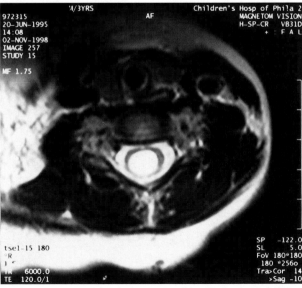

Figure 54–3. Midsagittal T2-weighted MRI (A) reveals a type II Chiari malformation with caudal displacement of the cerebellar vermis and medulla below the plane of the foramen magnum associated with a large cervicothoracic syrinx also seen in the axial plane (B).

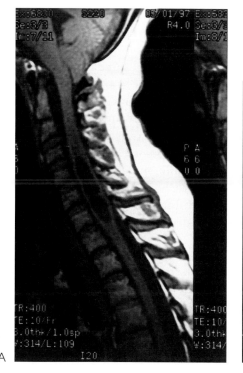
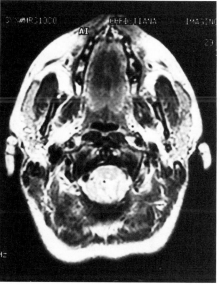

Figure 54–4. Midsagittal T1-weighted MRI (A) reveals a type I Chiari malformation with caudal displacement of the cerebellar tonsils below the plane of the foramen magnum associated with a moderate cervical syrinx. An axial MRI (B) at the level of the odontoid base reveals the presence of both the spinal cord anteriorly and the cerebellum posteriorly within the canal diameter.

Diagnosis

Clinical examination and radiographic evaluation are essential for diagnosis of Chiari malformations. The presence of scoliosis in the young girl prompted imaging that identified a type I Chiari malformation and syrinx. The presence of a large syrinx may have been a contributing factor to her scoliosis. The male infant initially developed apnea and bradycardia, which are common signs in infants with type II Chiari malformations. After symptoms recurred and progressed despite a functioning shunt, MRI of the cervicomedullary junction revealed persistent compression and a large cervicothoracic syrinx. Although he had previously undergone a suboccipital decompression, the infant had recurrent brain-stem symptoms with imaging evidence of cervicomedullary compression and syrinx, indicating the type II Chiari malformation was responsible. The MRI in case 3 performed for evaluation of intractable headaches identified a type I Chiari malformation with an associated cervical syrinx.

Surgical Management

Surgical management of Chiari malformations is necessary if symptoms persist despite treatment of associated hydrocephalus. After induction of general anesthesia and infusion of intravenous antibiotics, the patient is positioned prone and the head secured in a Mayfield head holder. Standard pin fixation is used for older children and adults, whereas young children are placed on a padded horseshoe headrest. Neck flexion facilitates exposure. The scalp is shaved from the inion down to the neck and prepped with Betadine. A midline skin incision from the inion to the upper cervical spine is followed by a subperiosteal dissection of the occiput and upper cervical laminae. The pericranium is preserved for use as a dural graft. The posterior arch of C1 is detached from ligaments and removed. Laminectomy is performed to the lowest level of caudal hindbrain displacement. A 3-cm suboccipital craniectomy is performed to decompress the width of the foramen magnum; decompression can be performed with a drill or rongeurs, but the latter is preferable in children.

In addition to bony decompression, a constricting dural band is also often found compressing the brain stem at the craniocervical junction. This band should be divided sharply, allowing dural expansion. In the second case, bradycardia immediately resolved upon releasing the band. The dura is often sufficiently translucent to assess whether the subarachnoid space has been reexpanded. If this does not occur or a syrinx is present, a duroplasty can be performed. The dura is opened with a scalpel in a Y-shaped incision, with the rostral limbs over the posterior fossa dura. Incising the occipital dura must be done cautiously to avoid bleeding from a poorly defined venous lake called the occipital sinus. Moreover, the small posterior fossa seen in patients with type II Chiari malformations is associated with a low transverse sinus. Hemostasis is facilitated by clipping or plicating the dural leaves together. The dural edges are reflected and sutured aside both to aid in visualization as well as to facilitate closure with a dural patch graft.

Although syringomyelia often resolves with decompression, the syrinx in case 2 was treated with a syringopleural shunt given the large focal spinal cord cavity. A complete cervical laminectomy was performed and the caudal syrinx was identified by ultrasound. After dural incision, a midline myelotomy was made over the translucent dorsal cord and a Silastic T-tube was inserted into the cavity. A subcutaneous tunnel was extended to the posterolateral thorax through which the distal catheter was tunneled and inserted into the pleural cavity. Prior to closing, the pleural opening was irrigated while the lungs are expanded by the anesthetist to prevent a postoperative pneumothorax. Once cerebrospinal fluid (CSF) flow has been restored, dural closure can be performed with an artificial dural substitute, pericranium, or nuchal ligament using 4-0 nonabsorbable suture. The fascia and subcutaneous tissues are closed in layers utilizing absorbable sutures, whereas the skin is closed with a running suture.

Postoperative Management

The patient is monitored in an intensive care unit after surgery with frequent neurologic examinations. The patient is mobilized and diet resumed within a few days once nausea and vomiting resolve; these common early postoperative complaints are managed with antiemetics. Although opiates can be used for pain relief in adults monitored in the intensive care unit, children rarely require medication more potent than acetaminophen. Muscle relaxants such as diazepam can also help manage postoperative cervical pain. After brief intensive care unit monitoring, the patient returns to normal activity and pain is managed with oral medications. Follow-up MRI is often reserved for evaluation of persistent or recurrent symptoms.

Discussion

Although Chiari malformation and syringomyelia have been studied for many decades, the etiology, pathophysiology, and treatment are still not understood. Prominent theories regarding the etiology and pathophysiology examine primary or secondary alterations in CSF flow dynamics. The Chiari malformation describes the caudal displacement of the hindbrain below the level of the foramen magnum. A type I malformation is a caudal displacement (4–6 mm) of the cerebellar tonsils below the plane of the foramen magnum. Although syringomyelia is present in 20 to 40% of all patients with type I Chiari malformations, 60 to 90% of symptomatic patients have this associated abnormality. A type II malformation is a caudal displacement of the cerebellar vermis, the fourth ventricle, and lower brain stem below the plane of the foramen magnum. Other associated anomalies include callosal dysgenesis and heterotopias. Moreover, nearly all have a myelomeningocele. Syringomyelia is present in 50 to 90% of patients with type II Chiari malformations, whereas hydrocephalus occurs in only 10% of patients with a type I and 85% of those with a type II Chiari malformation. In contrast, type III Chiari malformations are usually fatal and result from caudal displacement of the cerebellum into a high cervical meningocele.

The clinical presentation of patients with Chiari malformations is quite variable and age dependent. Symptoms may be related to compression of the upper cervical spinal cord, the cerebellum, and the medulla at the craniocervical junction, hydrocephalus, or associated syringomyelia. The cause of symptoms can be difficult to differentiate when several associated abnormalities exist.

Symptoms in children with type I malformations usually begin during adolescence from syringomyelia, including spastic quadriparesis, a dissociated sensory loss, upper limb atrophy, truncal ataxia, or scoliosis. In contrast, adults with type I malformations develop headache or neck pain exacerbated by the Valsalva maneuver. Less commonly, symptoms include vertigo, spastic quadriparesis, and dissociated sensory loss from syringomyelia. Symptomatic syringomyelia portends a poorer prognosis as a result of susceptibility to painless injuries or neurogenic arthropathies.

In contrast, type II Chiari malformations commonly become symptomatic in infancy. Although initially asymptomatic, 5 to 33% will develop symptoms that will stabilize and often improve after 1 year. Symptoms include nystagmus accompanied by a weak or absent cry. Inspiratory stridor may progress to apnea and bradycardia. Corticospinal tract signs as well as bulbar dysfunction including decreased gag reflex, facial paresis, and retrocollis may also be observed. Symptoms after infancy frequently include spastic quadriparesis or appendicular ataxia; these symptoms progress slowly but can be severe with bulbar signs of recurrent aspiration, gastroesophageal reflux, decreased cough or gag reflex, and even apnea. However, adolescents have similar symptoms to those with type I malformations.

MRI provides the best evaluation of a Chiari malformation. The degree of caudal cerebellar displacement into the spinal canal as well as the presence of syringomyelia

(60 to 90% in symptomatic patients) can be determined. CSF flow patterns can also be assessed in atypical patients to determine who might benefit from decompression. Enhanced images with gadolinium are recommended in patients with syringomyelia without a Chiari malformation to rule out a spinal cord neoplasm. In addition, radiographs of the spinal axis may identify frequently associated skeletal abnormalities (25%), including basilar impression, Klippel-Feil malformation, scoliosis, and atlanto-occipital assimilation. Finally, hydrocephalus (10% in type I and 85% in type II malformations) can be diagnosed with either computed tomography or MRI.

Surgical treatment requires identification and assessment of several associated diseases that are treated sequentially. Neonatal myelomeningocele should be closed shortly after birth. Hydrocephalus accentuates caudal cerebellar displacement and should be treated with a ventriculoperitoneal shunt. Persistent hydrocephalus despite placement of a shunt implies shunt malfunction, requiring shunt revision. Finally, treatment is directed at decompressing the hindbrain via a suboccipital craniectomy and cervical laminectomy to the lowest level of herniation. A duroplasty can be performed to ensure adequate decompression in the presence of an associated syrinx.

Alternative Methods of Management

Medical management alone for Chiari malformations is ineffective, unless treatment addresses headaches as the sole manifestation of a type I Chiari malformation in an adult. Given the pathophysiology of this entity, nonsurgical treatments are unlikely to provide additional benefit. Most surgeons treat symptomatic Chiari malformations with a suboccipital craniectomy and duroplasty after ensuring adequate treatment of hydrocephalus, if present. However, additional surgical treatments remain controversial. Some advocate opening the dura but preserving the arachnoid layer. Others have recommended various intradural manipulations including opening the fourth ventricle, resecting the tonsils, lysing arachnoid adhesions, plugging the obex, shunting the fourth ventricle, and/or stenting the fourth ventricle. Recent advances in fetal medicine, fetal surgery, and obstetrics may reduce the frequency of Chiari malformations by prenatal closure of a myelomeningocele.

Various treatment methods have been suggested for an associated syrinx. Many surgeons do not treat the syrinx unless symptoms persist after treatment of the hindbrain herniation has restored CSF flow dynamics. If a patient is still symptomatic from syringomyelia despite treatment of hydrocephalus and adequate decompression with duroplasty, then treatment of the syrinx itself is recommended. Percutaneous aspiration offers temporary drainage, whereas laminectomy and syringostomy with a syringosubarachnoid shunt may prolong the duration of decompression. However, shunting of the syrinx to the pleural or peritoneal cavity may be preferred to maintain a functional decompression. Moreover, a syrinx extending to the conus medullaris can be treated with a terminal ventriculostomy by sectioning of the filum at its junction with the conus medullaris.

Type of Management	Advantages	Disadvantages	Comments
Suboccipital craniectomy alone	Rapid decompression, preservation of dural barrier	Impedance to CSF flow may persist	May be sufficient in mild cases with dural band incision
Additional dural opening with arachnoid preservation	Arachnoid barrier to infection and CSF leak remains	Difficult to preserve thin arachnoid	Somewhat improves the craniocervical volume
Additional duroplasty	Greatest enlargement of the craniocervical volume	Risk of CSF leak, reaction to dural substitute	Preferred in the presence of syringomyelia
Additional maneuvers including tonsil resection, obex plugging, ventricular stenting	May offer additional ways to improve CSF flow dynamics	Significant risks of medullary, cranial nerve, or vascular injury	Typically not necessary for successful treatment

CSF, cerebrospinal fluid.

PEARL
• An associated syrinx often resolves after treatment of hydrocephalus and decompression of the craniocervical junction.

PITFALL
• Failure to address the associated abnormalities in sequence (hydrocephalus, craniocervical junction CSF flow obstruction, syringomyelia) may result in progression or persistent symptoms.

Complications

Surgical complications include infection and bleeding. Dural and arachnoid opening introduces the risk of CSF leak, aseptic meningitis, and pseudomeningocele. Medullary, lower cranial nerve (IX, X, XI), or vascular (posterior inferior cerebellar artery) injury from manipulation may cause a variety of neurologic complications. In addition, cerebellar herniation through an excessively large defect may occur. Cervical laminectomy, particularly in children with a syrinx, can result in a postlaminectomy kyphosis. Therefore, some surgeons recommend fusion at the time of decompression. Moreover, occipitocervical instability may be exacerbated or produced in patients with associated skeletal abnormalities. Finally, alteration in CSF flow can cause hydrocephalus.

Suggested Readings

Gardner WJ, Goodall RJ. The surgical treatment of Arnold-Chiari malformation in adults. An explanation of its mechanism and importance of encephalography in diagnosis. J Neurosurg 1950; 7:199–206.

Hall PV, Lindseth RE, Campbell RL, et al. Myelodysplasia and developmental scoliosis. A manifestation of syringomyelia. Spine 1976; 1:48–56.

Menezes AH. Chiari I malformations and hydromyelia—complications. Pediatr Neurosurg 1991; 17:146–154.

Oldfield EH, Muraszko K, Shawker TH, et al. Pathophysiology of syringomyelia associated with Chiari I malformation of the cerebellar tonsils: implications for diagnosis and treatment. J Neurosurg 1994; 80:3–15.

Williams B. The distending force in the production of communicating syringomyelia. Lancet 1969; 2:189–193.

Case 55
Diastematomyelia
James S. Harrop, Leslie N. Sutton, and Gregory J. Przybylski

History and Physical Examination

A 26-year-old woman described 6 years of low back pain, which recently began radiating to her left great toe. She noted significant increase in pain after the birth of her first child 3 months earlier. She had no bowel or bladder dysfunction other than a history of frequent urinary tract infections. However, she had a known scoliosis diagnosed at age 10 that was not treated. Physical examination revealed reproducible tenderness at the thoracolumbar junction. No cutaneous lesions or abnormalities were present. She had a positive straight leg raise on the left that reproduced her S1 radiculopathy. Neurologic examination revealed normal strength and muscle tone. She had diminished pinprick sensation in the S1 dermatome bilaterally. Her reflexes were symmetric and her rectal tone and perianal sensation were normal.

Radiologic Findings

Plain radiographs demonstrated a thoracolumbar scoliosis with butterfly vertebrae and bifid lower thoracic spinous processes. Magnetic resonance imaging (MRI) of the thoracolumbar spine revealed a low-lying conus displaced posteriorly at the L5 vertebral body. A thickened filum terminale with an associated small lipoma was

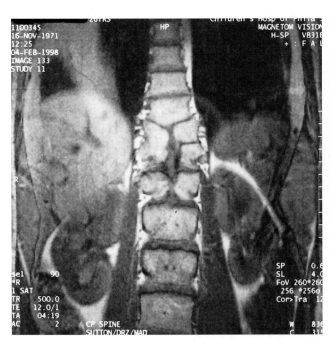

Figure 55–1. Coronal magnetic resonance imaging (MRI) image reveals butterfly vertebrae at the thoracolumbar junction.

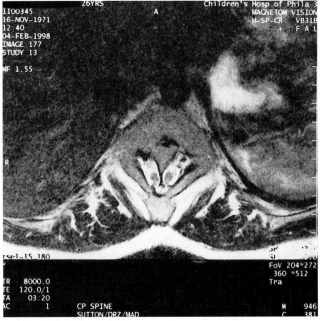

Figure 55–2. Axial T2-weighted MRI reveals spinal cord duplication with separation by an anterior bony septum within the dural sac.

observed. Coronal images demonstrated a widened spinal canal with butterfly vertebrae from T11 to L3 as well (Fig. 55–1). Axial T2-weighted images (Fig. 55–2) showed a duplicate spinal cord from T11 through L3 levels and separated by an anterior bony spur superiorly and a membranous septum inferiorly. Both duplicate spinal hemicords were located in a common dural sac.

Diagnosis

The symptoms of back pain and radiculopathy are early manifestations of a tethered cord syndrome. Two specific causes of tethering in this patient include a split cord malformation (SCM) and a thickened filum terminale with a low-lying conus medullaris. MRI demonstrated a combination of both types of SCM. The first consists of a midline bony spur that divides two separate hemicords within individual dural tubes (type I), whereas the second consists of a cartilaginous septum between the hemicords contained in a single dural tube (type II). The short, thickened filum terminale tethers the conus medullaris, causing tension on the spinal cord inferiorly, further contributing to the traction of the SCM superiorly. The low-lying conus medullaris at the L5 level with the posterior displacement of the conus associated with a split cord malformation confirmed the diagnosis in this patient.

Surgical Management

Preoperative evaluation may include urodynamic studies. The patient was given intravenous antibiotics and corticosteroids, and neurophysiologic monitoring of both somatosensory and motor evoked potentials was begun prior to induction of general anesthesia and continued until surgical closure of the wound. After an indwelling bladder catheter was placed, the patient was positioned prone on an Andrew's frame in a kneeling position to reduce intraabdominal pressure, thereby possibly decreasing epidural bleeding. Pressure points were padded and the patient was secured to the table to facilitate table rotation for improved visualization during the procedure. Both the thoracolumbar junction and the lumbar areas were prepped with a Betadine solution and draped.

A midline incision with subperiosteal dissection was performed at the thoracolumbar junction with localization of the malformation by an intraoperative radiograph. Dissection should be performed along normal laminae inferior or superior to the malformation because the vertebrae around the SCM are often anomalous. A laminectomy from T10 to L2 was performed, revealing a widened region of the dura and spinal canal. The dura was incised in the midline inferior to the widened region, allowing initial exposure over a normal spinal cord region. The durotomy was extended cephalad, revealing the cord splitting into two distinct hemicords, each with atrophic medial roots. Although a membranous septum divided the cord caudally, a transition into a midline bony septum was observed superiorly.

The inferior membranous septum was excised after multiple adhesions of the medial hemicords to the septum were dissected free with the aid of an intraoperative microscope. Rostrally, the bony spur was covered by a layer of dura that was incised. Microdissection to release adhesions facilitated removal of the bony spur with a rongeur without retracting neural tissue. Despite the dura excision over the bony spur, adherence of the dura to the vertebrae anteriorly minimizes the risk of cerebrospinal fluid leak.

Although both hemicords were now freely mobile, the caudal spinal cord remained tethered by the filum terminale. A second laminectomy of L5 exposed the filum terminale at the conus. The filum was displaced posterior to the cauda equina; identification was confirmed by direct electrical stimulation. Coagulation and section of the filum caused superior migration of the conus, thereby releasing the inferior tethering. Postlaminectomy instability of the spine is unlikely with preservation of the facet joints and capsular ligaments.

The dura was closed with 6-0 nonabsorbable suture and integrity checked by increasing intradural pressure with the Valsalva maneuver. The lumbodorsal fascia and subcutaneous tissues were closed in layers with absorbable suture, whereas the skin was closed with a running locked nylon suture. The patient was returned to a supine position and anesthesia was reversed.

Postoperative Management

The patient was neurologically monitored in an intermediate intensive care unit overnight. Bladder catheterization was discontinued the following day and the patient was allowed out of bed. She had no voiding difficulties and preserved perineal sensation. If the patient had urinary retention, postvoid residual volumes should be checked and intermittent catheterization begun. Postoperative ileus was treated with intravenous fluids, diet restriction, and nasogastric suction. The patient recovered with preserved neurologic function and resolution of preoperative symptoms of back pain and radiculopathy.

Discussion

This patient had symptomatic spinal cord tethering from a SCM and a hypertrophied, noncompliant filum terminale. Both SCM and a thickened, posteriorly displaced filum terminale cause stretching and traction of the spinal cord. Subsequent reduction in blood flow causes a decrease in neuronal oxidative metabolism. As a result, neuronal function becomes impaired, resulting in symptoms of muscle weakness, sensory loss, and/or dysfunction of bowel or bladder control. The pathophysiology of neurologic worsening from tethering is likely related to medullary rather than radicular dysfunction. Although split cord malformations can cause spinal cord tethering, other spinal dysraphic conditions can produce tethered cord syndrome including spina bifida, myelomeningocele, a thickened filum terminale, a spinal cord lipoma, a dermoid or epidermoid tumor, or a neuroenteric cyst.

Patients are diagnosed with SCM in a bimodal distribution, with epidemiologic differences between childhood and adult variants. In adults the female to male ratio is 3:1, and patients describe pain or urologic dysfunction; in contrast, children develop painless sensorimotor deterioration. Tethered cords in children are often discovered incidentally during imaging for scoliosis or suspected spinal dysraphism. Both forms of SCM occur in the thoracolumbar region. Patients often have cutaneous or limb abnormalities including hypertrichosis, subcutaneous lipoma or hemangioma over the involved spinal segment, scoliosis, pes cavus, and hammer toes.

Split cord malformations are congenital disorders that develop during the embryologic stage of neurulation through an abnormal inclusion of the mesodermal layer. It is these mesenchymal cells that evolve into the bony spur or membranous septum that separates the developing nervous tissue. During subsequent development, the vertebral column grows more rapidly than the spinal cord, causing the conus to ascend cephalad within the spinal canal. A hypertrophied or lipomatous filum terminale as well as an SCM may anchor the caudal spinal cord. As a result, the greater growth of the vertebral column causes severe traction on the spinal cord, reducing perfusion and therefore nutrition to the neurons. Tethering at the filum terminale is identified on MRI, which demonstrates the posteriorly displaced conus caudal to the L2/L3 interspace.

The nomenclature of spinal cord duplications can be confusing because these lesions were previously considered distinct. Diplomyelia described two spinal cords within one dural sac without any midline structures separating them, whereas diastematomyelia described two separate hemicords, each within its own dural tube, separated by a bony septum. A theory of common embryogenesis proposed by Pang classified SCM into two types. The first type, similar to diastematomyelia, involves two hemicords within individual dural sacs, separated by a midline cuff of dura that surrounds a bony or fibrocartilaginous spur. The second type involves a single dural tube with two hemicords separated by a thin fibrous septum. These types represent a continuum rather than distinct entities. The findings in the patient presented here support a common embryologic origin given the features from both types concurrently.

The surgeon treating SCM must address not only the adherence and tethering at the bony septum, but also the anchoring of the filum terminale, both of which can tether the spinal cord. However, the septum should be excised prior to release of the filum terminale. Otherwise, the caudally released spinal cord could rebound cephalad and become impaled by the bony septum. In addition, care must be exercised during dural opening because the conus is often displaced posteriorly against the dura. Moreover, the filum terminale can be difficult to distinguish from posteriorly displaced nerve roots. The filum appears as a thickened cord terminus, which can be distinguished from nerve roots by electrical stimulation; a response in any small nerve roots adherent to the filum allows separation of the nerve roots prior to filum section, thereby reducing the risk of neurologic injury.

In summary, the goal in treating SCM is to prevent further neurologic loss. Although the majority of patients will experience only modest recovery of impaired function, relief of radiculopathy or back pain can be substantial. In fact, the return of neurologic function is usually limited to abilities most recently lost. However, urologic dysfunction rarely improves substantially.

Alternative Methods of Management

Because the pathophysiology of this disorder is related to spinal cord traction, treatment requires surgical untethering of the SCM and section of the filum. There is no medical therapy that benefits this condition. Moreover, observation is also not recommended, because acute neurologic deterioration may be difficult to recover. Consequently, these malformations should be treated when diagnosed, as prolonged delay may result in irreversible loss of neurologic function.

Type of Management	Advantages	Disadvantages	Comments
Septum resection and untethering	Only treatment to address the structural restriction	Risk of iatrogenic neurologic injury	Should be performed before filum terminal release
Observation	Some identified incidentally	Fails to address the mechanical tethering	Loss of neurologic function is difficult to recover

PEARL
• Successful treatment includes both resection of the bony or cartilaginous septum as well as section of the filum terminale.

PITFALL
• Section of the filum terminale before resection of the bony or cartilaginous septum may cause neurologic deterioration.

Complications

Although the most common postoperative problem is a superficial wound infection that usually resolves with oral antibiotics, the dural opening adds a risk of meningitis, which must be considered in febrile patients. A constellation of fever, neck pain, photophobia, lethargy, or radicular pain should be evaluated by lumbar puncture. To avoid inadvertent transmission of infection intradurally, the lumbar puncture should not be performed within the previous exposure. Therefore, it may be necessary to perform a fluoroscopically guided cisterna magna or C1/C2 puncture to obtain spinal fluid.

Many patients with tethered cord syndrome have urologic dysfunction. Even with normal preoperative urodynamics, surgical manipulation and general anesthesia may cause postoperative urinary retention, which usually subsides with a short course of intermittent bladder catheterization. Persistent postoperative dysfunction requires further urologic evaluation and treatment.

Some patients with tethered cord syndrome have concurrent spinal deformities including scoliosis and spina bifida. Patients undergoing extensive laminectomies should be assessed for spinal instability. Although few patients will require an instrumented arthrodesis, patients should be examined for postlaminectomy kyphosis formation. A laminoplasty may reduce this risk in younger patients.

Despite tether release, a few patients develop late recurrent symptoms similar to their initial complaints. Retethering of the spinal cord from scar formation and adhesion of the conus medullaris and cauda equina to the durotomy site may require a second operation to release adhesions. Alternatively, the filum terminale may not have been released despite an initial recovery of spinal cord function. MRI can help differentiate these conditions.

Suggested Readings

Pang D. Split cord malformation. Part II: clinical syndrome. Neurosurgery 1992; 31:481–500.

Pang D. Tethered cord syndrome. In: Wilkins R, Rengachary S, eds. Neurosurgery, pp. 3465–3496. New York: McGraw-Hill, 1996.

Pang D, Dias MS, Ahab-Barmada M. Split cord malformation. Part I: a unified theory of embryogenesis for double cord malformations. Neurosurgery 1992; 31:451–480.

Yamada S. Tethered Cord Syndrome. Park Ridge, IL: American Association of Neurological Surgeons Publishing Committee, 1996.

Case 56
Spinal Deformity in Myelodysplasia— Lumbar Kyphectomy

Mohammad E. Majd, Richard T. Holt, and Joseph L. Richey

History and Physical Examination

A 15-year-old Caucasian boy who had a T10 complete paraplegia owing to myelodysplasia was referred for evaluation for his spinal deformity. The patient was under the care of a neurosurgeon since birth and had multiple reconstructive surgeries consisting of resection of his myelomeningocele, shunt placement, and closure of skin defects.

The patient was confined to a wheelchair. He had no sensation in his lower extremities. He had no bladder control. He had surgeries in the past for a dislocated hip and clubfeet. He had an old midline scar from approximately the T9 level down to the sacrum, with a severe spinal deformity in both the sagittal and coronal planes. The profound gibbus deformity in the lumbar region attenuated the overlying soft tissue to the point of near skin breakdown (Fig. 56–1). The skin was red and shiny over the apex of the deformity. The patient had marked lordosis of the thoracic spine. He had a 35-degree flexion contracture of the left hip and a 25-degree flexion contracture of the right hip. He also had a 20-degree flexion contracture in both knees. The patient had strong arms and a fairly good anteroposterior (AP) chest diameter with good chest expansion.

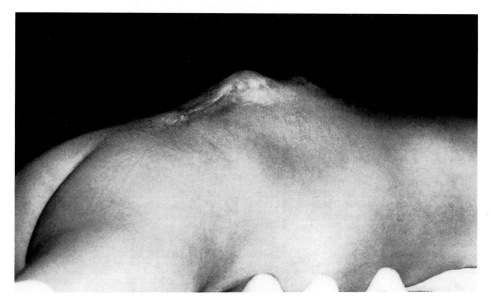

Figure 56–1. Marked magnitude of gibbus formation at the thoracolumbar spine with tenuous skin in a patient with myelodysplasia. Positioning is difficult due to the severity of the deformity.

Radiologic Findings

The sitting AP and lateral X-rays of the thoracolumbar spine revealed a moderate lordosis of the thoracic spine that was greatest at the lower thoracic region, with a severe kyphosis of the upper lumbar spine.

The Cobb measurement of the X-rays demonstrated more than a 130-degree kyphosis of the lumbar spine with a greater than 90-degree scoliosis of the thoracolumbar spine (Fig. 56–2). The spine X-ray also showed absence of the posterior elements in the lumbar spine. The flexion-extension films revealed no change in the spinal deformity, and the maximum traction X-ray demonstrated a 15-degree correction of scoliosis.

Diagnosis

Complete T10 paraplegia owing to myelodysplasia. The spinal deformity was classified as neuromuscular kyphoscoliosis with a prominent kyphosis of the lumbar spine. In addition to the spine deformity, the patient had bilateral hip and knee flexion contractures and a neurogenic bowel and bladder.

Surgical Management

Lumbar kyphectomy is performed with the patient in the prone position. Because of the severe thoracolumbar deformity, operative positioning is extremely difficult (Fig. 56–3A). Jelly rolls or a modified Wilson frame is used for positioning. Body warmers are strongly suggested because of the length of the spine exposed, the

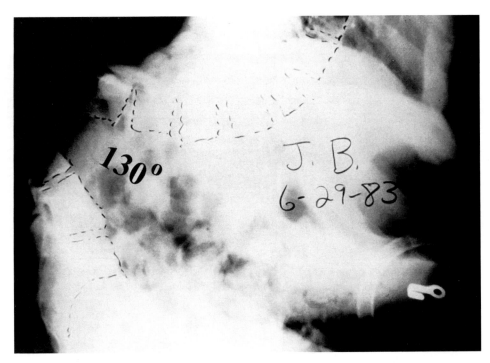

Figure 56–2. Lateral X-ray shows profound kyphosis at the thoracolumbar spine. Sitting on the pelvis is impossible.

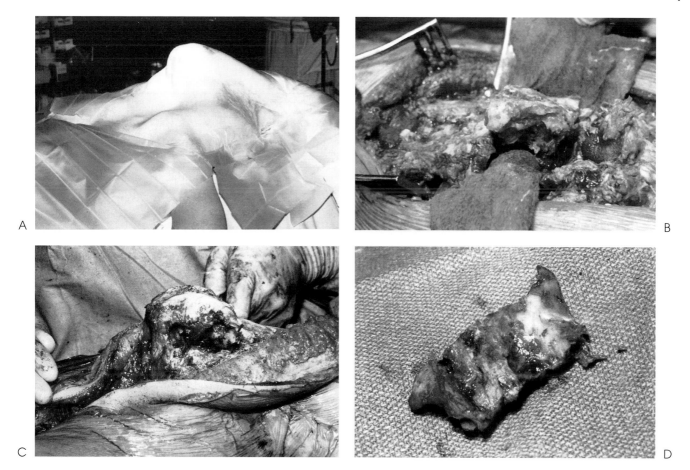

Figure 56–3. (A) Positioning of patient before kyphectomy. Preoperative scar for repair of myelodysplasia and significant kyphosis is observed. (B) Exposure of kyphosis. The front aspect of the vertebra is exposed subperiosteally and a sponge is passed under the kyphosis segment. (C) Complete elevation of the periosteum and detachment of kyphosis from the anterior structure and posterior muscles. (D) After resection of kyphosis, the bone can be used as bone graft.

amount of fluid replacement required, and, occasionally, the length of time of the case. Cell-Saver is also beneficial to conserve and replace the patient's own blood.

Exposure of the spine is performed in the standard fashion through a posterior midline incision. Care is taken to protect the fragile skin overlying the previous myelomeningocele repair. Thick skin and tissue flaps are developed to protect against poor wound healing.

The remnant dural sac is mobilized and transected cephalad to the level of the bony resection. As the vestigial neural elements are elevated from the vertebrae, venous sinusoids and nutrient foramen are encountered. Hemostasis is obtained by rubbing Gelfoam moistened with thrombin into the bleeding points; bone wax is avoided.

The apical vertebral segment (may be more than one body) is freed of its soft tissue attachments by subperiosteal circumferential dissection (Fig. 56–3B,C). Hall and Poitras (1999) described the placement of bone graft anterior to the spine during the posterior approach. They placed bone graft in the periosteal sleeve anterior to the spine and documented solid fusion mass in this anterior envelope by radiographs.

The intervertebral discs above and below the apical vertebral segment are removed. The discs are incised with a scalpel and removed using a combination of pituitary rongeurs and long-handled curettes. This discectomy aids in mobilization of the spine and fusion of the bone mass. Power tools such as the Midas Rex or the Hall drill are avoided to prevent accidental injury to the surrounding soft tissue and excessive removal of potential local bone graft.

Once the apical vertebrae are isolated by subperiosteal dissection and the discs are removed, the vertebrae can be safely and efficiently excised using osteotomes, large rongeurs, and Kerrison rongeurs (Fig. 56–3D). The periosteal sleeve provides protection for the abdominal contents. Preoperative planning using lateral radiographs indicates the amount of apical resection necessary to achieve an appropriate straightening of the kyphosis.

The cephalad segment is now reduced to the caudal segment (Fig. 56–4). Fixation is obtained using posterior instrumentation. The length of fusion includes approximately two levels above and three levels below the deformity, usually including the sacrum or pelvis. A combination of internal fixation techniques is often useful depending on the nature of the pathologic condition. Contoured Luque rods attached with sublaminar wires provide the majority of the correction and fixation. To this construction, cancellous bone screws are attached in the lower lumbar and sacral vertebral bodies (Fig. 56–5). These sacral and lumbar bone screws become a "steel pedicle" to which the Luque rods and wires can be solidly attached. In some patients, pelvic augmentation utilizing the Galveston technique is required.

Bone from the resected wedge can be placed posterolaterally over the posterior elements. If needed, additional allograft bone in the form of demineralized bone can supplement autologous bone material.

The skin flaps are closed over the vertebral column. Excising the bony kyphosis aids in closing the often tenuous, thin, scarred, and now redundant skin. Care should be taken to avoid excising too much redundant skin owing to postoperative scar shrinkage. The wound is closed over a medium Hemovac to prevent the formation of a hematoma.

Discussion

There are two types of spinal column deformities seen in patients with myelomeningocele: (1) developmental or paralytic, and (2) congenital anomalies of the vertebral column such as rigid lumbar kyphosis, which is present at birth. Raycroft and Curtis (1972) found that 20% of their patients with myelomeningocele had miscellaneous congenital anomalies with associated spinal deformities. These spinal deformities included scoliosis, lordosis, and kyphosis. All of the developmental curves appeared before adolescence.

The type of deformity is related to the level of neural tube defect. If the lesion is at the thoracolumbar junction, the majority of patients develop scoliosis. If the lesion is at the lumbosacral junction, scoliotic curvatures are less prevalent. Untreated, progressive scoliosis may cause pelvic obliquity, trunk decompensation, pressure sores, pain, cardiorespiratory and gastrointestinal compromise, and loss of functional ability. A collapsing C-shaped scoliosis is caused by muscle weakness, which is associated with high-level paraplegia. Usually, scoliosis deformity in myelodysplasia is associated with lordosis, but the collapsing type of scoliosis is associated with kyphosis.

Hall and colleagues (1979) found that with successful shunt insertion in patients with scoliosis and hydromyelia or hydrosyringomyelia, the degree of progression of scoliosis decreased, especially in patients with curves of less than 50 degrees.

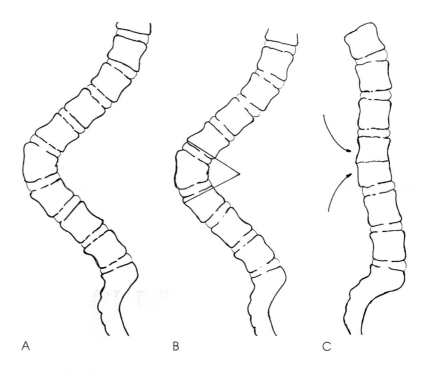

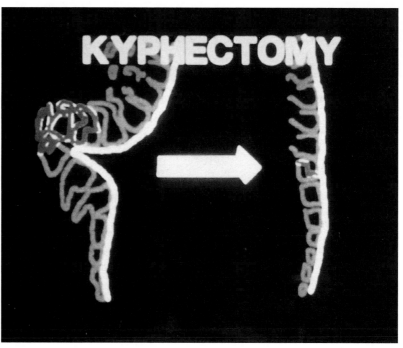

Figure 56–4. (A) Schematic view of lumbar kyphosis with apex at the L2 body. (B) Preoperative templating for resection of kyphosis. (C) After resection of kyphosis. (D) Schematic view of pre- and postoperative kyphectomy.

Another common curve in this patient population is an **S**-shaped scoliosis with a right thoracic and left lumbar curve. This curve pattern is mainly seen in the ambulatory patient and is similar to an idiopathic curve. These patients may also manifest symptoms of tethered cord syndrome, which is often associated with intraspinal pathologic conditions such as a dermoid tumor, lipoma, or diastematomyelia, often resulting

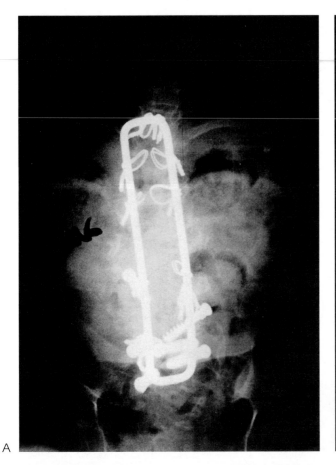
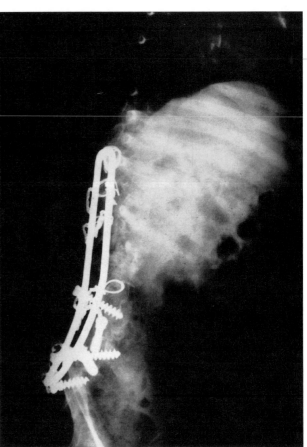

A   B

Figure 56–5. (A) Postoperative posteroanterior (PA) X-ray following correction of the scoliosis with a balanced spine. (B) Lateral X-ray of the same patient after kyphectomy, posterior spinal fusion (PSF), and instrumentation. The spine is balanced and the lumbar spine is straight with no kyphosis.

in scoliosis. Often the scoliotic curve is located in the thoracolumbar or lumbar region and is associated with marked lumbar lordosis. Release of the tethered cord usually stops the progression of the curve. In patients with scoliotic curves greater than 50 degrees, an associated spinal fusion is recommended at the time of cord release.

Indications for surgery in patients with myelodysplasia are based on the spinal curve magnitude, changes in functional status, the presence of decubitus ulcers, intractable back pain, cardiorespiratory and abdominal organ compromise, and difficulties with hygiene because of the abnormal posture. The goal of spine surgery in myelomeningocele patients is to obtain a solid fusion with a balanced spine, level pelvis, normal sagittal contour, and improved function.

Because of the presence of hypoesthetic or anesthetic skin, bracing is often an unacceptable option in this patient population. Occasionally, in a young patient, bracing may slow the rate of progression, allowing time for further trunk growth that will allow for greater sitting height.

A custom-molded thoracolumbar sacral orthosis or oyster-shell brace is used frequently as the patient develops to skeletal maturity. If curve progression occurs significantly during bracing or if the curve has a large magnitude at the first visit and the patient is immature, we would consider subcutaneous expandable rod placement without fusion to assist in controlling the spinal curvature without stunting truncal growth (Fig. 56–6).

PEARLS

- Plan to fuse nonambulatory children who have significant deformity to the sacrum. The probability of development of a severe deformity below a short fusion is high.
- If the sacral-pelvic fixation is tenuous, immobilize the spine with a spica cast or brace.

PITFALLS

- Be careful to avoid prominent implants under insensate skin. Otherwise, skin breakdown is likely.
- Y incisions are not needed and probably lead to more problems such as skin necrosis and breakdown as compared to straight incisions.
- When the residual meningocele is resected, expect bleeding from the venous sinusoids and be ready to treat them with Gelfoam moistened with thrombin.
- Beware of the location of the great vessels. Ordinarily, they are tethered across the deformity. However, they may follow the spine and be vulnerable with resection of the apical segments.

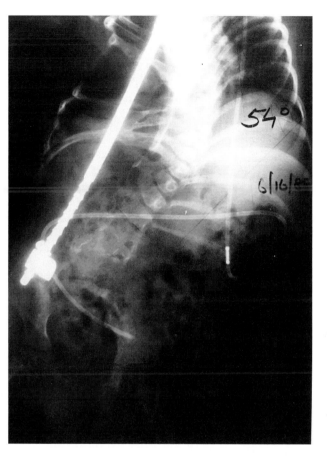

Figure 56–6. Postoperative X-ray of a young patient with a spinal deformity due to myelodysplasia. The patient underwent subcutaneous Harrington growing rod insertion for prevention of progression of the deformity and procrastination of the final arthrodesis.

Significant kyphosis at birth is the most common deformity found in children with thoracic myelodysplasia. The kyphotic deformity is often progressive owing to structural deficiencies in the posterior bone and soft tissue elements. In children with lumbar kyphosis who sit on the posterior aspect of their sacrum, skin problems over the prominent lumbar kyphosis are common.

Kyphotic deformity of the lumbar spine is a frequent and serious deformity in children with myelomeningocele. Although scoliosis is more common than kyphosis, the presence of a kyphotic deformity may be present in up to 21% of children with myelomeningocele. The kyphosis is most likely caused by abnormal development of the vertebrae, resulting in an anteriorly wedged vertebral body. Another significant factor in the development of the lumbar kyphosis is the lateral displacement of the spinous processes that convert the erector spinae muscles from extensors to flexors. Over time, the resulting muscle forces will overcome other soft tissue stabilizers of the spine and accentuate the kyphosis.

The apex of the kyphosis is usually the third lumbar vertebra, which is wedge-shaped anteriorly. The kyphosis generally begins in the lower thoracic spine and extends to the sacrum. The kyphosis is a major deformity in up to 15% of patients with myelomeningocele, often measuring 80 degrees or more at birth and then progressing to reach more severe proportions as the child grows.

We prefer to delay spinal fusion until the child is older to allow for maximum spinal growth. It is also technically easier to place internal instrumentation in a larger spine. Experience has also shown that the reduction will more likely be maintained in an older patient than in a younger one.

Alternative Methods of Management

Type of Management	Advantages	Disadvantages	Comments
Orthosis	Easy to apply	Pressure sores over the gibbus and increased pressure on the abdominal content	The orthotic device must push over the apex posteriorly and against the abdomen anteriorly; the abdominal pressure decreases the child's appetite and pulmonary reserve and increases the rate of complications
Sharrad technique	Preservation of the neuroelements	Technical difficulty; high complication rate; high recurrence rate	Excision of $1\frac{1}{2}$ vertebral bodies from the apex is not adequate to correct the deformity, and fixation with sutures, pins, staples, and screws is not rigid enough
Harrington instrumentation	Surgical technique is easy	Two endpoint fixation; hook dislodgment	Using Harrington rods usually augmented by an anterior strut graft provides good short-term results, but, in the long term, the recurrence and failure rate is high
McCarthy technique	Removal of disc anteriorly and laterally through posterior approach	The spine is not shortened; therefore, the chance of trauma to aorta and vena cava is significant; insertion of crosswise Steinmann pins through the vertebral body is difficult	With this method of disc evacuation, the chance of trauma to the tethered aorta and vena cava is high; Steinmann pin insertion through the body is not risk free
Dunn technique	The spine is shortened; correction of deformity is good; fixation is rigid	Required anterior approach to remove the disc space and endplate of all deformed vertebrae; passing the contoured Luque rod through the foramen of L5 and attachment to the anterior aspect of sacrum jeopardizes the vascular structures	Biomechanically, this technique provides all the necessary corrective forces; fixation is rigid enough to mobilize the patient postoperatively
Lindseth technique	Spinal alignment is close to normal; spine is shortened; fixation is rigid; early mobilization of patient is feasible	No fixation point at the level of the posterior-deficient vertebrae	With this technique, there is not enough fixation points at the posterior deficient spine region; the long lever arm of Luque rod, attached to the pelvis, increases the chances of loosening of the rod and fatigue fracture

Complications

In our series of four patients two significant complications occurred, both to the same patient. This patient had a deep wound infection that required operative irrigation and drainage 2 weeks after her initial kyphectomy procedure. During the initial operative procedure, a silicone pad covering the posterior instrumentation had been placed subfacially to protect the patient's thin tissue flaps. This synthetic pad was removed at the time of the irrigation and drainage. In retrospect, we think that this large foreign body might have contributed to the infection. We have not used this pad in any other patients.

The second complication was a loss of fixation of the distal bone screws and subsequent loss of reduction of the kyphosis. Possibly because of the infection, the distal screws failed by pullout. This patient returned to the operating room for revision of the distal instrumentation 6 weeks after the initial kyphectomy. The distal bone screws were revised, and the distal rods were converted to a Galveston technique. The patient's infection has resolved, her hardware has remained stable, and her reduction has been maintained. She has done well since.

Suggested Readings

Banta JV. The natural history of scoliosis in myelomeningocele. Orthop Trans 1986; 10:18.

Dias MS, McLone DG. Spinal dysraphism. In: Weinstein SL, ed. The Pediatric Spine. Principles and Practice, pp. 343–368. New York, Raven Press, 1994.

Dunn HK. Kyphosis of myelodysplasia. Operative treatment based on pathophysiology. Orthop Trans 1983; 7:19.

Eckstein HB, Vora, RM. Spinal osteotomy for severe kyphosis in children with myelomeningocele. J Bone Joint Surg 1972; 54B(2):328–333.

Eyring EJ, Wanken JJ, Sayers MP. Spine osteotomy for kyphosis in myelomeningocele. Clin Orthop 1972; 88:24–30.

Hall P, Lindseth R, Campbell R, et al. Scoliosis and hydrocephalus in myelocele patients: the effect of ventricular shunting. J Neurosurg 1979; 50(2):174–178.

Hull WJ, Moe JH, Winter RB. Spinal deformity in myelomeningocele: natural history, evaluation and treatment, abstract. J Bone Joint Surg 1974; 56B:1767.

Khoury MJ, Erickson JD, James LM. Etiologic heterogeneity of neural tube defects: clues from epidemiology. Am J Epidemiol 1982; 115:538–548.

Lindseth RE, Stelzer L Jr. Vertebral excision for kyphosis in children with myelomeningocele. J Bone Joint Surg 1979; 61A(5):699–704.

Lintner SA, Lindseth RE. Kyphotic deformity in patients who have myelomeningocele. J Bone Joint Surg 1994; 76A(9):1301–1307.

Majd ME, Muldowny DS, Holt RT. Natural history of scoliosis in the institutionalized adult cerebral palsy population. Spine 1997; 22(13):1461–1466.

McLaughlin TP, Banta JV, Gahm NH, et al. Intraspinal rhizotomy and distal cordectomy in patients with myelomeningocele. J Bone Joint Surg 1986; 68A:88–94.

Raycroft J, Curtis BH. Spinal Curvature in Myelomeningocele: Natural History and Etiology. St. Louis: CV Mosby, 1972.

Sharrard WJ, Drennan JC. Osteotomy-excision of the spine for lumbar kyphosis in older children with myelomeningocele. J Bone Joint Surg 1972; 54B(1): 50–60.

Case 57
Adult Scoliosis
David B. Cohen and John P. Kostuik

History and Physical Examination

A 40-year-old woman presented to the clinic with complaints of midlumbar pain. She states that her back pain started a few years ago as a pain that would

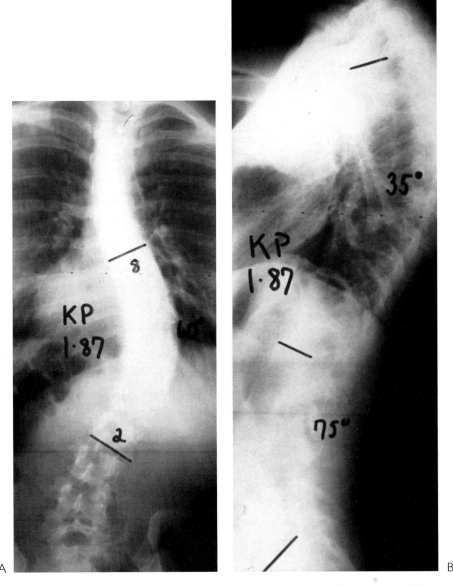

A   B

Figure 57–1. A 40-year-old woman with complaints of pain in area of spinal curve. (A) Preoperative anteroposterior (AP) scoliosis radiograph with 60-degree curve and 5 cm of lateral imbalance. (B) Lateral preoperative radiograph.

PEARL
• In these patients it is important to determine if a patient's leg complaints represent referred back pain or radicular symptoms that can occur as degenerative changes occur. Computed tomography (CT) myelogram is our study of choice to evaluate these radicular complaints because the standard magnetic resonance imaging (MRI) planes do not track scoliotic curves well.

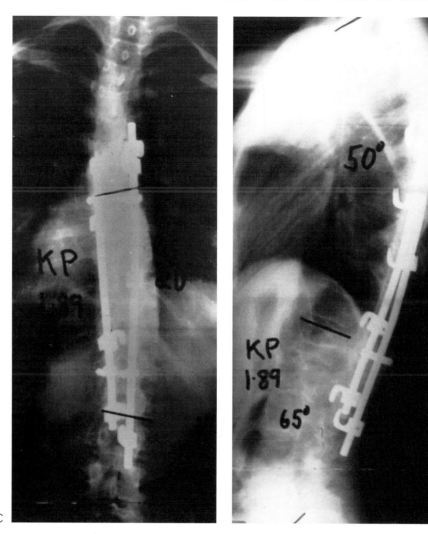

Figure 57–1 (Continued). *Postoperative AP (C) and postoperative lateral (D) radiographs.*

begin at the end of the day, but over the years it has become more constant throughout the day. She has used occasional nonsteroidal antiinflammatory drugs (NSAIDs) to give her marginal relief of pain, and she works on daily lower back stretching and strengthening exercises, which used to provide her significant relief but have gradually become less effective. She denies any alteration in her bowel or bladder function, but does notice that the back pain goes down her posterior buttock to the level of the knee. The patient reveals that she has noticed that her shape has changed over the last few years, as there has been a change in how her clothes fit her.

On physical examination, the patient stands with a slightly forward flexed posture leaning slightly to the side. She has a visible spinal deformity with a right-sided lower thoracic rib hump and a fullness present in the left portion of the lumbar spine. The patient measures 5'2" in height today, but she reports that she was 5'4" when she graduated from high school. Her legs are of equal length and her calves and thighs are of equal girth.

Radiologic Findings

Three-foot anteroposterior (AP) and lateral standing radiographs reveal a right-sided thoracolumbar scoliosis with an apex at T12 (Fig. 57–1A,B). The Cobb angle from T8 to L2 measures 60 degrees. There is no junctional thoracolumbar kyphosis present, but the patient demonstrates 5 cm of truncal imbalance. The L2/L3 disc space and lower disc spaces are well preserved.

Diagnosis

Right-sided thoracolumbar scoliosis from T8 to L2 of 60 degrees with mild compensatory lower lumbar and upper thoracic curves and a lateral truncal shift.

Surgical Management

This patient underwent a posterior instrumentation and fusion from T7 to L2 utilizing iliac crest bone grafting and a CD (Cotrel–Debousset) hook-rod segmental construct. Facet joints were excised during surgery to enhance the curve mobility. A claw construct was used to anchor the right-hand rod proximally and then compressive forces placed along the convexity of the curve. A distracting rod was placed along the concavity of the curve using a combination of proximal pedicle hooks and supralaminar hooks distally. The rods were cross-linked proximally and distally and a posterior and posterolateral fusion performed after the laminae, transverse processes and pars interarticularis were "petaled" using an osteotome (Fig. 57–1C,D). The wound was closed over suction drains.

Postoperative Management

The patient was admitted to the intensive care unit (ICU) overnight and then transferred to the spinal unit on postoperative day 1. Physical therapy for ambulating was started that day. Surgical drains and intravenous (IV) antibiotics were discontinued on day 2 and the patient's diet slowly started with the return of bowel function. During the hospitalization warfarin was used to maintain an INR of 1.5 to 2.0. The patient was discharged when ambulating independently and tolerating a regular diet. For the first 6 weeks postoperation the patient was encouraged to gradually increase the length and frequency of ambulation. From 6 to 12 weeks the patient restarted cardiovascular exercise (walking or riding an exercise bicycle). From 3 to 6 months other exercises including abdominal exercises were started. However, excessive bending and twisting is avoided until 6 months postoperation, when all restrictions are lifted. During the entire postoperative period no external bracing is utilized.

Discussion

Patients with adult scoliosis often differ greatly from patients with adolescent scoliosis. In adults, the most common surgical indication is related to pain due to either mechanical instability or nerve root compression. Adolescent scoliosis surgery, on the other hand, is often performed to correct a curvature that shows significant curve progression and magnitude despite nonsurgical treatments. Scoliotic curves do progress during adult life as disc degeneration can lead to curve progression and either sagittal or coronal imbalance. Thus, in the patient with adult scoliosis, the treatment must focus on restoring mechanical stability (alignment and balance) as well as addressing particular pain generators (discogenic pain or neural compression).

Alternative Methods of Management

The alternatives to the posterior spinal instrumentation and fusion for adult scoliosis include nonoperative management, bracing, posterior instrumentation and fusion, anterior spinal instrumentation and fusion, combined anterior/posterior spinal instrumentation and fusion, spinal decompression, and spinal decompression combined with one of the fusion procedures or spinal osteotomies.

The nonoperative management of patients with adult scoliosis is often helpful in the initial stages of a patient's physical complaints. Exercises to enhance trunk stability, stretches for spinal flexibility, and the use of NSAIDs or acetaminophen can often give the patient significant symptomatic relief for a variable period of time; however, we have found that it is unlikely to offer the patients a permanent solution.

The use of external spinal braces plays no role in the treatment of adult scoliosis. Unlike adolescent scoliosis, where curves remain flexible and can be braced in an improved position while further growth occurs, in adult scoliosis the curve rigidity and lack of remaining growth make bracing futile. The amount of force needed to effect a rigid curve makes the braces uncomfortable and exposes the patients to risks of skin ulceration.

Posterior spinal instrumentation and fusion has been the mainstay of surgical treatment of adolescent scoliosis for many years. In adults who have small progressive curvatures that are not completely rigid, this treatment offers a good alternative for the patient. However, we have found posterior instrumentation and fusion to be insufficient if either an extensive decompression must be performed or the fusion must include the sacrum. In these cases we have found the rates of pseudarthrosis to be unacceptable, and we prefer to obtain fusion in the anterior spine. As well, in cases of large deformity or significant sagittal or coronal imbalance the limited correction obtained with posterior instrumentation and fusion alone often requires either a spinal osteotomy or an additional anterior spine fusion.

Anterior spinal instrumentation and fusion can be useful alone in a certain proportion of adult scoliotic patients. If the patient has a fairly rigid major curve segment with fairly flexible compensatory curves, then anterior spinal instrumentation and fusion can allow the treating surgery to spare on average between two and four spinal motion segments for the patient. The complete excision of the annulus can afford the patient excellent corrections (Fig. 57–2). However, these surgeries are technically demanding and can result in significant vascular and pulmonary morbidity in inexperienced hands. As well, the anterior-only surgery does not allow for adequate neural decompression in cases where it is required.

Combined anterior and posterior spinal instrumentation and fusion offers the surgeon the most flexibility in treating the widest variety of patients. Excellent corrections can be obtained in many cases of sagittal or coronal imbalance. Fusion rates in the range of 95 to 97% can be seen even when a wide decompression or fusion to the sacrum is needed. However, these combined surgeries place the patient at risk of significant morbidity. For patients under 60 years of age, we

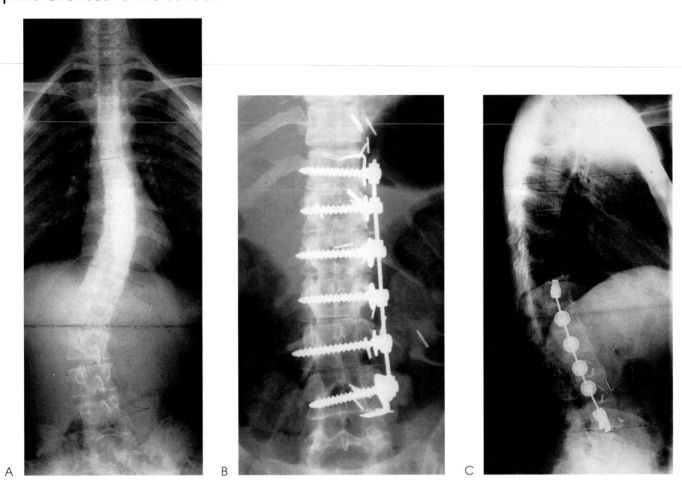

A   B   C

Figure 57–2. A 42-year-old with lumbar major curve and flexible thoracic curve. (A) Preoperative AP scoliosis radiograph. (B) AP lumbar radiograph showing curve correction. (C) Lateral postoperative scoliosis radiograph.

perform these surgeries as a single-day procedure. If the patient is older than 60, we routinely stage the surgeries 7 to 10 days apart and provide the patient with IV hyperalimentation between the surgeries. Even using these extreme precautions, we have found that combined anterior/posterior surgery is associated with between a 40 and 80% rate of mild complication (including urinary tract infection, atelectasis, and wound complications) and a 1 to 2% rate of major complication (including pulmonary embolism (PE), myocardial infarction, cerebrovascular accident, and death).

Spinal osteotomy plays a role in the most difficult cases of adult scoliosis. It can be used in conjunction with instrumentation and fusion to regain sagittal and coronal alignments in the most severe cases (Fig. 57–3). It can be utilized to correct kyphosis or flatback syndrome in patients with prior fusions as well. We currently prefer to perform a pedicle subtracting osteotomy in most cases. Up to 30 degrees of lordosis can be achieved through a single level. However, osteotomies raise significant risks for the patient. Extensive blood loss is often seen until the osteotomy is closed down. Additionally there have been reported serious neural complication rates in the range of 2 to 10% by most reports.

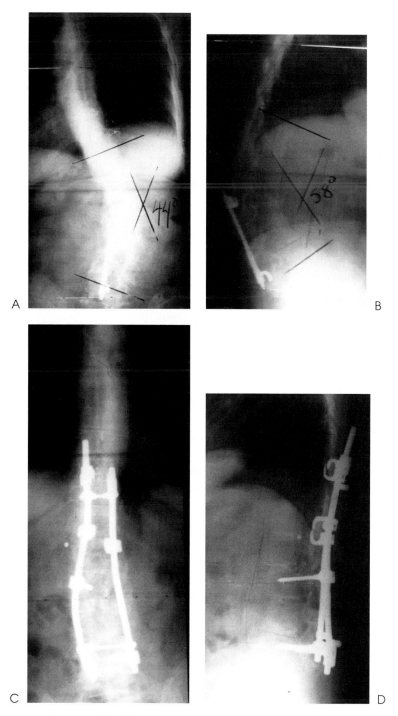

Figure 57–3. A 65-year-old with junctional and lumbar kyphosis following lumbar Harrington rod fusion. (A) AP preoperative radiograph shows coronal imbalance. (B) Lateral preoperative radiograph shows 58 degrees of lumbar kyphosis. Following combined AP fusion and osteotomy, the patient is rebalanced on AP (C) and lateral (D) radiographs.

Type of Management	Advantages	Disadvantages	Comments
Nonoperative management	Minimal risk to patient	Unlikely to provide long-term solution	Can be useful in the early stages
Bracing therapy	None	Skin injury and poor compliance	Of no use in adults
Posterior instrumentation and fusion	Limited morbidity for patient; familiar for most surgeons	Limited amount of correction; pseudarthrosis risks	Good for curves that still have some flexibility; if fusion to sacrum, must also go anteriorly
Anterior instrumentation and fusion	Spare spinal segments improved correction	Surgical risks to patient in inexperienced hands	Useful if curve is rigid but compensatory curves correct
Combined anterior/posterior instrumentation and fusion	High rates of fusion Can treat difficult cases	High patient morbidity	Needs a specialized center and team to do these cases
Spinal decompression surgery	Can address neural pain and compression	Curve will progress	Plays no role alone; stabilization needed
Spinal osteotomy	Can treat flat-back and severe imbalance	High blood loss; neurologic risks	Not needed in this case

PITFALL
- Spinal decompression alone plays virtually no role in the treatment of adult scoliosis. Although many patients complain of either neurogenic claudication or radicular symptoms, simple decompression often leads to disaster with rapid progression of the patient's deformity and return of pain. If a laminectomy or multiple level laminectomies need to be performed in the scoliotic patient, then a minimum of a posterior instrumentation and fusion is needed and quite possibly a combined anterior and posterior fusion.

Complications

The potential complications of a posterior spinal instrumentation and fusion for adult scoliosis in the case presented can occur at several time periods. Intraoperatively, the correction of the deformity can cause a stretch phenomenon on the spinal cord leading to spinal cord injury. Fortunately, these are rare, and the use of intraoperative spinal cord monitoring can allow the surgeon to release any excessive stress being placed on the spine. Perioperatively, patients are at risk of normal complications such as urinary tract infections, strokes, myocardial infarct, atelectasis, pneumonia, and wound infection. However, the spinal patient who has had a decompression or hook/screws placed is also at particular risk for an epidural hematoma and cauda equina syndrome. Early detection of any neurologic compromise through the vigilant monitoring of neural and rectal examination can allow for the rapid surgical treatment of the hematoma and maximize the patient's chance for recovery.

In the late stages of this patient's care the major risk of complication is that of pseudarthrosis formation. Unlike adolescent patients, adults with scoliosis have a significant chance of pseudarthrosis. This risk can be decreased by modifying patient factors (nutrition, smoking), performing a good fusion procedure with adequate iliac crest bone graft and fixation, as well as performing a fusion in the anterior spine.

Suggested Readings

Abitbol JJ, Kostuik JP, et al. Adult scoliosis. In: Herkowitz HN, Garfin SR, Balderston RA, et al, eds. Rothman-Simeone, The Spine, 4th ed., pp. 809–835. Philadelphia: WB Saunders, 1999.

Bridwell KH. Degenerative scoliosis. In: Bridwell KH, DeWald RL, eds. The Textbook of Spinal Surgery, 2nd ed., pp. 777–797. Philadelphia: Lippincott-Raven, 1997.

Kostuik JP. Adult scoliosis. In: Frymoyer J, ed. The Adult Spine, pp. 1579–1622. Philadelphia: Lippincott-Raven, 1977.

Case 58
Adult Isthmic Spondylolisthesis
Geoffrey J. Coldham and Edward N. Hanley, Jr.

History and Physical Examination

A 49-year-old woman presented with complaints of lumbar and bilateral lower extremity pain. Symptoms consistent with mechanical lower back pain had been present for the preceding 10 years, and for the past 2 years there was associated lower extremity pain radiating to the dorsum of both feet. Leg pain was initiated by standing for more than 15 minutes or walking 100 yards. Lower extremity pain was relieved by bending forward or by sitting. Lower back pain was constant and aggravated by hyperextension maneuvers. Pain had become incapacitating to the point that she was unable to perform normal activities of daily living. She experienced no sensory disturbances or subjective motor weakness and had normal bladder and bowel function. She was otherwise medically well.

Examination revealed a palpable step-off in the lower lumbar spine with accentuation of lumbar lordosis. Tenderness was elicited on palpation over the lumbosacral junction. There was minimal lower back pain felt on forward flexion; however, extension produced significant lower back pain. Motor examination was normal except for grade 4/5 extensor hallux longus bilaterally. Deep tendon reflexes and sensation were normal. Straight leg raising was negative to 90 degrees bilaterally.

Radiologic Findings

Anterior/posterior and lateral lumbar spine radiographs were performed. The lateral (Fig. 58–1) demonstrated a 45% subluxation of L5 on S1, equating to a grade II spondylolisthesis (Table 58–1 and Fig. 58–2). The L5/S1 joint was steep, measuring 60 degrees from the horizontal plane, with a sacral inclination of 60 degrees, indicating a relatively horizontal sacrum. Slip angle was 0 degrees (Fig. 58–3).

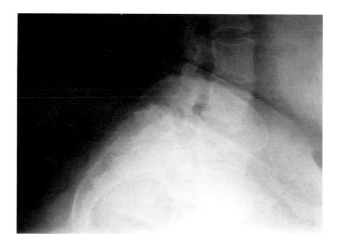

Figure 58–1. Lateral radiograph demonstrating grade II spondylolisthesis. Note the early anterior erosion of the sacrum.

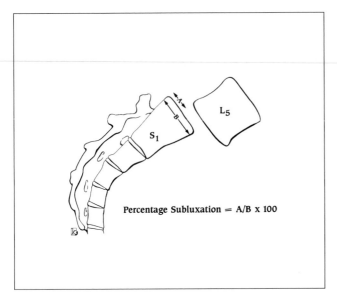

Figure 58–2. Measurement of subluxation.

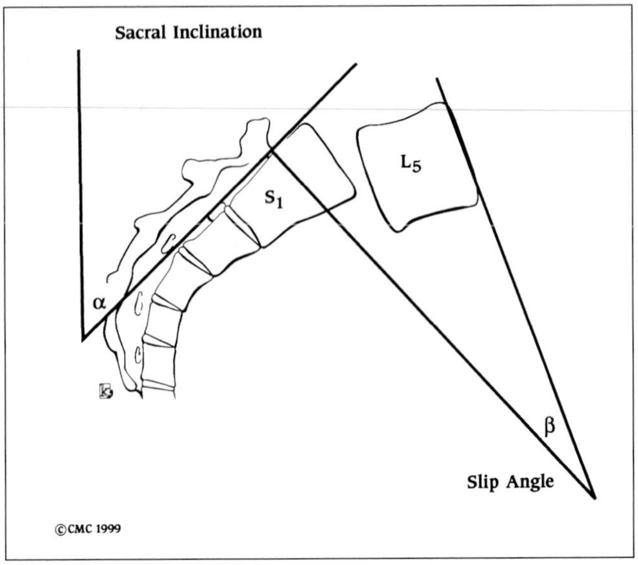

Figure 58–3. Measurement of sacral inclination (α) and slip angle (β).

Computed tomography (CT) scan of the lumbar spine confirmed isthmic defects of the L5 pars interarticularis bilaterally (Fig. 58–4). A redundant annulus was noted at the L5/S1 level, with the L5 interarticularis roots not visualized in the foramina (Fig. 58–5).

Diagnosis

Grade II lytic/isthmic spondylolisthesis of L5 on S1 with bilateral L5 nerve root stenosis.

Nonsurgical Management

The patient's symptoms had not improved after conservative treatment that included antiinflammatories and simple analgesics and a back-strengthening program. Due to the predominance of left leg pain on initial presentation, the patient underwent a left L5 nerve root block with local anesthetic and steroid. This substantially improved her left lower extremity symptoms for 1 month and thus was repeated with similar effect on the right L5 root. However, symptoms recurred and surgery was recommended.

Table 58–1
Grading of Spondylolisthesis

Grade I	0–25% subluxation
Grade II	26–50% subluxation
Grade III	51–75% subluxation
Grade IV	76–100% subluxation
Grade V	>100% (spondyloptosis

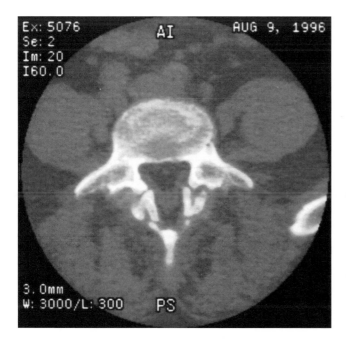

Figure 58–4. Axial computed tomography (CT) scan of L5 vertebra demonstrating bilateral sclerotic pars interarticularis defects.

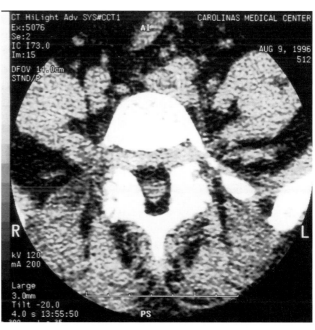

Figure 58–5. Axial CT scan of the interior aspect of the L5 vertebral body demonstrating redundant L5/S1 annulus. L5 nerve roots are not visualized.

Surgical Management

Under general anesthetic with intravenous cephalosporin administered a half-hour prior to surgery and with an indwelling catheter in place, the patient was positioned on a kneeling frame. A midline incision was made over the lumbar spine and soft tissues elevated to expose the posterior elements. A lateral localizing radiograph was taken using a Kocher clamp in the interspinous space to confirm the correct level. The L5 lamina "rattler" was clearly mobile and was resected en bloc (Fig. 58–6). The L5 pedicles were identified bilaterally to localize the L5 nerve roots. Fibrous cartilaginous pseudarthrosis material overlying both L5 nerve roots was resected with Kerrison rongeurs until the roots were visualized passing freely out of the neuroforamina. Both L5 pedicles were dysplastic and appeared to be impinging on the L5 roots, leading to the need for partial resection of the pedicles. Bilaterally, using anatomic land-

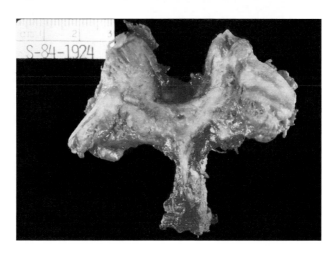

Figure 58–6. Excised posterior elements of L5 ("rattler").

473

marks, 6.25 × 40 mm pedicle screws were inserted into the L4 pedicle, whereas at the sacrum direct palpation of the pedicle of S1 allowed placement of two 7 × 35 mm pedicle screws. Initial purchase in the sacrum was poor, and these screws were exchanged for 8-mm screws with bicortical purchase (Fig. 58–7). Slotted connectors and $\frac{1}{4}$-inch rods were applied. No attempt was made to insert pedicle screws in the partially resected L5 pedicles or to correct the displacement of L5 on S1. The sacral alae, transverse processes of L4 and L5, and lateral aspects of the superior facets of L5 and L4 were decorticated, and bone graft harvested from a separate incision over the left iliac crest was onlaid. Check radiographs were performed intraoperatively to confirm pedicle screw position. Wounds were closed over drains.

Postoperative Management

The patient stood by the bed on the night of surgery and was subsequently mobilized without a brace. Hemovacs were removed once drainage ceased at 24 hours, and intravenous antibiotics were administered for 24 hours. The patient was discharged on postoperative day 2. Follow-up at 2 weeks revealed a healed wound with substantial improvement of lower extremity symptoms but persistent lower back pain. At 6 months leg pain was resolved with walking tolerance extended to beyond 1 mile. Plain radiographs at the 6-month follow-up demonstrated consolidation of the fusion mass.

Discussion

Isthmic spondylolisthesis is the forward slip of one vertebra on another due to either a defect or elongation in the pars articularis. Isolated cases of spondylolysis have been documented in children aged 6 weeks to 10 months, but the condition is generally rare before walking age. Wiltse (1969) noted a 5% incidence of spondylolysis in children aged 5 to 7 years of age increasing to 6 to 7% by age 18. The largest increase in frequency occurs between the ages of 11 and 15 years, corresponding to the growth spurt.

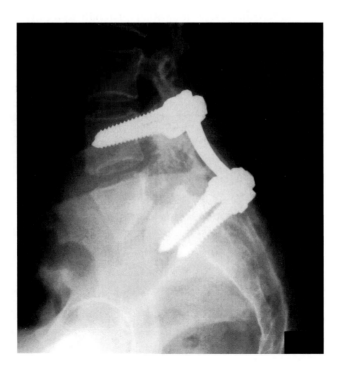

Figure 58–7. Postoperative lateral radiograph. Instrumentation L4 to sacrum. Note: No reduction in slip attempted.

Gender and racial differences occur, with African-American women having the lowest rates (1.1%) and Caucasian men the highest (6.4%). The highest prevalence is found in gymnasts (50%) and weight lifters (36%), with a likely biomechanical etiology of repetitive flexion and forcible hyperextension and rotation acting on a hereditary weakness or dysplasia. Other associations include lumbar Scheuermann's disease and spina bifida.

In the lumbar spine isthmic spondylolisthesis occurs at the L5/S1 level in 82.1% of cases. Fredrickson and colleagues (1984) noted that no patient in their study complained of pain during the development of the lytic defect and that in all patients slip occurred concomitantly with the development of the defect. In general, 90% of slippage will occur prior to presentation in adolescence, with most slippage occurring during the early teens. Most children with spondylolysis and spondylolisthesis remain asymptomatic. The likelihood of slip progression is low, with risk factors including adolescence, high grade of slip, female gender, and L4/L5 spondylolisthesis. In general, once skeletal maturity is obtained, slip progression is unlikely and minimal when present. The only exception is at the L4/L5 level, which may continue to be unstable until the third and fourth decades.

The question then is, Why do patients develop back and leg pain later in life? Magnetic resonance imaging (MRI) scans have shown no difference in disc degeneration between patients younger than 25 years of age who had spondylolisthesis and those who did not. Beyond 25 years of age markedly greater disc degeneration was noted, with up to 70% degeneration in the 25- to 45-year age group. It is thought that repetitive torsional and shear forces associated with spondylolisthesis accelerates disc degeneration. However, as patients age, the rate of disc degeneration rises in the general population. MacNab (1990) thought that in the patient younger than 25 years of age with back pain and isthmic spondylolisthesis, it was highly likely (18.9%) that this lesion was responsible for the pain, whereas in the patient older than 40 it was seldom the cause of back pain (5.2%). This last finding emphasizes the importance of a thorough workup, including MRI scan with or without discography in the patient presenting with back pain and radiographic evidence of a lytic spondylolisthesis. Patients with high-grade slips (greater than 25%) are noted to have rates of lower back pain greater than those of the general population but radiologic disc space narrowing and degenerative changes do not correspond to lower back pain.

The etiology of leg pain in association with lytic spondylolisthesis is usually local compression or irritation of the L5 root by the fibrocartilaginous mass at the level of the pars interarticularis. The defect tissue has been noted to be rich in sensory and sympathetic fibers and vascular tissue. The delay in presentation to middle age is thought to represent accumulation of scar tissue and progressive nerve root irritation rather than slip progression. Disc herniation at the same level is a rare cause of radicular symptoms, whereas herniation at an adjacent level should be excluded prior to considering surgery. In the patient with low back pain and lytic spondylolisthesis who has failed conservative treatment and is a candidate for surgery, MRI scan is the investigation of choice to exclude pathology at adjacent levels. Provocative discography may play a role if the MRI findings of adjacent levels are equivocal, particularly if fusion is to be undertaken.

Alternative Methods of Management

Alternative methods of management include both conservative and operative methods. The conservative methods include analgesics, physical therapy, bracing, nerve root injection, epidural injections, and a host of other modalities. Surgical alternatives to posterior decompression, fusion, and instrumentation are listed in the table below.

PEARLS

- Reserve fusion for lower back pain for those patients who have failed conservative treatment and have radiologic confirmation of isolated single-level disease.
- The inferior aspect of the pedicle of L5 may need to be removed to adequately decompress the L5 nerve root.
- Due to either dysplastic pedicles or pedicles that have had to be partially resected, or in those patients with high-grade slips, fusion and instrumentation may need to extend to the vertebra one level more cephalad than the slip.

PITFALLS

- Do not assume that lower back pain is due to lytic spondylolisthesis in the patient older than 45 years of age.
- Reduction of spondylolisthesis is seldom indicated in the adult and carries high risk of neurologic compromise.
- Identify associated spina bifida preoperatively to avoid thecal sac injury during exposure.

Posterolateral fusion alone, either by a midline incision or Wiltse approach, is the treatment of choice for skeletally mature patients with low back pain alone and for adolescent patients with lower back pain plus or minus minor neurologic symptoms, including hamstring tightness. Addition of internal fixation may improve the fusion rates, but clinical outcomes may not be improved. The L5/S1 isthmic lesion is thought to have greater mechanical stability than that at the L4/L5 level. Thus, in the former, fusion alone will often suffice, whereas in the latter, instrumentation is often added. In patients with higher grade (III, IV, and V) slips, the fusion mass between L5 and S1 is almost horizontal and pedicles of L5 are often inaccessible or dysplastic. This leads to extension of fusion and instrumentation to the L4 level, thus obtaining more rigid fixation and an element of axial compression in the bone graft. A steep lumbosacral joint and horizontal sacrum, as noted in this patient, and high slip angle are risk factors for postoperative slippage, and thus instrumentation may be indicated. High rates of fusion have been documented without instrumentation in grade I and II spondylolisthesis.

Although many authors have noted that, in the adult, as in the adolescent, radicular symptoms may improve with fusion alone, most surgeons advocate the addition of decompression if root compression symptoms are present. Gill and colleagues (1955) advocated removal of the entire loose neural arch, including the fibrocartilaginous mass, without fusion. However, progression of slip has been noted in up to 15% of patients, particularly in adolescents. Thus, fusion is usually added. The removal of the posterior arch allows visualization and complete decompression of the L5 nerve root from its takeoff to the far lateral region. Resection of the inferior aspect of the pedicle may be required to ensure that the L5 root is not under tension.

Posterior lumbar interbody fusion has been advocated in lower grade (grade I) slips. Theoretically, this achieves decompression of the neural elements, distraction of the disc space, and stabilization of the segment. However, the risks are significant, and complications, including neurologic injury and epidural scarring, are not uncommon. Posterior lumbar interbody fusion alone has been noted to further destabilize the segment, and supplementation with posterior instrumentation may be required.

With the advancement of laparoscopic procedures and the development of titanium-threaded cages, use of anterior lumbar interbody fusion has undergone resurgence. Theoretical advantages include placement of graft under compression versus posterior grafting being under tension. Use of anterior lumbar interbody fusion in lytic spondylolisthesis is limited to the grade I slip with no neurologic symptoms (i.e., low back pain alone). In patients with high-grade slips, the surface area for anterior bone graft is further reduced, and that procedure alone is not recommended.

Combined anterior interbody grafting and posterior fusion plus or minus decompression and instrumentation has an important role. It is definitely indicated in failed posterior fusions and may have a role in grade III and IV slips.

Direct repair of the pars articularis defect is seldom successful in the presence of spondylolisthesis in the older patient. Reduction of spondylolisthesis is rarely indicated in the adult patient.

For those patients who have lower back pain due to lytic spondylolisthesis, options include posterolateral fusion alone, posterolateral fusion plus instrumentation, posterior lumbar interbody fusion, anterior lumbar interbody fusion, or anterior and posterior surgery combined. The authors' preference in this select group is posterolateral fusion with the use of instrumentation, depending on the magnitude of slippage and the slip angle. Anterior lumbar interbody fusion (i.e., cages) may be an option in the carefully selected grade I spondylolisthesis patient with verified incapacitating low back pain and no lower extremity pain.

Type of Management	Advantages	Disadvantages	Comments
Posterolateral fusion alone	Avoid risks of instrumentation Shorter surgery	Does not directly decompress nerve root compression	Younger/adolescent patient with back pain ± radicular symptoms or patient with back pain alone
Posterolateral fusion and instrumentation (pedicle screws)	Immediate stability Increased fusion rates	Risks of instrumentation Does not directly decompress nerve roots	Grade III and IV slip with back pain alone Indications for instrumentation in grade I and II controversial Vertical lumbosacral joint L4/L5 slip
Microdecompression of nerve root/roots	Minimally invasive	Risk of development of lower back pain	Patient with unilateral radicular symptoms and no back pain
Gill laminectomy alone	Direct decompression of nerve roots	Risk of slip progression Incidence of persistent lower back pain	Seldom indicated alone Older patient with predominant radicular pain
Posterior decompression and posterolateral fusion	Direct decompression of neural elements Motion segment stabilization high (80%) rates of fusion	Reduced fusion rates vs. instrumentation	Grade I and II with leg ± back pain
Posterior decompression, posterolateral fusion, and instrumentation	Direct decompression of nerve roots Immediate stability ?Increased fusion rates (90%)	Longer operation Risks of instrumentation	Grade III and IV slip with back and leg pain Indication for instrumentation in grade I–II controversial Vertical lumbosacral joint L4/L5 level
Posterior lumbar intervertebral fusion (soft, hard, cages)	Decompresses neural elements Distracts disc space Achieves anterior interbody fusion	Root traction injuries Epidural scarring	Option in grade I with back and leg symptoms
Anterior lumbar intervertebral fusion (tricortical autograft, allograft dowels, cages, etc.)	Minimally invasive laparoscopic procedure or minilaparotomy Achieves interbody fusion	High rates of collapse if graft alone Long-term results of interbody cages unknown Vascular injuries Difficult salvage of cages	Limit use to grade I spondylolisthesis with back pain alone and imaging studies confirming single-level pathology
Combined anterior interbody fusion and posterior decompression and fusion	Increased fusion rates	Prolonged surgery	Role in failed surgery and symptomatic pseudarthrosis

Suggested Readings

Fredrickson BE, Baker D, McHolick WJ, et al. The natural history of spondylolysis and spondylolisthesis. J Bone Joint Surg 1984; 66A:699–707.

Gill GG, Manning JG, White HL. Surgical treatment of spondylolisthesis without fusion. J Bone Joint Surg 1955; 37A:493–520.

Kuslich SD, Ulstrom CL, Griffith SL, Ahern JW, Dowdle JD. The Bagby and Kuslich method of lumbar interbody fusion: history, techniques, and 2-year follow-up results of a United States prospective, multicenter trial. Spine 1998; 23:1267–1279.

MacNab I. Backache, 2d ed, p. 84. Baltimore: Williams & Wilkins, 1990.

Wiltse L. Spondylolisthesis: classification and etiology. In: American Academy of Orthopaedic Surgeons, eds. Symposium on the Spine, pp. 143–168. St. Louis: CV Mosby, 1969.

Case 59
Achondroplasia—Cervical Postlaminectomy Kyphosis

Jeffrey L. Bush, David Horn, and Alexander R. Vaccaro

History and Physical Examination

A 15-year-old boy with achondroplasia presented to another facility with pain, weakness, and occasional numbness of his upper and lower extremities. His symptoms began approximately 1 year prior to this visit, starting with weakness and pain in his arms and legs. His ability to walk became progressively diminished to the point that ascending and descending stairs became very difficult. There was no loss

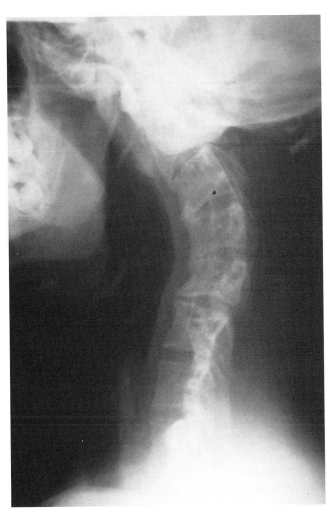

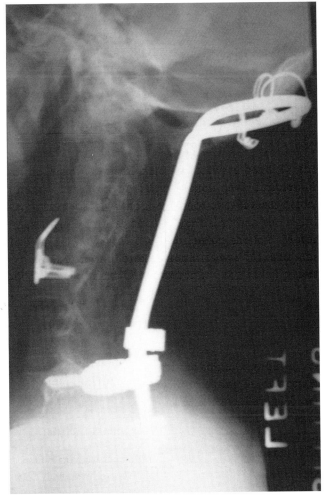

Figure 59–1. Lateral plain radiograph revealing a postlaminectomy cervical kyphotic deformity.

Figure 59–2. A lateral plain radiograph following an anterior cervical decompression and fusion followed by a posterior occipital to thoracic stabilization procedure.

of bowel or bladder function and no history of trauma. Other than achondroplasia, he had no significant medical history and no prior surgeries.

On examination, the patient was afebrile with stable vital signs and appeared to be in no distress. He had the normal appearance of a person with achondroplasia, with a large head, short limbs, and a waddling gait. His height was measured at 50 inches. He was alert, oriented, and cognition appeared to be normal. Cranial nerves II through XII were intact. In the upper extremities sensation was diminished to light touch and pin prick. Strength was 4/5 bilaterally and hyperreflexia was present. In the lower extremities, sensation was diminished to both pin prick and light touch. Strength was 4/5 bilaterally. Deep tendon reflexes showed hyperreflexia. Babinski signs were positive bilaterally.

Radiologic Findings

Computed tomography (CT) scan revealed significant spinal stenosis from C1 to C6.

Diagnosis

Achondroplasia.

Surgical Management

The patient subsequently underwent a posterior cervical laminectomy from C1 to T1 with marked improvement in strength, sensation, and the ability to walk. Approximately 3 years after surgery, his symptoms began to reappear. Over the next several years, his function gradually diminished. By the age of 21, he had developed a postlaminectomy cervical kyphosis and become quadriparetic, with decreased strength in all extremities. He was incontinent to both stool and urine. Physical exam revealed significant weakness, atrophy, and decreased sensation in his upper and lower extremities. Hyperreflexia was present and Babinski signs were again positive.

Radiographic analysis revealed evidence of a postlaminectomy cervical kyphosis (Fig. 59–1) with a ribbon (severe flattening) spinal cord on CT myelography.

Following a period of low weight traction without any effect on cervical alignment, the patient underwent a multilevel anterior cervical corpectomy fusion with iliac crest allograft followed by posterior occiput to thoracic fusion with thoracic pedicle screws and occipital wiring (Fig. 59–2). Postoperatively, the patient recovered most of the sensation and strength in his arms and legs. His bowel and bladder function returned to normal and he now ambulates with the use of a cane.

Discussion

Achondroplasia is the most common type of dwarfism, with an incidence of approximately 1/26,000 live births. It is inherited as an autosomal dominant trait, although the majority of cases (80%) are due to spontaneous mutations. The short stature is the result of rhizomelic shortening of the limbs, in which proximal segments are shortened more than distal segments.

Histologically, achondroplasia results in the thinning of the epiphyseal growth plate and a decreased amount of endochondral bone. Within the growth plate,

PEARLS

- When evaluating a patient with cervical spinal stenosis, it is very important to evaluate for compression of the foramen magnum. Sleep studies are often necessary to rule out associated sleep apnea when analyzing foraminal compression.
- When performing a cervicomedullary decompression, intraoperative ultrasound can be used to assess the need for decompression of the dura as well as the surrounding bone.
- In the surgical treatment of lumbar spinal stenosis, it is important that a laminectomy, and not a laminoplasty, be performed because the stenosis is primarily the result of a narrowed interpedicular distance that is not adequately compensated for with a laminoplasty.
- When a cervical and thoracolumbar decompression is needed, the cervical stage should be done first to minimize potential complications if a cerebrospinal fluid leak occurs during the thoracolumbar stage.

PITFALLS

- During a cervicomedullary decompression, excess bone removal around the condyles should be avoided. Excessive removal in this area can weaken the support of the cerebellum and cause a posterior herniation.
- Consider a fusion procedure in all cases of a cervical laminectomy to avoid the potential of a postlaminectomy deformity.

the zone of proliferating cartilage is very narrow, and bone still undergoes calcification but at a reduced rate. A transverse bar of bone eventually seals off the growth plate, leaving the bone substantially shortened compared to a normally developed bone.

The bones in affected individuals are abnormally short and thick. The head appears large and the spine is of normal length, although it contains various structural abnormalities. Mean heights for males and females, respectively, are 131 cm (51 inches) and 125 cm (49 inches). The typical patient has a small face with a bulging forehead (frontal bossing) and a depressed nasal bridge. Nasal passages are narrow, and the nose has a fleshy tip with up-turned nostrils. Patients tend to have an exaggerated lumbar lordosis and tilted pelvis, leading to a waddling gait and often causing flexion contractures of the hips. Despite the potential for serious medical problems, especially early in life, most patients can expect an average life span and normal mental function. In addition to the heterozygous autosomal dominant and sporadic forms, a homozygous form of the disease also exists. It is very severe, with a reported incidence of death in the first year of life as high as 80%.

There are numerous complications associated with achondroplasia, the most serious of which are narrowing of the foramen magnum and cervical spinal canal, leading to compression of the medulla oblongata and spinal cord. Such compression can cause respiratory and neurologic symptoms, occasionally severe enough to cause sudden infant death. Cervicomedullary decompression may need to be performed to alleviate such symptoms and reduce the risk of respiratory failure and death.

Affected infants have delayed motor milestones, most likely related to the altered center of gravity caused by the large, heavy head and shortened limbs. The ability to control the head, stand, and walk are all substantially delayed. Developmental neurologic reflexes, however, are intact and occur at appropriate times.

Patients tend to experience chronic otitis media during infancy and childhood, which can lead to hearing loss and delayed development of speech and language skills. Dental development can also be delayed due to altered bone growth. Affected individuals have straight legs at birth but eventually develop tibial bowing. The bowing is associated with genu recurvatum and lateral torsion of the knee and may be caused by relative excessive growth of the fibula compared to the tibia.

Ninety percent of infants with achondroplasia are reported to have a transient thoracolumbar kyphosis that usually resolves spontaneously as they begin to walk. The kyphosis is caused by the combination of the large head, ligamentous laxity, and hypotonia associated with achondroplasia. The child slumps forward when placed in a sitting position, leading to vertebral remodeling and the development of a thoracolumbar kyphosis.

Hydrocephalus is common in achondroplasia as the head rapidly increases in size during infancy. It is usually communicating and is caused by the impaired flow of cerebrospinal fluid through the foramen magnum and cervical spinal column. Symptoms of hydrocephalus, however, are usually not significant enough to warrant surgical intervention.

Lumbar spinal stenosis is very common in achondroplasia and can lead to compression of the cord, nerve roots, and blood vessels. Adult patients often experience the gradual development of back and leg pain, claudication, weakness, paresthesias, and even paralysis. Decompression of stenotic areas of the spine is occasionally necessary to alleviate and prevent worsening of symptoms.

Cervical spinal stenosis can also occur in the patient with achondroplasia, as in the case above. The stenosis is usually asymptomatic until adulthood. Symptoms including pain, weakness, paresthesias, respiratory depression, and paralysis can be severe enough to warrant cervical laminectomy, as in this case. To prevent instability following a cervical laminectomy, preservation of greater than 50% of the zygoapophyseal joints are necessary. Some surgeons recommend a concomitant fusion following a posterior decompression in all cases of cervical myelopathy due to the adverse consequences of spinal cord lengthening in the setting of myelomalacia.

In the case presented, the patient developed a postlaminectomy kyphotic deformity, which resulted in a progressive neurologic deficit. The goals of surgical treatment were to decompress the compromised neural tissues, correct spinal alignment, and confer adequate spinal stability through a circumferential reconstructive procedure.

Alternative Methods of Management

Type of Management	Advantages	Disadvantages	Comments
Nonoperative treatment	None	Continual neurologic decline from progression of deformity	No role in the treatment of a postlaminectomy cervical deformity
Cervical traction followed by a posterior instrumented fusion	Avoids morbidity of an anterior decompression and reconstructive procedure	Frequently biomechanically inadequate; often results in late instability	May be effective in the early development of a cervical deformity
Anterior posterior decompression and stabilization procedure	Improved ability to correct malalignment; optimum cervical stability; lessened risk of neurologic embarrassment with anterior decompression	Prolonged surgical procedure; technically challenging	Preferred surgical treatment

Suggested Readings

Hunter GW, Bankier A, Rogers JG, Sillence D, Scott CI Jr. Medical complications of achondroplasia: a multicentre patient review. J Med Genet 1998; 35:705–712.

Hurko O, Pyeritz R, Uematsu S. Neurological considerations in achondroplasia. In: Nicoletti B, Kopits SE, Ascani E, McKusick VA, eds. Human Achondroplasia: A Multidisciplinary Approach, pp. 153–162. New York: Plenum Press, 1988.

Kopits SE. Orthopaedic aspects of achondroplasia in children. In: Nicoletti B, Kopits SE, Ascani E, McKusick VA, eds. Human Achondroplasia: A Multidisciplinary Approach, pp. 189–197. New York: Plenum Press, 1988.

Murdoch JL, Walker BA, Hull JG. Achondroplasia: a genetic and statistical survey. Ann Hum Genet 1970; 33:227–235.

Netter FH. The Ciba Collection of Medical Illustrations, Volume 8: Musculoskeletal System, Part II: Developmental Disorders, Tumors, Rheumatic Diseases, and Joint Replacement. Summit, NJ: Ciba-Geigy, 1990.

Oberklaid F, Danks DM, Jensen F, Stace L, Rosshandler S. Achondroplasia and hypochondroplasia: comments on frequency, mutation rate, and radiological features in skull and spine. J Med Genet 1979; 16:140–146.

Pauli RM, Breed A, Horton VK, Glinski LP, Reiser CA. Prevention of fixed, angular kyphosis in achondroplasia. J Pediatr Orthop 1997; 17:726–733.

Pauli RM, Horton VK, Glinski LP, Reiser CA. Prospective assessment of risks for cervicomedullary-junction compression in infants with achondroplasia. Am J Hum Genet 1995; 56:732–744.

Ryken TC, Menezes AH. Cervicomedullary compression in achondroplasia. J Neurosurg 1994; 81:43–48.

Shiller AL. Bones and joints. In: Rubin E, Farber JL, eds. Pathology, pp. 1272–1345. Philadelphia: Lippincott, 1994.

Uematsu S, Wang H, Kopits SE, Hurko O. Total craniospinal decompression in achondroplastic stenosis. Neurosurgery 1994; 35:250–258.

Yamada Y, Ito H, Otsubo Y, Sekido K. Surgical management of cervicomedullary compression in achondroplasia. Child's Nerv Syst 1996; 12:737–741.

Yasui N, Kawabata H, Kojimoto H, et al. Lengthening of the lower limbs in patients with achondroplasia and hypochondroplasia. Clin Orthop Rel Res 1997; 344:298–306.

Case 60
Postradiation Spinal Deformity
Alan S. Hilibrand

History and Physical Examination

A 53-year-old woman presented to the outpatient center complaining of progressive lower extremity weakness with difficulty walking. A plain X-ray and magnetic resonance imaging (MRI) obtained prior to her evaluation was felt to be suspicious for tumor involving the T12 vertebral body (Fig. 60–1). A fine-needle computed tomography (CT)-guided biopsy of the vertebral body described a carcinoma that was not felt to be of primary spinal origin. The patient then underwent an extensive workup in search of a primary neoplasm, which could not be determined. Due to her persistent pain and the pathologic findings from biopsy, she underwent 3 weeks of radiation therapy locally to the T12 region, with relief of her back pain.

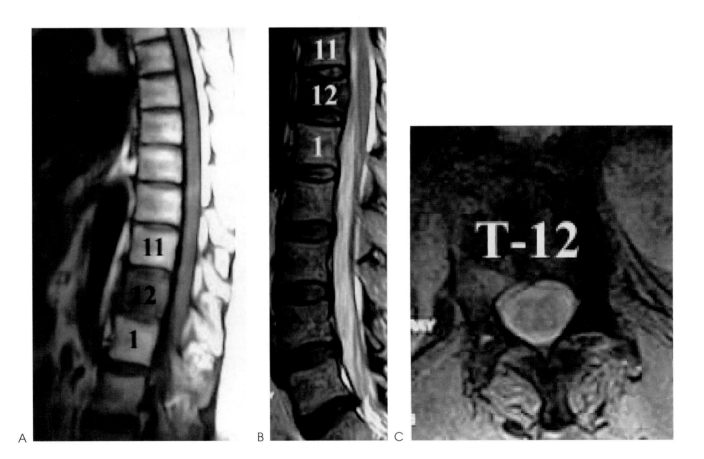

Figure 60–1. Magnetic resonance imaging (MRI) of the thoracolumbar spine from 1 year prior to initial evaluation, demonstrating decreased marrow signal on T1 (A) and intermediate signal on T2 (B). There is no significant kyphotic deformity or canal compromise (C). A course of radiation therapy was delivered to the T12 lesion shortly after these images were obtained.

One year later, during the month prior to presentation at our outpatient facility, the patient developed progressive lower extremity weakness with difficulty walking, as well as numbness in both feet and recurrent low back pain. Plain films demonstrated collapse with kyphosis at the previously irradiated T12 vertebral body, with the development of sagittal decompensation on long-cassette radiographs (Fig. 60–2).

On examination, the patient was able to ambulate on her heels and on her toes. She was able to perform a straight-line gait test. She had a palpable deformity at the thoracolumbar junction, with "leathery" skin changes throughout the radiated site. Lumbar flexion and extension were painful, although she was unable to assume a straight sagittal posture and keep her head over her pelvis. Neurologically she had minimal diffuse weakness in all lower extremity muscle groups. She had diffuse sensory changes below the knees in both lower extremities. She had generally decreased amplitude reflexes at both patellae and ankles, and a down-going Babinski reflex bilaterally.

Radiologic Findings

Anteroposterior (AP) and lateral plain radiographs demonstrate the T12 fracture with near-complete loss of anterior height, partial loss of posterior vertebral body height, and 30 degrees of segmental kyphosis at the level of the fracture (Fig.

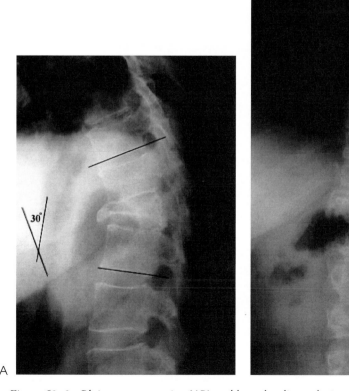

Figure 60–2. Plain anteroposterior (AP) and lateral radiographs 1 year after external beam irradiation for suspected neoplasm of the T12 vertebral body (see text). Lateral film (A) demonstrated 30 degrees of kyphosis, with maintenance of coronal alignment on the AP radiograph (B).

60–2). There are postradiation changes evident with sclerosis of the affected verte-bral bone.

Repeat MRI scans were also obtained to evaluate the lesion (Fig. 60–3). These demonstrate postradiation necrosis of the T12 vertebral body, with retropulsion of fragments from the middle column into the spinal canal, impinging upon the conus medullaris. There did not appear to be involvement of any of the other vertebral bodies above or below the T12 level.

Diagnosis

Postradiation thoracolumbar deformity with sagittal decompensation secondary to pathologic fracture of T12 vertebral body with 30-degree segmental kyphosis.

Surgical Management

Because of the patient's progressive deformity and progressive neurologic loss, we recommended operative intervention. The goals in surgery were to obtain further diagnostic tissue, decompress the neural elements, and restore sagittal balance. In general, these goals may be achieved through either anterior or posterior surgery. In the case of a flexible deformity with no posterior ligamentous disruption, anterior

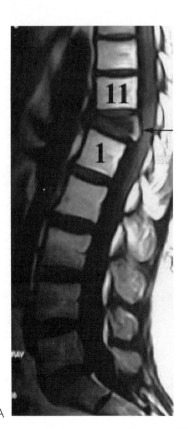
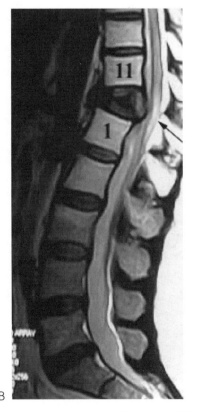
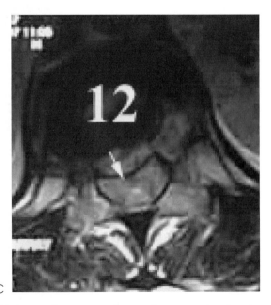

A   B   C

Figure 60–3. Repeat MRI obtaining following initial evaluation. T1 (A) and T2 (B) images demonstrate decreased marrow signal and complete collapse of the vertebral body, with retropulsion of bone on the axial images (C).

surgery with a femoral strut graft and instrumentation can restore sagittal balance while facilitating anterior spinal canal decompression. On the other hand, if the deformity is rigid, then either a combined anterior decompression and grafting with a posterior fusion is necessary, or the surgeon may attempt a posterior procedure involving an "eggshell" or pedicle subtraction osteotomy.

In the present case, the patient's deformity was rigid, with no motion on flexion/extension bilateral views (Fig. 60–4). In consideration of our goals of 30-degree kyphosis correction and neural element decompression, we recommended a posterior-only approach, with a transpedicular vertebrectomy/osteotomy at the T12 level. In this procedure, cancellous bone in the vertebral body is removed through the pedicles, leaving an eggshell vertebra. The decompression of the anterior aspect of the thecal sac is accomplished using curved curettes to pull the posterior vertebral body fragments into the cavitated vertebral body, away from the spinal cord. Once the posterior compression is removed, a closing-wedge osteotomy is performed. The pedicles and facets at the osteotomy level are resected, leaving one large neural foramen for the T11 and T12 nerve roots. The lateral walls of the vertebral body are

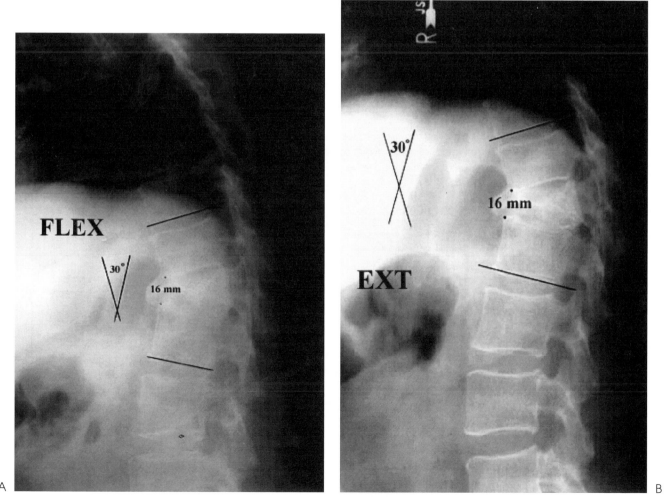

Figure 60–4. Dynamic lateral radiographs (A,B) demonstrating a fixed kyphotic deformity with no change in segmental sagittal alignment between flexion and extension.

- Review the entire metastatic workup and repeat any portions, if appropriate, to identify a possibly vascular lesion, such as renal cell carcinoma, which may benefit from preoperative embolization.
- Obtain three-foot-long standing AP and lateral radiographs to determine whether such a deformity is resulting in any sagittal or coronal decompensation. The center of the C7 vertebrae should be centered over the apex of the sacrum on the lateral view, and should be bisected by the median sacral line on the AP radiograph.
- To assess anterior column stability of this deformity, flexion/extension lateral views should be obtained. The finding of anterior column instability should lead to treatment by combined anterior/posterior techniques.
- The use of a lordosing table such as the Jackson table can greatly facilitate the postural reduction from a posterior approach.
- These procedures should be performed under electrophysiologic monitoring whenever deformity correction is planned and/or instrumentation is to be applied above L2. For the most reliable feedback, both sensory- and motor-evoked potentials should be monitored.
- To prevent collapse of the decancellated vertebral body prior to completion of the "eggshell" procedure, we recommend the prior application of internal fixation with at least one rod, followed by the controlled correction of the kyphosis by slowly loosening the internal fixation.

cracked with a small curette and gentle pressure is applied to the spine to shorten the posterior aspect of the spine. Lordotic correction occurs as the posterior column shortens while the anterior vertebral body height is maintained on the rigid anterior hinge. Achievement of sagittal balance required a 30-degree correction in overall alignment, which was achieved (Fig. 60–5). The reduction was stabilized with internal fixation, using bone screws inserted into the vertebral pedicles at T10, T11, L1, and L2. The wounds were drained subfascially and the patient was placed in a thoracolumbosacral orthosis (TLSO).

Postoperative Management

The patient was kept in a TLSO for a total of 3 months postoperatively. She was ambulated on postoperative day 2, although, because of her significant weakness, she required assistance with a walker, and was subsequently transferred to a rehabilitation hospital for further intensive rehabilitative efforts. The patient healed with much improved sagittal alignment (Fig. 60–6), but failed to recover any further neurologic function and remains ambulatory only with the use of assisting devices.

Discussion

The development of spinal deformity following irradiation of vertebral bodies has been described in experimental animal models as well as in clinical follow-up studies of children treated with radiation therapy for malignancies. Engel (1939) pro-

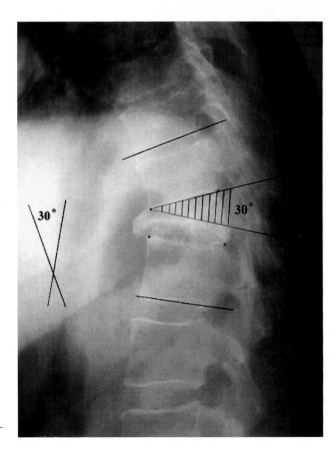

Figure 60–5. Planned wedge resection of bone through the T12 vertebral body, with the anterior hinge based at the anterior longitudinal ligament.

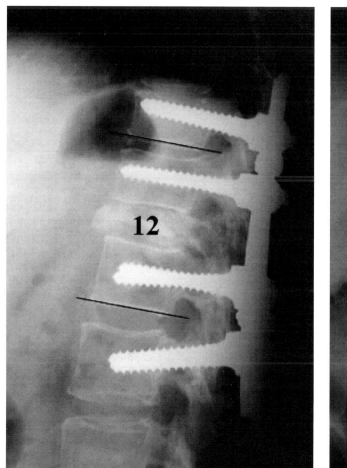
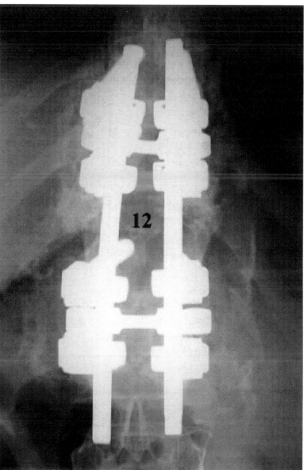

Figure 60–6. Three-month postoperative lateral (A) and AP (B) radiographs demonstrating restoration of neutral sagittal alignment and consolidation of the posterolateral fusion mass.

duced scoliotic deformities in a variety of laboratory animals following the unilateral insertion of radium needles into the paraspinal musculature. Arkin and Simon (1950) produced scoliosis in rabbits by irradiating one side of the epiphyseal plate. In both cases the radiation caused an ipsilateral "stunting" of growth resulting in the development of an experimental scoliosis. Yoshizawa and Ueda (1973) reported that external irradiation resulted in delayed ossification of caudal vertebrae in the mouse fetus, with the degree of the delay inversely related to the radiation dose. In mature mice, these effects were manifested as congenital anomalies and stunting of growth.

External beam irradiation has been shown to affect all aspects of physeal metabolism. Rubin and colleagues (1959) observed a greater impact upon enchondral than periosteal bone formation, whereas Kember (1967) described a direct relationship between the degree of physeal disruption and the dose of radiation delivered. Similarly, other authors have described weaker bone formation with lower activities of alkaline phosphatase and lower levels of calcium and phosphate with increasing radiation doses.

Clinically, abnormalities in immature vertebral column growth following external beam radiation have been reported. Lokajicek and colleagues (1969) described the

- When the pathologist is unable to make a firm diagnosis given ample tissue, a second review by a bone pathologist at another institution is essential.
- Avoid irradiation to the spinal column, even in adults, if there is any uncertainty regarding the actual diagnosis of metastatic cancer.
- Patients with neural element compression and progressive neurologic deficits may not recover function following decompression, especially in the setting of long-standing spinal cord compression, prior irradiation to the spinal cord, or other cause of vascular compromise. Patients must understand this possibility before giving informed consent for surgery.

development of irregularities in vertebral body shape progressing to gross spinal deformity following irradiation for intraabdominal malignancies in children. Bedrook (1969) described a high incidence of spinal deformity in paralytic children who had undergone irradiation of an intraspinal malignancy. Probert and Parker (1975) catalogued the clinical and radiographic postirradiation changes to include subcortical osteoporosis, endplate irregularities, maturational arrest, and the subsequent development of deformity.

In the adult patient, the development of spinal deformity following external beam irradiation is rare, and multiple searches of all Medline databases produced only two original reports of such a phenomenon in the English-language literature. Lord and Herndon (1986) reported three cases of pathologic vertebral fractures of the thoracolumbar spine due to metastatic disease. All three patients had undergone external beam radiation of the involved vertebral body, and subsequently developed kyphotic deformity with progressive neurologic deficits. Bone biopsy at the time of surgery revealed necrotic bone in all three cases, as was observed in the present report.

In the present case, the kyphotic deformity that developed in the T12 vertebral body following radiation therapy was most likely the result of necrosis of the irradiated vertebral bone, with subsequent resorption and structural collapse. Because the irradiation predated the onset of myelopathy and deformity by almost 1 year, the subsequent vertebral body collapse appears to have been an indolent process that was most likely the result of ischemic necrosis caused by the external beam irradiation.

Alternative Methods of Management

Alternative methods of management may also be used to treat a postradiation kyphotic deformity as described in this chapter, based on the patient's medical condition, the degree of the deformity, and the surgeon's experience with different approaches. In the patient with minimal deformity and no neurologic deficits, or in the case of a medically unstable patient, nonoperative treatment in a brace followed by progressive ambulation and postural training in physical therapy may be appropriate. Although this avoids the potential risks and complications of operative management, it does not correct the deformity nor the neural element compression, and may lead to deformity progression.

Anterior decompression and fusion with or without internal fixation is the most common approach used to treat these deformities. It allows a restoration of anterior column support, facilitates direct decompression of the neural elements, and provides ample specimen for biopsy.

A posterior approach to decompression and fusion will allow stronger internal fixation than an anterior approach using the pedicles and lamina for hardware attachment. In addition, use of a lordosing frame (such as the Jackson table) may facilitate postural reduction of the deformity. However, decompression of the anterior aspect of the vertebral canal from the posterior approach is much less reliable than with an anterior approach. Furthermore, restoration of anterior column support is substantially more difficult.

The combined procedure of anterior decompression and grafting followed by posterior stabilization combines the advantages of the anterior and posterior techniques.

Type of Management	Advantages	Disadvantages	Comments
Nonoperative/bracing	Avoids surgical risks and complications	No neural decompression No deformity correction Further progression?	If minimal deformity and no neurologic deficits If surgery contraindicated
Anterior decompression and fusion	Restores anterior column Direct neural decompression Ease of biopsy	Deformity recurrence? Difficult postural reduction Osteoporosis—poor fixation?	Most common approach
Posterior decompression and fusion	Rigid internal fixation Postural reduction easier	Anterior column support? Neural decompression?	Avoid laminectomy above L2 Usually not performed as a stand-alone procedure
Anterior/posterior decompression and fusion	Restores anterior column Direct neural decompression Rigid internal fixation Ease of biopsy	Two surgical exposures Increased surgical risks	Most definitive technique Appropriate in medically stable patient
Posterior decompression with decancellation osteotomy and fusion	Eliminates anterior defect Restores sagittal alignment Single surgical approach	Technically difficult Limited indications (see comments)	Inappropriate for deformity with >30 degrees kyphosis or unstable anterior column

Suggested Readings

Arkin AM, Simon N. Radiation scoliosis. J Bone Joint Surg 1950; 32A:396.

Bedbrook GM. Intrinsic factors in the development of spinal deformities with paralysis. Paraplegia 1969; 6(4):222–232.

Bhalla S, Reinus WR. The linear intravertebral vacuum: a sign of benign vertebral collapse. AJR 1998; 170(6):1563–1569.

Blackburn J, Wells AB. Radiation damage to growing bone: the effect of x-ray doses of 100 to 1000 r on mouse tibia and knee-joint. Br J Radiol 1963; 36:505–513.

Engel D. Experiments on production of spinal deformities by radium. AJR 1939; 42:217.

Kember NJ. Cell survival and radiation damage growth cartilage. Br J Radiol 1967; 40:496–505.

Lokajicek ML, Stasek V, Palecek L, Kolar J. Interdependence among some factors of importance in the development of radiation changes in children. Neoplasma 1969; 16:111–114.

Lord CF, Herndon JH. Spinal cord compression secondary to kyphosis associated with radiation therapy for metastatic disease. Clin Orthop Rel Res 1986; 210:120–127.

MacEwen GD. Experimental scoliosis. Clin Orthop Rel Res 1973; 93:69–74.

Mayfield JK. Postradiation spinal deformity. Orthop Clin North Am 1979; 10(4):829–844.

Probert JC, Parker BR. The effects of radiation therapy on bone growth. Radiology 1975; 114:155–162.

Riseborough EJ, Grabias SL, Burton RI, et al. Skeletal alterations following irradiation for Wilms' tumor with particular reference to scoliosis and kyphosis. J Bone Joint Surg 1976; 58A(4):526–536.

Rubin P, Andrews JR, Swarm R, et al. Radiation induced dysplasias of bone. AJR 1959; 82:206–216.

Woodard HQ, Laughlin JS. The effect of x-rays of different qualities on the alkaline phosphatase of living mouse bone. II. Effects of 22.5-Mevp x-rays. Radiat Res 1957; 7:236–252.

Yoshizawa Y, Ueda K. Effects of radiation on growth of caudal vertebrae of mouse fetus. J Radiat Res 1973; 14:1–8.

Section VII

Miscellaneous

Case 61

Persistent Spinal Fluid Leakage Following Spinal Surgery

Jeffrey D. Coe

History and Physical Examination

A 38-year-old woman underwent spinal implant removal 23 months after undergoing an instrumented posterolateral fusion from L4 to the sacrum for a grade II isthmic spondylolisthesis at L5/S1. During this procedure, while exposing the transverse connector overlying the L5 laminectomy defect with electrocautery, a leakage of clear fluid was detected caudal to the transverse connector device. The area of the leakage was gently packed with cotton pledgets. The remainder of the instrumentation was removed. When attention was redirected to the area of the clear fluid leakage, it was apparent that there were two linear 2-mm midline dural tears separated by a bridge of intact dura measuring 1.5 to 2.0 mm in length. Gentle dissection of the scar tissue from the edges of the dural tear was carried out. Each tear was repaired with a figure-of-eight 5-0 prolene suture. The repair was intact to 40 mm of water Valsalva airway pressure produced by the anesthesiologist. The wound was then closed in layers. No subfascial or subcutaneous drain was employed. Postoperatively, the patient was kept in a supine or lateral position for 24 hours and then ambulated. She was discharged late on the first postoperative day. At the time of discharge, she had no complaints other than minimal incisional low back pain.

Beginning the fourth postoperative day, however, the patient began to complain of nausea and headaches, which initially were not affected by position. Upon exam-

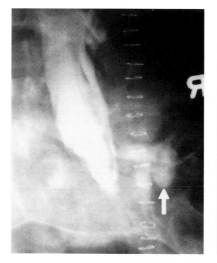

Figure 61–1. An oblique myelogram view demonstrates clearly the presence of extradural contrast appearing to emanate from the caudal-dorsal dura (arrow).

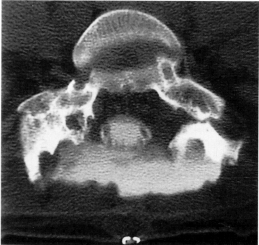

Figure 61–2. This postmyelogram computed tomography (CT) cut demonstrates a large subfascial collection of extradural contrast material.

- Prevention of inadvertent durotomies is the key. At the time of decompression, some surgeons recommend placing cotton pledgets over the exposed dura and passing the cotton pledgets ventral to the lamina prior to the removal of the lamina with the Kerrison rongeurs. With very tight stenosis in the lumbar spine, this may be quite difficult. Others surgeons suggest that this technique may in fact lead to a false sense of security. They argue that it is best to directly visualize the dura to minimize the risk of dural tears. Their alternative approach is to pass a Penfield no. 3 elevator ventral to the lamina to ensure that there are no adhesions between the dura and the ventral surface of the lamina, and then use a larger-size Kerrison rongeur to take several bites. These steps are repeated until the laminectomy has been completed. Whether or not one uses cotton pledgets, it is important to pull slowly away with the Kerrison rongeur after taking a bite. If a dural adhesion or the dura itself is captured in the jaw of the Kerrison, an inadvertent durotomy can be avoided, or the size of the tear minimized.
- When using a high-speed drill to either decorticate or thin the lamina, the drill should not be activated until the tip of the drill is within several millimeters of the point of application. The drill should be held with both hands, and one or both hands should be gently resting on the patient at the wound edge for precise control. The drill should be moved from medial to lateral to minimize the possibility of inadvertent durotomy and the more potentially devastat-

ination her wound was noted to be healing well without any evidence of deep or subcutaneous swelling or edema. There was no drainage noted. By the 10th postoperative day, however, she was complaining of lethargy, nausea, and positional headaches exacerbated by upright posture and relieved partially by supine positioning. Physical examination revealed no wound drainage with good initial primary wound healing. There was fullness of the deep tissues without evidence of subcutaneous fluid collections or erythema. Neurologic examination was normal. Nerve root tension signs were absent.

Radiologic Findings

A myelogram and a postmyelogram computed tomography (CT) scan were obtained on the 12th postoperative day. Both the myelogram and postmyelogram CT scan demonstrated an extradural collection of contrast (Figs. 61–1 and 61–2). The postmyelogram CT scan demonstrated that all of the cerebrospinal fluid (CSF) collection was subfascial (Fig. 61–2).

Diagnosis

Persistent spinal fluid leak secondary to disruption of primary repair of a small dural laceration.

Surgical Management

The patient was returned to the operating room later the same day that the myelogram was performed (12th postoperative day). Upon reexploration, no subcutaneous fluid was found; however, after removal of the deep fascial sutures, a substantial collection (approximately 30 cc) of clear but very slightly blood-tinged fluid was observed. Upon reexploration of the initial dural tears, it was noted that the cephalad suture had loosened and that the two small tears had become one tear by virtue of disruption of the intervening bridge of dura between the tears.

Further dissection of the scar tissue from the dural edges was carried out. A running 5-0 prolene suture was used to repair the dura; 5 cc of homologous fibrin glue was used to reinforce the repair. The repair was intact to 40 cm water Valsalva (both before and after application of the fibrin glue). The wound was then closed without subcutaneous or subfascial drainage.

Postoperative Management

Postoperatively, the patient was maintained in a supine or lateral position for 48 hours. She was discharged late on the second postoperative day. Her wound healed without complication. She noted complete relief of her headaches and nausea, and at 6-month follow-up had no complaints related to her spinal fluid leakage.

Discussion

Inadvertent durotomy is one of the most common complications in spinal surgery. The incidence of dural tears ranges between 4 and 14% of all spinal procedures that

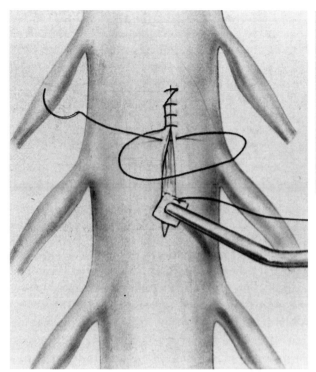

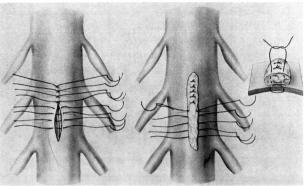

Figure 61–4. Application of a fat or muscle graft. First the dural tear is primarily repaired with interrupted sutures that are left with needles attached at both ends. Then the sutures are passed through the piece of fat (or muscle) and tied down securing the graft over the repaired tear to assist in achieving a watertight closure. (From Eismont FJ, Wiesel SW, Rothman RH. Treatment of dural tears associated with spinal surgery. J Bone Joint Surg 1981; 63A:1132–1136. With permission.)

Figure 61–3. Illustration of dural repair using a running-locked suture. As illustrated, the suction should be applied through a small cotton pledget to protect the exposed nerve rootlets. (From Eismont FJ, Wiesel SW, Rothman RH. Treatment of dural tears associated with spinal surgery. J Bone Joint Surg 1981; 63A:1132–1136. With permission.)

ing complication of nerve root laceration or avulsion. When decorticating after a laminectomy, it is helpful to protect the dura with either cotton pledgets or surgical sponges, and/or have the assistant hold a large Cobb elevator or malleable retractor and "shadow" the tip of the drill as guided by the surgeon. With this technique, if the drill were to "kick" medially, dural and/or neurologic injury would be prevented.

PITFALLS

• Dural adhesions in primary cases are relatively rare except ventral to the sacral lamina where there is very little mo-

involve lumbar decompression as a major component of the procedure. Generally, primary repair is the appropriate acute management of dural tears (Fig. 61–3). Suture material for dural repair includes dural silk, dural nylon, and prolene. The recommended size range is 4-0 to 7-0 using the smallest available needle. Adequate lighting is essential and, in most cases, loupe magnification should be considered. More extensive tears may be treated by interrupted dural sutures incorporating a fat graft or muscle graft (Fig. 61–4). If a dural tear results in a defect that is too large to permit primary closure, it can be repaired with a fascial patch graft (either fascia lata or lumbar fascia, depending on the size of the defect) (Fig. 61–5). Ventral and lateral tears remain the most challenging tears to repair by direct suturing. A "pull-through" fat or muscle graft can be used to repair this type of tear (Fig. 61–6).

Recently, Surgical Dynamics Inc. has developed the DuraClose dura clip applier that allows for more rapid closure of simple durotomies. It does not, however, necessarily permit closure of lateral durotomies that could not otherwise be primarily repaired because this device requires direct accessibility to the region of the tear (Fig. 61–7). In general, successfully repaired dural tears result in few long-term sequelae.

Another major advancement in the management of CSF leaks has been the development of fibrin glue. This is produced when equal amounts of thrombin and cryoprecipitate solution are mixed, forming a virtually instantaneous clot when ap-tion. Moreover, the lordosis of the lower lumbosacral spine can often lead the surgeon to misjudge the angle of the Kerrison foot.

- The surgeon should always be aware of the possibility of spina bifida occulta or a S1/S2 dorsal interlaminar defect. It is surprisingly easy to violate the dura during exposure because the dura at this sacral region may be relatively subcutaneous, particularly in thin patients.

- Gaining exposure in revision cases is particularly difficult. It is generally best to follow the surgical principle of identifying the normal anatomy first. This is accomplished by exposing the cephalad and caudad aspect of the spine first, then carrying the dissection laterally, identifying the facets and remaining pars interarticularis. One can then very carefully dissect medially to identify the medial border of the previous laminectomy defect. With this technique, using small angled cup or ring curettes, the scar tissue can be separated from the medial border of the residual lamina, pars, and facets, thereby exposing the nerve roots and gaining access to the neural foramen. Once all osseous landmarks have been identified, the scar overlying the dorsal aspect of the dura can be thinned. In most cases, it is not necessary to completely excise the remaining midline scar because central stenosis in these revision cases is usually not an issue. Great care should be taken when thinning the midline scar to minimize the possibility of entering into an unrecognized pseudomeningocele.

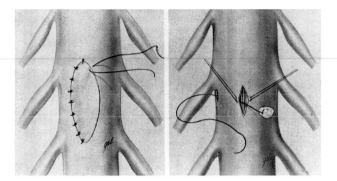

Figure 61–5. Application of a fascial patch graft with multiple interrupted fine sutures. (From Eismont FJ, Wiesel SW, Rothman RH. Treatment of dural tears associated with spinal surgery. J Bone Joint Surg 1981; 63A:1132–1136. With permission.)

plied directly to the dura. Homologous cryoprecipitate is usually used for fibrin glue, but its use carries the risk of viral transmission, specifically the human immunodeficiency virus (HIV) and hepatitis viruses. Use of single-donor homologous cryoprecipitate has reduced, but not eliminated, this risk. Autologous cryoprecipitate can be collected in anticipation of its use for fibrin glue; however, this results in an additional possibly unnecessary expense in these patients because this cryoprecipitate would be used only in the event of inadvertent durotomy. Recently, Baxter Healthcare Corp. began marketing a homologous cryoprecipitate (Tisseel VH) that has been rendered free of potential viruses by a two-step vapor heating process. The manufacturer's literature states that there have been 5 million applications of this product in Europe with no confirmed cases of viral transmission. This product, however, has been approved by the United States Food and Drug Administration (FDA) only for use as a hemostatic agent in cardiac surgery and general surgery, and, as of the date of this writing, has not yet been approved for use in spinal surgery.

Persistent spinal fluid leaks can be subdivided into two categories—those with cutaneous fistulas and those without. The major risk of persistent spinal fluid leaks

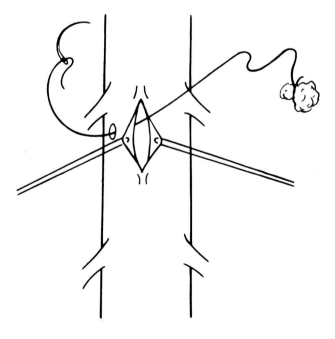

Figure 61–6. A small lateral dural tear can be plugged by creating a midline durotomy and pulling a small piece of muscle or fat attached to a suture that is threaded through the defect. For small tears, hydrostatic pressure is sufficient to keep the graft in place. One or two anchoring sutures may be required for larger defects. (From Mayfield FH, Kurokawa K. Watertight closure of spinal dural mater: technical note. J Neurosurg 1975; 43:639–640. With permission.)

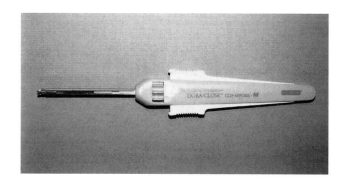

Figure 61–7. The Dura-Close clip applier. Three different sizes of titanium clips are available: 1.4, 2.0, or 3.0 mm.

with cutaneous fistula is that of infection, specifically meningitis. Treatment of these leaks must be addressed on an urgent, if not emergent, basis. Generally, the diagnosis of CSF cutaneous fistulas is not difficult. The patient will have positional headaches in association with a persistent, usually clear, drainage from the wound; most noticeably the headache is markedly exacerbated by standing or sitting and relieved—in some cases completely—by supine or lateral positioning. Valsalva maneuver may increase the amount and rate of drainage. The patient must be evaluated for signs of infection, and appropriate evaluation (to include lumbar puncture and immediate treatment with appropriate antibiotics) must be carried out if meningitis is suspected. In some cases the diagnosis may be in question, even in the presence of a CSF fistula. Magnetic resonance imaging (MRI) or myelogram with postmyelogram CT scanning is appropriate in these instances. These studies may also be appropriate as a preoperative planning tool in certain cases in which questions remain as to the anatomic location and extent of the dural tear. Immunofixation of B2 (beta-2) transferrin of the draining fluid has been described as a diagnostic procedure that can confirm the diagnosis of CSF fistula.

Persistent spinal fluid leaks without cutaneous fistula with subcutaneous or subfascial CSF collections, although often significantly symptomatic, do not carry the same relative level of urgency for management. In patients in whom there is a suspicion of a CSF leakage without fistula, either MRI or myelogram and postmyelogram CT is generally indicated to identify the location of the leak and confirm the diagnosis. Pseudomeningoceles are large CSF collections resulting from chronic, often unrecognized, dural leaks. Neural tissue may migrate into pseudomeningoceles, potentially resulting in neurologic deficit. Pseudomeningoceles may also produce neurologic deficit by compression of the thecal sac or exiting nerve roots.

Management of CSF cutaneous fistula consists of wound reexploration and direct repair with supplemental fat graft application, or fascial graft application as indicated by the extent of the tear. We recommend the use of fibrin glue in surgical reexplorations for persistent spinal fluid leak. If a pseudomeningocele is identified at the time of reexploration, care should be taken to carefully reduce any displaced nerve roots into the thecal sac prior to repair or grafting. The patient is to be kept from sitting or standing for up to 4 days.

Alternative Methods of Treatment

Kitchel and colleagues (1989) have recommended the use of closed lumbar drainage for treatment of persistent CSF leak. This technique consists of percutaneous intradural placement of a standard 25-gauge epidural catheter into the thecal sac; 200

to 300 cc of spinal fluid is drained per day, with the amount of drainage controlled by elevation of the collection bag. Daily laboratory assessment of the CSF drainage is mandatory to include culture, cell count and differential, and determination of glucose and protein levels. Four days of treatment is recommended, but success was reported in this series in one of the two cases with early catheter removal. Of the 17 patients in their series in whom the catheter remained in place for 4 days, 14 had successful resolution of their CSF leak. The remaining three patients underwent successful surgical repair.

Autologous blood patch has also been employed in patients with persistent CSF leak following lumbar surgery. This technique is probably best suited for very small dural tears in patients who have undergone either laminotomy or single-level laminectomies.

Type of Management	Advantages	Disadvantages	Comments
Surgical exploration with repair	Addresses the problem at its source	Requires a surgical procedure; persistent leakage possible	The "gold standard" treatment for persistent cerebrospinal fluid leak
Surgical exploration with repair supplemented with fibrin glue	A "belts and suspenders" technique, may allow earlier mobilization of patient	Potential for viral disease transmission	Fibrin glue should be considered a reinforcement rather than a substitute for direct dural repair
Closed lumbar drainage	Surgery potentially avoided	Requires 4 days of hospitalization; risk of meningitis; careful monitoring by physician and nursing staff mandatory; not universally successful	Ideally suited for patients with small, closed, persistent leaks and leaks that are in surgically inaccessible regions
Blood patch	Simple procedure to perform	Lowest success rate of all management techniques; not suited for patients with extensive laminectomies	Best suited for patients with 1–2 mm persistent tears in wounds without extensive dead space

Complications

Complications of persistent CSF leak include nerve root entrapment or compression, infection (including meningitis), persistent positional headache, and nausea. Nerve root entrapment or nerve root compression is generally addressed by surgical correction and reduction of the nerve roots. Meningitis is best treated with appropriate antibiotic treatment based on CSF culture obtained at the time of lumbar puncture. Clinical suspicion and early diagnosis is critical. The headaches and nausea of persistent CSF leakage are treated by positioning the patient in such a manner as to minimize the amount of leakage. Generally, patients with lumbar CSF leaks are best relieved by supine or supine positioning with log-rolling. Analgesics may be helpful, but are usually inadequate without appropriate positioning. Associated nausea may respond to treatment with antiemetics.

Suggested Readings

Eismont FJ, Wiesel SW, Rothman RH. Treatment of dural tears associated with spinal surgery. J Bone Joint Surg 1981; 63A:1132–1136.

Jane JA. Neurosurgical application of fibrin glue: augmentation of dural closure in 134 patients. Neurosurgery 1990; 26:207–210.

Kitchel SH, Eismont FJ, Green BA. Closed subarachnoid drainage for management of cerebrospinal fluid leakage after an operation on the spine. J Bone Joint Surg 1989; 71A:984–987.

Mayfield FH, Kurokawa K. Watertight closure of spinal dural mater: technical note. J Neurosurg 1975; 43:639–640.

McCormack BM, Zide BM, Kalfas IH. Cerebrospinal fluid fistula and pseudomeningocele after spine surgery. In: Benzel EC, ed. Spine Surgery: Techniques, Complication Avoidance, and Management, 1st ed., pp. 1465–1474. Philadelphia: Churchill Livingstone, 1999.

Morris GF, Marshall LF. Cerebrospinal fluid leaks: etiology and treatment. In: Herkowitz HN, Garfin SR, Balderston RA, et al, eds. Rothman-Simeone: The Spine, 4th ed., pp. 1733–1738. Philadelphia: WB Saunders, 1999.

Wang JC, Bohlman, HH, Riew KD. Dural tears secondary to operations on the lumbar spine. Management and results after a two-year-minimum follow-up of eighty-eight patients. J Bone Joint Surg 1998; 80A(12):1728–1732.

Case 62
Syringomyelia and Scoliosis
Kirkham B. Wood and Francis Denis

History and Physical Examination

A 5-year-old girl presented for examination of a spinal deformity first noticed by her mother 3 months earlier. She had been born of a normal pregnancy and vaginal delivery, and had developed appropriately for her age. There was no family history of spinal deformity. Her past medical history was significant only for recurrent otitis. There were no complaints of back pain, leg numbness, or tingling, nor had there been any urinary or bowel problems. On physical examination, her height was 109 cm and her weight 18 kg. She ambulated normally without limp. Examination of her back revealed the right shoulder to be elevated 2 cm with her

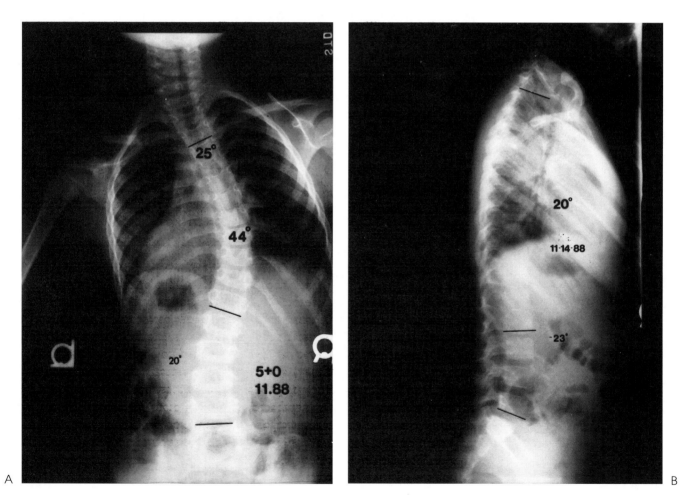

A   B

Figure 62–1. Posteroanterior (PA) (A) and sagittal (B) radiographs demonstrating 44 degree scoliosis convex to the right (A). Note severity of truncal shift despite relatively mild axial plane vertebral rotation. These are characteristics somewhat more suggestive of neuropathic causes as opposed to idiopathic scoliosis. Note negative T1 tilt.

head decompensated 1 cm to the left of the natal cleft. On forward bending, the right thorax was 2 cm prominent. There were no hairy patches, nevi, dimples, or café-au-lait spots. Her feet were symmetrical without evidence of cavovarus deformity; however, the left calf measured 1 cm less circumferentially than the right. The ankle reflex on the right was 1+; however, it was absent on the left. Motor strength in all muscle groups of the upper and lower extremities was 5/5, and sensation was intact to light touch and pinprick. Distal extremity and radial pulses were equal.

Radiologic Findings

Standing posteroanterior (PA) and lateral radiographs of the spine (Fig. 62–1) revealed a right thoracic scoliosis from T6 to T12, apex T9, measuring 44 degrees. A compensatory curve extended from C5 to T6 convex to the left measuring 25 degrees. The sagittal radiograph revealed a kyphosis of 20 degrees. Magnetic resonance imaging (MRI) examination of the brain stem and spinal cord revealed a multiloculated central cyst within the spinal cord extending from C2 to T9, associated with caudal herniation of the cerebellar tonsils through the foramen magnum (Fig. 62–2). Void artifact within many of the spinal cord cavities suggests continued pulsatile flow enlarging the defect.

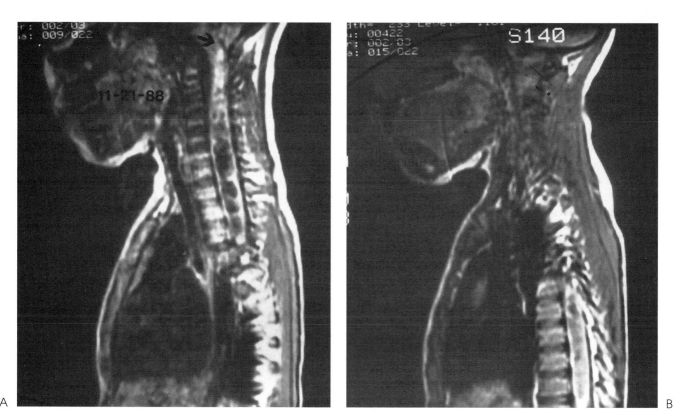

Figure 62–2. Magnetic resonance imaging (MRI) of the hindbrain and spinal cord reveals a Chiari I malformation of the hindbrain with herniation of the cerebellar tonsils through the foramen magnum (large arrow, A) and a cavitated syrinx extending through the cervical into the thoracic spinal cord (B). The void artifact seen within the syrinx suggests pulsatile flow.

- The diagnosis of central nervous system pathology associated with spinal deformity almost always requires a careful and systematic physical examination with particular attention to the neurologic exam and reflexes. Frequently, as in the case presented here, the only clue to neuropathology might be a subtle change in the size of a limb, or the strength of a particular muscle when compared with its counterpart. Asymmetries or absence of the abdominal reflexes are many times the only sign that a central nervous system disorder exists.
- The scoliotic curves associated with various central neuropathies often display features that may distinguish them from similar albeit more common idiopathic curves. Viewed in the coronal plane, they will often appear to be somewhat longer or more sweeping—a "spasm character"—than the idiopathic variety, frequently with more shoulder and truncal imbalance, yet interestingly with less vertebral rotation—features commonly associated with more paralytic or neuromuscular deformities. The tilt of T1 may also be particularly negative (Fig. 62-1), something not commonly seen in true idiopathic curves.
- Left thoracic curves have traditionally been associated with syringomyelia and prompted evaluation with MRI. This right thoracic curve associated with a syrinx reminds us to increase our index of suspicion beyond the typical left thoracic deformity.

Diagnosis

Right thoracic scoliosis secondary to syringomyelia associated with Arnold-Chiari I malformation. The right thoracic curve pattern is similar to that of idiopathic scoliosis; however, some features are reminiscent of neuromuscular or paralytic-type scoliosis. As the herniation of the cerebellar tonsils is through the foramen magnum, it is classified as an Arnold-Chiari type I malformation. Chiari type II malformation would include caudal displacement of the cerebellar vermis, fourth ventricle, and lower brain stem below the foramen magnum typically associated with myelodysplasia. The syringomyelia is felt to be a result of a disturbance of normal cerebrospinal fluid (CSF) dynamics due in large part to the displaced hindbrain at the cervical medullary junction.

Surgical Management

Under general endotracheal anesthesia with the patient in the prone position in a Craig headrest, a midline incision was made from the occiput to the midcervical spine. The suboccipital bone and the posterior arches of C1 and C2 were exposed and removed with the suboccipital craniectomy measuring $1 \times 2\frac{1}{2}$ cm. The dura was opened, resulting in an abundant outflow of spinal fluid. At the C1/C2 level the tips of the cerebellar tonsils were seen markedly herniating through the foramen magnum. The cisterna magna was opened at the level of the foramen magnum and the tonsillar tips were separated by tacking them up to the dura, resulting in opening of the foramen of Magendie. With excellent CSF flow with the tonsils tacked back, it was not felt to be necessary to shunt the syrinx. The dura was closed with a patch graft from the deep fascia. The wound was closed in multiple layers of absorbable suture and the skin was approximated with running nylon suture.

Postoperative Management

The patient tolerated the procedure well and was up and ambulating in the hospital in 3 days and discharged on postoperative day 4. The nylon sutures were removed on postoperative day 7.

As early as 4 months after her cervicomedullary decompression, her shoulders were nearly level, and her right thoracic prominence was only 1.5 cm. Her motor and sensory exams were normal, although the left ankle reflex remained absent. PA radiograph of the spine revealed the right thoracic scoliosis now measuring 25 degrees, with 15 degrees of residual cervicothoracic compensatory curve (Fig. 62–3). At 1 year postdecompression, her right thoracic prominence was only 1 cm, and her scoliosis measured 17 degrees (Fig. 62–4). A repeat MRI revealed significant diminution of her syringomyelia (Fig. 62–5). At 10 years postdecompression, age 15 years 5 months, she was active with no musculoskeletal complaints. Her physical examination revealed level shoulders, negligible thoracic prominence, and a normal motor, sensory, and reflex examination. Standing PA radiographs reveal a right thoracic curve measuring 10 degrees (Fig. 62–6). Follow-up MRI of the spine reveals near complete collapse of the syrinx, now measuring only 1 to 2 mm from C5 to the midthoracic spine (Fig. 62–7).

• If surgery is performed for scoliosis associated with syringomyelia, a few points bear mentioning: (1) As the cord itself is frequently dilated, the placement of hooks or sublaminar wires into the canal should be minimized. (2) Care should be exercised when decorticating the posterior structures as the protective layer of CSF is less than normal and spinal cord concussion may ensue. (3) Spinal cord monitoring is encouraged and a wake-up test should be performed. (4) If possible, titanium instrumentation should be used so as to follow the syrinx with MRI postoperatively. (5) Associated tight filum terminale or other signs of conus medullaris tethering mechanisms should be ruled out.

Discussion

Frequently, treatment of scoliosis associated with syringomyelia involves definitive treatment of the central nervous system pathology itself. The therapeutic surgical treatment addresses the very etiology of the syrinx, that is, the Arnold-Chiari I malformation. The hydrodynamic theory of hydrosyringomyelia suggests that because the normal outlets of the ventricles have been obstructed, pulsatile flow is redirected down the central canal, causing it to dilate. In most cases, such as the one presented here, with a syrinx and Chiari I malformation, surgery will involve occipitocervical decompression and correction of the cerebellar tonsil herniation so as to restore normal CSF hydrodynamics.

Provided the scoliosis is reasonably flexible, and sufficient growth potential remains, it will normally regress spontaneously following neurosurgical decompression of a Chiari I malformation/syringomyelia. If not, then the scoliosis treatment is similar to that for idiopathic scoliosis, including orthotic containment and or surgery.

Finally, it is important to make sure that other etiologic possibilities of the syringomyelia have been either ruled out or treated. Children often present with many factors contributing to the production of the cyst, and if unrecognized, the treatment, operative or not, may fail. An example would be an individual with scoliosis, a syrinx, hydrocephalus, a Chiari malformation, and a tight filum terminale.

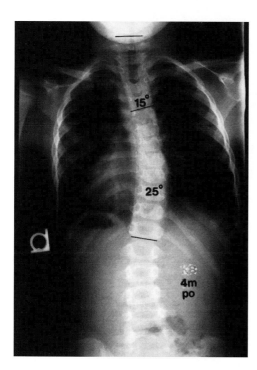

Figure 62–3. PA radiograph at 4 months postdecompression reveals reduction of the thoracic scoliosis to 25

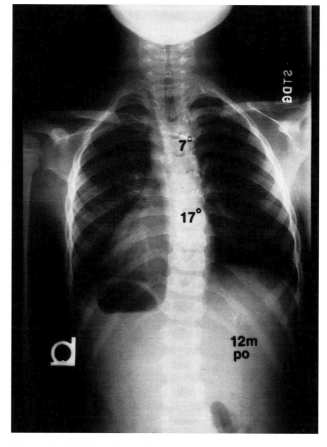

Figure 62–4. PA radiograph at 12 months postdecompression reveals the thoracic scoliosis to now measure 17 degrees.

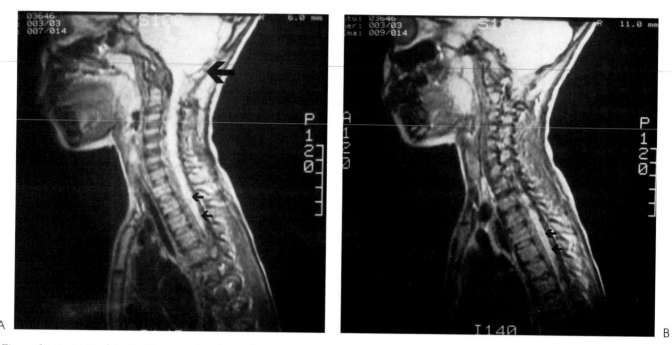

Figure 62–5. MRI of the hindbrain and spinal cord at 12 months postdecompression reveals the cerebellar tonsils well placed above the foramen magnum (large arrow, A), and the spinal cord syrinx to be dramatically reduced in size (small arrows, B).

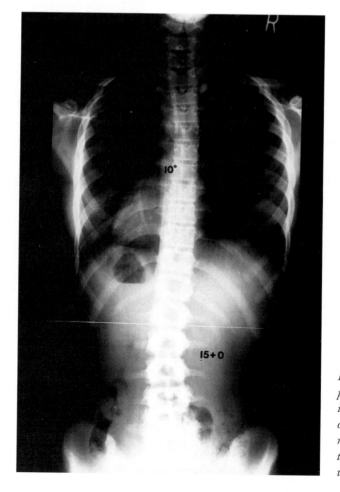

Figure 62–6. At 10 years postdecompression the subject is without symptoms. PA radiographs reveal mild right thoracic curvature of 10 degrees; the patient is well balanced with level shoulders.

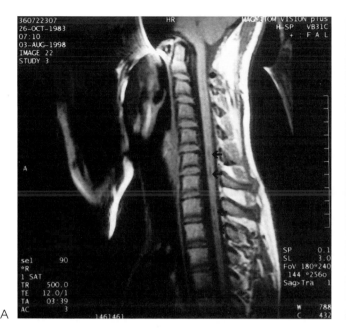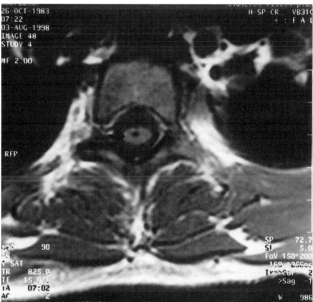

Figure 62–7. Final MRI examination at 10 years postdecompression reveals maintenance of the neurosurgical correction (A). Axial images show only 1 to 2 mm of cystic cavitation (B).

This patient may require multiple surgical approaches prior to the resolution of the syrinx.

Alternative Methods of Management

As the primary abnormality is a structural one (i.e., the craniocervical compression), there are no medical options for its correction. If the scoliosis is rapidly progressive, it may be braced as in idiopathic scoliosis or surgically corrected if it worsens much past 45 or 50 degrees.

As for the syringomyelia, if the patient is asymptomatic, with minimal scoliosis (i.e., <20 degrees) clinical observation is possible; however, it should be closely monitored, for the natural history of many patients with cystic cavitation of the spinal cord can be progressive loss of neurologic function over years.

Following craniocervical junction decompression, if it appears at all likely that less than normal CSF flow has been restored, or there is any evidence of persisting syringomyelia, insertion of a syringosubarachnoid shunt should be considered. Whenever hydrocephalus is present, it may have to be promptly addressed with ventriculoperitoneal shunting.

Type of Management	Advantages	Disadvantages	Comments
Nonoperative	Minimal risk	Scoliosis may progress; neurologic symptoms typically worsen over time	Natural history of spinal deformities associated with neural axis pathology unknown
Occipital-cervical decompression	Corrects the neuropathology; scoliosis may resolve spontaneously	Risk of injury to the structures of the cerebellum, hindbrain, cranial nerves	Primary goal is the restoration of normal cerebrospinal fluid dynamics
Syringosubarachnoid shunt	May deflate the syrinx	Palliative procedure may need revision	Frequently leads to painful paresthesias due to myelostomy
Scoliosis correction: instrumentation and fusion	Immediate correction; three dimensional	Risk of injury to the neural structures is heightened	Tethering of the cord, if present, must be released primarily

Complications

Complications associated with decompression of the cerebrocervical junction for Chiari malformation include infection, postoperative meningocele, postoperative CSF leak, and bulbar nerve palsy. Infection (meningitis) is managed by the use of appropriate prophylactic antibiotics pre- and postoperatively as well as meticulous surgical technique. Postoperative meningocele or pseudomeningocele as well as postoperative CSF leakage are prevented by carefully sizing an appropriate dural fascia graft and obtaining watertight closure. Bulbar nerve palsy is a rare complication and may be due to excessive removal of occipital bone during the decompression, allowing descent of the hindbrain with resultant traction on the lower cranial nerves. Most cases, however, are temporary and resolve with observation.

Suggested Readings

Denis F. Spinal deformities associated with syringomyelia. Spine: State of the Art Rev 1998; 12(1):21–31.

Dyste GN, Menezes AH. Presentation and management of pediatric Chiari malformations without myelodysplasia. Neurosurgery 1988; 23:589–597.

Nohria V, Oakes WJ. Chiari I malformation: a review of 43 patients. Pediatr Neurosurg 1992; 16:222–227.

Case 63
Vascular Malformations of the Spinal Cord

James S. Harrop and Gregory J. Przybylski

History and Physical Examination

A 65-year-old woman was hospitalized for acute severe paraparesis. She had years of low back pain with an initial gradual decline in lower limb strength over 18 months. She was diagnosed with neurogenic claudication from lumbar stenosis. However, over several recent months she developed brief episodes of sudden leg weakness not associated with neurogenic claudication that spontaneously resolved over minutes to hours. During these events, she sustained multiple falls and described a change in the quality of her back pain. The episodes became more frequent and lasted longer until her paraparesis persisted. Moreover, she had urinary incontinence and fecal urgency. Examination revealed severe paraparesis, with less than antigravity strength in all muscles except the quadriceps. Sensation was diminished below the midthoracic region inferiorly. She was hyporeflexic with bilateral flexor plantar responses. Her rectal tone was diminished. She had no cutaneous lesions or bruits over the spine.

Radiologic Findings

Plain anteroposterior and lateral radiographs of the thoracic and lumbar spine demonstrated lumbar spondylosis. Abnormal signal in the conus medullaris on T2-weighted magnetic resonance imaging (MRI) of the lumbar spine prompted thoracic imaging, which revealed serpiginous, serpentine flow voids (Fig. 63–1). These

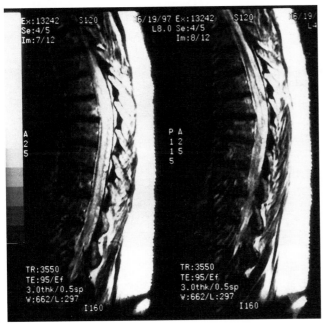

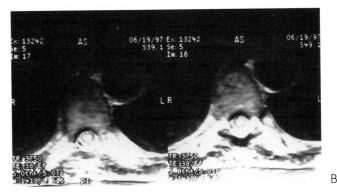

Figure 63–1. Sagittal (A) and axial (B) T2-weighted magnetic resonance imaging (MRI) of the thoracic spine demonstrates increased spinal cord signal intensity and serpiginous flow voids representing dilated extramedullary veins.

represent dilated extramedullary veins, whereas increased signal intensity in the spinal cord results from venous hypertension. Selective angiography failed to identify the site of the suspected arteriovenous fistula. An anteroposterior myelogram confirmed the serpiginous vessels (Fig. 63–2A), but additionally demonstrated a single draining vein toward the right at T6 (Fig. 63–2B). Axial computed tomography (CT) after myelography likewise demonstrated the single draining vein (Fig. 63–3).

Diagnosis

The patient was diagnosed with a spinal arteriovenous malformation (AVM), also termed a dural arteriovenous malformation. Preoperative imaging demonstrating a single draining vein suggested a diagnosis of a type IA spinal AVM, whereas a fistula with multiple draining veins would be classified as type 1B. The remaining spinal AVMs (types II–IV) are intradural malformations, which are much less common.

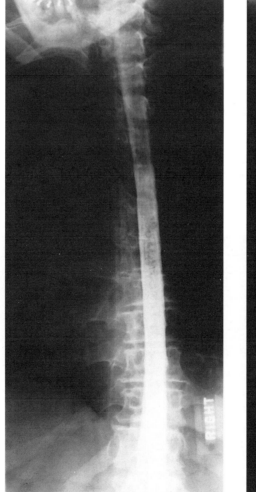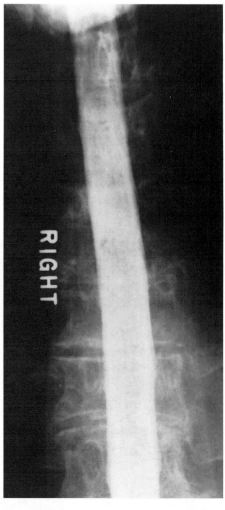

A   B

Figure 63–2. Anteroposterior thoracic myelography (A) demonstrates serpiginous flow voids representing dilated extramedullary veins. A magnified view (B) shows a single draining vein to the right at T6.

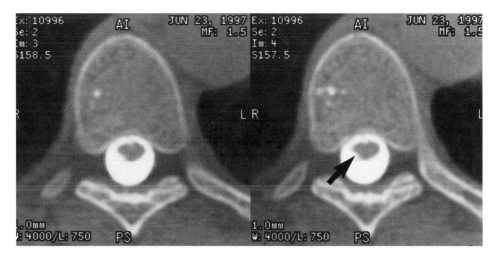

Figure 63–3. Postmyelographic axial computed tomography (CT) demonstrates a single draining vein (arrow) leaving the spinal cord at the T6 level.

Surgical Management

Preoperative management included intravenous steroid infusion and a thorough urologic examination with urodynamic testing. The patient was given perioperative intravenous antibiotics. Neurophysiologic monitoring of both somatosensory and motor evoked potentials was begun prior to induction of general anesthesia and continued until closure of the surgical wound. The patient was then positioned prone on longitudinally oriented, padded rolls and her head was supported in a Mayfield headrest. The entire thoracic spinal region was prepped with Betadine in case additional levels of venous drainage were identified.

A midline incision with subperiosteal dissection laterally to the facet joints was completed to expose the dorsal elements from T5 to T8 as identified by an intraoperative anteroposterior radiograph. A four-level en block laminectomy was performed by drilling troughs at the lateral laminar border and detaching the flaval ligament at the rostral and caudal ends with a curette. In the absence of angiographic confirmation, this additional bony exposure was performed to be certain to identify additional adjacent draining veins that the myelogram might not have demonstrated. Thin strips of Surgicel were placed in the epidural space underneath the medial facets to assist with hemostasis after the intrathecal pressure is reduced by dural opening.

The dura was incised in the midline and edges were sutured laterally, thereby exposing the dorsal spinal cord. The arachnoid layer was opened separately. There were many large arterialized veins observed on the dorsal surface of the spinal cord (Fig. 63–4). The operating microscope was utilized to facilitate microdissection. An arterialized vein at the T6 level extending to the right was identified and traced back laterally to the dural edge, where the site of the fistula was observed. Sharp dissection was performed to avoid avulsion of the veins, which might impair normal spinal venous drainage. As with most of these malformations, the fistula was intradural at the root sleeve. A temporary aneurysm clip was placed on the arterialized vein while evoked potentials were carefully monitored for changes in amplitude or latency. Such an alteration implies that the occluded vessel represents a radicular artery rather than an arterialized draining vein; temporary occlusion should be dis-

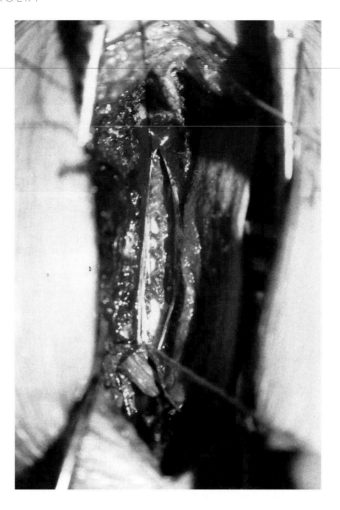

Figure 63–4. Intradural exposure reveals many dilated, arterialized veins on the spinal cord surface.

continued and a further search for the fistula must commence. The site of the fistula and the arterialized draining vein were obliterated with bipolar cautery and division.

A gradual change in the color of surface veins on the spinal cord from bright to dark red accompanied by a reduction in turgor was observed over a 10-minute interval. If this change is not seen after dividing the vein, then additional vessels contributing to the fistula must be present and should be treated similarly. Once venous hypertension has been eliminated, dural closure with a running, locked 4-0 neurolon suture is completed. A laminoplasty was performed and the fascial, subcutaneous, and skin layers were individually closed.

Postoperative Management

A neurologic examination was performed after completion of general anesthesia. Her neurologic condition was monitored overnight in an intermediate intensive care unit. She was mobilized out of bed on the second postoperative day. The patient perceived immediate improvements in sensation and motor function. Physical therapy was begun and continued in a rehabilitation center. She recovered lower limb strength and ambulated independently by 5 months after treatment. However, bowel and bladder function remained impaired at 17 months. Postoperative MRI (Fig. 63–5) at 16 months demonstrated resolution of the abnormal cord signal and serpiginous vessels. If the fistula had been angiographically demonstrated, an immediate intraoperative or postoperative angiogram would have been performed to confirm obliteration of the fistula.

Discussion

Spinal AVMs are broadly classified by intradural and extradural location. The latter malformation, as seen in this patient, has a slow-flow arteriovenous fistula. Venous hypertension causes the neurologic dysfunction. A single draining vein is characteristic of a type IA spinal AVM, whereas multiple fistula sites are termed type IB. The fistulas are acquired during life and are most commonly seen in men older than 40. Their clinical course is marked by episodic paraparesis superimposed on progressive lower limb weakness and numbness as well as bowel and bladder dysfunction. The fistulas are usually located in the thoracolumbar region.

In contrast, the less common intradural vascular malformations are high-flow malformations. These typically occur in younger patients and are likely congenital lesions. Acute neurologic deterioration is observed after hemorrhage. These spinal AVMs are located throughout the spinal cord and occur with equal frequency in males and females.

The pathophysiology of the spinal arteriovenous fistula (type I spinal AVM) is related to venous hypertension and associated neuronal edema. Persistent venous hypertension can progress to cause vascular thrombosis and a necrotic myelopathy termed Foix-Alajouanine syndrome. Therefore, the treatment objective is to eliminate the venous hypertension by obliterating the arteriovenous fistula. This type of malformation is formed by an abnormal anastomosis between the dural branch of a radicular artery and a medullary vein of the spinal cord, causing direct transmission of intraarterial pressure to the spinal cord through the vein.

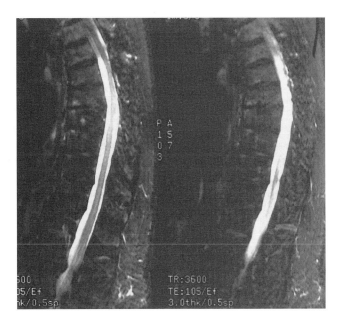

Figure 63–5. Postoperative sagittal T2-weighted MRI reveals resolution of the abnormal spinal cord signal intensity and absence of dilated serpiginous vessels.

MRI can demonstrate the serpiginous vessels and spinal cord edema that can occur with spinal AVMs. Although selective spinal angiography may identify the location of the fistula, the small diameter of the radicular arteries may impede successful catheterization during angiography. Alternatively, a double-contrast spinal myelogram may also identify the site of the fistula.

Successful treatment of the fistula requires interruption of the flow of high pressure arterial blood through the medullary vein. Typically, the dural fistula only drains via the intradural medullary vein and can be managed by coagulation and division of the vein as it enters the dura. Although the dilated medullary veins were once considered pathologic and were dissected off the cord, some patients sustained neurologic injury from resection of these normal venous drainage channels. Currently, the dilated arterialized veins are considered to be a response to the fistula, and they return to their normal size and function after obliteration of the fistula alone. When resecting the fistula, the surgeon must be careful to identify the function of the arterial branch to avoid spinal cord infarction. Preoperative arteriography may help identify the normal arterial supply of the spinal cord. Moreover, intraoperative temporary occlusion with electrophysiologic monitoring can help determine whether the artery can be sacrificed. Otherwise, only the venous component of the fistula should be resected. Patients with intradural and extradural venous drainage require either obliteration of both components or resection of the fistula site. After obliteration of the fistula, the dilated, bright red medullary veins should gradually darken as arterialized blood flow disappears.

The damage of nervous tissue from the venous hypertension is progressive. Patients treated earlier have the best outcome. Therefore, it is imperative to have a high index of suspicion to diagnose these lesions to maximize neurologic recovery.

Alternative Methods of Management

Direct surgical exposure and resection may be avoided in angiographically demonstrated fistulas. Endovascular techniques can occlude the fistula through direct microcatheterization and embolization. However, this technique requires angiographic identification of the fistula by selective microcatheterization of the arterial supply, which does not directly flow to the spinal cord. Inadvertent embolization of an arterial supply to the spinal cord may cause infarction and irreversible paraplegia. However, endovascular treatment enables the surgeon to identify and eliminate the fistula without open surgical exposure. Additional levels of the fistula can be similarly treated, and obliteration can be confirmed angiographically at the end of the procedure. Medical management with intravenous corticosteroids alone is ineffective because the venous hypertension from the fistula will continue to cause progressive spinal cord damage. Another treatment option being investigated involves the use of stereotactic radiosurgery for the obliteration of the lesion. This has been used for certain intradural AVMs (types 2 and 3), but has not been used for the more common type I arteriovenous fistula.

Type of Management	Advantages	Disadvantages	Comments
Open obliteration	Direct visualization; easier identification of multiple sites	Additional associated complications	Obliteration confirmed by direct inspection
Endovascular obliteration	Minimally invasive	Requires angiographic demonstration; selective catheterization difficult	Works well for angiographically demonstrated type IA arteriovenous malformation
Stereotactic radiosurgery	Minimally invasive	Investigational; risk of spinal cord injury	Used for types 2 and 3
Steroid therapy	Noninvasive	Provides transient improvement only	Should not be performed alone

Complications

Complications of any open surgical technique include infection and bleeding. Moreover, meningitis is an additional infectious risk related to dural opening. Cerebrospinal fluid leak and pseudomeningocele formation may occur. Although these risks are absent from endovascular techniques, femoral hematoma and arterial dissection are additional complications of this treatment method. Incomplete obliteration may result from failure to treat multiple sites of fistula formation. Inadvertent obliteration of the arterial supply to the spinal cord may cause infarction if the collateral circulation is insufficient. Both intradural and extradural venous drainage should be identified and eliminated to prevent recurrence of the fistula through a different drainage pathway.

Suggested Readings

Afshar JK, Doppman JL, Oldfield EH. Surgical interruption of intradural draining vein as curative treatment of spinal dural arteriovenous fistula. J Neurosurg 1995; 82:196–200.

Criscuolo GR, Oldfield EH, Doppman JL. Reversible acute and subacute myelopathy in patients with dural arteriovenous fistulas. J Neurosurg 1989; 70:354–359.

Niimi Y, Berenstein A, Setton A, Neophytides A. Embolization of spinal dural arteriovenous fistulae: results and follow-up. Neurosurgery 1997; 40:675–683.

Oldfield EH, Doppman JL. Spinal arteriovenous malformations. Clin Neurosurg 1988; 34:161–183.

Index

Achondroplasia cervical postlaminectomy
        kyphosis, 479–483
    diagnosis, 480
    management, 482
        alternative methods, 482
        surgical, 480
    patient history, 479–480
    physical examination, 479–480
    radiologic findings, 480
Acupuncture, for axial low back pain, 82
Adolescent idiopathic scoliosis, 401–410
    complications of, 409–410
    diagnosis, 402
    management, 409
        alternative methods, 408
        postoperative, 405
        surgical, 402–405
    patient history, 401–402
    physical examination, 401–402
    radiologic findings, 402
Ankylosing spondylitis, cervical osteotomy,
        215–219
    anesthesia with spinal cord, nerve
            monitoring, segmental internal
            fixation, 218
    complications of, 218–219
    diagnosis, 216
    management, 218
        alternative methods, 218
        nonoperative, 218
        surgical, 216
    patient history, 215
    physical examination, 215
    radiologic findings, 215–216
Antibiotics, gunshot wounds, cervical spine,
        thoracic spine, lumbar spine, 340
Arachnoid cyst, intradural disc herniation,
        lumbar spine, 154–155
Arachnoiditis, intradural disc herniation,
        lumbar spine, 155
Arthritis cranial–C1/C2 disease, 189–198
    atlantoaxial subluxation, 191
    diagnosis, 190
    external fixation—halo, 197
    internal posterior fixation—wiring, 197
        with transarticular screws, 197
    management, 196
        alternative methods, 196–197
        nonoperative, 192
        surgical, 192–196
    nonoperative therapy, 196
    observation, 196
    odontoid, superior migration of, 191–192
    patient history, 189
    patterns of involvement, 191–192
    physical examination, 189
    radiologic findings, 189–190
Arthroscopic microdiscectomy, recurrent
        lumbar disc herniation, 148
Astrocytomas, 384

Atlantoaxial rotatory deformity, traumatic,
        fixed, 305–312
    anterior decompression, with transoral
            approach, 311
    arthrodesis in situ, 311
    closed cervical reduction
        external immobilization, 311
        posterior arthrodesis, with internal
                fixation, 311
    collar immobilization, 311
    diagnosis, 306–307
    halo-Ilizarov distraction cast, 311
    halo immobilization, 311
    management, 311
        alternative methods, 310–311
        nonsurgical, 307
        postoperative, 308
        surgical, 308
    open reduction, with lateral approaches, 311
    patient history, 305–306
    physical examination, 305–306
    radiologic findings, 306–307
Axial back pain
    lumbar degenerative disc disease
        anterior approach, 84–92
        anterior lumbar interbody fusion
                with allograft dowels, 92
                with cages, 92
        circumferential fusion, with anterior graft,
                fixation posteriorly, 92
        diagnosis, 85
        management, 92
            alternative methods, 91–92
            conservative, 92
            postoperative, 86–89
            surgical, 85–86
        patient history, 84–85
        physical examination, 84–85
        PLIF with bone dowels, rectangular
                grafts, 92
        posterolateral fusion, with, without
                pedicle fixation, 92
        radiologic findings, 85
    minimally invasive laparoscopic approach,
            136–142
        antiinflammatory medication, 141
        circumferential fusion, anterior, posterior,
                141
        complications of, 142
        diagnosis, 137
        management, 141
            alternative methods, 141–142
            postoperative, 140
            surgical, 137–139
        patient history, 136
        pedicle screws, 141
        physical examination, 136
        physical therapy, 141
        radiologic findings, 137
        spinal injections, 141

Axial back pain (*continued*)
  nonoperative approach, 78–83
    acupuncture, 82
    diagnosis, 79
    magnets, 82
    management, 79–80, 82
      alternative methods, 82
    manipulation, 82
    patient history, 78–79
    physical examination, 78–79
    prolotherapy, 82
    radiologic findings, 79
Axial neck pain, 3–9
  active assisted, 9
  cervical collar, 9
  cervical manipulation, 9
  cold, 9
  diagnosis, 4
  electrical stimulation, 9
  heat, 9
  management, 8–9
    nonoperative, 4–5
      clinical assessment, 5–6
      diagnostic tests, 6–7
      physical measures, 7–8
      treatment, 7
  manual traction, 9
  massage, 9
  mechanical traction, 9
  medications, 8–9
  modalities, 9
  muscle relaxants, 9
  narcotics, 8
  nonoperative approach, 3–9
  nonsteroidal antiinflammatory drugs, 8
  oral steroids, 8
  passive, 9
  patient history, 304
  physical measures, 9
  physical therapy, 9
  plain X-ray, 4
  radiologic findings, 4
  strengthening, 9
  tricyclic low-dose antidepressant, 9
  ultrasound, 9

Back pain
  axial, lumbar degenerative disc disease,
      anterior approach, 84–92
    anterior lumbar interbody fusion
      with allograft dowels, 92
      with cages, 92
    circumferential fusion, with anterior graft,
      fixation posteriorly, 92
    diagnosis, 85
    management, 92
      alternative methods, 91–92
      conservative, 92
      postoperative, 86–89
      surgical, 85–86
    patient history, 84–85
    physical examination, 84–85
    PLIF with bone dowels, rectangular
      grafts, 92

    posterolateral fusion, with, without
      pedicle fixation, 92
    radiologic findings, 85
  low, axial
    lumbar degenerative disc disease,
      minimally invasive laparoscopic
      approach, 136–142
      antiinflammatory medication, 141
      circumferential fusion, anterior,
        posterior, 141
      complications of, 142
    diagnosis, 137
    management, 141
      alternative methods, 141–142
      postoperative, 140
      surgical, 137–139
    patient history, 136
    pedicle screws, 141
    physical examination, 136
    physical therapy, 141
    radiologic findings, 137
    spinal injections, 141
  nonoperative approach, 78–83
    acupuncture, 82
    diagnosis, 79
    magnets, 82
    management, 79–80, 82
      alternative methods, 82
    manipulation, 82
    patient history, 78–79
    physical examination, 78–79
    prolotherapy, 82
    radiologic findings, 79
Back surgery, failed, syndrome, 172–177
  anterior spinal fusion, with instrumentation,
    178
  bracing, with, without exercise, 178
  diagnosis, 173
  management, 178
    alternative methods, 177
    postoperative, 174
    surgical, 173–174
  patient history, 172–173
  physical examination, 172–173
  posterior spinal fusion, with
    instrumentation, 178
  radiologic findings, 173
Biphosphonates, Pagetoid disease of spine,
    236–237
Bowel program, spinal cord injury, 286
Bridging plate, cervical spondylosis—
    myelopathy, 43
Buttress plate, cervical spondylosis—
    myelopathy, 44

Calcitonin, Pagetoid disease of spine, 236, 237
Cervical collar, with axial neck pain, 9
Cervical facet joint dislocation, bilateral,
    without neurologic deficit, 297–304
  anterior cervical discectomy followed by
    posterior then anterior cervical fusion,
    303
  anterior cervical discectomy with fusion,
    302

diagnosis, 298
halo immobilization, 302
management, 302–303
    alternative methods, 302–303
    nonsurgical, 298
    surgical, 299–300
patient history, 297
physical examination, 297
posterior cervical fusion
    with interspinous wiring, 302
    with lateral mass plates and screws, 302
    with pedicle screws, 302
radiologic findings, 297–298
Cervical manipulation, with axial neck pain, 9
Cervical osteotomy, ankylosing spondylitis, 215–219
    anesthesia with spinal cord, nerve monitoring, segmental internal fixation, 218
    complications of, 218–219
    diagnosis, 216
    management, 218
        alternative methods, 218
        nonoperative, 218
        surgical, 216
    patient history, 215
    physical examination, 215
    radiologic findings, 215–216
Cervical spine
    gunshot wound, 336–341
        antibiotics, 340
        bracing, 340
        management, 340
            alternative methods, 340
            postoperative, 338
            surgical, 337
        patient history, 336–337
        physical examination, 336–337
        radiologic findings, 337
        steroids, 340
        surgical decompression, 340
        surgical stabilization, 340
        tetanus prophylaxis, 340
        timing of surgery, 340
    metastatic disease, 366–377
        anterior/posterior procedures, 374
        anterior procedures, 373
        clinical presentation, 371–372
        complications of, 376
        diagnosis, 368
        management, 372–373, 375
            alternative methods, 375
            anterior, 375
            postoperative, 369–370
            surgical, 368–369
        patient history, 366
        physical examination, 366
        posterior, posterolateral management, 375
        posterior procedures, 373–374
        radiologic findings, 367–368
    osteomyelitis, 199–208
        anterior debridement
            with autogenous bone grafting, 207

with grafting, posterior instrumentation, 207
        complications of, 207
        diagnosis, 200, 202
        laminectomy, 207
        management, 207
            alternative methods, 206–207
            nonoperative, 207
            postoperative, 201–202, 205–206
            surgical, 200, 202–204
        patient history, 199, 202
        physical examination, 199, 202
        posterior debridement, 207
        radiologic findings, 199, 202
    primary tumor, 345–353, 354–359
        anterior approach, posterior, combined, 358
        anterior surgical approach, 358
        diagnosis, 346, 355
        en bloc laminectomy, posterior spinal instrumentation, 346–347
        en block corpectomy, reconstruction, spinal column, 347–348
        management, 351, 358
            alternative methods, 351, 358
            surgical, 346, 355–356
        nonoperative treatment, 358
        patient history, 345, 354–355
        physical examination, 345, 354–355
        piecemeal resection, 351
        posterior surgical approach, 358
        radiologic findings, 345–346, 355
Cervical spondylosis
    myelopathy
        anterior approach, 35–44
        bridging plate, long, anterior, 43
        buttress plate, short, anterior, 44
        corpectomy, fusion with, without instrumentation, 43
        diagnosis, 36
        discectomy
            with fusion, with, without instrumentation, anterior, 43
            without fusion, anterior, 43
        dynamic plate, long, anterior, 44
        management, 43–44
            alternative methods, 41–44
            posterior, 43
            postoperative, 39–40
            surgical, 37–39
        no instrumentation, 43
        physical examination, 35–36
        posterior fusion, instrumentation, 43
        radiologic findings, 36
    posterior approach, 45–51
        diagnosis, 46
        laminectomy, 51
            with fusion, 51
        laminoplasty, 51
        management, 50–51
            alternative methods, 50–51
            postoperative, 48
            surgical, 46–48
        patient history, 45–46

Cervical spondylosis, posterior approach
  (*continued*)
    physical examination, 45–46
    radiologic findings, 46
  soft disc herniation
    anterior approach, 18–26
    anterior cervical discectomy
      with fusion, 24
      without fusion, 24
    complications of, 24–25
    diagnosis, 19
    grafting, 23
    management, 24
      alternative methods, 24
      postoperative, 21
      surgical, 19–21
    patient history, 18–19
    posterior laminotomy, 24
    radiologic findings, 19
  posterior approach, 27–34
    anterior cervical discectomy
      with fusion, 33
      without fusion, 33
    complications of, 33–34
    diagnosis, 28
    management, 33
      alternative methods, 32–33
      postoperative, 30
      surgical, 28–30
    physical examination, 27–28
    posterior laminoforaminotomy, 33
    radiologic findings, 28
Cervical spondylosis—myelopathy, anterior
  approach, patient history, 35–36
Cervical spondylosis—soft disc herniation
  anterior approach, 18–26, 24
    anterior cervical discectomy
      with fusion, 24
      without fusion, 24
    foraminotomy, 24
    physical examination, 18–19
  posterior approach, 27–34
    anterior cervical discectomy
      with fusion, 33
      without fusion, 33
    complications of, 33–34
    diagnosis, 28
    management, 33
      alternative methods, 32–33
      postoperative, 30
      surgical, 28–30
    patient history, 27–28
    posterior laminoforaminotomy, 33
    radiologic findings, 28
Chemonucleolysis
  microdiscectomy, arthroscopic discectomy,
    chymopapain injection, 135
  recurrent lumbar disc herniation, 148
Chiari malformations, 443–449
  complications of, 449
  diagnosis, 445
  management, 449
    alternative methods, 448–449
    postoperative, 446–447
    surgical, 445–446

  patient history, 443–444
  physical examination, 443–444
  radiologic findings, 444
Chymopapain injection, microdiscectomy,
    arthroscopic discectomy, 129–135
  automated percutaneous discectomy, 135
  chemonucleolysis, 135
  conservative treatment, 132–133, 135
  diagnosis, 130–131
  lumbar disc herniations in special situations,
    133–134
  management, 135
    alternative methods, 135
    postoperative, 132
    surgical, 131–132
  manual percutaneous discectomy, 135
  microdiscectomy, 135
  open discectomy, 135
  patient history, 129–130
  physical examination, 129–130
  radiologic findings, 130
  surgery, 133
Circumferential fusion, lumbar degenerative
    disc disease, axial low back pain, 141
Circumferential surgery, ossification of
    posterior longitudinal ligament,
    cervical spine, 239–246
  anterior corpectomy and fusion with or
    without plates, 244
  anterior plates, 243
  complications of, 243–244
  CT, 243
  fusion, 244
  halo immobilization, 243
  laminectomy with or without posterior
    wiring and fusion, 245
  laminoplasty, 244
  management, 244–245
    alternative methods, 244–245
  MRI, 243
  neurologic status, 243
  operative time, 244
  patient history, 239
  physical examination, 239
Cold, with axial neck pain, 9
Continuous pulse oximetry, spinal cord injury,
    286
Corpectomy, myelopathy, cervical spondylosis,
    anterior approach, fusion with,
    without instrumentation, 43
Costotransversectomy, thoracic disc herniation,
    60
Cranial arthritis, C1/C2 disease, 189–198
  atlantoaxial subluxation, 191
  diagnosis, 190
  external fixation—halo, 197
  internal posterior fixation—wiring, 197
    with transarticular screws, 197
  management, 196
    alternative methods, 196–197
    nonoperative, 192
    surgical, 192–196
  nonoperative therapy, 196
  observation, 196
  odontoid, superior migration of, 191–192

patient history, 189
patterns of involvement, 191–192
physical examination, 189
radiologic findings, 189–190

Deformity
    achondroplasia, cervical postlaminectomy
        kyphosis, 479–483
    Chiari malformations, 443–449
    diastematomyelia, 450–454
    Klippel-Feil syndrome, 435–442
    kyphectomy, lumbar, myelodysplasia, spinal
        deformity in, 455–463
    kyphosis
        postlaminectomy, 420–425
            cervical, achondroplasia, 479–483
            round-back deformity, 411–419
        myelodysplasia, lumbar kyphectomy, spinal
            deformity in, 455–463
        obliquity, pelvic, fixed, 426–434
        postlaminectomy kyphosis, cervical,
            achondroplasia, 479–483
        postradiation spinal deformity, 484–495
        round-back deformity, 411–419
        Scheuermann's kyphosis, 411–419
        scoliosis
            adult, 464–470
            congenital, 391–400
            idiopathic, adolescent, 401–410
        spondylolisthesis, isthmic, adult, 471–478
Degenerative condition
    axial low back pain, nonoperative approach,
        78–83
    axial neck pain, 3–9
    cervical spondylosis—myelopathy
        anterior approach, 35–44
        posterior approach, 45–51
    cervical spondylosis—soft disc herniation
        anterior approach, 18–26
        posterior approach, 27–34
    failed back surgery syndrome, 172–177
    intradural disc herniation—lumbar spine,
        150–156
    Iatrogenic lumbar instability, 163–171
    lumbar degenerative disc disease, axial back
        pain
        anterior approach, 84–92
        minimally invasive laparoscopic approach,
            136–142
        posterior approach, 93–99
    lumbar degenerative scoliosis, with spinal
        stenosis, 119–128
    lumbar degenerative spondylolisthesis,
        109–128
    lumbar disc herniation, recurrent, 143–149
    lumbar spinal stenosis, without instability,
        100–108
    microdiscectomy, arthroscopic discectomy,
        chymopapain injection, 129–135
    neck pain, axial, 3–9
    perineural cysts, 157–162
    sacroiliac joint dysfunction, 179–185
    spinal meningeal cyst, 157–162
    thoracic disc herniation
        anterior approach, 52–60

posterior approach, 61
thoracic disc herniations, minimally invasive
    approach, 68–77
whiplash injuries, 10–17
Diastematomyelia, 450–454
    complications of, 454
    diagnosis, 451
    management, 454
        alternative methods, 453–454
        postoperative, 452
        surgical, 451–452
    patient history, 450
    physical examination, 450
    radiologic findings, 450
Discectomy
    percutaneous lumbar, recurrent lumbar disc
        herniation, 148
    with posterolateral lumbar fusion, recurrent
        lumbar disc herniation, 148
Discitis, lumbar, postoperative, 208–214
    anterior decompression, fusion, 213
    anterior/posterior decompression, fusion,
        213
    antibiotics, 213
    bracing, 213
    diagnosis, 209
    hospital readmission, 209
    management, 213
        alternative methods, 213
        postoperative, 211–212
        surgical, 209–211
    patient history, 208
    percutaneous biopsy, closed
        treatment/bracing, 213
    physical examination, 208
    posterior decompression, fusion, 213
    radiologic findings, 208
Dynamic plate, cervical spondylosis—
    myelopathy, 44

Electrical stimulation, with axial neck pain, 9
Electromagnetic fields, pulsed, for whiplash
    injury, 15
Ependymoma, 384
    intradural disc herniation, lumbar spine, 153
Epidermoid tumor, intradural disc herniation,
    lumbar spine, 154
Exercise regimen, home, for whiplash injury,
    15
Extramedullary tumor, 378–387
    astrocytomas, 384
    biopsy, 385
    chemotherapy, 385
    complications of, 386
    diagnosis, 379
    differential diagnosis, 383
    ependymomas, 384
    filum ependymomas, 382
    hemangioblastomas, 384
    intradural-extramedullary tumors, 381–383
    intramedullary metastic tumors, 385
    intramedullary neoplasms, 383
    lipomas, 384–385
    management, 383–384, 385
        alternative methods, 385

Extramedullary tumor, management (*continued*)
    postoperative, 379–380
    surgical, 379
  meningiomas, 382
  nerve sheath tumors, 382
  neurologic deficit, exacerbation of, 386
  patient history, 378–379
  physical examination, 378–379
  radiation therapy, 385
  radiologic findings, 379
  specific tumor types, 384–385
  surgical resection, 385
  surgical therapy, 382–383

Failed back surgery syndrome, 172–177
  anterior spinal fusion, with instrumentation, 178
  bracing, with, without exercise, 178
  diagnosis, 173
  management, 178
    alternative methods, 177
    postoperative, 174
    surgical, 173–174
  patient history, 172–173
  physical examination, 172–173
  posterior spinal fusion, with instrumentation, 178
  radiologic findings, 173
Filum ependymomas, 382
Fixed pelvic obliquity, 426–434
  complications of, 433
  diagnosis, 427
  management, 432
    alternative methods, 432
    postoperative, 428–429
    surgical, 427–428
  patient history, 426–427
  physical examination, 426–427
  radiologic findings, 427
Foley catheter, spinal cord injury, 286
Fracture
  lumbar, low, with, without neurologic deficit, 320–328
    anatomic fracture reduction, 326
    anterior decompression, fusion, 327
    complications of, 328
    correction maintenance, 326
    diagnosis, 322
    fixation length, minimizing, 327
    management, 327
      alternative methods, 327
      nonoperative, 323, 326, 327
      postoperative, 324
      surgical, 323–324, 326–327
    neural elements, decompression, 326–327
    patient history, 320
    physical examination, 320
    posterior instrumented reduction, fusion, with/without decompression, 327
    radiologic findings, 320–321
    sagittal alignment, 327
  osteoporotic, 262–268
    anterior fusion, 267
      posterior, combined, 267
    complications of, 267

diagnosis, 263
management, 267
  alternative methods, 266–267
  nonoperative, 267
  postoperative, 264
  surgical, 263–264
patient history, 262
physical examination, 262
posterior fusion, 267
radiologic findings, 263
spine, 262–268
  anterior, posterior fusion, combined, 267
  anterior fusion, 267
  complications of, 267
  diagnosis, 263
  management, 267
    alternative methods, 266–267
    nonoperative, 267
    postoperative, 264
    surgical, 263–264
  patient history, 262
  physical examination, 262
  posterior fusion, 267
  radiologic findings, 263
sacral, 329–336
  complications of, 335
  decompression
    early, 335
    late, 335
  diagnosis, 330
  management, 335
    alternative methods, 334
    nonoperative, 335
    postoperative, 332
    surgical, 331–332
  open reduction, internal fixation, 335
  patient history, 329
  physical examination, 329
  radiologic findings, 329

Genitourinary management, spinal cord injury, 286
Gunshot wounds, cervical spine, thoracic spine, lumbar spine, 336–341
  antibiotics, 340
  bracing, 340
  management, 340
    alternative methods, 340
    postoperative, 338
    surgical, 337
  patient history, 336–337
  physical examination, 336–337
  radiologic findings, 337
  steroids, 340
  surgical decompression, 340
  surgical stabilization, 340
  tetanus prophylaxis, 340
  timing of surgery, 340

Heat, with axial neck pain, 9
Hemangioblastomas, 384
Herniated disc/stenosis, posterior longitudinal ligament with, transthoracic, transabdominal approach to T9 to T12 ossification, 247–254

Herniation
    cervical spondylosis, soft disc, posterior
        approach, 27–34
    cervical spondylosis—soft disc,
        laminoforaminotomy, posterior
        approach, 33
    intradural disc, lumbar spine, 150–156
    lumbar disc, 133–134
        recurrent, 143–149
        anterior lumbar interbody fusion, 148
        arthroscopic microdiscectomy, 148
        chemonucleolysis, 148
        diagnosis, 144
        front/back fusion, 148
        laminotomy/discectomy with
            posterolateral lumbar fusion, 148
        management, 148
            alternative methods, 147–149
            postoperative, 146
            surgical, 144–146
        patient history, 143–144
        percutaneous lumbar discectomy, 148
        physical examination, 143–144
        posterior lumbar interbody fusion, 148
        radiologic findings, 144
    soft disc, cervical spondylosis
        anterior approach, 18–26
        posterior approach, 27–34
    spinal cord, 360–365
        complications of, 364
        diagnosis, 361
        management, 364
            alternative methods, 363–364
            postoperative, 362
            surgical, 361–362
        patient history, 360
        physical examination, 360
        posterolateral approach, 364
        radiologic findings, 360–361
        transthoracic approach, 364
    thoracic disc
        anterior approach, 52–60
        minimally invasive approach, 68–77
        posterior approach, 61
Home exercise regimen, for whiplash injury, 15
Hyperostosis
    diffuse, idiopathic, 255–261
        anterior approach, 260
            posterior, combined, 260
        complications of, 260
        diagnosis, 256
        management, 260
            alternative methods, 259–260
            postoperative, 258
            surgical, 256–257
        patient history, 255–256
        physical examination, 255–256
        posterior approach, 260
        radiologic findings, 256
    idiopathic, skeletal, diffuse, 255–261
        anterior, posterior approach, combined,
            260
        complications of, 260
        diagnosis, 256
        management, 260

    alternative methods, 259–260
        anterior, 260
        posterior, 260
        postoperative, 258
        surgical, 256–257
    patient history, 255–256
    physical examination, 255–256
    radiologic findings, 256

Immobilization, for whiplash injury, 15
Infection
    inflammatory disorders, postoperative,
        220–228
    longitudinal ligament, posterior, T9 to T12
        ossification, with herniated
        disc/stenosis, transthoracic,
        transabdominal approach,
        250–251
    postoperative spinal wound, 220–228
    spinal wound, postoperative, 220–228
        antibiotic-impregnated beads, with
            closed-suction drainage, wound
            closure over, 226
        closed suction drainage, primary wound
            closure over, 226
        complications of, 227
        diagnosis, 221
        management, 226
            alternative methods, 226
            postoperative, 224
            surgical, 221–224
        patient history, 220–221
        physical examination, 220–221
        radiologic findings, 221
        suction-irrigation catheter systems,
            wound closure over, 226
    thoracolumbar trauma, 319
Inflammatory disorders
    ankylosing spondylitis cervical osteotomy,
        215–219
    lumbar discitis, postoperative, 208–214
    osteomyelitis—cervical spine, thoracic spine,
        lumbar spine, 199–208
    rheumatoid arthritis cranial–C1/C2 disease,
        189–198
    spinal wound infections, postoperative,
        220–228
Injections, for whiplash injury, 15
Intradural disc herniation, lumbar spine, 150–156
    arachnoid cyst, 154–155
    arachnoiditis, inflammatory mass, 155
    complications of, 156
    diagnosis, 150
    ependymoma, 153
    epidermoid tumor, 154
    management, 155
        alternative methods, 155
    meningiomas, 153
    neurilemoma, 153–154
    neurofibroma, 152–153
    observation, 155
    patient history, 150
    physical examination, 150
    radiologic findings, 150
    surgery, 155

Intradural tumor, 378–387
  astrocytomas, 384
  biopsy, 385
  chemotherapy, 385
  complications of, 386
  diagnosis, 379
  differential diagnosis, 383
  ependymomas, 384
  filum ependymomas, 382
  hemangioblastomas, 384
  intradural-extramedullary tumors, 381–383
  intramedullary metastic tumors, 385
  intramedullary neoplasms, 383
  lipomas, 384–385
  management, 383–384, 385
    alternative methods, 385
    postoperative, 379–380
    surgical, 379
  meningiomas, 382
  nerve sheath tumors, 382
  of neurologic deficit, exacerbation, 386
  patient history, 378–379
  physical examination, 378–379
  radiation therapy, 385
  radiologic findings, 379
  specific tumor types, 384–385
  surgical resection, 385
  surgical therapy, 382–383
Intramedullary tumor, 378–387
  astrocytomas, 384
  biopsy, 385
  chemotherapy, 385
  complications of, 386
  diagnosis, 379
  differential diagnosis, 383
  ependymomas, 384
  filum ependymomas, 382
  hemangioblastomas, 384
  intradural-extramedullary tumors, 381–383
  intramedullary metastic tumors, 385
  intramedullary neoplasms, 383
  lipomas, 384–385
  management, 383–384, 385
    alternative methods, 385
    postoperative, 379–380
    surgical, 379
  meningiomas, 382
  nerve sheath tumors, 382
  neurologic deficit, exacerbation of, 386
  patient history, 378–379
  physical examination, 378–379
  radiation therapy, 385
  radiologic findings, 379
  surgical resection, 385
  surgical therapy, 382–383
  tumor types, 384–385
Isthmic spondylolisthesis, adult, 471–478
  diagnosis, 472
  grading of, 472
  management, 477
    alternative methods, 475–477
    nonsurgical, 472
    postoperative, 474
    surgical, 473–474

patient history, 471
physical examination, 471
radiologic findings, 471–472

Klippel-Feil syndrome, 435–442
  diagnosis, 435–437
  management, 441
    alternative methods, 441
    postoperative, 438
    surgical, 437
  patient history, 435
  physical examination, 435
  radiologic findings, 435
Kyphectomy, lumbar, myelodysplasia, spinal
      deformity in, 455–463
  complications of, 462–463
  diagnosis, 456
  management, 462
    alternative methods, 462
    surgical, 456–458
  patient history, 455
  physical examination, 455
  radiologic findings, 456
Kyphosis, postlaminectomy, 420–425
  achondroplasia, cervical, 479–483
    diagnosis, 480
    management, 482
      alternative methods, 482
      surgical, 480
    patient history, 479–480
    physical examination, 479–480
    radiologic findings, 480
  complications of, 424
  diagnosis, 421
  management, 423
    alternative methods, 423
    surgical, 421
  patient history, 420
  physical examination, 420
  radiologic findings, 421
Kyphosis—round-back deformity, 411–419
  diagnosis, 413
  management, 418
    alternative methods, 417–418
    postoperative, 414
    surgical, 413–414
  patient history, 411–412
  physical examination, 411–412
  radiologic findings, 412
  surgical indications, 416
  technical aspects, 416–417

Laminectomy
  en bloc, cervical spine, primary tumor,
      posterior spinal instrumentation,
      346–347
  lumbar degenerative scoliosis, with spinal
      stenosis, 127
  postlaminectomy, achondroplasia cervical,
      kyphosis, 479–483
  spondylolisthesis, lumbar degenerative, 117
Laminoforaminotomy, cervical spondylosis—
      soft disc herniation, posterior
      approach, 33

Laminotomy
    lumbar degenerative scoliosis, with spinal
        stenosis, 127
    posterior, cervical spondylosis—soft disc
        herniation, anterior approach, 24
    spondylolisthesis, lumbar degenerative, 117
Laminotomy/discectomy with posterolateral
        lumbar fusion, recurrent lumbar disc
        herniation, 148
Iatrogenic lumbar instability, 163–171
    anterior, posterior fusion, for iatrogenic
        instability, 170
    biomechanics of, 167
    decompression
        with fusion for spinal stenosis, 170
        without fusion for spinal stenosis, 170
    diagnosis, 165
    indications, for fusion, 169
    management, 170
        alternative methods, 169–170
        postoperative, 166
        surgical, 165–166
    patient history, 163–164, 167
    physical examination, 163–164, 167
    posterolateral fusion, for iatrogenic
        instability, 170
    radiographic diagnosis of, 167–168
    radiologic findings, 164
    risk factors for, 168–169
Leakage, spinal fluid, persistent, following
        spinal surgery, 495–501
    alternative methods of treatment, 499–500
    complications of, 500
    diagnosis, 496
    management, 500
        postoperative, 496
        surgical, 496
    patient history, 495–496
    physical examination, 495–496
    radiologic findings, 496
Lipomas, 384–385
Longitudinal ligament, posterior
    cervical spine, circumferential surgery for
        ossification of, 239–246
        anterior corpectomy and fusion with or
            without plates, 244
        anterior plates, 243
        complications of, 243–244
        CT, 243
        fusion, 244
        halo immobilization, 243
        laminectomy, with, without posterior
            wiring, fusion, 245
        laminoplasty, 244
        management, 244–245
            alternative methods, 244–245
        MRI, 243
        neurologic status, 243
        operative time, 244
        patient history, 239
        physical examination, 239
    T9 to T12 ossification, with herniated
        disc/stenosis, transthoracic,
        transabdominal approach, 247–254

anterior surgery only, 252
costotransversectomy, 253
exposure, 249
extracavitary management, 253
follow-up MRI/CT studies, 250
grafting, 250
indications, 253
infection, 250–251
intubation period, 250
laminectomy, 253
management, 253
    alternative methods, 253
    surgical, 248–251
operative approach, 249
other specialists involved, 249
patient history, 247–248
physical examination, 247–248
radiologic findings, 248
timing of surgery, 250
transthoracic-transabdominal, 253
Low back pain, axial
    lumbar degenerative disc disease, minimally
        invasive laparoscopic approach,
        136–142
        antiinflammatory medication, 141
        circumferential fusion, anterior, posterior,
            141
        complications of, 142
        diagnosis, 137
        management, 141
            alternative methods, 141–142
            postoperative, 140
            surgical, 137–139
        patient history, 136
        pedicle screws, 141
        physical examination, 136
        physical therapy, 141
        radiologic findings, 137
        spinal injections, 141
    nonoperative approach, 78–83
        acupuncture, 82
        diagnosis, 79
        magnets, 82
        management, 79–80, 82
            alternative methods, 82
        manipulation, 82
        patient history, 78–79
        physical examination, 78–79
        prolotherapy, 82
        radiologic findings, 79
Low lumbar fracture, with, without neurologic
        deficit, orthosis, 327
Lumbar degenerative disc disease, axial back
        pain, 136–142
    anterior approach, 84–92
        anterior lumbar interbody fusion
            with allograft dowels, 92
            with cages, 92
        circumferential fusion, with anterior graft,
            fixation posteriorly, 92
        diagnosis, 85
        management, 92
            alternative methods, 91–92
            conservative, 92

Lumbar degenerative disc disease, axial back
pain, anterior approach; management
(continued)
postoperative, 86–89
surgical, 85–86
patient history, 84–85
physical examination, 84–85
PLIF with bone dowels, rectangular
grafts, 92
PLIF with cages, 92
posterolateral fusion, with, without
pedicle fixation, 92
radiologic findings, 85
minimally invasive laparoscopic approach,
136–142
antiinflammatory medication, 141
circumferential fusion, anterior, posterior,
141
complications of, 142
diagnosis, 137
management, 141
alternative methods, 141–142
postoperative, 140
surgical, 137–139
patient history, 136
pedicle screws, 141
physical examination, 136
physical therapy, 141
posterior lateral instrumented fusion, 141
radiologic findings, 137
spinal injections, 141
posterior approach, 93–99
anterior lumbar interbody fusion
with allograft dowels, 99
with cages, 99
circumferential fusion, with anterior graft,
fixation posteriorly, 99
diagnosis, 94
management, 99
alternative methods, 99
conservative, 99
postoperative, 95–97
surgical, 94–95
patient history, 93–94
physical examination, 93–94
PLIF with bone dowels, rectangular
grafts, 99
PLIF with cages, 99
posterolateral fusion, with, without
pedicle fixation, 99
radiologic findings, 94
Lumbar degenerative scoliosis, with spinal
stenosis, 119–128
complications of, 128
decompression
alone, 126
with fusion, 127
diagnosis, 120–121
fusion, alone, 127
laminectomy, 127
laminotomy, 127
management, 126–127
alternative methods, 126–127
anterior, 127
instrumented, 127

nonoperative, 126
posterior, 127
postoperative, 124
surgical, 121–124
uninstrumented, 127
osteotomy, 127
patient history, 119–120
physical examination, 119–120
posterior lumbar interbody fusion, 127
radiologic findings, 120
Lumbar degenerative spondylolisthesis,
109–128
complications of, 118
decompression, with fusion, 117
decompression management, 117
diagnosis, 110
laminectomy, 117
laminotomy, 117
management, 117
alternative methods, 116–117
instrumented, 117
nonoperative, 117
postoperative, 114–115
surgical, 110–113
uninstrumented, 117
patient history, 109–110
physical examination, 109–110
radiologic findings, 110
Lumbar disc herniation, recurrent, 143–149
anterior lumbar interbody fusion, 148
arthroscopic microdiscectomy, 148
chemonucleolysis, 148
diagnosis, 144
front/back fusion, 148
laminotomy/discectomy with posterolateral
lumbar fusion, 148
management, 148
alternative methods, 147–149
postoperative, 146
surgical, 144–146
patient history, 143–144
percutaneous lumbar discectomy, 148
physical examination, 143–144
posterior lumbar interbody fusion, 148
radiologic findings, 144
Lumbar discitis, postoperative, 208–214
anterior decompression, fusion, 213
anterior/posterior decompression, fusion,
213
antibiotics, 213
bracing, 213
diagnosis, 209
hospital readmission, 209
management, 213
alternative methods, 213
postoperative, 211–212
surgical, 209–211
patient history, 208
percutaneous biopsy, closed
treatment/bracing, 213
physical examination, 208
posterior decompression, fusion, 213
radiologic findings, 208
Lumbar fracture, low, with, without neurologic
deficit, 320–328

anatomic fracture reduction, 326
anterior decompression, fusion, 327
complications of, 328
correction maintenance, 326
diagnosis, 322
fixation length, minimizing, 327
management, 327
    alternative methods, 327
    nonoperative, 323, 326, 327
    postoperative, 324
    surgical, 323–324, 326–327
neural elements, decompression, 326–327
patient history, 320
physical examination, 320
posterior instrumented reduction, fusion,
    with/without decompression, 327
radiologic findings, 320–321
sagittal alignment, 327
Lumbar kyphectomy, myelodysplasia, spinal
    deformity in, 455–463
complications of, 462–463
diagnosis, 456
management, 462
    alternative methods, 462
    surgical, 456–458
patient history, 455
physical examination, 455
radiologic findings, 456
Lumbar spinal stenosis, without instability,
    100–108
complications of, 107
diagnosis, 101, 103
indications, 102
levels to decompress, 103
management, 107
    alternative methods, 107
    conservative, 101–102, 107
    surgical, 102–103
microdecompression, 107
midline decompression, 107
patient history, 100–110
percutaneous procedures, 107
physical examination, 100–110
radiologic findings, 101
surgery, 103
Lumbar spine, primary tumor, 345–353
diagnosis, 346
en bloc laminectomy, posterior spinal
    instrumentation, 346–347
en block corpectomy, reconstruction, spinal
    column, 347–348
management, 351
    alternative methods, 351
    surgical, 346
patient history, 345
physical examination, 345
radiologic findings, 345–346
tumor, piecemeal resection of, 351
Lumbar spine gunshot wound, 336–341
antibiotics, 340
bracing, 340
management, 340
    alternative methods, 340
    postoperative, 338
    surgical, 337

patient history, 336–337
physical examination, 336–337
radiologic findings, 337
steroids, 340
surgical decompression, 340
surgical stabilization, 340
tetanus prophylaxis, 340
timing of surgery, 340
Lumbar spine metastatic disease, 366–377
anterior/posterior procedures, 374
anterior procedures, 373
clinical presentation, 371–372
complications of, 376
diagnosis, 368
management, 372–373, 375
    alternative methods, 375
    anterior, 375
    postoperative, 369–370
    surgical, 368–369
patient history, 366
physical examination, 366
posterior, posterolateral management,
    375
posterior procedures, 373–374
radiologic findings, 367–368
Lumbar spine osteomyelitis, 199–208
anterior debridement
    with autogenous bone grafting, 207
    with grafting, posterior instrumentation,
        207
complications of, 207
diagnosis, 200, 202
laminectomy, 207
management, 207
    alternative methods, 206–207
    nonoperative, 207
    postoperative, 201–202, 205–206
    surgical, 200, 202–204
patient history, 199, 202
physical examination, 199, 202
posterior debridement, 207
radiologic findings, 199, 202

Magnets, for axial low back pain, 82
Manipulation, axial low back pain, 82
Manual traction, with axial neck pain, 9
Marsupialization, spinal meningeal, perineural
    cysts, 162
Massage, with axial neck pain, 9
Mechanical traction, with axial neck pain, 9
Meningiomas, 382
intradural disc herniation, lumbar spine,
    153
Metabolic disease
hyperostosis, skeletal, diffuse idiopathic,
    255–261
longitudinal ligament, posterior
    in cervical spine, ossification of,
        circumferential surgery for, 239–246
    herniated disc/stenosis, transthoracic,
        transabdominal approach, T9 to T12
        ossification, 247–254
osteogenesis imperfecta, spinal deformity in
    presence of, 269–278
osteoporotic fractures, spine, 262–268

Metabolic disease (*continued*)
  Pagetoid disease of spine, 231–238
Metastatic disease, cervical spine, thoracic
    spine, lumbar spine, 366–377
  anterior management, 375
  anterior/posterior procedures, 374
  anterior procedures, 373
  clinical presentation, 371–372
  complications of, 376
  diagnosis, 368
  management, 372–373, 375
    alternative methods, 375
    postoperative, 369–370
    surgical, 368–369
  patient history, 366
  physical examination, 366
  posterior, posterolateral management, 375
  posterior procedures, 373–374
  radiologic findings, 367–368
Microdiscectomy, arthroscopic discectomy,
    chymopapain injection, 129–135
  automated percutaneous discectomy, 135
  chemonucleolysis, 135
  conservative treatment, 132–133, 135
  diagnosis, 130–131
  lumbar disc herniations in special situations,
    133–134
  management, 135
    alternative methods, 135
    postoperative, 132
    surgical, 131–132
  manual percutaneous discectomy, 135
  microdiscectomy, 135
  open discectomy, 135
  patient history, 129–130
  physical examination, 129–130
  radiologic findings, 130
  surgery, 133
Muscle relaxants
  with axial neck pain, 9
  with whiplash injury, 15
Myelodysplasia—lumbar kyphectomy, spinal
    deformity in, 455–463
  complications of, 462–463
  diagnosis, 456
  management, 462
    alternative methods, 462
    surgical, 456–458
  patient history, 455
  physical examination, 455
  radiologic findings, 456
Myelopathy, cervical spondylosis
  anterior approach, 35–44
    bridging plate, long, anterior, 43
    buttress plate, short, anterior, 44
    corpectomy, fusion with, without
      instrumentation, 43
    diagnosis, 36
    discectomy with fusion, with, without
      instrumentation, anterior, 43
    discectomy without fusion, anterior, 43
    dynamic plate, long, anterior, 44
    management, 43–44
      alternative methods, 41–44
      postoperative, 39–40

      surgical, 37–39
    no instrumentation, 43
    physical examination, 35–36
    posterior fusion, instrumentation, 43
    posterior management, 43
    radiologic findings, 36
  posterior approach, 45–51
    diagnosis, 46
    laminectomy, 51
    laminectomy with fusion, 51
    laminoplasty, 51
    management, 50–51
      alternative methods, 50–51
      postoperative, 48
      surgical, 46–48
    patient history, 45–46
    physical examination, 45–46
    radiologic findings, 46

Narcotics
  with axial neck pain, 8
  with whiplash injury, 15
Nasogastric tube, with spinal cord injury,
    286
Neck pain, axial, 3–9
  active assisted, 9
  cervical collar, 9
  cervical manipulation, 9
  cold, 9
  diagnosis, 4
  electrical stimulation, 9
  heat, 9
  management, 8–9
    nonoperative, 4–5
      clinical assessment, 5–6
      diagnostic tests, 6–7
      physical measures, 7–8
      treatment, 7
  manual traction, 9
  massage, 9
  mechanical traction, 9
  medications, 8–9
  modalities, 9
  muscle relaxants, 9
  narcotics, 8
  nonsteroidal antiinflammatory drugs, 8
  oral steroids, 8
  passive, 9
  patient history, 304
  physical measures, 9
  physical therapy, 9
  plain X-ray, 4
  radiologic findings, 4
  strengthening, 9
  tricyclic low-dose antidepressant, 9
  ultrasound, 9
Neoplasm
  cervical spine
    metastatic disease, 366–377
    primary tumor, 345–353, 354–359
  extramedullary tumor, 378–387
  herniation, spinal cord, 360–365
  intradural intramedullary tumor, 378–387
  lumbar spine
    metastatic disease, 366–377

primary tumor, 345–353
thoracic spine
metastatic disease, 366–377
primary tumor, 345–353
Nerve sheath tumors, 382
Neurilemoma, intradural disc herniation, lumbar spine, 153–154
Neurofibroma, intradural disc herniation, lumbar spine, 152–153
Neurologic classification system, 286
Nonsteroidal antiinflammatory drugs
with axial neck pain, 8
for whiplash injury, 15
NSAIDS. *See* Nonsteroidal antiinflammatory drugs

Obliquity, pelvic, fixed, 426–434
complications of, 433
diagnosis, 427
management, 432
alternative methods, 432
postoperative, 428–429
surgical, 427–428
patient history, 426–427
physical examination, 426–427
radiologic findings, 427
Occipitocervical junction, traumatic injuries of, 288–296
complications of, 294–295
diagnosis, 289
halo immobilization, 294
management, 294
alternative methods, 292–294
postoperative, 292
surgical, 289–291
occipitocervical fusion
with plates/rods, screws, 294
with wire, 294
occipitocervical fusion with wire, 294
patient history, 288–289
physical examination, 288–289
radiologic findings, 289
in situ bone grafting, 294
in situ onlay bone grafting, 294
Oral steroids, with axial neck pain, 8
Ossification, posterior longitudinal ligament, in cervical spine, circumferential surgery for, 239–246
anterior corpectomy and fusion with or without plates, 244
anterior plates, 243
complications of, 243–244
CT, 243
fusion, 244
halo immobilization, 243
laminectomy with or without posterior wiring and fusion, 245
laminoplasty, 244
management, 244–245
alternative methods, 244–245
MRI, 243
neurologic status, 243
operative time, 244
patient history, 239

physical examination, 239
Osteogenesis imperfecta, spinal deformity with, 269–278
bracing, 274–275, 277
diagnosis, 269
halo traction, 274, 277
management, 277
alternative methods, 277
nonoperative, 269–270
surgical, 270–272
patient history, 269
physical examination, 269
posterior spinal fusion, 275–276, 277
radiologic findings, 269
Osteomyelitis, cervical spine, thoracic spine, lumbar spine, 199–208
anterior debridement
with autogenous bone grafting, 207
with grafting, posterior instrumentation, 207
complications of, 207
diagnosis, 200, 202
laminectomy, 207
management, 207
alternative methods, 206–207
nonoperative, 207
postoperative, 201–202, 205–206
surgical, 200, 202–204
patient history, 199, 202
physical examination, 199, 202
posterior debridement, 207
radiologic findings, 199, 202
Osteoporotic fracture, 262–268
anterior, posterior fusion, combined, 267
anterior fusion, 267
posterior, combined, 267
complications of, 267
diagnosis, 263
management, 267
alternative methods, 266–267
nonoperative, 267
postoperative, 264
surgical, 263–264
patient history, 262
physical examination, 262
posterior fusion, 267
radiologic findings, 263
Osteotomy
cervical, ankylosing spondylitis, 215–219
anesthesia with spinal cord, nerve monitoring, segmental internal fixation, 218
complications of, 218–219
diagnosis, 216
management, 218
alternative methods, 218
nonoperative, 218
surgical, 216
patient history, 215
physical examination, 215
radiologic findings, 215–216
lumbar degenerative scoliosis, with spinal stenosis, 127

Pagetoid disease of spine, 231–238

Pagetoid disease of spine (*continued*)
  biphosphonates, 236–2370
  calcitonin, 236, 237
  CT-guided biopsy, 237
  management, 237
    alternative methods, 237
    nonoperative, 231
  medical management, 236–237
  patient history, 231
  physical examination, 231
  radiologic findings, 231, 233–236
Pedicle screws, lumbar degenerative disc
      disease, axial low back pain, 141
Pelvic obliquity, fixed, 426–434
  complications of, 433
  diagnosis, 427
  management, 432
    alternative methods, 432
    postoperative, 428–429
    surgical, 427–428
  patient history, 426–427
  physical examination, 426–427
  radiologic findings, 427
PEMF. *See* Pulsed electromagnetic fields
Peptic ulcer prophylaxis, spinal cord injury,
      286
Physical therapy
  with axial neck pain, 9
  with whiplash injury, 15
Posterior longitudinal ligament, T9 to T12
      ossification, with herniated
      disc/stenosis, transthoracic,
      transabdominal approach, 247–254
  anterior surgery only, 252
  costotransversectomy, 253
  exposure, 249
  extracavitary management, 253
  follow-up MRI/CT studies, 250
  grafting, 250
  indications, 253
  infection, 250–251
  intubation period, 250
  laminectomy, 253
  management, 253
    alternative methods, 253
    surgical, 248–251
  operative approach, 249
  other specialists involved, 249
  patient history, 247–248
  physical examination, 247–248
  radiologic findings, 248
  timing of surgery, 250
  transthoracic-transabdominal, 253
Postlaminectomy kyphosis, 420–425
  achondroplasia, cervical, 479–483
    diagnosis, 480
    management, 482
      alternative methods, 482
      surgical, 480
    patient history, 479–480
    physical examination, 479–480
    radiologic findings, 480
  complications of, 424
  diagnosis, 421
  management, 423

    alternative methods, 423
    surgical, 421
  patient history, 420
  physical examination, 420
  radiologic findings, 421
Postoperative lumbar discitis, 208–214
  anterior decompression, fusion, 213
  anterior/posterior decompression, fusion, 213
  antibiotics, 213
  bracing, 213
  diagnosis, 209
  hospital readmission, 209
  management, 213
    alternative methods, 213
    postoperative, 211–212
    surgical, 209–211
  patient history, 208
  percutaneous biopsy, closed
      treatment/bracing, 213
  physical examination, 208
  posterior decompression, fusion, 213
  radiologic findings, 208
Postoperative spinal wound infections, 220–228
  antibiotic-impregnated beads, with closed-
      suction drainage, wound closure over,
      226
  closed suction drainage, primary wound
      closure over, 226
  complications of, 227
  diagnosis, 221
  management, 226
    alternative methods, 226
    postoperative, 224
    surgical, 221–224
  patient history, 220–221
  physical examination, 220–221
  radiologic findings, 221
  suction-irrigation catheter systems, wound
      closure over, 226
Postradiation spinal deformity, 484–495
  diagnosis, 486
  management, 491
    alternative methods, 490–491
    postoperative, 488
    surgical, 486–488
  patient history, 484–485
  physical examination, 484–485
  radiologic findings, 485–486
Primary tumor, cervical spine, 354–359
  anterior approach, posterior, combined,
      358
  anterior surgical approach, 358
  diagnosis, 355
  management, 358
    alternative methods, 358
    surgical, 355–356
  nonoperative treatment, 358
  patient history, 354–355
  physical examination, 354–355
  posterior surgical approach, 358
  radiologic findings, 355
  thoracic spine, lumbar spine, 345–353
    diagnosis, 346
    en bloc laminectomy, posterior spinal
        instrumentation, 346–347

en block corpectomy, reconstruction,
spinal column, 347–348
management, 351
alternative methods, 351
surgical, 346
patient history, 345
physical examination, 345
radiologic findings, 345–346
tumor, piecemeal resection of, 351
Prolotherapy
axial low back pain, 82
sacroiliac joint dysfunction, 183
Pulsed electromagnetic fields, for whiplash
injury, 15

Radiation, spinal deformity following,
484–495
Recurrent lumbar disc herniation, 143–149
Rheumatoid arthritis cranial–C1/C2 disease,
189–198
atlantoaxial subluxation, 191
diagnosis, 190
external fixation—halo, 197
internal posterior fixation—wiring, 197
with transarticular screws, 197
management, 196
alternative methods, 196–197
nonoperative, 192
surgical, 192–196
nonoperative therapy, 196
observation, 196
odontoid, superior migration of, 191–192
patient history, 189
patterns of involvement, 191–192
physical examination, 189
radiologic findings, 189–190
Round-back deformity, 411–419
management, 418
alternative methods, 417–418
postoperative, 414
patient history, 411–412
physical examination, 411–412
radiologic findings, 412
surgical indications, 416
technical aspects, 416–417

Sacral fractures, 329–336
complications of, 335
decompression
early, 335
late, 335
diagnosis, 330
management, 335
alternative methods, 334
nonoperative, 335
postoperative, 332
surgical, 331–332
open reduction, internal fixation, 335
patient history, 329
physical examination, 329
radiologic findings, 329
Sacroiliac joint dysfunction, 179–185
anterior SI fusion, 183
antiinflammatory medications, conditioning
program, 183

diagnosis, 179–180
management, 183
alternative methods, 183–184
postoperative, 181–182
surgical, 180–181
patient history, 179
percutaneous screw fixation, 183
physical examination, 179
prolotherapy, 183
radiologic findings, 179
Scheuermann's kyphosis, 411–419
diagnosis, 413
management, 418
alternative methods, 417–418
postoperative, 414
surgical, 413–414
patient history, 411–412
physical examination, 411–412
radiologic findings, 412
surgical indications, 416
technical aspects, 416–417
Scoliosis, 502–509
adolescent, idiopathic, 401–410
complications of, 409–410
diagnosis, 402
management, 409
alternative methods, 408
postoperative, 405
surgical, 402–405
patient history, 401–402
physical examination, 401–402
radiologic findings, 402
adult, 464–470
complications of, 470
diagnosis, 466
management, 470
alternative methods, 467–470
postoperative, 466
surgical, 466
patient history, 464–465
physical examination, 464–465
radiologic findings, 466
complications of, 508
congenital, 391–400
diagnosis, 394
management, 400
alternative methods, 399–400
postoperative, 394–395
surgical, 394
patient history, 391–392
physical examination, 391–392
radiologic findings, 392
diagnosis, 504
management, 508
alternative methods, 507–508
postoperative, 504
surgical, 504
patient history, 502–503
physical examination, 502–503
radiologic findings, 503
syringomyelia, 502–509
Soft disc herniation, cervical spondylosis
anterior approach, 18–26
anterior cervical discectomy
with fusion, 24

Soft disc herniation, cervical spondylosis,
        anterior approach (*continued*)
    without fusion, 24
    complications of, 24–25
    diagnosis, 19
    grafting, 23
    management, 24
        alternative methods, 24
        postoperative, 21
        surgical, 19–21
    patient history, 18–19
    posterior laminotomy, 24
    radiologic findings, 19
    posterior approach, 27–34
        anterior cervical discectomy
            with fusion, 33
            without fusion, 33
        complications of, 33–34
        diagnosis, 28
        management, 33
            alternative methods, 32–33
            postoperative, 30
            surgical, 28–30
        physical examination, 27–28
        posterior laminoforaminotomy, 33
        radiologic findings, 28
Spasticity management, with spinal cord
        injury, 286
Spinal cord herniation, 360–365
    complications of, 364
    diagnosis, 361
    management, 364
        alternative methods, 363–364
        postoperative, 362
        surgical, 361–362
    patient history, 360
    physical examination, 360
    posterolateral approach, 364
    radiologic findings, 360–361
    transthoracic approach, 364
Spinal cord injury, 281–287. *See also* Spinal
        cord herniation
    adjunctive treatment, 283–286
    bowel program, 286
    cardiovascular management, 286
    continuous pulse oximetry, 286
    diagnosis, 282
    distal extremities, splinting of, 286
    DVT prophalaxis, 286
    extremities, splinting of, 286
    fluid monitoring, 286
        DVT prophalaxis, 286
    Foley catheter, 286
    gastrointestinal management, 286
    genitourinary management, 286
    management, 286
        alternative methods, 286
        nonoperative, 282
    musculoskeletal management, 286
    nasogastric tube, 286
    neurologic classification system, 286
    neurologic management, 286
    patient history, 281–282
    peptic ulcer prophylaxis, 286
    pharmacologic management, 282–283, 286

physical examination, 281–282
    pulmonary toilet, 286
    radiologic findings, 282
    range of motion, 286
    respiratory management, 286
    skin management, 286
    spasticity management, 286
    steroids, 286
    surveillance, 286
    turning, 286
    vital capacity, 286
Spinal deformity, with presence of osteogenesis
        imperfecta, 269–278
    bracing, 274–275, 277
    diagnosis, 269
    halo traction, 274, 277
    management, 277
        alternative methods, 277
        nonoperative, 269–270
        surgical, 270–272
    patient history, 269
    physical examination, 269
    posterior spinal fusion, 275–276, 277
    radiologic findings, 269
Spinal fluid leakage, persistent, following
        spinal surgery, 495–501
    alternative methods of treatment, 499–500
    complications of, 500
    diagnosis, 496
    management, 500
        postoperative, 496
        surgical, 496
    patient history, 495–496
    physical examination, 495–496
    radiologic findings, 496
Spinal meningeal, perineural cysts, 157–162
    diagnosis, 158
    excision, 162
    management, 162
        alternative methods, 161–162
        surgical, 158
    marsupialization, 162
    partial excision, oversewing edges with
            suture, muscle graft, 162
    patient history, 157
    physical examination, 157
    radiologic findings, 157–158
Spinal wound infections, postoperative,
        220–228
    antibiotic-impregnated beads, with closed-
            suction drainage, wound closure over,
            226
    closed suction drainage, primary wound
            closure over, 226
    complications of, 227
    diagnosis, 221
    management, 226
        alternative methods, 226
        postoperative, 224
        surgical, 221–224
    patient history, 220–221
    physical examination, 220–221
    radiologic findings, 221
    suction-irrigation catheter systems, wound
            closure over, 226

Spondylolisthesis
  isthmic, adult
    diagnosis, 472
    grading of, 472
    management, 477
      alternative methods, 475–477
      postoperative, 474
      surgical, 473–474
      nonmanagement, surgical, 472
  lumbar degenerative, 109–128
    complications of, 118
    decompression, with fusion, 117
    decompression management, 117
    diagnosis, 110
    instrumented management, 117
    laminectomy, 117
    laminotomy, 117
    management, 117
      alternative methods, 116–117
      nonoperative, 117
      postoperative, 114–115
      surgical, 110–113
    patient history, 109–110
    physical examination, 109–110
    radiologic findings, 110
    uninstrumented management, 117
Steroids
  with gunshot wounds, 340
  with spinal cord injury, 286
Syringomyelia, 502–509
  complications of, 508
  diagnosis, 504
  management, 508
    alternative methods, 507–508
    postoperative, 504
    surgical, 504
  patient history, 502–503
  physical examination, 502–503
  radiologic findings, 503
  scoliosis and, 502–509

Tetanus prophylaxis, with gunshot wounds, 340
Thoracic disc herniation
  anterior approach, 52–60
    costotransversectomy, 60
    diagnosis, 53–54
    lateral extracavitary, 60
    management, 60
      alternative methods, 60
      postoperative, 55
      surgical, 54–55
    patient history, 52–53
    physical examination, 52–53
    radiologic findings, 53
    thoracoscopic management, 60
    transpedicular management, 60
  minimally invasive approach, 68–77
    complications of, 76
    costotransversectomy, 75
    diagnosis, 69
    laminectomy, 75
    lateral extracavitary management, 75
    management, 75
      alternative methods, 74–75
      postoperative, 73

      surgical, 69–73
    patient history, 68
    physical examination, 68
    radiologic findings, 68–69
    surgical approaches, 74
    transpedicular management, 75
    transthoracic management, 75
  posterior approach, 61
    diagnosis, 62
    lateral extracavitary management, 67
    management, 67
      alternative methods, 66–67
      postoperative, 63
      surgical, 62–63
    patient history, 61–62
    physical examination, 61–62
    radiologic findings, 62
    thoracoscopic management, 67
    transpedicular management, 67
    transthoracic management, 67
Thoracic spine
  gunshot wound, 336–341
    antibiotics, 340
    bracing, 340
    management, 340
      alternative methods, 340
      postoperative, 338
      surgical, 337
    patient history, 336–337
    physical examination, 336–337
    radiologic findings, 337
    steroids, 340
    surgical decompression, 340
    surgical stabilization, 340
    tetanus prophylaxis, 340
    timing of surgery, 340
  metastatic disease, 366–377
    anterior management, 375
    anterior/posterior procedures, 374
    anterior procedures, 373
    clinical presentation, 371–372
    complications of, 376
    diagnosis, 368
    management, 372–373, 375
      alternative methods, 375
      postoperative, 369–370
      surgical, 368–369
    patient history, 366
    physical examination, 366
    posterior, posterolateral management, 375
    posterior procedures, 373–374
    radiologic findings, 367–368
  osteomyelitis, 199–208
    anterior debridement
      with autogenous bone grafting, 207
      with grafting, posterior
        instrumentation, 207
    complications of, 207
    diagnosis, 200, 202
    laminectomy, 207
    management, 207
      alternative methods, 206–207
      nonoperative, 207
      postoperative, 201–202, 205–206
      surgical, 200, 202–204

Thoracic spine, osteomyelitis (*continued*)
    patient history, 199, 202
    physical examination, 199, 202
    posterior debridement, 207
    radiologic findings, 199, 202
  primary tumor, 345–353
    diagnosis, 346
    en bloc laminectomy, posterior spinal
      instrumentation, 346–347
    en block corpectomy, reconstruction,
      spinal column, 347–348
    management, 351
      alternative methods, 351
      surgical, 346
    patient history, 345
    physical examination, 345
    radiologic findings, 345–346
    tumor, piecemeal resection of, 351
Thoracolumbar trauma, with, without
    neurologic deficit, 313–319
  anterior surgery, 318
  bracing, 318
  complications of, 318–319
  decubiti, 319
  diagnosis, 314
  hardware failure, 319
  infection, 319
  management, 318
    alternative methods, 317–318
    nonoperative, 317, 318
    postoperative, 316
    surgical, 314–315
  neurologic complications of, 319
  operative management, 317–318
  patient history, 313
  physical examination, 313
  posterior surgery, 318
  pulmonary complications of, 318
  radiologic findings, 314
  reduction, casting, 318
  treatment options, 317
  vascular complications of, 319
Trauma
  atlantoaxial rotatory deformity, traumatic,
    fixed, 305–312
  cervical facet joint dislocation, bilateral,
    without neurologic deficit, 297–304
  cervical spine, gunshot wound, 336–341
  lumbar fracture, low, with, without
    neurologic deficit, 320–328
  lumbar spine, gunshot wound, 336–341
  occipitocervical junction, traumatic injuries
    of, 288–296
  osteogenesis imperfecta, spinal deformity in
    presence of, 269–278
  osteoporotic fractures, spine, 262–268
  sacral fractures, 329–336
  skeletal hyperostosis, diffuse, idiopathic,
    255–261
  spinal cord injury, pharmacologic,
    management, nonoperative, 281–287
  thoracic spine, gunshot wound, 336–341
  thoracolumbar trauma, with, without
    neurologic deficit, 313–319

Tricyclic low-dose antidepressant, with axial
    neck pain, 9
Tumor. *See also under specific tumor type*
  intradural, intramedullary, extramedullary,
    378–387
    astrocytomas, 384
    biopsy, 385
    chemotherapy, 385
    complications of, 386
    diagnosis, 379
    differential diagnosis of intramedullary
      spinal cord tumors, 383
    ependymomas, 384
    filum ependymomas, 382
    hemangioblastomas, 384
    intradural-extramedullary tumors,
      381–383
    intramedullary metastic tumors, 385
    intramedullary neoplasms, 383
    lipomas, 384–385
    management, 385
      alternative methods, 385
      postoperative, 379–380
      surgical, 379
    management decisions regarding
      intramedullary spinal cord tumors,
      383–384
    meningiomas, 382
    nerve sheath tumors, 382
    neurologic deficit, exacerbation of, 386
    patient history, 378–379
    physical examination, 378–379
    radiation therapy, 385
    radiologic findings, 379
    surgical resection, 385
    surgical therapy, 382–383
    types, 384–385
  primary, cervical spine, 354–359
    anterior approach, 358
      posterior, combined, 358
    diagnosis, 355
    management, 358
      alternative methods, 358
      surgical, 355–356
    nonoperative treatment, 358
    patient history, 354–355
    physical examination, 354–355
    posterior surgical approach, 358
    radiologic findings, 355
    thoracic spine, lumbar spine, 345–353
      diagnosis, 346
    en bloc laminectomy, posterior spinal
      instrumentation, 346–347
    en block corpectomy, reconstruction,
      spinal column, 347–348
    management, 351
      alternative methods, 351
      surgical, 346
    patient history, 345
    physical examination, 345
    radiologic findings, 345–346
    tumor, piecemeal resection of, 351
Turning of patient, schedule, with spinal cord
    injury, 286

Ultrasound, use of with axial neck pain, 9

Vascular malformation, spinal cord, 509–515
   complications of, 515
   diagnosis, 510
   management, 515
      alternative methods, 514–515
      postoperative, 512–513
      surgical, 511–512
   patient history, 509
   physical examination, 509
   radiologic findings, 509

Whiplash injury
   clinical classification, disorders, 12

immobilization, 15
injections, 15
management, 15
   alternative methods, 15
   nonoperative, 13–14
narcotics, 15
nonoperative approach, 10–17
nonsteroidal antiinflammatory drugs, 15
patient history, 10–12
physical examination, 10–12
physical therapy, 15
prognosis, 14
pulsed electromagnetic fields, 15
radiologic findings, 11, 12–13
symptoms, 12